RM
258.5
.U83
2003

CLEARI

Chicago Public Library

User's guide to nutritional supplements

User's Guide to *Nutritional* Supplements

D1307684

OCT -- 2003

Chicago Public Library
Clearing Branch
6423 West 63rd Place
Chicago, Illinois 60638-5005

User's Guide to *Nutritional* Supplements

Jack Challem, Editor

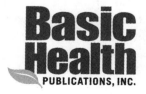

Basic Health
PUBLICATIONS, INC.

The information contained in this book is based upon the research and personal and professional experiences of the authors. It is not intended as a substitute for consulting with your physician or other health care provider. Any attempt to diagnose and treat an illness should be done under the direction of a health care professional.

The publisher does not advocate the use of any particular health care protocol but believes the information in this book should be available to the public. The publisher and authors are not responsible for any adverse effects or consequences resulting from the use of the suggestions, preparations, or procedures discussed in this book. Should the reader have any questions concerning the appropriateness of any procedures or preparation mentioned, the authors and the publisher strongly suggest consulting a professional health care advisor.

Editor: Jack Challem
In-house editors: Carol Rosenberg and Roberta W. Waddell
Typesetter and book designer: Gary A. Rosenberg
Cover designer: Mike Stromberg

Basic Health Publications, Inc.
8200 Boulevard East
North Bergen, NJ 07047
1-800-575-8890

Library of Congress Cataloging-in-Publication Data

User's guide to nutritional supplements / Jack Challem, editor.
   p. cm.
Includes bibliographical references and index.
   ISBN 1-59120-067-9
1. Dietary supplements. I. Challem, Jack.
RM258.5.U83   2003
613.2—dc21
                                        2002154607

Copyright © 2003 by Basic Health Publications, Inc.

All rights reserved. No part of this publication may be reproduced, stored in a retrieval system, or transmitted, in any form or by any means, electronic, mechanical, photocopying, recording, or otherwise, without the prior written consent of the copyright owner.

Printed in the United States of America

10   9   8   7   6   5   4   3   2   1

CONTENTS

R0179856225

Chicago ~~~~ ~~~~
Clearing Branch
6423 West 63rd Place
Chicago, Illinois 60638-500~

INTRODUCTION

All of us hear about wonderful, sometimes miraculous research on the health benefits of nutritional supplements: for example, how vitamin E can reduce your risk of developing heart disease and some types of cancer, how chromium can help you lose weight, and how ginkgo can sharpen your memory and perhaps help prevent Alzheimer's disease.

And then we hear the other side, that none of these things actually work. Confused? Exasperated? Not sure who or what to believe? It's not surprising you sometimes feel that way. But that's what this book is intended to remedy.

The *User's Guide to Nutritional Supplements* describes, in simple terms, the scientific research and likely benefits of the most popular vitamin, mineral, and herbal supplements sold. And in doing so, it explains how you can reduce your chances of developing a range of ailments, from bothersome aches and pains to debilitating and life-threatening catastrophic diseases.

Among the pearls of information you'll learn are these:

- Vitamin E can reduce your risk of cardiovascular diseases—and which are the best types of vitamin E to take.

- Selenium can slash your chances of developing some types of cancer.

- Ginkgo can improve your memory and recall, and how much you should take.

- Chromium can help lower your risk of diabetes.

- Glucosamine and chondroitin can prevent osteoarthritis.

- Calcium and magnesium work together to build strong bones.

- Coenzyme Q_{10} can boost your energy levels and strengthen your heart.

- Ginseng and other supplements can increase your exercise stamina.

What Are Nutritional Supplements?

Nutritional supplements are concentrated forms of nutrients, typically in a capsule or tablet, that are either essential to, or likely beneficial to, your health. Nearly all of these nutrients would be found in a wholesome, diverse diet—

and therein lies part of the problem. Most of us don't eat the way we should.

With our fast-paced, stress-filled lives, fewer people have the luxury of cooking meals from scratch. Worse, more of us end up relying on fast foods and microwave, convenience, or snack foods. These foods may satisfy our hunger pangs, but they are highly processed—meaning that most of their original nutritional value has been removed.

As a consequence, many people do not consume all of the vitamins and minerals they need for optimal health, which means their bodies break down and become susceptible to disease earlier than they should. Countless studies have found that many of us are shortchanged when it comes to vitamin C, vitamin E, many B vitamins, calcium, magnesium, and many other essential nutrients. In a very real sense, as other people have astutely observed, we are starving on full stomachs.

Even when we eat healthy foods, many things can sabotage how our bodies use nutrients. For example, tobacco products deplete vitamins C and E. Antibiotics disrupt the gut's ability to absorb B vitamins. Antacids interfere with calcium and other minerals. Cholesterol-lowering "statin" drugs lower the body's production of coenzyme Q_{10}, a vitaminlike nutrient needed for energy and normal heart function.

When you consider these factors, as well as that our individual genetic differences may affect absorption, it becomes clear that we would be better off to "err" on the side of nutritional insurance. At the very least, I believe, every person should take a moderately high-potency daily vitamin and mineral supplement. Many of us could likely benefit from larger amounts of other supplements, tailored to our diets and lifestyles.

Nutrients Are Not Drugs

You might be wondering how nutritional supplements and drugs differ. After all, both usually come in capsules and tablets. Their differences are important to keep in mind. Drugs are "foreign" substances to the body, and they work by forcefully altering the body's normal biochemical processes. They are, as some brave physicians have pointed out, low doses of poisons—with side effects that often outweigh their benefits.

How dangerous are prescription drugs? Consider a couple of examples. Are you really better off if an antidepressant drug improves your mood but leaves you with erectile dysfunction? Or is it worthwhile to take hormone-replacement therapy to relieve hot flashes, when such drugs will increase your risk of heart attack and cancer? Such issues should concern everyone who takes a drug. According to an article in the *Journal of the American Medical Association*, prescription drugs cause the deaths of more than 100,000 hospitalized Americans each year, making them a leading cause of death.

At best, drugs only mask the symptoms of diseases while failing to treat their underlying causes. Sometimes, they even make a disease worse. For example, ibuprofen and some other nonsteroidal anti-inflammatory drugs (NSAIDs) can temporarily relieve the pain of osteoarthritis, but over the long term, they speed the breakdown of joint cartilage, the very cause of osteoarthritis.

In contrast, vitamins, minerals, and the nutritional substances in herbs are substances normally found in the body. They foster the myriad normal biochemical processes that literally do everything, such as burn food for energy, beat your heart, enable your eyes to see, fight infections, further thinking processes, and much more. I have heard many physicians and their patients speak of surprising "side benefits" after taking a nutritional supplement, when more than the intended health problem is resolved.

Why You Have to Educate Yourself

So, if nutritional supplements are so good, why don't most physicians recommend and prescribe them? There are two major reasons why doctors shun safe, comparatively inexpensive supplements in favor of drugs. Physicians are generally not taught very much about nutrition and health in medical school. Their classes emphasize anatomy, diagnosis, surgery, and medications—virtually nothing about diet and nutritional supplements.

As a consequence of this training, the majority of physicians believe there is little scientific evidence to support the health benefits of vitamin, mineral, and herbal supplements. The late Nobel laureate Linus Pauling, Ph.D., observed that "If a doctor isn't 'up' on something, he is 'down' on it."

After medical school, the drug companies take over physicians' ongoing education—and these drug companies promote their patented high-profit products, not inexpensive nutritional supplements. Each year, drug companies spend billions of dollars on advertising to physicians and consumers, and they also influence how many so-called scientific studies are conducted and published.

One more example will convey how drug companies influence what physicians and their patients hear. A recent headline-grabbing study found that the herb St. John's wort

was ineffective in treating depression. But few journalists reported that the study was funded and organized by the maker of one of the most widely prescribed prescription drugs. Buried deep in the report, published in a major medical journal, was an acknowledgment that the herb actually did have benefits. But few physicians or journalists read far enough to notice this critical bit of information.

All this means, unfortunately, that you often have to fend for yourself when trying to make important decisions about maintaining or regaining your health. But it is easy to make educated decisions.

Huge Body of Research

Thousands of articles on nutrition are published each year in scientific and medical journals. In fact, in a typical year, more than 5,000 articles are published on vitamins. Over the past thirty-five years, more than 150,000 articles on vitamins were published in these journals, with about a third of them published during the 1990s. In truth, more research—and most of it positive—has been published on nutrients than most drugs! The problem is not a lack of vitamin research. The problem is keeping up with all of the research.

That, in a nutshell, is what the *User's Guide to Nutritional Supplements* will help you do: to bring you up to date with the most important findings on vitamins, minerals, and herbs.

As a health writer and lecturer, as well as someone who has published original research, I have spent nearly thirty years delving into the relationship between nutrition and health. In my mind, the evidence supporting the benefits of vitamins, minerals, and herbs is overwhelming and persuasive. And on a very personal level, I have seen how dietary changes and supplements have greatly improved my own health, helping me lose weight and dramatically reverse a dangerous course toward diabetes.

In this book, Basic Health Publications and I have brought together some of the best health writers—physicians, herbalists, nutritionists, and other experts—who understand nutritional supplements the way few people do. They describe in simple terms the research you need to know and what it really means to you and your well-being. Together, we cover all of the major vitamin, mineral, and herbal supplements, describing fascinating research and providing practical advice that nearly everyone can benefit from.

Whether you read this book from cover to cover, skim it, or simply refer to the sections most important to your health concerns, I believe you will find it to be a trove of useful and sound information. Join me in enjoying the best of health and all that life offers us.

—Jack Challem, The Nutrition Reporter™
www.nutritionreporter.com

PART ONE

Vitamins & Minerals

Jack Challem & Liz Brown

Vitamins. They captivate. And, yes, they often do cure. Few newspaper headlines grab a person's attention faster than those describing the seemingly miraculous benefits of vitamins. Almost every week we hear reports that they can reverse heart disease, ease the aches and pains of arthritis, and reduce the risk of cancer.

Vitamins sound almost too good to be true. And you're probably wondering if vitamins are as good as they've been cracked up to be.

The answer, in a nutshell, is a resounding "yes." For years, doctors dismissed the value of vitamins, preferring to prescribe expensive drugs or to perform surgery. Now, each year, medical journals publish thousands of scientific articles describing the health benefits of vitamins, minerals, and other nutrients. And more doctors are recognizing the impressive health benefits of vitamins.

If you're one of the six out of ten Americans who take vitamin supplements, this book will give you a better understanding of how they work to maintain and improve health. If you are thinking about taking vitamins, this book can help you decide what to take.

Vitamins are natural substances found in wholesome foods, and they have many advantages over drugs. They work in tandem with your body to promote health. They're safe. They're relatively inexpensive. They help keep you well. But with all the research and all the confusing headlines on vitamins, it's also easy to be overwhelmed.

This part of the *User's Guide to Nutritional Supplements* is meant to clear the confusion by providing simple, straightforward answers to your questions about vitamins and minerals. In the first chapter, you'll learn some vitamin basics: why they are important to your health and why supplements are necessary even if you're eating a healthy diet. The following sections in this book will describe the benefits of specific vitamins or family of vitamins, such as vitamin A; the B vitamins; and vitamins C, D, E, and K.

The second half of this book focuses on minerals, which are nutritionally related to vitamins. Minerals are just as important for health, and you're probably already familiar with at least some of them, such as calcium. You'll also learn about the health benefits of magnesium, chromium, selenium, and other minerals. Finally, the last chapter gives you important tips on how to buy and use vitamins and minerals.

Read on. Be well. And take your vitamins and minerals.

What Vitamins Can Do for Your Health

Your body requires relatively small amounts of vitamins compared with protein or carbohydrate. Still, many people do not obtain enough vitamins, either because they don't eat the right foods or because of absorption problems.

Low levels of vitamins interfere with health, and many people go through life believing their health problems are a normal part of life or aging. When people take vitamin supplements for the first time, they often discover just how dramatically vitamins can improve health.

What Are Vitamins and Minerals?

If you ask a scientist, he or she will tell you that vitamins are organic compounds (containing at least one carbon atom) that promote virtually all biochemical processes in the body. This simple definition actually belies their powerful and diverse roles in health. For example, vitamin C is needed for the formation of skin and all other tissues, as well as for normal functioning of the immune system. Your body cannot make most vitamins, at least not in any substantial amount, so you have to get them from foods or supplements.

In contrast, minerals are elements, meaning that they cannot be broken down into simpler substances. However, minerals that have nutritional roles are found in the form of compounds, meaning they are combined with something else. Calcium citrate and chromium picolinate are examples of the many mineral compounds.

To keep things simple, think of vitamins and minerals as essential ingredients in a recipe—in this case, a recipe for your health. Basically, you need vitamins and minerals to grow, produce energy, fight disease, repair injured tissue, and maintain normal health. Recent scientific studies have even shown that many vitamins and minerals influence the behavior of genes in a positive way. You don't need much of most vitamins and minerals compared with, let's say, dietary protein or carbohydrate. Yet many people do not obtain adequate amounts of these important nutrients.

> **What do vitamins do?** *Vitamins initiate and promote virtually all of the body's biochemical activities needed for life and health.*

The thirteen essential vitamins are divided into two groups. One group consists of water-soluble vitamins that need to be replenished daily because they are rapidly excreted. These vitamins include vitamin C and the B-complex family of vitamins.

The second group consists of fat-soluble vitamins, which the body is capable of storing for weeks or months. The fat-soluble vitamins are vitamins A, D, E, and K.

There are also many vitaminlike nutrients that are not officially recognized as vitamins, though their functions are similar. Coenzyme Q_{10}, alpha-lipoic acid, beta-carotene and other carotenoids, and quercetin and other flavonoids are among these vitaminlike nutrients.

You'll learn more about minerals starting on page 17.

Vitamins Can Do a Lot for You

Whether you're young or old, male or female, work hard physically or have a desk job, vitamin supplements can often have an amazing effect on your health.

First and foremost, vitamins are essential nutrients that help your body function normally. They can help reduce your risk of developing many serious diseases, such as heart disease, cancer, Alzheimer's disease, and arthritis.

Secondly, many doctors also use vitamins to treat diseases. For example, several large studies with people (not laboratory rats, mind you) have found that vitamin E supplements dramatically reduced the risk of coronary heart disease. Other studies have found that vitamin C reduces symptoms of the common cold and flu by one-third—basically meaning that the vitamin cuts down your sick time by a couple of days.

Still other studies have found that high intakes of vitamins reduce the risk of diabetes, arthritis, and many different types of cancer. It practically goes without saying that most people prefer to be healthy than to be sick and miserable. Vitamins can keep you healthy.

One of the most amazing things that happens with vitamin supplementation is what some nutritionally oriented physicians call "side benefits." The term is in sharp contrast to drugs, which tend to have side effects. These doctors have found over and over again that a vitamin supplement prescribed for one condition, such as arthritis, produces unexpected benefits, such as improvements in sleep or mood.

Vitamins Often Reverse Health Problems

Many people who start taking vitamin supplements quickly discover that they can correct and reverse long-standing health problems. For example, British researchers recently gave natural vitamin E supplements (400–800 IU/day) to men and women who had suffered a heart attack. After an average of eighteen months, people getting vitamin E had 77 percent fewer heart attacks than those given a dummy pill.

Here's another example: Abram Hoffer, M.D., Ph.D., of Victoria, Canada, has been treating terminal cancer patients with a high-potency vitamin/mineral regimen. He started doing this years ago to treat their depression and anxiety related to the cancer diagnosis. Hoffer has found that 30 percent of his early cancer patients (that is, long-term users of supplements) have lived at least ten years longer than comparable patients who receive only conventional treatment—a phenomenal success rate. So the answer is yes, vitamins can reverse very serious diseases. We'll tell you more about Hoffer's regimen later in this book.

Vitamins Are Good for Healthy People, Too

Vitamins and minerals can certainly correct a lot of damage and reverse or slow the course of many diseases. But you don't have to be a dietitian to figure out that it's far better to prevent diseases. The reason is very simple: it's more difficult to reverse a disease than to prevent it.

You can prevent—or at least reduce the risk of—disease by eating a diet high in fruits and vegetables, exercising, and taking vitamin and mineral supplements. If you're very healthy now, it may take a few years before you see benefits from vitamins. But as the years go by, you'll probably notice that you aren't getting sick as often as people who don't take vitamins and minerals, that your cholesterol and blood pressure aren't creeping up as much as theirs, and that you don't have as many aches and pains.

Are Vitamins a Fountain of Youth?

They may be. Before you dismiss this as too wild of a claim, consider what happens during the aging process. Aging is the result of damage to the 100 trillion cells that compose your body. All of the damage makes these cells less and less efficient with age. An old heart doesn't pump blood as well as a young heart. An old stomach doesn't digest food as well as a young stomach. Old wrinkled skin isn't as supple as baby's skin.

Vitamins function a lot like biological spark plugs that energize your cells and protect them from damage. They promote the myriad biological activities of your cells—and in doing so, they keep them functioning more like younger cells. Numerous studies have shown that vitamin supplements extend life expectancy. Some supplements have age-reversing effects in animals, suggesting that they are likely to have the same effect on people.

Vitamins Are Not the Same as Drugs

Vitamin supplements and drugs might appear similar, but they are very different. Vitamins are not drugs. They are natural substances that should be normally found in the diet, and they work by promoting normal biological processes. Because of poor eating habits (such as too many junk foods or some types of very restrictive diets), many people do not obtain enough vitamins. Scientific studies have found that many people don't consume adequate amounts of vitamins A, C, and E and other nutrients.

In contrast, drugs work by interfering with natural processes in the body, often acting like a chemical sledgehammer to change something. For example, you don't develop a headache because of an aspirin deficiency. However, there are scientific reports showing that vitamin B_2 deficiency can sometimes cause migraine headaches. As another example, antiviral drugs are sometimes used to treat serious viral infections, but these drugs are extremely toxic. In contrast, vitamin C naturally stimulates the activity of the body's own immune cells to fight infections.

Vitamins Are Very Safe

Vitamin supplements are extraordinarily safe. There are only two vitamins—vitamins A and D—that pose some risk in very high doses because the body stores them. However, it is unlikely that most people will ever overdose on them. The more common problem is that people don't get enough of them.

In general, it's important to follow the usage directions on bottles of these vitamins, which will typically recommend RDA (Recommended Dietary Allowance) or Daily Value (DV) levels of vitamins A and D (5,000 IU and 400 IU, respectively). However, higher doses are often warranted. For example, a recent study, published in the *New England Journal of Medicine*, found that vitamin D deficiency was fairly common among people who seemed to be getting enough of the vitamin. You'll read more about the appropriate uses of high-dose vitamins A and D later in this book.

Vitamins Are More Than Catalysts

At one time, doctors and researchers believed that vitamins worked as catalysts to stimulate normal chemical reactions in the body. In chemistry, catalysts promote chemical reactions.

Modern research has changed and broadened this view

of vitamins. The building blocks of your body and its biochemicals are nutrients, which include protein, carbohydrate, fats, minerals, and vitamins. In a sense, vitamins help cement together your heart, lungs, skin, brain, and other organs. Vitamins are also needed for your body to make enzymes, hormones, energy, new cells (such as blood and skin cells), and even deoxyribonucleic acid (DNA), which is what your genes are made of.

The latest research on vitamins shows that they protect genes from damage and "turn on" good genes and "turn off" bad genes. The health of your genes is important because they influence your health and your risk of developing cancer. So by helping your body function in a normal way, vitamins enhance health and prevent disease.

You Don't Get Enough Vitamins in Food

We've all heard that Americans are the best fed people in the world. We're also one of the most overfed people in the world, because almost two-thirds of all Americans are now overweight. That situation points to a severe dietary imbalance, and vitamins frequently get shortchanged.

IU, mg, and mcg
Each is a measurement of vitamins by potency or weight. All three are extremely small amounts. For example, 400 mcg is about $1/70,000$ of an ounce.

One reason is that many people don't select very nutritious foods. Fruits and vegetables are particularly high in most vitamins, and the U.S. Department of Agriculture recommends that people eat three to five servings of fruits and vegetables daily. Yet several studies have found that only 9 to 32 percent of Americans eat five daily servings of fruits and vegetables, which means that 68 to 91 percent do not! It's easy to be tempted by burgers, fries, fried chicken, and super-sized drinks—and to skip salads and broccoli—and to miss a lot of vitamins.

Another reason people often don't get enough vitamins is that the American diet has undergone tremendous changes in processing over the past 100 years. In the nineteenth century, people ate whole-grain breads rich in vitamin E. Around 1900, technological changes in the milling of grains removed the vitamins, leaving white starch for bread making. Even though bread is "enriched" with a few vitamins, far more nutrients are removed from bread than are added back in.

In addition, soils deficient in some minerals limit a plant's production of vitamins. Synthetic fertilizers (in contrast to plain old manure) don't solve the problem. Several years ago, U.S. Department of Agriculture researchers found that conventional nitrogen fertilizer reduced vitamin C levels in some food crops by as much as one-third. Additional nutrient losses have been documented during the transportation, storage, and processing of produce and during cooking. So even if your intentions are good, it's often hard to buy nutritious foods.

The Average Diet Is Pretty Bad

Nutritional surveys have found that half of Americans consume less than 50 mg and 25 percent consume less than 39 mg of vitamin C daily—far below the Recommended Dietary Allowance (RDA) of 90 mg. Other studies have found that half of the population consumes only 950 IU of vitamin A (19 percent of the RDA) and 4 IU of vitamin E (18 percent of the RDA) or less daily.

The same pattern applies to the consumption of other micronutrients as well, meaning that large numbers of people simply aren't getting enough vitamins. These numbers look even worse if you consider that the RDA is a very conservative number, and that typical requirements are probably higher.

Furthermore, even a good diet is no guarantee that your body is doing a good job absorbing nutrients. Sherry Rogers, M.D., of Syracuse, New York, makes the point that "you are what you absorb." Many things can interfere with normal absorption. For example, high-sodium (salt) diets impair calcium absorption, and grains interfere with vitamin D. Sometimes, people have subtle genetic defects that limit vitamin utilization.

Some People Need More Vitamins

The very concept of an RDA may be flawed. In the 1950s, Roger Williams, Ph.D., developed the concept of "biochemical individuality." Williams was one of the most eminent vitamin researchers of the twentieth century.

> **Biochemical Individuality**
> Each person is genetically and biochemically unique, meaning we all have varying nutritional requirements in order to maintain health.

Biochemical individuality means that each of us is a nutritional, biochemical, genetic, and anatomical individual. Just as we look different on the outside, each of us requires different amounts of various vitamins. For one person, 100 mg daily of vitamin C might be sufficient for health; for another, 3,000 would be needed.

These differences stem from our genetic individuality, as well as from different conditions when we were in the womb and different conditions as we grew up. As one example, people's stomachs come in all shapes and sizes, and some people produce far more digestive enzymes than do others. The person with good digestion will absorb nutrients better than the person with poor digestion. These differences exist on a very minute level in the body, but they have profound effects on our health and risk of disease.

The bottom line is that everyone needs vitamins and minerals, but different people need different vitamins and minerals in different amounts. One size does not fit all.

Isn't 100 Percent of the RDA Adequate?

The RDA and the DV are extremely conservative estimates of the amounts of vitamins and minerals people need. They are largely designed to prevent the most serious deficiency diseases. The RDA and the DV are not intended as guidelines for optimal intakes for achieving the best health.

The predecessor to today's RDA was designed as a guideline for "practically all healthy persons" by the federal government during World War II. But many prominent nutrition researchers have questioned whether Americans can be considered healthy—and, therefore, whether RDA levels of vitamins are really adequate.

Paul LaChance, Ph.D., of Rutgers University, has pointed out that 30 percent of Americans smoke, and many drink too much alcohol. Others suffer from diabetes, high cholesterol levels, or hypertension. An article in the *Journal of the American Medical Association* recently reported that 45 percent of Americans suffered from at least one chronic condition. "After age 45, most people are not 'healthy' in the strict sense of the word and relatively few qualify as having no chronic or acute problem," LaChance explained in the journal *Nutrition Reviews*.

For example, vitamin B_6, folic acid (another B vitamin), and vitamin E are three of the vitamins most important for a healthy heart. A study by Harvard University researchers found that folic acid and vitamin B_6 protect against coronary heart disease. However, the most beneficial dose was three or more times the RDA. Similarly, vitamin E seems to offer the most protection to the heart at 400 IU daily—18 times the RDA.

By the way, don't be scared off by a vitamin product that contains 400 percent of the RDA. This amount is 4 times, not 400 times, the RDA.

There's Great Scientific Support for Vitamins

The scientific research supporting the roles of vitamins in health is far better than the research on most drugs. On average, journals publish about 500 to 600 studies a year on vitamin E and about an equal number on vitamin C. In a typical year, more than 5,000 studies are published on vitamins in medical and scientific journals. Over the past thirty-five years, more than 150,000 studies on vitamins have been published, with more than one-third of them published during the 1990s.

If you scrutinize all this research, you'll notice two trends, regardless of whether the studies are on people, animals, or cells. One trend is that higher levels of vitamins and minerals are almost always associated with health. The other is that lower levels of these nutrients are almost always associated with disease.

In the 1940s and 1950s, when a handful of physicians started using vitamins to treat diseases, no one really understood how these nutrients worked. Today, researchers have gained a better understanding of vitamins. For example, vitamin E helps the cardiovascular system by maintaining normal blood vessel flexibility, by reducing the heart-damaging effects of cholesterol, and by blocking the activity of disease-promoting compounds.

Vitamins Protect against Free Radicals

Radicals are hazardous molecules that age us and cause diseases. Bear with us for a few brief paragraphs, because this is about as technical as this book gets: Atoms are the smallest building blocks of everything, living or not. Each atom has electrons circling around its center, much the way planets revolve around the sun. Normally, electrons come in pairs. But when an atom is short one electron (or has one too many), it's called a free radical.

Free Radical
A harmful molecule produced by the body and pollutants. They have one electron too few or one too many, making them highly unstable.

The radical is "free" in the sense that it's cruising around aggressively and looking for a partner. If it grabs a replacement electron from an atom that's part of a healthy cell in your body, it damages that cell. Oxygen, which you need to breathe, is the source of most free radicals, so the damage is called "oxidation."

Free radical oxidation is also what makes iron rust and butter turn rancid. Although free radicals are found in air pollution, cigarette smoke, and other nasty compounds, they are also formed when the body burns food for energy. Free radicals are pretty powerful—your body also makes them to kill germs. Too much exposure to sunlight also generates free radicals, which is why sun worshipers tend to have older looking skin.

It helps to think of free radicals as dominoes. One free radical creates another and another and another—until the cascade of free radicals is quenched by an antioxidant vitamin.

Antioxidants to the Rescue

Antioxidants are the flip side of the free radical coin, because they quench (or neutralize) free radicals. Many vitamins and vitaminlike nutrients function as antioxidants, and in doing so, they limit the damage caused by free radicals. Vitamins E and C are antioxidants, as are beta-carotene, lutein, coenzyme Q_{10}, and alpha-lipoic acid.

You Need More Than One Antioxidant

Your health will benefit from taking a single antioxidant supplement, such as vitamin E or vitamin C. However, you'll do much better by taking a combination of antioxidants.

Researcher Al L. Tappel, Ph.D., of the University of California, Davis, has shown that a diverse selection of antioxidants may be more important than high doses of just one or two. That doesn't mean you have to swallow handfuls of antioxidant tablets and capsules. For reducing your long-term risk of disease, consider taking an antioxidant "cocktail" containing four to ten different antioxidants. If you're already taking a high-potency multivitamin, you may be getting enough antioxidants.

Lester Packer, Ph.D., has described this antioxidant interaction, or synergism, as the "antioxidant network." Many antioxidants—vitamins E and C, coenzyme Q_{10}, glutathione—work together as a team, helping one another out. Keep in mind, though, that not all vitamins function as antioxidants.

Antioxidant
A molecule that donates electrons to stabilize damaging free radicals. Vitamins E and C are two of the most powerful vitamin antioxidants.

What about Megadosing with Vitamins?

So, what exactly is a megadose of a vitamin? Dietitians, who are generally conservative when it comes to supplements, tend to feel that anything above RDA levels amounts to a megadose. However, the trend in nutrition research is toward developing recommendations that are higher than the current RDAs—that is, more optimal.

A growing number of researchers and physicians believe that vitamin levels roughly three times the RDA are often optimal doses. In an experiment, Mark Levine, M.D., Ph.D., of the National Institutes of Health, Bethesda, Maryland, found that 200 mg of vitamin C daily—more than twice the RDA—was the ideal intake for young, healthy men. But Levine's study didn't look at women or sick people (about half the population), or people who smoked or were under a lot of stress, so he was reluctant to extrapolate his recommendations to them.

Many others, particularly practicing physicians, have had great success treating patients with so-called megadoses of vitamins. Some of these doctors, such as Hugh Riordan, M.D., of Wichita, Kansas, use laboratory tests to carefully document that patients have low levels of vitamins—and that their improvement follows taking vitamin supplements. Other physicians have developed protocols based on their clinical experiences. Robert Cathcart III, M.D., of Los Altos, California, recommends large amounts of vitamin C (and other vitamins and minerals) to patients with severe infections, ranging from colds and flus to mononucleosis and AIDS.

Why Don't More Doctors Recommend Vitamin Supplements?

Actually, more and more doctors are taking and recommending vitamin supplements. For example, a recent survey found that 44 percent of cardiologists took antioxidants, though only 37 percent also recommended them to patients. Still, physicians do not generally see vitamins as being therapeutic. According to Richard Kunin, M.D., of San Francisco, nutrients are the most dynamic driver of body chemistry.

Other physicians, such as Peter Langsjoen, M.D., a cardiologist in Tyler, Texas, point out that drug companies influence much of a physician's education after medical school. Drug companies are going to market and sell their products, not low-cost natural alternatives. A number of studies have found that physicians tend to prescribe what they hear about the most—just as the average shopper tends to buy the big brand names over the little ones.

Are Excess Vitamins "Expensive Urine"?

There are still some physicians who totally dismiss the use of vitamin supplements, and some have said that excess vitamins lead only to expensive urine. But it's really nothing more than a mean-spirited, irrational argument.

Here's why: If you drink an expensive bottle of wine, you'll also have expensive urine. Ditto for a prime steak—your body will use part of it and turn the rest into expensive stools. Should you then eat and drink the cheapest foods possible? Of course not, you should eat the most nutritious foods possible.

Your body will never absorb 100 percent of any of the food or nutrients you consume. If it did, you'd never have to go to the bathroom. You actually absorb a relatively small portion of what you eat, and it's no different with vitamins. When you take large doses of vitamins, your absorption becomes less efficient—but you'll still absorb more overall than if you took a smaller amount. So, don't pay attention to the critics. After reading this book, you'll probably know more about vitamins and health than they do.

Communicate with Your Physician

Nutritionally oriented physicians usually recommend that patients work with a physician if they want to use vitamins to treat a specific disease. This is good advice. But many people don't take it, perhaps because it's too hard to find a doctor who knows something about vitamins or because their insurance won't reimburse for that doctor's care.

As a consequence, many people end up treating themselves with vitamins, which isn't really all that bad. Vitamins are very safe, and people have a right to treat themselves. (For example, vitamins are safer than aspirin, which many people take to treat headaches without a physician's involvement.) If you have a serious chronic disease, you should, at the very least, let your doctor know you're taking vitamins, even if he or she doesn't believe vitamins have any benefits. You may have to assert yourself and tell your doctor that you intend to take vitamins unless he or she can come up with a good reason why you shouldn't.

It's wise to read up on anything you take, whether it's a vitamin or a prescription drug. While this book is a starting point, there are others that go into more depth about vitamins and how to use them. Some of these books and websites are listed in the Other Books and Resources section toward the end of this book. You can buy many of these books at bookstores and health food stores or borrow them from a public library.

VITAMIN A AND THE CAROTENOIDS

Vitamin A is an essential nutrient found in animal foods, and the carotenoids are found in fruits and vegetables. Beta-carotene, one of the most common carotenoids, can be converted to vitamin A in the body. The carotenoids lutein and lycopene play important roles in health, but the body cannot convert them to vitamin A. Vitamin A has weak antioxidant activity, whereas beta-carotene, lutein, and lycopene are powerful antioxidants with vitaminlike actions.

Carotenoids
Fat-soluble antioxidants produced by plants that protect cells from free radical damage.

Vitamin A for Eyes and More

If you've heard that vitamin A is good for the eyes, you heard right. Vitamin A helps convert light to signals that your brain can read, enabling you to see things and distinguish colors. Inadequate intake of vitamin A causes night blindness—a condition in which the eyes have difficulty adjusting to the dark or to bright lights. For this reason, night blindness impairs the vision of drivers. If it takes you more than a minute to adjust your eyes in a darkened theater, you probably have this condition.

Treating night blindness is relatively easy and fast acting. Simply increase your intake of vitamin A–containing foods, such as liver, or take daily supplements—up to 10,000 IU daily. Increasing your intake of fruits and vegetables or taking beta-carotene capsules can help, but these approaches take longer than pure vitamin A.

Emphysema
A lung disease caused by damage to the wall of the lungs, which creates large spaces that trap air, causing low blood oxygen levels, shortness of breath, and other problems.

Vitamin A is essential for the body's production of epithelial cells, which line most tissues and the skin. Many people find it helpful in skin disorders, such as cystic acne. One recent study found that a form of vitamin A might reverse emphysema in lab rats, but human studies are lacking.

In addition, vitamin A also has hormonelike effects in that it controls the growth and normal differentiation of cells. Differentiation is a normal process that turns new cells into heart cells or lung cells or bone cells. Cancer cells, on the other hand, are *undifferentiated*. In other words, vitamin A helps make normal cells.

Vitamin A protects against infection by strengthening the epithelial cell barrier to attacking bacteria and viruses. For years, children in developing nations died from measles, a respiratory disease that has been almost completed eliminated in Western nations. In the mid-1970s, it was discovered that these children were severely deficient in vitamin A and that brief high-dose supplements could cut the death rate from measles by one-third. The preventive dosage is 100,000 IU of vitamin A daily for two days, followed by 100,000 IU one month later.

Some studies have found high doses of vitamin A helpful in other respiratory infections, such as chicken pox and pneumonia. The key is high doses taken for a very short time, such as two days—not long-term, high-dose consumption.

Supplementing with Vitamin A Safely

There is a remote risk of toxicity with vitamin A. That's why recommendations for treating respiratory (lung) infections are high doses for only two days. While the dose—100,000 IU—is very high, it is taken for too short a time to cause side effects (which include hair loss and headaches).

In general, it's quite safe for people to take 10,000 IU of vitamin A daily for many years. Pregnant women, or women who plan to become pregnant, should probably take no more than 8,000 IU of vitamin A daily, because there is a slight risk of birth defects among pregnant women taking very large doses of this vitamin.

Beta-carotene is safe, even at very high doses. In some people, very high doses will turn the skin (particularly hands and feet) a yellow-orange color, but this is not dangerous, and it goes away shortly after supplementation is stopped. Only a small portion of beta-carotene is converted to vitamin A, so you can't create toxic levels of vitamin A by taking a lot of beta-carotene.

Understanding the Carotenoids

The carotenoids are fat-soluble antioxidants that plants produce to protect themselves from the damaging effects of free radicals. Free radicals are one of the basic causes of cancer, heart disease, and other degenerative diseases. Fourteen of the more than 600 carotenoids in nature show up in the blood, indicating that they are absorbed.

The principal dietary carotenoids appear to be beta-carotene (found in carrots), alpha-carotene (also found in carrots), lutein (found in kale, broccoli, and spinach), and lycopene (found in tomatoes). Other important—though minor—carotenoids are zeaxanthin and cryptoxanthin. When we eat foods containing carotenoids, we benefit from their antioxidant properties.

For example, in addition to being a source of vitamin A, beta-carotene quenches a type of free radical called "singlet oxygen." Several studies have reported that beta-carotene increases lung capacity—basically the amount of oxygen you can breathe in and out. The more oxygen you can take in with a single breath, the healthier you are. This

is because all of our cells need adequate oxygen to do their jobs well. Lung capacity generally decreases with age.

Beta-Carotene Research Results

Two studies found that beta-carotene slightly increased the risk of lung cancer among current smokers, particularly if they also drank alcohol. But these studies used synthetic beta-carotene. The synthetic form does not contain the powerful antioxidant found in natural beta-carotene supplements, which comes from *Dunaliella salina* algae. Even so, one of these studies found that former smokers taking beta-carotene had a lower risk of developing lung cancer.

Many studies have reported that beta-carotene taken with other antioxidants, such as vitamin E and selenium, is good for health. Beta-carotene seems to work best as part of an antioxidant team rather than by itself. Taking supplements containing "mixed carotenoids" and additional antioxidant vitamins as opposed to beta-carotene alone is recommended.

Several studies have found that a combination of beta-carotene supplements (taken orally) and conventional sunscreens (applied to the skin) work better than sunscreens alone. In a sense, beta-carotene helps provide inside-out protection against the ultraviolet (UV) radiation in sunlight. It most likely works by improving the skin's natural and internal defenses against UV damage.

Carotenoids for Eye and Prostate Health

The macula is the center of the eye's retina, acting kind of like a theater screen, and its premature breakdown is the leading cause of blindness among Americans over age sixty-five. Two carotenoids, lutein and zeaxanthin, seem to help preserve the macula. Together, they form the yellowish macular pigment that filters out damaging ultraviolet light and protects lipid-rich membranes from free radical damage.

A study published in *The Journal of the American Medical Association* (*JAMA*) found that people who eat foods rich in lutein—particularly kale and spinach—were less likely to develop macular degeneration. Studies have reported that consuming lutein-rich foods or supplements increases the thickness of the macular pigment. Lutein supplements may not reverse macular degeneration, but researchers believe it can slow the progression of this disease.

Zeaxanthin is also important to the macula, but it appears that the body can convert some lutein to zeaxanthin. There is evidence that lutein and zeaxanthin (both found in the eye lens) may also help slow the development of cataracts, but it's unclear whether these two carotenoids could actually reverse cataracts.

Recent studies on lutein and zeaxanthin have found that supplements increase the thickness of the macular pigment and, conse-

Cataract
Clouding over of the normally transparent eye lens, impairing vision. It is often associated with aging and diabetes.

quently, should reduce the long-term risk of macular degeneration. These nutrients work, in part, like polarizing sunglasses—they filter out stray light particles so they do not damage the eye.

Lycopene May Benefit the Prostate Gland

Some carotenoids, especially lycopene and beta-carotene, appear to benefit the prostate. In a study in the *Journal of the National Cancer Institute*, Edward Giovannucci, M.D., of Harvard University, reported that men eating large amounts of tomato sauce (more than ten servings weekly) were 45 percent less likely to develop prostate cancer. Raw tomatoes provided some benefit, but tomato juice didn't help at all.

Cooking tomatoes (for example, for spaghetti or pizza sauces) breaks down the cell walls containing lycopene, making more of this nutrient available for digestion and absorption. Such sauces are also made with olive oil, which aids lycopene absorption (because it is fat-soluble). Raw tomatoes are typically eaten with either salad dressing or meat, so the oil or fat in these foods aids absorption. Tomato juice is not cooked; nor does it contain additional oil.

Another Harvard University study found that, among men not eating fruits and vegetables, beta-carotene supplements reduced the risk of prostate cancer by one-third. High dietary intakes of lutein and zeaxanthin have also been associated with reduced prostate cancer risk.

THE B-VITAMIN COMPLEX

Together, the eleven B vitamins influence many aspects of health. For example, the B vitamins affect energy levels, mood, behavior, and risk of degenerative diseases, including heart disease and cancer. This section covers some of the ways B vitamins can improve your health.

Stress Relief and Improved Mood

The B vitamins have long been regarded as antistress vitamins. They are important for normal nerve and brain function, so inadequate levels of them interfere with the nervous system. According to David Benton, Ph.D., a researcher and professor at the University of Wales Swansea, the first signs of vitamin deficiencies are psychological problems. Among these are irritability, anger, and difficulty dealing with pressures at home or work.

To help combat stress, consider taking a B-complex supplement. Look on the label to make sure that it contains 10 mg of vitamin B_1, also known as thiamine—this is a clue to the relative amounts of the other B vitamins in the supplement. If you don't sense any improvement after thirty days, either triple the dose or buy a B-complex supplement with 25 mg of vitamin B_1.

Vitamin B_1 can also improve mood. Benton gave healthy students either a high-potency multivitamin (containing ten times the RDA of most vitamins) or a placebo (dummy pill) for a year. When he reevaluated the mood of the students, Benton found that the multivitamin group described themselves as more agreeable, and the women said their moods had improved significantly, according to his article in *Biological Psychology/Pharmacopsychology*.

While all of the vitamins seemed to help, vitamin B_1 stood out among the others. This may be because popular high-carbohydrate diets reduce vitamin B_1 activity. In a follow-up study that Benton conducted, female university students taking vitamin B_1 described themselves as more clearheaded, self-composed, and energetic after two months of supplementation. They also had faster reaction times.

Another B vitamin, folic acid, seems to improve mood, too. Low levels of this vitamin have been found in a significant percentage of adults suffering from depression. Supplementing with therapeutic amounts of folic acid has improved depression in many patients, according to recent research.

Lowering Cholesterol with Niacin

The niacin form of vitamin B_3 has been known since 1955 to lower cholesterol levels, which results in decreased heart disease risk. This was discovered by Abram Hoffer, M.D., Ph.D., one of the pioneers in the medical use of vitamins. Other forms of vitamin B_3, such as niacinamide, do not have this cholesterol-lowering effect.

Before you take niacin, be aware of its principal side effect. After taking it, you will have a body-wide flushing, or tingling, sensation. Your skin will turn beet red and you'll feel itchy all over. This reaction can be a little unsettling, but it is not harmful. The warm, flushing sensation (which some people even like) passes after about an hour.

If you continually take niacin three times a day, the flushing reaction will lessen and eventually stop. Hoffer recommends taking 500 mg of niacin three times daily. Vitamin C supplements—1,000 mg daily—can also sometimes reduce blood cholesterol levels, without flushing.

Vitamin B_3 for Schizophrenia

Schizophrenia is a mental disorder characterized by delusions (such as extreme paranoia) and hallucinations (seeing or hearing things that aren't there); it is not the same as split personality. In the early 1950s, Abram Hoffer, M.D., Ph.D., and Humphry Osmond, M.D., theorized that some types of schizophrenics were producing a hallucinogen in their own bodies. The hallucinogen was an oxidized form of adrenaline.

Based on their knowledge of biochemistry, these researchers believed that high doses of vitamin B_3 (either niacin or niacinamide) and vitamin C would neutralize this hallucinogen. They turned out to be right. The researchers published the first double-blind trial in the field of psychiatry in the *Bulletin of the Menninger Clinic.*

Hoffer usually gives schizophrenic patients 3,000 mg of vitamin B_3 and 1,000–3,000 mg of vitamin C daily. He has pointed out that patients with a recent onset of schizophrenia respond better to vitamin therapy than do patients who have suffered from schizophrenia for a very long time. Also, some schizophrenic patients respond better to high doses of vitamin B_6 and zinc, an essential dietary mineral.

Vitamins for Carpal Tunnel Syndrome Relief

Carpal tunnel syndrome is characterized by extreme pain or numbness in the wrist and hand. It is caused by the stress of a repetitive hand motion. Supermarket cashiers, typists, and factory workers are prone to it.

Some thirty years ago, John Ellis, M.D., of Mount Pleasant, Texas, found that vitamin B_6 could help patients with carpal tunnel syndrome. He found that patients with this disorder had low levels of vitamin B_6 and that taking 100 mg daily would restore normal levels after ninety days. Other researchers have also found strong associations between low vitamin B_6 levels and carpal tunnel syndrome. It's likely that the repetitive stress increases vitamin B_6 requirements.

It's unusual, however, for a person to be deficient in just one nutrient, and the B vitamins work together as a family of related nutrients. A better regimen for carpal tunnel might be 100 mg of vitamin B_6, plus a B-complex supplement containing all members of this family.

Normalizing Homocysteine Levels

Homocysteine is a byproduct of protein found in the blood. High blood levels of homocysteine cause free radical damage to blood vessel walls and set the stage for cholesterol deposits. Eventually, these deposits, or "plaques," can obstruct blood flow, increasing the risk of coronary heart disease.

Unlike cholesterol, homocysteine is not found in foods. Homocysteine levels rise when a person consumes too much protein (especially red meat) relative to B vitamins. A number of B vitamins are involved in breaking down homocysteine or recycling it back to protein. Folic acid appears to be the most important of these, but vitamins B_6 and B_{12} are also involved.

Homocysteine
An amino acid found in the blood and a byproduct of protein metabolism. At high levels, it damages blood vessel walls, increasing the risk of heart disease.

Research has also pointed to a likely relationship between elevated homocysteine levels, B vitamins, and the risk of Alzheimer's disease. Low blood levels of vitamin B_{12} and/or folic acid, as well as elevated homocysteine levels, greatly increase one's risk of developing the disease, according to recent studies. Folic acid supplementation can also reduce the risk of neural tube defects (like spina bifida) in babies when taken by the mother prior to conception and during pregnancy.

Quick and relatively inexpensive ways to test homocysteine levels are now available. In general, the lower the homocysteine level, the better; a level of less than 6 micromoles per liter of blood is ideal. Heart disease risk increases with the level, and more than 13 micromoles per liter is considered very dangerous. Supplements of 400 mcg of folic acid daily should normalize elevated homocysteine levels. Again, it may be best to take this amount as part of a B-complex supplement.

Multiple Sclerosis and Vitamin B_{12}

Multiple sclerosis, or MS, is characterized by damage to the sheaths that protect neurons of the central nervous system. Muscle weakness, visual impairment, lack of coordination, and other problems can result. The cause of the disease and satisfactory treatment are unknown.

A number of studies have found that people with MS are consistently deficient in vitamin B_{12}. Low levels of folic acid may also be a problem, as these two vitamins work hand in hand.

Multiple Sclerosis
A disease in which the protective coatings around neurons in the central nervous system deteriorate, slowing and short-circuiting nerve impulse conduction.

Many people have trouble absorbing B_{12} through the gut. Injections of B_{12} administered by a doctor can get around this problem. So can sublingual tablets, which are small and meant to dissolve under the tongue (where absorption is very efficient).

More B-Vitamin Benefits

If you have arthritis, listen up. Years ago, doctors found that they could ease symptoms of rheumatoid arthritis by giving one of the B vitamins, then ease symptoms some more by giving another B vitamin. It might be faster and more effective to simply take a high-potency B-complex supplement, rather than trying the B vitamins one by one.

One study, reported in the *Journal of the American College of Nutrition,* found that daily supplements of folic acid (6,400 mcg) and vitamin B_{12} (20 mcg) relieved symptoms of osteoarthritis of the hands. A more recent study, in the German journal *Schmerz,* described the analgesic (pain-relieving) properties of vitamins B_1, B_2, and B_{12}. The researcher noted that the combination of these vitamins is more effective than any of them individually.

Two recent studies showed that vitamin B_2 may reduce the frequency of migraine headaches. About two-thirds of migraine patients given 400 mg of B_2 daily for at least three months improved significantly. Only a small number in a placebo group improved. (Vitamin B_2 can make urine bright yellow, but this is its natural color and not harmful.)

Women experiencing premenstrual syndrome, or PMS, might find relief with B vitamins as well. PMS is often caused by excess estrogen, a female hormone. Two B vitamins, choline and inositol, help convert estrogen into estriol, a form of the hormone that doesn't seem to cause problems. In addition, vitamin B_6 is a diuretic and can prevent water retention before your period. Again, if you take B_6 (50–100 mg daily), add a B-complex supplement.

Vitamin C

Vitamin C is abundant in fruits and vegetables, but most people do not eat as many of these foods as they should. Have you eaten your three to five (or, as some organizations recommend, five to nine) servings of fruits and vegetables today? Probably not. For this reason alone, you could likely benefit from vitamin C supplements.

The Vitamin C and Cold Connection

In 1970, Nobel laureate Linus Pauling, Ph.D., recommended large doses of vitamin C in his book *Vitamin C and the Common Cold.* According to scientific studies published since then, Pauling was on to something. Vitamin C can reduce the symptoms and the length of colds and flu. There's no evidence suggesting that it prevents them, though; washing your hands after contact with an infected person is probably more preventive.

There have been dozens of scientific studies investigating vitamin C's effects on the common cold. Harri Hemilä, Ph.D., a researcher at the University of Helsinki, Finland, analyzed these studies as a group and found that taking 2–6 g (2,000–6,000 mg) of vitamin C daily, beginning at the first symptoms of a cold, cut the length and severity of the cold by about 30 percent. The minimum effective dose appeared to be 1 g (1,000 mg) daily. Another recent review also found that taking relatively high doses of vitamin C at a cold's onset does appear to reduce symptom duration, at least modestly.

Vitamin C works by enhancing your immune system's ability to fight infections. It increases the activity of white blood cells, T cells, and antibodies—all of which help kill bacteria and viruses. It also cleans up excess free radicals, which your body produces to fight bacteria and viruses.

Robert Cathcart III, M.D., of Los Altos, California, has for years recommended high doses of vitamin C to patients with much more serious infections, including mononucleosis and HIV/AIDS. Cathcart has used extremely high doses—from 25–100 grams daily—to treat these severe infections.

Vitamin C and Cancer

In the 1970s, Ewan Cameron, M.D., of Scotland, treated ter-minal cancer patients with large doses of vitamin C. In general, they lived longer than did patients not given vitamin C. A small number of patients were considered "cured." Over the past ten years, Abram Hoffer, M.D., Ph.D., of Victoria, Canada, has treated terminal cancer patients with large doses of vitamin C combined with other vitamins and minerals. About one-third of his earliest patients, who were judged terminal, have lived more than ten years and are considered, by conventional criteria, to be "cured."

Some types of cancer respond better than others to vitamin C. For example, women with reproductive cancers, such as breast cancer, respond to vitamin therapy much better than people with lung cancer. Hoffer's cancer regimen includes the following nutrients on a daily basis; the doses may vary from patient to patient.

- Vitamin C: 12 g or more
- Coenzyme Q_{10}:   300 mg
- Vitamin B_3:   500 mg–3 g
- Vitamin B_6:   250 mg for some (not all) patients
- Folic acid: 5–10 mg (not mcg)
- Other B vitamins: 25 to 50 times the RDA
- Vitamin E: 800 IU in the "succinate" form
- Carotenoids: 25,000–50,000 IU
- Selenium: 200–600 mcg
- Zinc: 220 mg (or 59 mg zinc citrate)

Of course, if you have cancer, it's best to work with a physician instead of treating yourself. If you have already had surgery, chemotherapy, or radiation, these supplements can enhance your immune system so your body does a better job of fighting recurrent cancer.

Vitamin C and Rheumatism

Vitamin C can protect against arthritis and rheumatism, though it likely works best in combination with B-complex vitamins. In rheumatism and rheumatoid arthritis, weak capillaries (our tiniest blood vessels) leak blood cells into the joints. The immune system responds as if these blood cells were invading bacteria, triggering a painful inflammatory response.

Rheumatism
A painful disorder of the body's supporting structures, including bones, joints, and muscles. Rheumatoid arthritis involves inflamed joints.

Supplemental vitamin C strengthens capillary walls, as do antioxidant flavonoids (vitaminlike nutrients found in fruits and vegetables). In this way, they prevent leakage from blood vessels and the resulting inflammatory response. Vitamin C is also essential for the body's manufacture of collagen, a protein needed to form the soft tissue in bone joints and the skin.

In a recent issue of the French medical journal *Revue Du Rhumatisme*, Jean Léone, M.D., of the Robert Debré Teaching Hospital in Reims, describes how two patients with rheumatism were actually suffering from scurvy (rheumatism was a symptom of scurvy). Scurvy is a severe vitamin C deficiency disease characterized by bleeding gums and other abnormal bleeding, such as wounds that do not heal. (The bleeding is caused by weak capillary walls.) Léone's patients recovered after he gave them 1,000 mg of vitamin C daily for ten days.

Additional Potential Benefits

In a study directed by Allen Taylor, Ph.D., of Tufts University, Boston, vitamin C supplements dramatically reduced the risk of developing cataracts. A cataract is the clouding of the eye's lens, which impairs vision. It can be caused by excessive exposure to UV sunlight, medications, injury, and disease complications. While cataracts are easily corrected with surgery (in which the lens is removed and replaced by a plastic one), it's always best to avoid surgery. Also, cataracts may be a sign of other looming health problems.

In Taylor's study, he found that women who took at least 400 mg of vitamin C supplements daily—for more than ten years—were about 80 percent less likely to develop cataracts. Dietary vitamin C didn't offer this protection. The association between higher blood levels of vitamin C and decreased cataract risk has been supported by more recent research, too.

Vitamin C may even help allergies because it has a slight antihistaminic effect, like many allergy medications. During allergic reactions, the body releases a compound called histamine, which makes you red and itchy. Vitamin C does not have any of the negative side effects associated with antihistamine drugs. For example, it will not make you drowsy. It is also essential for normal immune function, and it likely corrects some of the immune defects involved in allergies.

Vitamin C might reduce the risk of gallbladder disease. Your gallbladder stores bile, a substance that helps digest fats. Gallstones are rich in cholesterol, and vitamin C limits their formation by activating an enzyme that breaks cholesterol down into bile acids. An estimated 20 million Americans suffer from gallstones, and the typical person with gallbladder disorders is an overweight, middle-aged woman.

Joel A. Simon, M.D., of the University of California, San Francisco, found that among 2,744 women, those consuming large amounts of vitamin C—particularly from supplements—had a 26 percent lower risk of developing gallbladder disease (of all types) and a 23 percent lower risk of having their gallbladders removed, compared with women consuming little vitamin C.

More recent research, based on data from the Third National Health and Nutrition Examination Survey, supports these findings. This time, vitamin C supplements on their own were associated with a 34 percent lower prevalence of gallstones in women. Total vitamin C intake was linked to a 39 percent lower risk among women. Vitamin C did not influence gallstone risk among men.

Taking Vitamin C Supplements

Most people can benefit from 1,000–2,000 mg of vitamin C daily. Even 500 mg is better than nothing. If you're willing to take higher dosages, follow Cathcart's concept of adjusting the dose to "bowel tolerance." He recommends increasing your vitamin C dose (divided up several times daily) until your stools become loose, and then lowering the dose slightly.

Cathcart has found that the sicker a person is, the more vitamin C he or she can tolerate without diarrhea. For example, if you get an average cold, your vitamin C tolerance may increase to 10 grams a day. If you get a very bad cold, your vitamin C tolerance may increase to 25 grams a day. As you start to get better, your vitamin C requirements will decrease. For example, when you're in good health, you may be able to tolerate only 1–3 grams of vitamin C a day.

For most people, the ideal dose of vitamin C is just under the amount that causes loose stools and diarrhea. Divide your dosage so you take a little of it two to four times per day. This increases absorption and decreases the likelihood of developing diarrhea.

Some evidence suggests that many people don't get enough vitamin C. Early signs of a deficiency include tiredness and irritability; advanced signs include bleeding gums, bruising, sores that take a long time to heal, frequent colds, and extreme fatigue. Vitamin C is considered very safe for nearly everyone in the general population at levels up to 2 grams daily, according to The Food and Nutrition Board of the Institute of Medicine of the United States and Canada. One study, published in 1998, reported that 500 mg of vitamin C damaged DNA, but the subsequent experiments by the researchers found just the opposite: that vitamin C protected DNA.

VITAMINS D AND K FOR HEALTHY BONES

It's often assumed that people get adequate quantities of vitamin D, but low intake may be fairly common. The vitamin works with calcium, an essential mineral, to help build strong bones and teeth. Thus, it plays an important role in preventing osteoporosis, the disease in which bones become porous, fragile, and susceptible to fracture.

The Calcium Helper

You probably already know that calcium is important for building and maintaining strong bones. But calcium needs vitamin D to do its job. That's because vitamin D enhances the absorption of calcium.

Research results have shown that treating vitamin D deficiency results in a significant reduction of hip fractures in patients with osteoporosis. In a separate study, reported in the *New England Journal of Medicine,* a combination of calcium (500 mg daily) and vitamin D (700 IU daily) increased bone density in several hundred elderly men and women.

Osteoporosis and osteoarthritis are not the same problem, but vitamin D may play a role in both. In one study, Timothy E. McAlindon, M.D., of the Boston University Arthritis Center, found that patients were more likely to have osteoarthritis of the knees if they did not consume 400 IU of vitamin D daily. Vitamin D has hormonelike roles in the body, so it probably influences the growth of cells involved in healthy joints.

"D" for Deficiency

Children might get enough vitamin D from milk, but not all milk is fortified with vitamin D and many adults don't drink much milk. Your body can make its own vitamin D with the sun's help. Spending at least fifteen minutes in the sun at least three or four times each week is considered adequate. Yet many people with office jobs and elderly people restricted to their homes don't get outside much or may face cloudy weather when they do.

Elderly, frail people are especially susceptible to vitamin D deficiency. In a study of 290 patients, Melissa K. Thomas, M.D., Ph.D., of Massachusetts General Hospital, Boston, found that 164 patients over age sixty-five were deficient in vitamin D, and 22 percent were severely deficient. Even many younger subjects turned out to be deficient in vitamin D. Thomas found that 42 percent of men and women, ranging from the late thirties to the late fifties in age, were low in vitamin D.

Supplementation can ensure that you get enough vitamin D. Very high doses for extended periods can be toxic, but getting 400–800 IU daily is safe for adults. (The RDA is 400 IU daily.) Some experts recommend 800 IU daily for those over age sixty-five and 400 IU daily for younger people.

And What about Vitamin K?

Vitamin K, also called phylloquinone, is a fat-soluble vitamin needed to help blood platelet cells clot after a cut or incision. Without vitamin K, you would bleed to death from the slightest scratch. It is also essential for brain development. According to M. J. Shearer, Ph.D., of St. Thomas's Hospital, London, babies who were deficient in this vitamin during the first six months of their lives risk permanent brain damage or death.

Recent research has emphasized the role of vitamin K in bone formation. Osteocalcin is one of the proteins involved in bone development. To build bone, osteocalcin must be loaded by chemical structures known as carboxyl groups. Your body uses vitamin K to help attach these carboxyl groups to osteocalcin. In a study of nine healthy women at Tufts University, Boston, James A. Sadlowski, Ph.D., found that vitamin K supplements increased the attachment of carboxyl groups to osteocalcin, setting the stage for bone formation.

Sadlowski's study used 420 mcg of vitamin K daily, which is about four times the RDA. Some study findings suggest that vitamin K intakes much higher than current recommendations improve bone health. In addition, researchers found that low vitamin K intake may increase hip fracture risk in women, based on results from the Nurses' Health Study cohort. This has led some experts to suggest that vitamin K requirements be reassessed.

According to an article in the *Journal of Nutrition,* the vitamin K content of most foods is low. Leafy green vegetables are excellent dietary sources. However, absorption of vitamin K from foods is poor, so supplements may be beneficial. If you take a multivitamin, make sure there's some vitamin K in it.

VITAMIN E FOR HEART AND MIND

Years ago, doctors dismissed vitamin E as the "sex vitamin" and a "cure in search of a disease." Yet time has been on this amazing vitamin's side. Studies have found that vitamin E supplements can reduce your risk of coronary heart disease and stroke. It can slow the progression of Alzheimer's disease and maybe prevent it. It can even help your immune system.

Vitamin E and Heart Health

In the 1940s, Evan Shute, M.D., and his brother Wilfrid Shute, M.D., of Canada, pioneered the use of vitamin E supplements in the prevention and treatment of coronary heart disease. Even *Time* magazine wrote about their work in 1946. But most doctors believed vitamins cured only vitamin-deficiency diseases, not conditions like heart disease. So while the Shutes went on to treat tens of thousands of patients with vitamin E over the years, most doctors felt vitamin E was worthless.

Meanwhile, researchers conducted basic research on vitamin E and found it to be a powerful antioxidant and the body's principal fat-soluble antioxidant. In the early 1990s, researchers at Harvard University reported that supplements of vitamin E greatly reduced the risk of heart disease and heart attacks. A 1996 study published in the journal *Lancet* showed that vitamin E supplements—400–800 IU daily—reduced the incidence of heart attack by 77 percent.

Since then, vitamin E has practically become a standard part of mainstream medicine. Many physicians take vitamin E and recommend it to their patients. An analysis of the five largest trials investigating vitamin E for heart health, published in the journal *Current Opinion in Lipidology* in 2001, concluded that alpha-tocopherol (the most common form of vitamin E) was beneficial in patients with preexisting heart disease. (The one study showing no benefit was criticized for design flaws.)

Vitamin E's antioxidant power helps explain how it keeps cholesterol from damaging your blood vessels. Low-density lipoprotein, the so-called "bad" form of cholesterol commonly referred to as LDL, is actually needed to transport vitamin E and the carotenoids through the bloodstream. When there is insufficient vitamin E in the LDL, that LDL is prone to oxidation, or free radical damage.

Oxidized LDL builds up on blood vessel walls over time, limiting normal blood flow. In studies with people, Ishwarlal Jialal, M.D., of the University of Texas Southwestern Medical Center, Dallas, found that vitamin E supplements protect LDL from oxidation, thus preventing LDL deposits in blood vessels and reducing the risk of coronary heart disease.

LDL
Low-density lipoprotein, or LDL, transports proteins, triglycerides (fats), cholesterol, and fat-soluble vitamins through the blood to body cells.

Vitamin E can benefit even those eating a diet high in fat, but eating healthfully is best, of course. In a study described in the *Journal of the American Medical Association*, Gary D. Plotnick, M.D., of the University of Maryland School of Medicine, Baltimore, found that high-fat foods prevent blood vessels from relaxing. The long-term effect is to increase blood pressure and the risk of heart disease. When Plotnick gave his subjects (men and women) 800 IU of vitamin E and 1,000 mg of vitamin C, their blood vessels behaved normally after eating a high-fat, high-carbohydrate meal.

Vitamin E and Reproductive Health

When vitamin E was discovered in 1922, it was called the "fertility vitamin" because rodents deficient in vitamin E became sterile. Being infertile, of course, is different from being impotent. Still, people started referring to vitamin E as the sex vitamin.

Some men with impotency may improve with vitamin E, though the improvement won't happen overnight. This is because impotence is often related to cardiovascular disease. In impotency, the blood vessels of the penis become as damaged as those of the heart. So anything that improves cardiovascular disease—including vitamin E—might also help in impotency.

Vitamin E improves blood flow to all tissues, including those in the penis. Every condition improves with better blood flow. However, if you are impotent because of psychological reasons, like performance anxiety, vitamin E probably won't help.

Several studies, published in *Fertility and Sterility*, have reported that infertile men have high levels of free radicals and low levels of antioxidants in their semen. For this reason, many urologists recommend vitamin E and other antioxidants to infertile men. It takes at least three months for vitamins to have an effect, mainly because it takes that long for sperm to mature. Infertile couples should both take supplemental vitamin E and a high-potency multivitamin for several months before trying to conceive.

More Good News

The list of vitamin E benefits doesn't end with reproductive and heart health. Researchers have found that this incredible vitamin seems to slow the progression of Alzheimer's disease. This debilitating disease affects about 20 million people in the world, robbing them of healthy minds. There is currently no cure for Alzheimer's disease.

Mary Sano, Ph.D., of Columbia University's College of Physicians and Surgeons, New York, and her colleagues found that 2,000 IU of vitamin E (a very large dose) given to severe Alzheimer's patients for two years delayed the progression of end-stage Alzheimer's disease by eight months compared with the placebo group. After Sano's study was published in the *New England Journal of Medicine*, the American Psychiatric Association recommended that Alzheimer's patients receive vitamin E. Since then, the American Academy of Neurology and the Alzheimer's Association have officially encouraged physicians to use 1,000 IU of vitamin E, twice daily, to slow the progression of Alzheimer's disease.

Alzheimer's Disease
A degenerative brain disease caused by neuron dysfunction and death that causes problems with memory, feelings, thinking, and behavior.

There are a couple of reasons that vitamin E may slow Alzheimer's disease—and possibly even prevent or delay its onset. This nutrient is essential for normal functioning of cell membranes, or walls. These cell membranes have doors that allow vitamins and other nutrients in and waste products out. These membranes harden with age, but vitamin E seems to keep them younger and suppler. In addition, vitamin E limits free radical damage to brain cells, and high levels of free radicals are thought to be a major cause of Alzheimer's disease.

Several studies show that vitamin E can enhance resistance to infection. This is particularly important for older folks, because the immune system declines with age. In a study at Tufts University, Boston, researchers found that 200 IU of vitamin E daily improved immune responsiveness significantly, meaning that the immune system would be more likely to respond to infection during a bacterial attack. Subjects taking vitamin E had 30 percent fewer infections, too. Other studies have found that vitamin E (as well as the mineral selenium) can prevent dangerous mutations in the Coxsackie virus, which infects some 20 million Americans a year, causing sore throats and coldlike symptoms.

If you feel wiped out after a workout, consider upping your vitamin E intake. Your body's cells produce free radicals as a byproduct of normal activities, called metabolism. When you exercise, you speed up the process and generate more free radicals. So ironically, excessive exercise is bad. The solution is not to become a couch potato, but to take vitamin E and other antioxidants.

These vitamins prevent DNA (genetic) damage and oxidation of cell fats caused by overexercise. According to Lester Packer, Ph.D., a researcher at the University of California, Berkeley, and one of the foremost authorities on antioxidants, vitamin E can probably reduce exercise-induced fatigue. Quicker recovery from fatigue can improve exercise performance.

Vitamin E for Diabetes

People with diabetes taking insulin or hypoglycemic drugs should start taking vitamins at a low dose and gradually increase the dose, unless their physician asks them to take higher doses sooner. Because most vitamins are involved in converting blood sugar, or glucose, to energy, vitamins may speed up this process and lower glucose levels. So you have to exercise a little caution at first.

The good news is that anyone with diabetes can benefit from vitamin supplementation. Glucose generates large numbers of free radicals, and this gets out of hand in diabetic people because they have high glucose levels. These free radicals oxidize cholesterol and damage blood vessel walls; this is one reason why people with diabetes have an above-average risk of developing cardiovascular diseases.

Vitamin E and a vitaminlike antioxidant, alpha-lipoic acid, help control these excess free radicals and reduce the damage. Alpha-lipoic acid (300–600 mg daily for diabetes) may also lower glucose levels by 10 to 30 percent, but the glucose levels also stabilize, which is better for controlling diabetes. Other vitamins, such as vitamin C and the B-complex vitamins, also help control diabetes and diabetic complications.

Vitamin E and Heart Disease Patients

Even people who already have heart disease can benefit from boosting vitamin E intake. As mentioned earlier, authors of a recent analysis of large-scale trials of vitamin E supplementation found that four out of the five supported a benefit for vitamin E supplementation in patients who already had heart disease. (The fifth study was criticized for design flaws.) Subjects taking vitamin E (the alpha-toco-

pherol form) supplements in these studies had a dramatically reduced risk of nonfatal heart attack.

Substantial research shows that vitamin E and other antioxidant vitamins can reduce the risk of complications from heart surgery. Heart surgery is a major stress, and about 3 percent of people undergoing bypass surgery do not survive. It's crucial for heart disease patients to check with their doctors before supplementing with vitamin E, however. Large doses of vitamin E could potentially thin the blood too much in patients who already take prescription blood thinners like Coumadin.

During bypass surgery, blood flow is stopped so doctors can graft new arteries. When blood flow is replenished, large numbers of free radicals are generated, and these radicals can damage the heart. Some heart surgeons give their patients vitamin E supplements before surgery to limit this damage.

Taking Vitamin E

As Americans, our vitamin E requirements are very high, in part, because we eat large quantities of refined oils (for example, in salad dressing, French fries, and many other foods). These oils are very prone to oxidation, and vitamin E protects against their oxidation, in and out of the body. So the more fats you eat, the higher your vitamin E needs are.

Most experts seem to have settled on 400 IU of vitamin E daily as the best dose for heart health support and other benefits. Some studies have shown that levels as low as 100 IU provide some benefit and that higher doses (800 IU–1,200 IU) are safe, though probably unnecessary. It's virtually impossible to get 400 IU of vitamin E from diet alone. It's been estimated that you'd have to eat 1,000 almonds to get 400 IU of vitamin E—and all those almonds would contain 8,000 calories and more than a pound of fat.

d-alpha tocopherol
The form of natural vitamin E most abundant in our bodies and most often used in vitamin supplements. It supports reproduction and promotes good health.

Natural vitamin E (most of which comes from soybeans) is better for you than the synthetic form. Over the years, studies have found that natural vitamin E is about 36 percent more biologically active than the synthetic form. A recent study by Graham W. Burton, Ph.D., of Canada's National Research Council, found that natural vitamin E was absorbed twice as efficiently as the synthetic form.

It's easy to distinguish between synthetic and natural forms of vitamin E with a little detective work. Synthetic vitamin E will be identified by its chemical name, "dl-alpha tocopherol" or "dl-alpha tocopheryl acetate" on the nutrition facts panel of supplement bottle labels. In contrast, natural vitamin E is called "d-alpha tocopherol," "d-alpha tocopheryl acetate," or "d-alpha tocopheryl succinate." In other words, "dl" signifies synthetic and "d" denotes natural vitamin E.

There's a simple way to remember the difference. The "d" means that it is *delicious* to your body; conversely, your body *doesn't like* the "dl" (or synthetic) form as much. There are various vitamin E compounds, but the key is to look for the "d," which indicates natural.

Some experts believe that a "full-spectrum" vitamin E supplement is even better than d-alpha tocopherol alone. Unlike most vitamins, vitamin E has eight different forms, known as stereoisomers. Alpha-tocopherol is the most well known. The other forms are also important to health in ways that researchers are just beginning to understand. This is why Andreas Papas, Ph.D., one of today's foremost vitamin E experts, recommends that people seek out a supplement containing all eight forms of vitamin E, often listed on labels as "mixed tocotrienols" and "mixed tocopherols." Together, the thinking goes, the eight forms of vitamin E work as a team to keep us healthy. (Again, look for the natural form.)

WHAT MINERALS CAN DO FOR YOUR HEALTH

By now, you surely realize that vitamins offer amazing health benefits, but the story doesn't end there. There's another group of micronutrients that deserves your attention. This group is made up of essential minerals. They're referred to as essential because the body needs them to function correctly and we must get them from the diet; the body can't make them on its own. Minerals make up only about 4 percent of one's total body weight, but their importance is weighty indeed.

Minerals Defined

As we mentioned earlier, minerals are elements, which means that they cannot be broken down into simpler substances. Unlike vitamins, which come from living organisms, minerals come from nonliving matter. This is why we refer to minerals as inorganic, or nonliving.

Minerals are usually ingested as compounds (in combination with other minerals or organic compounds) as opposed to solitary elements, whether they be in food or supplement form. Minerals must be freed from their compounds during digestion so they can be absorbed and used by the body.

There are two groups of minerals that everyone needs: macrominerals (or major minerals) and microminerals (often called trace minerals). Macrominerals are considered the major minerals because they make up more body weight than the microminerals. The body requires each

macromineral in an amount greater than 100 milligrams per day from diet and supplement intake. Calcium, magnesium, chloride, sodium, potassium, phosphorus, and sulfur are macrominerals.

The remaining essential minerals—iron, zinc, selenium, manganese, chromium, cobalt, molybdenum, iodine, fluorine, and copper—are microminerals. These are usually required in amounts less than 100 milligrams per day—but that doesn't mean that they are any less crucial for good health. Other trace minerals—silicon and vanadium, for example—are essential in animals and thought to be essential in humans, too.

Macro- and Microminerals
Macrominerals are minerals that the body needs in amounts greater than 100 milligrams each day. Microminerals are those that the body requires in smaller amounts.

The Myriad Roles of Minerals

Minerals play an impressive array of roles in the body. Calcium, for one, helps make bones and teeth hard, regulates hormones, and is involved in muscle contractions, blood clotting, and more. Minerals regulate many body processes and are needed for brain function, fluid regulation, acid-base balance, bone growth, enzyme action, carrying oxygen in the blood, making fatty acids, digesting protein, and so on.

Some minerals act as electrolytes, which are salts found in body fluids that maintain electrical neutrality. Electrolytes called cations have a positive electrical charge, while anions are negatively charged. A proper ratio of cations to anions is needed to keep the body in balance at all times.

Like vitamins, many minerals are finally gaining attention for their incredible antioxidant powers. As you'll remember from earlier chapters, antioxidants neutralize pesky free radicals before they have a chance to wreak havoc on our cells. This is one way that minerals help protect us from heart disease, cancer, and other age-related diseases.

Mineral Intake Affects Disease Risk

Mineral intake affects the risk and course of many diseases. For example, researchers have determined that copper deficiency may contribute to high blood pressure, enhanced inflammation, anemia, and heart disease. Low magnesium levels are also associated with heart disease and irregular heartbeats called arrhythmias. Some researchers have compared deficiencies of zinc and some vitamins to harmful radiation because these deficiencies break DNA strands and cause oxidative damage that encourages disease.

As you might expect, sufficient mineral intake can often decrease disease risk and complications. Many studies have found that supplemental calcium decreases a person's risk of osteoporosis, a bone disease affecting millions

Osteoporosis
A condition of reduced bone density and increased bone brittleness that can lead to bones that break easily.

of people in the United States that causes pain, fracture, and deformity.

Zinc has inhibited prostate cancer cell growth and disease progression in recent studies. And it's very clear, based on research results from human clinical trials and other studies, that selenium protects against cancer. Chromium picolinate, the most effective form of the mineral chromium, improves insulin activity and blood glucose levels in people with type II diabetes, a disease characterized by high blood sugar levels and an increased risk of heart disease, kidney disease, and nerve function loss.

Supplements Can Boost Mineral Intake

You might be surprised to learn that mineral intake in the United States is often inadequate. Some of the reasons for this are the same as those that explain why people aren't getting enough vitamins: the lack of a truly balanced diet high in vitamins and minerals and lower nutrient levels in farmland soil, for starters.

The good news is that mineral supplements can help you get enough of these very valuable micronutrients. Certainly, supplements are no substitute for a healthy diet and lifestyle, but they can help fill in nutritional gaps and improve your health. Think of vitamin and mineral supplements as inexpensive insurance.

In the following pages, you'll read about the important functions of many essential minerals, the latest exciting research about their disease-fighting powers, ways to improve your intake, and where you can learn more about them. The topic of minerals is complex, but if you keep reading, you'll no doubt learn more about how minerals can help you live a long and healthy life.

CALCIUM, MAGNESIUM, AND POTASSIUM FOR HEALTHY HEART AND BONES

You probably already associate calcium with strong bones, but did you know that magnesium is also needed for bone health due to its role in calcium metabolism? Were you aware that calcium can alleviate premenstrual syndrome, that magnesium is recommended for migraine relief, and that potassium might help lower blood pressure? These three minerals have many functions in the body—some related to their common status as electrolytes. Their potential to fend off health problems is promising.

Calcium for Strong Bones and Teeth

Ninety-nine percent of the calcium you ingest is used to

mineralize bones and teeth, making them harder and stronger. But the other 1 percent of calcium plays many other roles in health. It helps clot blood, regulates contraction and relaxation in heart and skeletal muscles, frees up energy from food, helps the body use iron, and more.

We tend to view bones as static, solid structures. However, bone is constantly changing, remodeling itself throughout our lives. Calcium absorbed from the diet and supplements is deposited in bone, and old bone is resorbed (the opposite of absorbed) and excreted. Calcium is drawn from bone to normalize body fluid levels when necessary.

People generally reach skeletal maturity and homeostasis by around thirty years of age. This means that the amount of calcium deposited in bone is equal to the amount resorbed. After that, we begin to lose more bone than we gain. This age-related bone loss is associated with the loss of bone strength and density and increased susceptibility to fracture over time.

Adequate intake of calcium and other bone-building nutrients (vitamin D, vitamin K, and magnesium, for example) from childhood on encourages the formation of new bone, protecting us from the bone disease osteoporosis as we age. Ten million people in the United States have the disease, in which bones become porous, fragile, and susceptible to fracture. Eighteen million more are at risk for the disease due to low bone mass.

Menopausal and postmenopausal women are especially at risk for osteoporosis, as bone loss speeds up when estrogen levels decline in menopause. In fact, one in two women over age sixty-five will have an osteoporotic fracture. Building strong bones early in life with good nutrition and regular exercise is paramount to staving off osteoporosis down the road. Adequate calcium intake, in the presence of vitamin D, has been proven to prevent bone loss and reduce the risk of fractures in peri- and postmenopausal women.

Calcium is also useful in treating osteoporosis. In a recent research review of eleven well-designed studies, calcium was effective in treating the disease among populations with low intake who were given adequate supplementation. This mineral may also offer benefits in relation to disorders including hypertension, colorectal cancer, and obesity; but the scope of calcium's effects and the way it works in these disorders are not well understood.

Calcium Can Alleviate PMS

Premenstrual syndrome, or PMS, is one of the most common disorders in women, afflicting millions of premenopausal age. Fortunately, calcium has proven effective in significantly alleviating PMS. Clinical trials have found that calcium supplementation alleviates most mood and physical symptoms, such as cramps.

A study reported in the *American Journal of Obstetrics*

and *Gynecology* in 1998 found that 1,200 milligrams of elemental calcium daily taken as calcium carbonate was effective in squelching PMS symptoms. Several hundred healthy, premenopausal female subjects took the calcium supplements or placebo for the duration of three menstrual cycles. Those taking calcium experienced reduced total symptoms of PMS by 48 percent overall by the third cycle (the placebo group improved only 30 percent). Symptoms reduced included "negative effect," water retention, food cravings, and pain. Although 1,200–1,600 mg per day of calcium supplementation may alleviate PMS, women can take less if they eat diets high in calcium.

It isn't surprising that calcium and PMS are interrelated. Ovarian hormones affect the metabolism of calcium, vitamin D, and magnesium, and calcium metabolism and its intestinal absorption are regulated by estrogen. Fluctuating hormone levels throughout the menstrual cycle affect the regulation of calcium and these other nutrients. PMS shares several symptoms (anxiety and depression, for example) with hypocalcemia, a state of below-normal calcium levels. This has led some researchers to conclude that PMS represents the manifestation of calcium deficiency that can be reversed with supplementation.

Getting Enough Calcium

Most people associate calcium with dairy products, but it is also found in seafood, almonds, sesame seeds, mustard greens, corn tortillas, broccoli, dried fruits, beans, and other foods. Even so, you may not be getting enough calcium. It's one of the few nutrients still deficient in several industrialized countries, including the United States.

The average adult gets 500–700 mg of the recommended 1,000 mg per day for adults over age eighteen. A supplement of 300–700 mg per day may even be sufficient for optimal intake. A dosage of 1,200 mg per day is recommended for women over age fifty on estrogen replacement therapy (ERT), and 1,500 mg is recommended for women not taking ERT. In addition, 400–600 mg of vitamin D is recommended to ensure adequate calcium absorption.

Adolescents aged nine to eighteen should get 1,300 mg of calcium each day. Pregnant and lactating women should follow guidelines for their age group, according to Tori Hudson, N.D., a professor of gynecology at the National College of Naturopathic Medicine in Portland, Oregon. Calcium absorption increases during pregnancy, so higher intake for pregnant women may not be necessary. Up to 2,500 mg of calcium daily is considered safe.

Only about one-third of the calcium you ingest is actually absorbed, and absorption varies among different forms. Dollar for dollar, calcium citrate is the best-absorbed form. Avoid calcium from oyster shell or bone meal, as these can contain high levels of lead. The lowest lead levels are in refined calcium carbonate and calcium chelates. Citrate,

fumarate, malate, succinate, and aspartate are all chelate forms of calcium. Hudson advises taking half the recommended dosage if you're taking calcium citrate or malate, the most absorbable forms.

Antacids are not a good source of calcium for two reasons. One, the aluminum compound they contain may hinder calcium absorption, and two, they may reduce calcium absorption by making the stomach more alkaline. There is also concern that aluminum may be linked to the development of Alzheimer's disease. Research suggests that calcium-rich bottled mineral waters, however, are a good source and at least as well absorbed as that from dairy products.

Chelated Minerals
Minerals that are bound to other molecules that increase absorption by the body.

Too much calcium can interfere with absorption of zinc and other nutrients. For example, magnesium and calcium compete for absorption when there is an excess of either in the gut. Finding a well-formulated multivitamin and mineral supplement or bone health formula can help you get enough—but not too much—of each ingredient. Many experts recommend taking two parts calcium to one part magnesium. Calcium and phosphorus in a ratio of 2:1 in a formula is also often advised.

Magnesium—The Multifaceted Mineral

Magnesium is needed for proper calcium metabolism and deficiencies of it have been linked to osteoporosis. This trace mineral is involved in several hundred chemical reactions in the body and is required by every cell. Magnesium is needed to generate and use adenosine triphosphate, or ATP, your body's energy source. It is also involved in contracting heart and smooth muscle, mineral absorption, protein synthesis, blood clotting, and insulin function.

Sixty percent or more of magnesium in your body is found in bone, so it's not surprising that depleted magnesium levels negatively affect bone metabolism and are considered a risk factor in osteoporosis. Oral magnesium supplements suppressed bone turnover in healthy, young men in one recent study. Because increased bone turnover contributes to bone loss, magnesium supplementation may reduce bone loss associated with high bone turnover, such as in age-related osteoporosis.

Magnesium benefits more than bones. Deficiency of this mineral has been linked to insulin resistance, and supplementation has improved insulin sensitivity and insulin secretion among patients with type II diabetes. Insulin helps glucose (the sugar your cells use for fuel) go from blood into cells to be used for energy. This keeps the amount of glucose in blood within a normal range.

In diabetes, the body doesn't produce enough insulin, or cells aren't sensitive to the insulin it does produce. The result is dangerously elevated blood glucose levels. Theoretically, better insulin sensitivity and secretion resulting

Diabetes Mellitus

A condition caused by undersecretion of the hormone insulin (in type I diabetes) or cell insensitivity to insulin (in type II diabetes), leading to high blood glucose levels.

from magnesium supplementation could help regulate the amount of glucose in blood.

No beneficial effect of magnesium on blood glucose control in diabetic patients has yet been demonstrated, though. Still, there is also potential for magnesium to help people with diabetes by decreasing the risk of retinopathy (deterioration in the blood vessels of the retina) and high blood pressure (at least a little).

Many studies have shown that magnesium intake affects blood pressure. High blood pressure is a major risk factor for stroke, the third leading cause of death in the world. Magnesium, as well as potassium and fiber, appeared to decrease stroke risk in male subjects in one study, especially among those who were hypertensive (that is, those who had high blood pressure).

Another study found that diets high in magnesium and potassium were associated with reduced medication cost and better blood pressure control in elderly, hypertensive patients. These findings led researchers to recommend increased magnesium intake for hypertensive people. (Anyone with kidney problems should consult their doctor first.) Magnesium, along with calcium and potassium, encourages relaxation of vascular smooth muscle, helping to keep blood passageways open and blood pressure in check.

Ameliorating Migraines and More

Migraine is marked by extremely painful headaches, nausea, vomiting, increased sensitivity to light and sound, and reduced activity. Drugs used to treat migraine have side effects. Low brain levels of magnesium have been reported in migraine, and as many as 50 percent of patients have lowered levels of ionized magnesium during an attack.

In one recent study, two weeks of magnesium-rich mineral water intake improved intracellular (that is, within cells) magnesium status in migraine patients. Intravenous magnesium sulfate alleviates pain and other symptoms during migraine attacks, but a doctor must administer this form. Two well-controlled studies have suggested that regular oral magnesium supplementation might reduce the frequency of migraine headaches. These supplements are safe, inexpensive, and often recommended for migraine.

Magnesium may also benefit heart failure and heart attack patients, pregnant women with preeclampsia (also called toxemia), chronic fatigue patients, and others under a doctor's guidance. These topics are beyond the scope of this book, but the list does highlight the breadth of magnesium's impact.

Taking More Magnesium

It's difficult to measure a person's magnesium levels, because 99 percent of this mineral in your body is in soft tissue and bone as opposed to blood, which is easier to test. Even so, we know that deficiency is common in the general population. Low levels can result from low intake, diarrhea, vomiting, chronic diuretic use, some prescription medications, and too much sugar and fat in the diet.

Some good dietary sources of magnesium are nuts, legumes, soybeans, blackstrap molasses, vegetables, seafood, and brown rice. When it comes to supplements, look for magnesium in citrate, aspartate, or malate forms. These are better absorbed and tend to not have the laxative effect of magnesium sulfate and others.

The RDA for magnesium is 310–320 mg daily for adult females and 400–420 mg daily for adult men. Up to 700 mg a day may be recommended for specific health problems. Excess magnesium is unlikely to cause toxicity in healthy people. If you have diarrhea from magnesium supplementation, reduce the dosage. Those with kidney disorders should consult their doctors before taking magnesium, as should pregnant and nursing women.

Potassium—Keeping the Body in Balance

Potassium, sodium, calcium, magnesium, and chloride all act as electrolytes in body fluids. The molecules of electrolytes separate into charged ions when dissolved in water, and all electrolytes have either a negative charge (anions) or a positive charge (cations). They control water movement between body compartments, help maintain acid-base balance, and carry electrical current in the body. Potassium is the main cation (remember, a particle with a positive charge) in the fluid inside cells. We all need normal levels for the life of our cells.

Electrolytes

Substances that separate into charged ions when dissolved in water.

With sodium (another cation), potassium helps keep the body's acid-base balance, or pH, in check. The pH is a measure of hydrogen ion concentration in body fluids. Don't worry about the chemistry, just keep in mind that pH must be kept within a limited range to maintain the body's delicate balance, or homeostasis. Potassium also has a diuretic effect, meaning that it encourages your body to excrete water through urination. With sodium (which has the opposite effect), potassium helps balance body fluid levels.

In addition to its role in bone health, energy use, nerve function, normal heartbeat, and more, potassium is known for its ability to lower blood pressure, at least marginally. As noted earlier, dietary intake of potassium and magnesium are associated with keeping blood pressure in check among the elderly. A study published in the *American Journal of Hypertension* found that non-medicated, hypertensive subjects who increased dietary intake of potassium, magnesium, and calcium over ten weeks successfully decreased blood pressure.

Another recent study found that middle-aged male and female Chinese subjects—who tend to eat a diet high in salt and low in potassium—experienced significant reductions in blood pressure with moderate potassium supplementation for ten weeks. Additional study results, published in the journal *Circulation,* showed that potassium supplement use was inversely related to stroke risk among middle-aged men. Supplementation was especially protective in hypertensive men. Longer-term studies are needed to measure the benefit.

Potassium deficiencies are rare, but if you're taking diuretics, laxatives, or corticosteroid drugs or if you have diabetes, you may have depleted levels. Severe vomiting and diarrhea could lead to deficiencies, too. Striving for a ratio of five times as much potassium as sodium in your diet is advised by some experts. There is no RDA for this nutrient, but up to 4,500 mg per day has been recommended to offset high salt intake. You might want to cut back on salt intake, too.

REDUCE YOUR CANCER RISK WITH SELENIUM

Selenium was once regarded as toxic, but now it's considered as an essential dietary mineral. Selenium is a powerful antioxidant that protects against serious health problems, including cancer. It improves vitamin E activity in the body and helps the body hang on to this vital vitamin. Selenium shows promise in limiting heart disease risk (by protecting cholesterol from lipid peroxidation) and more.

Prostate Cancer Prevention

Prostate cancer protection is one of selenium's most well researched benefits. This disease is the second leading cause of cancer deaths in men, so finding a way to fend off this killer is a high public health priority. Selenium falls under the heading of chemopreventive agents, because it seems to ward off cancer before it strikes.

In a 1998 study published in the *British Journal of Urology,* 974 patients with a history of prostate cancer received either 200 micrograms of selenium or a placebo for four and a half years. After six and a half years from the beginning of the study, only thirteen prostate cancer cases in the selenium-treated group had developed, compared to thirty-five cases in the placebo group. The incidence of lung and colorectal cancer was also lower among the selenium-treated group. Another group of researchers determined that higher, long-term selenium intake was associated with reduced prostate cancer development in several thousand men aged forty to seventy.

Prostate Gland
The doughnut-shaped gland below the bladder in men that surrounds the upper part of the urethra and secretes a solution that aids in sperm movement and health.

Researchers have questioned whether the link between low selenium levels and prostate cancer may simply be due to cancer depleting selenium in the body. In other words, do low selenium levels encourage cancer, or vice versa? But results from many studies measuring long-term supplementation before the onset of cancer suggest that preexisting low selenium levels increased the risk of developing cancer.

More Cancer Protection

The Journal of the National Cancer Institute has reported that pretrial blood selenium levels were inversely associated with the later incidence of esophageal and gastric cardia cancer. Very low selenium status might also contribute to lung cancer risk, according to additional findings. High blood levels of selenium have even been associated with reductions in liver cancer risk among men with chronic hepatitis virus infection.

In a study published in the *European Journal of Clinical Nutrition* in 2001, sixty patients with gastric cancer undergoing chemotherapy were given 200 mcg of selenium daily and 21 mg of zinc daily as tablets for fifty days. The patients taking zinc and selenium had improved conditions (stable nutritional status and increased appetite, for example) by the study's end.

Selenium seems to fight cancer (both before it develops and after it has struck) in more ways than one. Selenomethionine, a common form of this mineral, induced apoptosis, or cell death, in human prostate cancer cells during in vitro studies. Normal human prostate cells were unharmed by selenium.

Other evidence suggests that selenium protects DNA, fats, and protein in the body from oxidative damage, due to its antioxidant action. Oxidative damage sets the stage for carcinogenesis, or cancer development. Many experts agree that selenium and other antioxidants (including vitamin E) may be beneficial in preventing prostate and other cancers.

Selenium Blocks Dangerous Viruses

Outbreaks of influenza, or flu, kill more than 20,000 Americans each year and hospitalize another 110,000 annually. New strains appear every year, so it's virtually impossible for the immune system to make a permanent defense against flu-causing viruses. But recent research suggests that adequate intake of selenium might prevent dangerous flu virus mutations.

A study conducted by Melinda A. Beck, Ph.D., and her colleagues found that mice eating a low-selenium diet that were exposed to a mild flu virus developed more serious infections than those eating diets with adequate selenium. This flu virus also mutated into another form, making lung infections worse in the selenium-deficient mice and causing infections in healthy mice. Beck and her colleagues had found, in earlier published studies, that mutations in the

Coxsackie's virus in Chinese citizens were stimulated by deficiencies in selenium.

Selenium and zinc supplementation boosted immune function in a two-year study of 725 French geriatric patients, published in *The Archives of Internal Medicine* in 1999. Subjects receiving low-dose zinc and selenium developed increased levels of infection-fighting antibodies and fewer respiratory tract infections. Subjects taking low-dose vitamin supplements instead didn't experience these benefits.

The effects of selenium on immunity help explain why the mineral may protect us from flu and cancer. Selenium is needed for the production of glutathione peroxidase, a powerful antioxidant and immune-system stimulant. Inadequate levels of selenium disable the body's antioxidant defenses. This breakdown seems to allow free radicals to mutate otherwise-stable DNA.

Natural-Killer Cells
A type of immune cell that targets and destroys tumor- or virus-infected cells.

Selenium deficiencies might also decrease the body's production of natural killer cells. These are a kind of lymphocyte, or immune cell, that targets and destroys tumor- or virus-infected cells. Selenium and zinc deficiencies among elderly people have been linked to low natural killer cell levels. This immune activity might explain why HIV and AIDS patients are thought to benefit from selenium supplementation.

Supplementing with Selenium

Bran, garlic (from selenium-rich soil), oatmeal, onions, mushrooms, broccoli, brown rice, and whole-grain products are plant sources of selenium. Eggs, tuna, seafood, chicken, and liver are good animal sources of the mineral. Even so, low soil levels of selenium and food processing can lead to inadequate amounts in the diet.

Supplements can help you get enough selenium. Both selenomethionine and high-selenium yeast are excellent supplements, and the high-selenium yeast has been found to reduce the risk of several types of cancer in people. A daily dosage of 200 mcg is considered safe and adequate for the average American adult.

Very high doses of selenium—more than 800 mcg daily or more for extended periods—could be hazardous. Follow recommended intakes to reap only the benefits of selenium. Deficiencies are more likely, and they can lead to nerve disorders, early aging, increased fragility of red blood cells, pancreatic degeneration, and weakened vision.

CHROMIUM OPTIMIZES INSULIN AND GLUCOSE FUNCTION

Chromium is a trace mineral that you need for normal sugar and fat metabolism. It improves the efficiency of insulin, a hormone that orchestrates the movement of sugar and fat into your body's cells to be used or stored for energy. When chromium levels are low, insulin can't perform well. This can set the stage for diabetes mellitus, obesity, and heart disease. Increasing daily intake of this essential element can help control diabetes and may aid in weight loss and lowering cholesterol levels.

Improving Insulin Efficiency

Several clinical studies have shown that chromium supplements improve insulin activity in people with diabetes. This

Insulin
A hormone that helps move sugar and fat from blood into body cells to be used or stored for energy.

is good news, because low insulin production and insulin insensitivity are serious problems in the all too common disorder. The most promising results have been in regard to type II (or non–insulin-dependent) diabetes. Unlike people with the type I (insulin-dependent) diabetes, those with type II diabetes produce enough insulin in their bodies. The problem is that their cells' insulin receptors aren't sensitive to insulin.

When the body doesn't produce enough insulin (as in type I) or cell receptors aren't sensitive to the hormone (as in type II), glucose can't be ushered into cells from the bloodstream. Instead, blood glucose levels remain dangerously high and cells don't receive the fuel they need. This leads to serious health problems.

Numerous studies have found that supplemental chromium, in the form of chromium picolinate, improves blood glucose, insulin, and cholesterol status among people with type II diabetes, who tend to have low chromium levels. No side effects have been documented among people with type II diabetes taking supplemental chromium.

A lack of chromium seems to increase the risk of insulin resistance, a condition also called Syndrome X. In Syndrome X the body can't process glucose normally, so it secretes more and more insulin. The insulin does not work efficiently, so it keeps circulating in the blood along with the elevated blood levels of glucose. Syndrome X, which is characterized by insulin resistance and abdominal obesity, greatly increases risk of heart disease and diabetes. Some experts estimate that 25 percent of the population suffers from Syndrome X, with most cases undiagnosed.

Insulin becomes less effective when we eat a lot of sugary foods and refined carbohydrates, like sweets, pasta, and white bread. When we eat too much of these foods, muscle cells temporarily switch off their insulin recognition system. As a result, blood sugar, or blood glucose, is redirected to fat cells and to the liver. Eventually, fat cells ignore insulin altogether; they become insulin-resistant.

When cells stop pulling glucose out of the blood, the glucose spills over into the urine. This is a typical sign of diabetes. However, a person can have trouble with insulin and insulin resistance, or Syndrome X, without being diabetic. Chromium deficiency is characterized by many of the signs of Syndrome X, including insulin resistance, poor glucose control, and high cholesterol and triglyceride levels.

Syndrome X
A disorder marked by high blood levels of insulin and glucose and associated with high cholesterol and other blood fat levels and with increased risk of heart disease and diabetes.

Several studies have found that chromium picolinate supplementation can play a major role in reducing symptoms of Syndrome X and diabetes. Again, chromium works by enhancing insulin function and the burning of blood sugar, or glucose. Chromium supplements alone are not a cure for Syndrome X, but they can help reverse this disorder.

Chromium and Lean Body Mass

Chromium is purported to spare or increase lean body mass and aid in fat loss. Some—but not all—research does support the theory that chromium may help those looking to increase (or keep) muscle and lose fat. Considering chromium's role in sugar and fat metabolism, it does seem plausible.

In a recent double-blind, placebo-controlled study, twenty overweight African-American women followed a modest diet and exercise regimen and received either placebo or 200 mcg of chromium (in the niacin-bound form) three times daily for two months. Then, they switched to the other regime for two months. Body weight loss was comparable with both regimens, but fat loss was greater and lean body mass loss was less with chromium intake compared to placebo. The women had lost more fat and less muscle by taking 600 mcg of niacin-bound chromium daily, experiencing no adverse effects.

In another double-blind study, 123 participants took either a patented natural dietary supplement containing chromium picolinate, inulin (a long-chain sugar molecule found in Jerusalem artichokes), capsicum, L-phenylalanine (a protein building block), and other potentially fat-fighting nutrients or placebo for four weeks. They all followed the same diet and exercise program throughout the study. At the end of the study, those taking the natural supplement had a faster rate of body fat loss and maintained more lean body mass than the placebo group.

Of course, this study didn't investigate the effects of chromium alone. And eating a healthy diet and exercising are crucial to any fat- and weight-loss plan, as they were in these studies. Even so, there appears to be potential for chromium to play a role in decreasing one's fat to muscle ratio. Future large-scale human trials should shed more light on the topic, as well as on the potential for chromium supplementation to decrease total and LDL, or "bad," cholesterol levels.

Choosing Supplements

Normal dietary intake of chromium is often less than optimal. Mushrooms, prunes, nuts, asparagus, organ meats, and whole-grain products are good sources, but levels of chromium in these foods vary. Chromium supplements have an excellent safety record and are relatively inexpensive.

The amount of chromium a person needs depends on age, activity level, and overall health. For example, a teenaged girl might benefit from 200–300 mcg daily, whereas 300–400 mcg daily may be best for a teenaged boy. Adults up to retirement age should get 400 mcg daily. Elderly people should take at least 200 mcg per day. The most dramatic and consistent results have been with 200 mcg of chromium picolinate for every 1,000 calories of food eaten.

Some studies have found that 1,000 mcg of chromium daily as chromium picolinate can help patients with diabetes. A daily intake of 200 mcg per day is thought to be enough to improve glucose tolerance in people who do not have full-blown diabetes. Anyone with diabetes should work with a doctor on this, however, because insulin or hypoglycemic drug requirements may need to be adjusted.

Chromium picolinate is made up of chromium combined chemically with picolinic acid in order to help the body use it most efficiently, so choose a supplement with this form. Chromium picolinate is sometimes referred to as "trivalent" because it is a chelate made of chromium attached to three picolinate molecules.

ZINC AND COPPER FOR IMMUNITY

Zinc is essential to many enzyme systems in the body. We need it to grow and develop, digest protein, produce energy, and absorb vitamin A efficiently, for starters. Prostate and reproductive health depend on adequate zinc status, too. But this mineral is perhaps most famous for its starring role in immune system function. High levels of copper, also an essential mineral, can suppress zinc levels.

Zinc for Immunity

The immune system needs zinc to fight infections. It is required for normal synthesis of deoxyribonucleic acid (DNA), which helps make new immune cells. It also promotes the activity of immune cells. Zinc deficiency leads to impaired immunity and, as a result, increased susceptibility to viral, bacterial, and fungal infections. Infections can even lead to death when the immune system is damaged.

Supplementation with zinc has repeatedly improved immunity in people with low levels. Studies have found that elderly people, who often have low zinc levels, experience a decreased risk of infection by taking the RDA of zinc for one to two months. Zinc and selenium supplements have improved immunity and decreased the risk of respiratory infections among elderly patients. Zinc also increases the survival rate of elderly people following infection.

Children need zinc for strong immunity, too. In a recent study, Indian researchers gave 609 children, ranging in age from six months to three years, daily supplements of zinc gluconate (containing 10 mg of elemental zinc) or a multivitamin without zinc. After four months of supplementation, zinc levels increased in children receiving zinc. Levels declined in the other group. Children taking zinc had a 45 percent reduction in acute lower respiratory infections.

Results with zinc lozenges for cold symptom relief have been mixed, but many have concluded that these lozenges in the gluconate or acetate forms reduce the symptoms and duration of colds. In one recent study, fifty patients who began taking zinc acetate lozenges (containing 12.8 mg of zinc) every two to three hours within twenty-four hours of the onset of cold symptoms reported symptom relief in less than five days, compared to eight days for symptom relief among the placebo group.

Zinc's role in immunity helps explain its ability to inactivate viruses (including some types of herpes). The immune-boosting mineral is sometimes recommended to patients with the AIDS virus (along with conventional drug therapy), who often have low levels and hindered immune function. It works by inactivating a protease that is essential for the proliferation of the AIDS virus HIV-1. Zinc may also offer protection against various forms of cancer, due in part to its positive effects on the immune system.

Prostate Cancer Protection and Then Some

Healthy prostate tissue has the highest zinc levels of any body soft tissue. This suggests that it plays a big role in the prostate. Cancer protection may be part of that role.

Zinc levels in prostate cancer are significantly decreased compared to levels in other tissues. A recent human cell culture study published in the journal *Prostate* revealed that zinc prompted self-destruction (apoptosis) and inhibited growth of human prostate cancer cells. Another study—this one with 697 men with prostate cancer—found that the subjects had low supplement intake of zinc and vitamins C and E individually over the two years before their cancer diagnosis. Researchers concluded that each of these three supplements might have a protective effect against prostate cancer. There is strong evidence that the loss of the ability to hang on to zinc is a factor in the development and progression of prostate cancer cells.

Zinc is needed for sexual maturation and reproduction, including the production of the hormone testosterone and sperm formation. Infertile males tend to have lower levels of zinc than fertile males, and low blood levels of testos-

terone have been linked to low zinc levels. What's more, this antioxidant mineral may work by scavenging free radicals produced by defective sperm in semen after ejaculation, according to study results. It is crucial in maintaining prostate and testicular tissue.

Atherosclerosis
A disorder characterized by the buildup of blood fats on the damaged lining of artery walls, leading to plaques that block blood flow.

Heart health is another promising area of zinc research. Zinc protects cell walls, and it appears to protect blood vessel walls from injury that can contribute to atherosclerosis, or hardening of the arteries. In addition, a dose of 25 mg of zinc daily for three months decreased oxidation of blood fats during a recent study of elderly Italian men and women. (Remember that oxidized blood fats can eventually lead to blockage of blood flow.) The researchers concluded that adequate intake could be important in preventing and regulating age-related diseases.

Another study found that zinc intake was positively associated with a healthier ratio of total cholesterol to HDL, or "good" cholesterol, among African-American male subjects. (A high ratio of HDL to total cholesterol is desirable.) Female African-American subjects with higher zinc intake had higher HDL values than subjects with low intake. In other words, zinc might protect against heart disease by improving cholesterol levels. Study results with European Americans have been mixed.

The effect of zinc supplementation in Wilson's disease is clearer. The FDA even approved zinc acetate for treatment of the disease, which results in the toxic buildup of copper in the body, liver disease, and neurological disorders. The two FDA-approved treatment drugs for Wilson's disease have side effects and may damage fetuses. In a recent study, zinc was found to be effective and safe for mothers and fetuses. (Consult your doctor first if you're pregnant or nursing.) It works by inducing intestinal metallothionein, which binds to copper and keeps it from entering the blood.

Ensuring Adequate Intake

There are some good sources of zinc in the food we eat—pumpkinseeds, turkey, whole grains, and raw oysters, for example. But you may need more. Researchers from the Centers for Disease Control and Prevention found that only slightly more than half of Americans surveyed in the Third National Health and Nutrition Examination Survey got adequate amounts of zinc from food and supplements. Children aged one to three years old, adolescent girls, and people over age seventy-one were at greatest risk of inadequate intake.

Some signs of zinc deficiency are growth retardation, loss of appetite, diarrhea, impotence, and increased risk of infectious diseases. The RDA is 8 mg per day for women and 11 mg per day for men, but some practitioners recommend up to 50 mg per day. Taking much more than that regularly can cause signs of toxicity, including diarrhea and upset stomach.

Look for citrate, gluconate, or protein chelate forms of zinc. When it comes to lozenges, opt for those supplying 15–25 mg of elemental zinc per lozenge. Choose a brand sweetened with glycine, as other sweeteners (sorbitol, mannitol, and citric acid) might limit absorption. Dissolve them in your mouth every couple of hours for up to seven days when you feel a cold coming on.

Be Sure to Get Some Copper

Copper activates key enzyme reactions and helps make ATP, the body's energy source. It is, along with zinc, part of an antioxidant enzyme called superoxide dismutase, or SOD, which keeps free radical damage in check. Copper is involved in making hormones and collagen, a protein that holds connective tissue together. It is also needed to make hemoglobin, the molecule that carries oxygen in the blood.

A potential benefit of copper supplementation is its ability to relieve inflammation and ease symptoms of rheumatoid arthritis. Animal studies have found that a copper-supplemented diet has an antiarthritic effect, but human studies are lacking. Increased body copper levels, which are associated with arthritis inflammation, were once thought to make the disease worse. But now they are thought to increase as part of the body's response to arthritis.

Getting enough copper may help your heart, too. Copper deficiency might hamper heart health by contributing to high blood pressure, increased inflammation, arteriosclerosis, and anemia. Inadequate copper reduces the effectiveness of many enzymes, so deficiencies can lead to negative changes in the heart, blood vessels, and circulating blood cells, according to authors of a research review published in the journal *Biofactors*.

Most people get enough copper because it is in so many foods. Multivitamin and mineral supplements also contain it. You should only take extra copper if your doctor recommends it, as toxicity can occur at high levels. People taking large amounts of zinc may need 1–2 mg of copper per day.

IRON, IODINE, AND MANGANESE

Several minor minerals play essential roles in health. Of these, iron and iodine are well known to most people, but manganese is not. This chapter describes some of their important roles in maintaining health.

Iron for Life—In Small Amounts

The micromineral iron is part of hemoglobin, the protein that transports oxygen in red blood cells to other body cells that need it. Iron is also part of myoglobin, which supplies oxygen to muscles. It is needed to make ATP, as well. People deficient in this mineral tire easily because their bodies' cells aren't getting the oxygen they need, or they aren't synthesizing enough ATP for energy.

Most of us grew up hearing about how important it is to get enough iron. Iron is essential to life itself, but it may surprise you to learn that most adults don't need supplemental iron. In fact, too much iron can cause oxidative damage.

This kind of damage can contribute to or worsen some diseases (including heart disease and rheumatoid arthritis) and speed up aging, so it's best not to supplement with iron unless you know that you're deficient. Some research results even suggest that iron overload, or hemochromatosis, may contribute to the risk of developing heart disease in men and women, due to the mineral's role in increasing oxidation.

Monthly blood losses of iron in premenopausal women actually protect against iron overload. After menopause, women no longer lose iron on a monthly basis, so they can end up with high levels. This relationship may help explain why postmenopausal women have a higher risk of heart disease than their younger counterparts.

Deficiency and Dosage

People who are deficient in iron usually lose large amounts or don't absorb iron well, as opposed to merely having a low intake. Pregnant and lactating women, infants and children, elderly people, endurance athletes, and people with hemorrhoids, ulcerative colitis, or other conditions might be at risk. Even these people should check with their doctors before starting an iron supplement routine beyond a multivitamin and mineral formula.

Anemia
A blood condition in which the amount of hemoglobin in red blood cells, or the number of red blood cells themselves, is below normal.

Women who have very heavy menstrual periods might have low iron levels, too. That's because iron is lost in menstrual blood every month. But the amount found in a multivitamin and mineral formula helps restore lost iron in these women.

Iron-deficiency anemia does sometimes result from iron deficiency. In this disorder, hemoglobin in blood cells, or the number of red blood cells themselves, is low. If you experience fatigue and have trouble breathing normally, consult your doctor to determine whether or not you have anemia and if it is caused by iron deficiency or another problem. Do not try to self-treat what you think may be anemia.

The most absorbable iron, called heme iron, is found in clams, oysters, red meat, and organ meats. Dark, leafy green vegetables, brewer's yeast, wheat germ, blackstrap molasses, and acidic foods cooked in iron pans are sources of non-heme iron. Vegetarians may have lower iron levels than meat-eaters because iron from plant sources is less absorbable; however, many non-meat foods, such as cereal, are fortified with iron. Vitamin C can aid iron absorption, too, so drinking orange juice with your cereal, for example, increases absorption.

If you're concerned about heart disease risk, consider taking an iron-free multivitamin and supplement formula. For premenopausal women, an iron-containing multivitamin and mineral formula is probably a good idea. Iron toxicity is very dangerous and especially serious in children, so stick to the RDA.

Iodine for Thyroid Health

Iodine and the amino acid tyrosine are required by the thyroid gland in order to secrete thyroid hormones, which regulate biochemical reactions. In the early 1900s, low iodine levels in soil and water led to hypothyroidism and goiter (enlarged thyroid) among people living in Michigan and other "goiter belt" states. Thanks to the addition of iodine to table salt, deficiencies are rare in the United States today.

Iodine deficiency and hypothyroidism are much more common in developing countries, where people don't consume iodized salt. A deficiency can result in mental retardation, goiter, abnormal development, and cretinism, a serious developmental disorder in infants. Some studies and clinical findings suggest a link between low iodine intake and fibrocystic breasts, a condition causing breast pain, discomfort, and/or lumpiness. Increased iodine intake and other natural remedies may improve fibrocystic breasts. Talk to a nutritionally minded doctor if this affects you.

The RDA for iodine is 150 mcg for adults, but the average intake in the United States is more than 600 mcg per day. It's best not to get more than 600 mcg per day on a regular basis, as high levels may hinder normal thyroid function.

Manganese Aids Cartilage Formation

Manganese is necessary for normal brain function, collagen formation, bone growth, energy metabolism, and more. It is only found in trace amounts in people—about 10–20 mg total in the average man. It is not related to magnesium.

There's a chance that this trace mineral may improve arthritis and diabetes in people with low levels, but more human studies are needed. Animal studies have found that manganese is involved in making chondroitin sulfate, a part of articular cartilage and a common supplement for arthritis relief. Deficiencies of manganese have caused a disorder of cartilage metabolism in farm animals. Whether or not low manganese intake contributes to arthritis, and whether

supplementation can alleviate arthritis in people, remains to be seen.

Manganese is part of the antioxidant enzyme MnSOD. (This is another form of SOD, which we mentioned earlier.) This enzyme is part of the body's defense against harmful free radical damage to pancreas beta cells, which normally produce insulin but don't work well in type I diabetes. Manganese is needed by SOD to protect against free radical damage to insulin-producing cells. (Low levels of MnSOD have been found in patients with osteoarthritis, too.)

In guinea pigs, manganese deficiency leads to diabetes and pancreas abnormalities in their offspring. Low levels of manganese are common in people with diabetes. Even so, future human studies are needed to find out whether or not manganese is effective as diabetes therapy.

Deficiencies of manganese are very rare and there is no RDA. A daily intake of 1.8 mg for women and 2.3 mg for men is considered adequate. Whole grains, fruits, nuts, and vegetables are high in manganese.

SULFUR, SILICON, AND VANADIUM

Relatively little is known about the minerals sulfur, silicon, and vanadium, but they do play crucial roles in health. For example, sulfur is one of the most abundant minerals in the body, but most nutrition textbooks do not discuss it at all. Without sulfur, life simply would not be possible. Why it has been so ignored is a mystery.

Sulfur for Skin and Maybe More

Sulfur is a component of amino acids and thiamine, biotin, lipoic acid, and some hormones, including insulin. It has been used therapeutically for thousands of years to treat skin disorders, such as eczema and psoriasis. Sulfur baths are still recommended to people with these conditions.

Like benzoyl peroxide, sulfur is an antiseptic, but it is gentler on the skin. The FDA has even approved sulfur for treating acne. Sulfur is also very safe. Look for topical products containing at least 3 percent sulfur for the best results. (Vitamin E, vitamin A, and other nutrients might alleviate acne, too.)

Low levels of sulfur have been found in arthritis sufferers. Some researchers speculate that increasing sulfur-rich foods in the diet might lessen the pain and swelling associated with arthritis. A study published in the journal *Rheumatology International* in 2000 found that sulfur baths prolonged the benefits of sun exposure and Dead Sea mineral-bath treatment (also available at health and natural food stores) among patients with psoriatic arthritis, a type of arthritis associated with the skin condition psoriasis.

A form of sulfur known as methylsulfonylmethane, or

MSM, has become popular in the last few years in supplement form, especially in joint health formulas. Stanley Jacob, M.D., of Oregon Health Sciences University, Portland, has found MSM supplements useful in reducing muscle and joint pain and interstitial cystitis (a type of very painful bladder inflammation). According to Jacob, MSM also eases symptoms of scleroderma, a chronic degenerative disease that scars skin, joints, and connective tissue.

Silicon—Micromineral Newcomer

Silicon is needed for normal growth and development of collagen, the "tissue cement" that literally holds together skin, nails, and all of the other tissues in the body. It also helps form cartilage and bone, the latter by speeding up the mineralization of bone.

Silicon, sometimes referred to as silica (silicon dioxide), is considered a sister element to carbon, which forms the basis of all life on Earth. Despite the relative obscurity of silicon, the body contains a higher level of it than it does iron, zinc, copper, and iodine.

Scientists realized, about a century ago, that high levels of silicon were found in tendons, connective tissue, and the eyes, and that it might protect blood vessels against disease. More recent research, while not conclusive, hints that it might lower blood fats and block aluminum absorption in the brain. Recently, researchers have found that the silica form of the mineral can reduce cracking and brittleness in fingernails and improve the appearance of hair.

Vanadium—Looking Ahead

Vanadium is involved in bone and teeth metabolism. It may be needed for good health by humans (as it is in animals). Good food sources include shellfish, spinach, parsley, whole grains, mushrooms, and soy. No deficiency in humans is known, and there's no RDA, so you don't have to take extra vanadium. Side effects and negative reactions are not likely to be a problem.

Over the last few years, vanadium has garnered attention for its potential to improve diabetes. Several animal and limited human studies testing this relationship have taken place, with promising results. In one study, a combination of vanadium and insulin regenerated beta cells (which make insulin) and relieved diabetes in insulin-dependent diabetic rats during a year of treatment and after treatment ended. Those rats that were given only insulin did not experience these benefits.

Vanadium has proven therapeutic in clinical studies with patients with type I diabetes and in others with type II diabetes, noted the authors of a recent review published in *The Journal of Complementary Medicine*. The mineral is considered an "insulin mimic," in that it can partially substitute for insulin and help metabolize blood sugar.

However, this benefit, which improves insulin function and lowers blood sugar levels, warrants caution. High-dose vanadium may be toxic, and it may trigger insulin resistance when supplementation is ceased. If you have diabetes, it would be best to discuss vanadium with your physician before you start supplementing with it.

HOW TO BUY QUALITY SUPPLEMENTS

There's no doubt that vitamin and mineral supplements are good for your health. But how do you know which ones to take, how much to take, and in what form? This chapter will steer you in the right direction.

Micronutrients Work as a Team

Vitamins and minerals are essential nutrients, and each performs myriad functions in the body. For example, vitamin C, vitamin E, and folic acid reduce the risk of coronary heart disease. But they protect the heart and blood vessels in different ways. Similarly, vitamin C and the B vitamins can ease arthritis, but they do so differently.

Various vitamins and minerals need other nutrients to do their jobs well. Vitamin D is essential for efficient calcium absorption. Vitamin C encourages iron absorption.

You can improve your health by taking vitamin C supplements, but you could improve it even more by also taking vitamin E supplements. The most sensible approach is to take all of the vitamins and essential minerals. If it's a hassle to take pills, stick with one high-potency multivitamin and mineral supplement.

Set Clear Goals

Set clear objectives that you want to achieve with supplements. If you are in your twenties, eat a reasonably good diet, and are in good health, your objective might be "dietary insurance." A high-potency multivitamin and mineral supplement may be enough. If you're in your thirties or forties and face a lot of stress at home or at work, "stress management" might be an objective. In this case, you might do well taking a high-potency B-complex supplement.

Reducing disease risk is a very clear objective. If people in your family have a high risk of developing heart disease or cancer, it's wise to start supplementing before the first signs of trouble. In addition to a multivitamin, vitamin E would probably be the most important vitamin for you.

If you have specific health problems, such as high blood pressure, hardening of the arteries, premenstrual syndrome (PMS), or osteoporosis, taking high doses of specific supplements may be in order. (Again, check with your doctor first if you have serious health problems or are taking medication.) By starting with specific objectives, you've got something against which to measure your improvement.

How Much and When?

Understanding supplement labels requires knowing a few measurement terms. Most stand for the weight of a given ingredient. For example, g stands for gram, mg for milligram, and mcg for microgram.

To put these weights into perspective, consider that there are about 454 grams in a pound; 1,000 mg in a gram; and 1,000 mcg in a milligram. So, in general, we're talking about very small quantities. For example, 400 mcg of folic acid is equivalent to about $1/70,000$ of an ounce—a very small quantity, but very important nonetheless. IU stands for international unit, which is a way of measuring vitamins A, D, and E. (Unfortunately, international units do not consistently correspond to milligrams.)

Specific recommendations for supplement dosage vary, but you might strive for something similar to the following in a high-potency multivitamin and mineral supplement. To get these amounts, you may have to take more than one tablet or capsule daily.

Vitamin A: 5,000 IU and/or natural beta-carotene: 10 mg or 16,000 IU

Vitamin B_1 (thiamine): 10–15 mg

Vitamin B_2 (riboflavin): 10–25 mg

Vitamin B_3 (niacinamide): 100–200 mg

Vitamin B_6 (pyridoxine): 10–20 mg

Vitamin B_{12}: 10–100 mg

Folic acid: 400 mcg

Pantothenic acid: 25–100 mg

Biotin: 30–50 mcg

PABA: 30–50 mg

Choline: 250 mg

Inositol: 250 mg

Vitamin C: 1,000–4,000 mg

Vitamin D: 400 IU

Vitamin E: 400 IU

Vitamin K: 100 mcg

Calcium (citrate or malate): 1,000 mg

Magnesium: 400 mg

Potassium: 99 mg

Selenium: 200 mcg

Chromium (picolinate): 200–400 mcg

Zinc (citrate or gluconate): 15–25 mg

Copper: 1–2 mg

Iron: 18 mg for menstruating women
(Men should take an iron-free supplement unless tests have indicated anemia.)

Iodine: 150 mcg

Manganese: 2–5 mg

These dosages are for adults. Tailoring vitamin and mineral supplements for children can be trickier because they weigh less. For general supplementation, one or two times the children's RDA (which is lower than the adult RDA) should be safe. Stick with RDA levels of vitamins A and D and minerals for children. An easy solution is one of the many children's supplements available at health food stores.

Most multivitamin and mineral formulas contain all of the vitamins and essential minerals, but there is great variation in dosage. Because the RDA is a conservative amount, look for a supplement that provides at least four times the RDA for the B vitamins, vitamin C, and vitamin E. However, stick with RDA levels for vitamins A and D and iron.

Vitamins and minerals are components of food, so in general they are best taken with food. It's a good idea to take them with breakfast so your body can use them while you're most active. If you take your vitamins before going to bed, you may have a restless night, due to their stimulatory effects. Sometimes, product labels recommend taking supplements two or three times a day, with each meal. Some minerals and mineral formulas advise taking them a couple of hours after meals so they won't hinder digestion. Follow label directions for the best results.

If you're taking large amounts of a single vitamin or mineral, it's best to divide the dose over the course of a day. Splitting up the dose improves the efficiency of absorption, so less is excreted. You don't have to take vitamin C with food because it's water-soluble and easily absorbed. Dividing the dose of vitamin C will also reduce the likelihood of loose bowels resulting from taking too much at one time.

Vitamins & Minerals during Pregnancy

If you're a pregnant woman already taking a high-potency multivitamin and mineral formula roughly equivalent to the one outlined above, you're probably fine, though you should show the bottle to your physician to make sure he or she agrees.

While the vitamin levels above are safe, you and your physician may wish to adjust or reduce some of the vitamin or mineral levels. If you are not already taking supplements, consider starting with a prenatal supplement. Ideally, the time to take such a supplement is before you become pregnant. That's because the risk of birth defects is greatest very early in a pregnancy, often before a woman even realizes she is pregnant.

Vitamins are essential for normal fetus development. For example, if the fetus does not have adequate folic acid through its mother's diet by the sixteenth week of pregnancy, its neural tube (spine) will not seal. The result will be a serious birth defect, such as spina bifida.

Also, a study described in the *Journal of the National*

Cancer Institute found that women who took vitamins while pregnant were less likely to have children with brain tumors. Of course, it's also important to seek prenatal medical care, eat a balanced diet, and not smoke or drink alcohol during pregnancy.

Natural versus Synthetic

Most vitamin supplements are synthetic duplicates of their natural counterparts in all respects. But there are big differences between natural and synthetic vitamin E and beta-carotene, with the natural form superior to the synthetic. The natural form of vitamin E (d-alpha tocopherol) is twice as well absorbed as the synthetic form (dl-alpha-tocopherol).

Natural beta-carotene supplements are derived from *Dunaliella salina* algae. (This should be listed on the label.) Natural beta-carotene consists of two forms that chemists call isomers. The synthetic form contains only one of these forms.

Vitamin C is produced from corn sugar (dextrose), and the B vitamins are produced through bacterial fermentation. This means that bacteria are cultivated to produce large amounts of B vitamins. Vitamins A, D, and K come from both natural and synthetic sources, but the differences are not significant.

Are Excipients Safe?

All tablets and capsules contain excipients, which are compounds with no nutritional value. They are added to improve the consistency of vitamin supplements during processing.

Excipients *Nonnutritive ingredients added to supplements to improve consistency and other characteristics.*

Before vitamins are pressed into tablets or poured into capsules, they are in powder form and are thoroughly mixed in vats. Some excipients, such as lubricants, promote consistent mixing, so you get the same amount of a vitamin in every tablet or capsule. Other excipients, such as cellulose, add bulk so vitamins can be pressed into tablets. Cellulose also absorbs water, so the tablet swells and breaks apart in your digestive tract.

All excipients are approved for use by the Food and Drug Administration and are safe. Some people, however, may have reactions to specific excipients, such as lactose (milk sugar). If this happens, buy a different product. If you're allergic to milk or you're lactose intolerant, avoid supplements containing lactose. The same goes for corn, yeast, and other potential allergens. In general, capsules contain fewer excipients compared with tablets, and health food store brands tend to have fewer excipients overall than pharmacy brands.

Finding the Best Form

Every supplement form—capsules, tablets, and liquids—has pros and cons. Choosing one over another depends on a variety of factors. Among these are availability, cost, ease of swallowing, digestive efficiency, and the number of excipients you're willing to ingest.

Most supplements are sold in tablet form. They're less expensive to make than capsules, but capsules are easier to swallow than tablets (especially large tablets). One drawback is that sometimes tablets pass through the gut without breaking down. If this happens to you consistently, switch to a capsule, or consider taking betaine hydrochloride or another digestive aid to improve your stomach acid. Tablets can be a good alternative for vegetarians avoiding gelatin capsules (but there are vegetarian capsules out there, too).

Some supplements, such as vitamin B_{12}, are available as sublingual tablets. These are meant to dissolve under the tongue; much the way nitroglycerin (a heart medication) is taken. A network of blood vessels under the tongue instantly absorbs vitamins and drugs. In addition, you'll also find some vitamins and minerals in liquid form. Because vitamins generally don't taste very good, some products contain a lot of sugar to mask the taste.

Time-release supplements are another option. The idea behind them is that they maintain steadier levels in the blood and less is excreted. The disadvantage is their cost; some are twice the cost of regular vitamin supplements. A less expensive approach would be to divide your vitamins into smaller doses that you take throughout the day.

Time-Release Supplements *A supplement manufactured for the slow release of its ingredient(s).*

Gauging Results

If you're taking a specific supplement to treat a condition—such as B vitamins to treat arthritis—you should see some benefits within about thirty days, assuming you're taking enough. If you don't see an improvement after thirty days, stop taking the supplement. It's possible that your improvement was very subtle and you won't notice it until you stop. Or maybe you would benefit from a different vitamin.

It's a little harder to assess the effects of vitamins and minerals if you are in good health and are trying to reduce your long-term risk of disease, such as heart disease. The benefits of vitamin and mineral supplements will become clearer the longer you take them. You'll find that you'll be in generally better health than people your age who don't take them.

Also, keep in mind that supplements are supplements to—not replacements for—good nutrition. They provide dietary insurance, they can compensate somewhat for some subtle biological defects, and they can prevent and treat many diseases. But they won't protect you from a fundamentally bad diet. Eat well, and take your supplements.

PART TWO

VITAMIN E

JACK CHALLEM & MELISSA DIANE SMITH

Could one single vitamin reduce your risk of developing heart disease, cancer, and Alzheimer's disease?

If the supplement is vitamin E, the answer is yes. Does this sound too incredible to be true? Read on, and you may change your mind.

Discovered in 1922, vitamin E was for years the butt of jokes that referred to it disparagingly as the sex vitamin. Amazingly, as far back as the 1940s, a team of Canadian physicians discovered that vitamin E could protect people from coronary heart disease. But because these doctors could not explain, in scientific terms, why vitamin E worked, they were dismissed as quacks and charlatans. And for many years to come, vitamin E would be regarded as a "cure in search of a disease" and nothing more than a waste of money.

Fast-forward to the present, and the view of vitamin E is strikingly different. Scientific research has caught up with this remarkable nutrient. Today, with thousands of studies to support it, vitamin E is quickly being recognized as the closest thing to a "magic bullet" in the prevention of Alzheimer's disease, cancer, heart disease, and many other disorders.

So, what exactly makes vitamin E so great? Scientists tell us that age-related diseases—and the risk of most diseases increases with age—are caused in part by hazardous molecules known as free radicals. Free radicals make iron rust and butter turn rancid. In a sense, they make your body more rusty and rancid with age.

Nature, however, provided a way to neutralize free radicals—with a group of beneficial molecules called antioxidants. Vitamin E stands out as one of the most powerful antioxidants found in foods. It scavenges free radicals in the body and limits their damage. In so doing, vitamin E slows the aging process and reduces the long-term risk of age-related degenerative diseases. It doesn't matter if you're a woman or a man—vitamin E can provide all people with important health benefits.

But, you might be wondering, don't we all get enough vitamin E in the foods we eat? And if vitamin E is so great, why don't doctors recommend it?

Over the past century, the Western diet has undergone tremendous changes. The foods most people eat are highly processed, and vitamin E (along with many other nutrients) is removed. The typical American is consuming only a small percentage of the vitamin E his or her grandparents consumed.

In addition, our nutritional requirements for vitamin E have increased. Most people are eating more fried foods and vegetable oil than people consumed in the past. These foods are prone to free radical damage and boost our need for vitamin E. Also, with more industrialization and the increased use of polluting automobiles, people have been exposed to unprecedented levels of air pollution. This also boosts our need for vitamin E.

As for doctors, they have slowly but steadily been catching on to the benefits of vitamin E. In recent years, the scientific research on this amazing nutrient has become an irresistible force in medicine. One recent survey found that almost half of all cardiologists were taking vitamin E supplements themselves, though they were a bit reluctant to recommend them to patients. When we ask physicians about vitamin E, they say that nearly every doctor takes the vitamin. The question, now, might be this: Why aren't you taking vitamin E?

In Part Two of the *User's Guide to Nutritional Supplements*, we will tell you the remarkable story of vitamin E and how it can reduce your risk of serious, degenerative diseases and how it may even help protect you against infections. First, we will explain how vitamin E prevents heart disease, the leading cause of death among Americans and most other Westerners. Then we'll describe the exciting research showing that vitamin E can probably reduce your long-term risk of cancer, including breast cancer in women and prostate cancer in men. Later we'll cover how vitamin E can protect you from numerous other diseases, including Alzheimer's and additional neurological disorders, cataracts, infertility, and menopausal hot flashes. Lastly, we'll explain how to shop for the best types of vitamin E, which, according to research, are the natural forms of this vitamin.

PROTECTING THE HEART

Heart disease is the leading cause of death among men and women in most Western nations. It has killed more Americans than all wars combined. Heart disease is complex and develops subtly and slowly. It has multiple causes, but a lack of vitamin E is paramount among the reasons it develops. In this chapter, we'll look at the causes of heart disease, some different aspects of this condition, and the many ways vitamin E helps prevent heart disease.

Vitamin E Reduces the Risk of Heart Disease

Research and the clinical experiences of physicians show beyond a doubt that vitamin E is good for the heart. Evidence supporting the role of vitamin E as a heart protector has been building for decades. In the past several years, the evidence has become so strong that most doctors can't ignore it.

For example, Harvard University researchers reported in the *New England Journal of Medicine* that vitamin E supplements dramatically reduced the risk of coronary heart disease in men and women. The amount of vitamin E used—more than 100 IU (international units)—was more than six times the Recommended Dietary Allowance (RDA) for vitamin E. This is an amount you can obtain only from supplements, not foods.

Vitamin E
The body's principal fat-soluble antioxidant that is incorporated into cell membranes and protects cells from free radical damage.

Even more impressive were the results of a blockbuster study reported in the British medical journal *Lancet*. Researchers from the University of Cambridge in England gave either 400 or 800 IU of natural vitamin E or placebos (dummy pills) daily to 2,000 patients with confirmed heart disease. The group taking vitamin E for an average of eighteen months had a remarkable 77 percent lower incidence of nonfatal heart attacks compared to the placebo group.

Those British researchers pronounced vitamin E more powerful in controlling heart attacks than aspirin or cholesterol-lowering drugs—and the benefits of vitamin E were evident within only six and one-half months after the subjects started taking it. So impressive were these results that the American Heart Association ranked vitamin E number four on its list of the top ten heart-related developments in 1996.

The encouraging research results with vitamin E for heart health continue. In an analysis of the five largest trials investigating vitamin E for heart health, published in the journal *Current Opinion in Lipidology*, the authors concluded that alpha-tocopherol (the most common form of vitamin E) was beneficial in patients with pre-existing heart disease. In the majority of these studies, those taking the alpha-tocopherol supplements had a reduced risk of a nonfatal heart attack.

The one study of the five showing no benefit was criticized for its poor design.

Additional recent research, also published in *Lancet*, has found that vitamin E helps prevent heart disease in kidney dialysis patients who are four times more likely to die of cardiovascular disease than healthy people. In the study, a dose of 800 IU of natural vitamin E or a placebo daily for an average of seventeen months was given to dialysis patients. Seventeen patients who took placebos had heart attacks during the study, but only five of the patients who took vitamin E had heart attacks during the study.

Occasionally you'll hear that a new study has found no protective effect of vitamin E on heart health or some other condition. That's a good time to take a critical look at the study's design. For how long did the subjects take vitamin E to gauge results? You probably need to take vitamin E for years to experience long-term benefits. Also, was natural vitamin E (far superior to synthetic) used in the study? Sadly, many published studies still don't even distinguish whether the natural or synthetic form was used. Yet these questions—even if they go unanswered in your search for information—highlight just a couple of the factors that affect research outcomes.

Understanding the Vitamin E Connection to Heart Health

It may be hard to believe, but it has been more than half a century since doctors first discovered that vitamin E could prevent heart disease. In the 1940s, Evan Shute, M.D., and his colleagues in London, Canada, reported that vitamin E could reverse many symptoms of heart disease. Although their findings were described in 1946 in the respected scientific journal *Nature*, as well as in *Time* magazine, the medical establishment largely rejected their findings.

Part of the reason was that most doctors at the time could not imagine how a mere vitamin would protect against the leading cause of death among Americans and Canadians. Over the years, vitamin E was ridiculed. Some people considered it a waste of money; others called it "a cure in search of a disease."

During the 1980s and 1990s, researchers quietly built a strong scientific case to support vitamin E. Simply put, vitamin E is a protective substance called an antioxidant. It neutralizes harmful substances called oxidants, or free radicals. During this time, the free radical theory of aging—and age-related diseases—gained momentum as well. So, as an antioxidant, vitamin E could be considered an antiaging and antidisease vitamin. The human studies of the 1990s clearly demonstrated its benefits—and proved Shute correct in his original observations that vitamin E was good for the heart.

Free radicals are molecules that have one unpaired electron. As a consequence, they're highly unstable. In an effort to become more stable, free radicals cruise around inside the body, aggressively seeking compounds with which they can react to gain an electron. They can damage anything they come across—fats, sugars, your cells and the DNA inside your cells, to name a few—in the process.

Antioxidants quench free radicals by donating electrons to make up for the missing ones in free radicals. This means that antioxidants scavenge free radicals before they cause harm to our cells. Think of antioxidants as body-guards that protect cells from damage by free radicals. This kind of damage is implicated in the development and spread of not just heart disease but all degenerative diseases, as you'll read many times throughout this book. Taking antioxidants such as vitamin E is important for protecting the whole body—not just the heart—against disease.

Free Radicals
Harmful molecules produced by the body and pollutants. They have one electron too few or one too many, making them highly unstable.

How Heart Disease Develops

Heart disease (sometimes referred to as coronary artery disease) develops slowly, usually without our knowledge, in a step-by-step progression of events. It begins when artery walls become damaged or injured by free radicals. "Smooth muscle cells" then begin to grow on artery walls and plaque forms.

Then a series of events occurs that cause artery walls to become clogged with fat and cholesterol. If the artery walls become too narrow and if the blood becomes sticky and blood clots form, blood flow can become restricted. Blood clots in arteries are sort of like a wad of hair caught in a drainpipe; blood (or water, in your bathroom sink) can't get past the blockage to where it's supposed to go.

When blood flow is restricted, the heart or brain doesn't receive the oxygen from blood that it needs to function. The result can be a heart attack or stroke. Heart tissue dies as a result of the blood supply being cut off (as in a heart attack), making the heart weaker. A heart attack can disrupt the heartbeat, which is controlled by rhythmic electrical activity within the heart itself. The most common form of stroke is called ischemic stroke, which results from decreased blood supply to the brain and leads to neurological problems. Often, a stroke is caused by cholesterol-containing deposits of plaque that block blood flow in the arteries supplying the brain.

Vitamin E, as an antioxidant, protects both the artery walls and the cholesterol found in our bloodstream from free radical damage. Both of these protections help prevent heart disease from developing and progressing. And, considering the serious consequences of this major killer, that's very good news.

Vitamin E's Protective Effects on Cholesterol

In discussing heart health, many people wonder how cholesterol is affected. Vitamin E won't actually lower high blood levels of cholesterol, but it does protect against heart disease by doing something more important—it prevents the low-density lipoprotein (LDL) form of cholesterol from being chemically changed and becoming toxic to arteries. LDL cholesterol is often referred to as "bad" cholesterol, but it isn't inherently bad. Low levels of LDL are actually needed to transport vitamin E and other fat-soluble vitamins through the bloodstream.

LDL becomes harmful to arteries when there is insufficient vitamin E in our system to prevent it from being oxidized, or damaged, by free radicals. This damage is called lipid peroxidation. Without enough antioxidants, circulating free radicals in the body damage the structure of LDL, making it appear foreign to the immune system. This system, attempting to protect us from foreign invaders, sends out immune cells to engulf the oxidized LDL.

These immune cells filled with lipids, called foam cells, clump together on blood vessel surfaces. This is plaque, which then builds up, limiting the flow of oxygen and other nutrients in the blood to the heart. Avoiding LDL oxidation is one of the central goals in current preventive and therapeutic natural approaches to staving off heart disease. Studies in animals and humans consistently show that 400–500 IU of vitamin E daily protects LDL from oxidation, thus preventing LDL deposits in blood vessels and reducing the risk of coronary artery disease.

LDL
Low-density lipoprotein, or LDL, transports proteins, triglycerides (fats), cholesterol, and fat-soluble vitamins through the blood to body cells.

In one such study, published in the journal *Arteriosclerosis, Thrombosis, and Vascular Biology*, forty-eight men and women aged forty-five to sixty-nine took either 271 IU of natural vitamin E, 500 mg of vitamin C, a combination of the two, or a placebo daily for three years. Both vitamin E and the combination of vitamins C and E made the LDL cholesterol in these men and women less prone to oxidation. (Vitamin C alone had no effect.) Another recent study found that people with coronary artery disease who took 400 IU of vitamin E per day for thirty days had significant decreases in lipid peroxidation compared with a placebo group. Others taking vitamin C or vitamin A or increasing their fruit intake also experienced decreased oxidative damage, but not as much as the vitamin E group did.

If you take cholesterol-lowering drugs, it's especially important for you to take vitamin E. These drugs cause vitamin E levels in LDL to drop and LDL, in turn, oxidizes more quickly than normal. Thus, although such drugs do lower cholesterol levels, they may actually increase the damage to blood vessel walls. (Supplementing with the vitaminlike antioxidant coenzyme Q_{10} is also a good idea for people taking cholesterol-lowering drugs.)

Vitamin E's Other Heart-Protective Benefits

Vitamin E works in a variety of ways beyond that of an antioxidant to slow or stop the development of heart disease and stroke. As you've read, it slows down the buildup of smooth muscle cells on artery walls that contribute to artery-clogging plaque. In some people, vitamin E also may increase levels of the high-density lipoprotein (HDL) form of cholesterol, the type that is called the "good" cholesterol, because it carries cholesterol from the bloodstream to the liver for elimination.

Vitamin E decreases excessive platelet aggregation, too. This is the tendency of blood platelets to stick together and promote the formation of blood clots, which increase the risk of heart attack and stroke because they restrict blood flow. The blood-thinning benefits of vitamin E make it particularly important for those with diabetes and women who take oral contraceptives, because these groups have an increased tendency for excessive platelet aggregation and higher risk of stroke.

Platelet Aggregation
The tendency of blood platelets to stick together, promoting blood clot formation.

In a recent study, Jane E. Freedman, M.D., and John F. Keaney, M.D., found that natural vitamin E was well absorbed by blood platelets in blood taken from healthy volunteers. The synthetic form was not well absorbed (you'll learn more about the advantages of natural over synthetic vitamin E later). The researchers determined that natural vitamin E reduced platelet aggregation by more than half! In other research, published in the journal *Atherosclerosis, Thrombosis, and Vascular Biology*, vitamin E supplements taken daily for two weeks decreased platelet aggregation and led to lower levels of free radicals in human subjects.

Keep in mind that reducing platelet aggregation, or stickiness, decreases the likelihood of blood clots and a resulting cardiac event. Interestingly, Freedman and Keaney found that the anticoagulant effect of vitamin E was not related to its antioxidant properties. Rather, it was because vitamin E inhibits protein kinase C, an enzyme that promotes blood clotting and breakdown of collagen tissue.

Vitamin E Protects against the Harmful Effects of Junk Foods

According to recent studies, vitamin E can even protect you from some of the cardiovascular effects of high-fat/ high-carbohydrate foods—a combination found in most convenience, microwave, and "fast" foods. Fatty meals normally trigger a chain of chemical reactions that tense up, or constrict, blood vessels, leading to reduced blood flow. This cardiovascular consequence is called endothelial dysfunction. A fascinating study by cardiologist Gary Plotnick, M.D., of the University of Maryland, found that vitamin E and vitamin C offer significant protection against the damaging effects of high-fat/high-carbohydrate meals.

Endothelial Dysfunction
A pronounced constriction of blood vessels that leads to a stiffening of blood-vessel walls and reduced blood flow, increasing the risk of heart disease.

In the study, twenty faculty members ate a popular, high-fat, fast-food breakfast consisting of eggs and sausage on a roll along with hash browns. As the researchers expected, the fat burden of this breakfast prevented the subjects' arteries from relaxing, or dilating, normally. Normal dilation is necessary for normal blood flow.

On another day, the same subjects ate the same breakfast, but about fifteen minutes before eating they also took 800 IU of vitamin E and 1,000 mg vitamin C. This combination offered remarkable protection. Their blood vessels behaved normally, as if they had eaten low-fat foods—and the benefits lasted for six hours.

Unfortunately, Plotnick blamed the endothelial dysfunction only on what he described as a meal high in saturated fat. While the fast-food breakfast was high in saturated fat, it was also high in hydrogenated vegetable oils, trans fatty acids (now known to be much worse than saturated fat), oxidized fats, and refined carbohydrates. So, rather than just indicating saturated fats, Plotnick actually showed the overall danger of a typical fast-food meal—and how vitamins E and C could blunt part of the damage.

Another study, conducted by David L. Katz, M.D., and his colleagues at the Yale University School of Medicine, echoed these findings. Fifty healthy, nonsmoking men and women had decreased blood flow in their forearms after drinking a milkshake made with ice cream, coconut cream and pasteurized eggs—a high-fat (and high-sugar) meal. On separate occasions, these same subjects were given—individually—either 800 IU of vitamin E in capsule form, oatmeal, or whole-wheat cereal, in addition to the milkshake. The vitamin E supplements and the oatmeal (independently) protected against any reduction in blood flow.

Once again, this researcher conducted a study that attempted to show the cardiovascular effects of a high-fat meal. But, in actuality, he demonstrated the hazards of a high-fat/high-carbohydrate meal because the ice cream eaten in this study contained large amounts of sugar. On the positive side, however, the vitamin E and the oatmeal offered some protection against this dietary disaster.

Taking vitamin C and E supplements and choosing healthier foods offers the best protection against heart disease. However, these studies show that if you do indulge in high-fat/high-carbohydrate foods, it's smart to take vitamin E and vitamin C right before, or with your meal.

Vitamin E Might Help Reverse Clogged Arteries

There is evidence from animal and human studies that vitamin E may help *reverse* heart disease. Researchers have found that in monkeys, our close biological relatives, clogged arteries induced by a high-fat diet can not only be prevented, but can also be reversed by modest amounts of vitamin E. In a six-year research project, Anthony J. Verlangieri, Ph.D., of the University of Mississippi's Atherosclerosis Research Laboratory, fed monkeys a high-fat diet that caused their arteries to become clogged and blocked.

When the monkeys were also given vitamin E, the extent of arterial blockage dropped 60 to 80 percent. More remarkable was the fact that arteries that were seriously clogged began to open up.

Similarly, Howard N. Hodis, M.D., of the University of Southern California School of Medicine, Los Angeles, monitored the condition of people who had undergone bypass surgery. He found that patients who took 100–450 IU of vitamin E daily developed smaller lesions, or cholesterol deposits, on their arteries, than other bypass patients who didn't take vitamin E supplements. So, even if you've already had bypass surgery, vitamin E can help you. And, as we noted earlier in this chapter, a recent analysis of five large-scale, published trials led to the conclusion that many patients with pre-existing heart disease who took alpha-tocopherol supplements had a reduced risk of a nonfatal heart attack.

Vitamin E and Bypass Surgery

It's never too late to start taking vitamin E. But if you're scheduled for heart surgery, you should discuss taking vitamin E with your heart doctor. There is substantial research showing that vitamin E and other antioxidant vitamins can reduce the risk of complications, not only from bypass surgery, but also from balloon angioplasty and other types of surgical procedures.

During bypass surgery, blood flow is temporarily stopped so surgeons can graft new arteries. When the flow of oxygen-rich blood is replenished, large numbers of free radicals are generated, and these radicals can damage the heart. To protect against the free radical damage that's common with surgery, an increasing number of heart surgeons give their patients supplements of vitamin E and other antioxidants, such as vitamin C and coenzyme Q_{10}, before surgery. But a word of caution here: Due to its blood-thinning action, it is not advisable to take vitamin E before surgery if you're also taking a prescription blood-thinner like warfarin (Coumadin), without the guidance of a doctor knowledgeable about vitamin E.

Antioxidants *Molecules, including vitamin E, that donate electrons to stablilize damaging free radicals.*

Doctors' Opinions about Vitamin E

A growing number of doctors are warming up to the idea of taking vitamin E and are recommending supplements to their patients. Years ago, doctors had no explanation for why vitamin E could prevent and effectively treat heart disease. Today, most doctors understand that vitamin E is an antioxidant that protects against heart-damaging free radicals.

In general, Western medicine has long been skeptical of the health benefits of vitamin supplements. It has taken a long time for doctors to adjust to the idea that high doses of vitamins might be good for health. For example, it's difficult for many surgeons to recommend a nonsurgical way to treat heart disease. They have been trained as surgeons, and that's how they make their living.

Another problem has been physician education. In medical schools, doctors learn a lot about anatomy, physiology, diseases, and treatments, but almost nothing about nutrition. Dietitians are schooled in nutrition, but even they often underestimate the health benefits of vitamin supplements in amounts beyond the too-conservative RDAs. After medical school, much of a physician's ongoing education is strongly influenced by large drug companies. These companies are interested in selling expensive, proprietary drugs, not inexpensive vitamins. So drugs, not vitamins, are what physicians hear about most, particularly from the drug representatives who visit frequently and inundate them with drug samples and reams of copy on the special qualities of their product.

Nobel laureate Linus Pauling, Ph.D., once said, "If a doctor isn't 'up' on something, he's 'down' on it." If your doctor tells you vitamin E is a waste of money, he or she is either uninformed, irresponsible, or behind the times in his or her medical knowledge. In a typical year, medical journals publish about 500 scientific reports on vitamin E research.

If you decide to stick with this doctor, and to entrust your health to him, it's up to you to educate him—and to protect your health by taking vitamin E. Bring up the subject in a polite, non-threatening way. You could even share this book with him.

Even though your doctor may be skeptical about a "popular" (rather than medical) book, point him to the scientific references at the back of this book. He'll be able to use these references to look up everything he needs to know about vitamin E. If your doctor doesn't want to look up the references, and isn't willing to have a two-way conversation with you, the handwriting is on the wall: This doctor isn't a good one. Find another one.

How Much Vitamin E Is Needed to Benefit the Heart?

In general, 400 IU of natural vitamin E should be an ideal dose for most people to prevent coronary artery disease. The natural form of vitamin E is superior to the synthetic form, and we'll explain more about the difference later. If you have very serious heart disease, or are taking prescription drugs for your heart, tell your doctor of your interest in vitamin E. Sometimes people can reduce their intake of prescription drugs after they start taking vitamin E, but this is best done with a physician's guidance.

Even if you eat a healthy diet, you're probably not getting enough vitamin E. The amount most commonly recommended to benefit the heart—400 IU—is impossible to get from foods alone. You'd have to eat 1,000 almonds (or one pound of sunflower seeds)—8,000 calories worth of food—to obtain this amount of vitamin E.

REDUCING THE RISK OF CANCER

We tend to think of cancer as a single disease, but there are more than 100 kinds of cancer. They can cause different symptoms and be brought on by various factors, but virtually all develop because of damage by free radicals, the same hazardous molecules that also cause heart disease.

The good news is that there are many preventive measures we can take to reduce our risk for cancer. One of the most important is to take vitamin E. In this chapter, we'll look at how cancer develops, the relationship between vitamin E and cancer prevention, some of the ways vitamin E is thought to protect against specific types of cancer, and the forms of vitamin E that may be the most protective.

Vitamin E Reduces Cancer Risk

The scientific evidence shows that vitamin E can reduce cancer risk. According to an article in *Cancer Causes and Control*, researchers analyzed fifty-nine human studies on vitamin/mineral supplements and cancer risk and found that, of all the supplements studied, vitamin E supplements were the most strongly associated with a reduced cancer risk. Many studies have also found that high levels of vitamin E in the body are associated with a lower risk of cancer, whereas low levels are associated with a greater risk. These trends have been identified with breast cancer, cervical cancer and cervical dysplasia, colon cancer, lung cancer, and throat cancer.

Although vitamin E can reduce the risk of cancer, do not view it as a treatment (though it may be helpful in conjunction with other treatments). In some studies that have found no anticancer benefits from vitamin E, the participants have smoked for years or eaten a poor diet. Smoking and an unhealthy diet are strong risk factors for cancer, so vitamin E isn't a magic bullet that can totally erase the deleterious, cumulative effects brought on by years of unhealthy living. It is, however, an essential nutrient the body needs to function properly and help ward off diseases.

How Cancer Develops

Cancer is a disease in which normal cell growth goes awry. It usually (but not always) develops very slowly. Most cancers begin when free radicals damage the deoxyribonucleic acid (DNA, or genetic material) within your cells. Malignant tumors can result from the buildup of cells dividing uncontrollably, then they tend to spread and cause new malignant growths.

DNA is a set of biological instructions that tells your cells how to function normally. When DNA becomes damaged, the instructions that tell cells to perform properly become garbled. Even when a cell becomes cancerous, the immune system can often destroy it before it replicates and becomes established as a cancer. But when free radical damage occurs in enough of your cells, cancerous cells can overwhelm the beleaguered immune system and can proliferate, accumulate, and spread.

Free radicals are byproducts of normal cellular processes, so they're a natural part of living. But free radicals also are generated by exposure to pollutants, radiation, and chemicals. Modern living, therefore, often tips the balance between free radicals and antioxidants (free radical quenchers) toward too many free radicals.

Tobacco smoke increases free radicals significantly, which is why smokers have a very high risk of most cancers (not just lung cancer). Because a big part of the process that leads to cancer involves damage from too many free radicals, the best way to protect your body against cancer is to supplement your diet with such antioxidants as vitamin E, and to avoid the unnecessary free radical production that such behavior as smoking causes.

How Vitamin E Protects against Cancer

Vitamin E protects against cancer in several ways. First and foremost, as a component of cell membranes, vitamin E helps prevent these membranes from becoming damaged by free radicals from a wide variety of sources, including chemicals, radiation, and toxins.

Vitamin E also can prevent nitrites (compounds found in smoked, cured, and pickled foods) from forming nitrosamines, which are strong tumor promoters. It may also assist or accelerate the body's metabolism of carcinogenic, or cancer-causing, substances. In other words, vitamin E may help the body get rid of potential cancer-causing agents in the body more quickly.

In addition, vitamin E appears to block the formation of blood vessels in tumors. This is significant because tumors need their own network of blood vessels for nourishment in order to grow. Creating these blood vessels is a process called angiogenesis. According to cell and rodent studies, vitamin E has anti-angiogenic properties.

This anti-angiogenic property is particularly true of the

"succinate" form (d-alpha-tocopheryl succinate) of vitamin E. In addition, there is growing evidence that vitamin E plays a role in normal gene expression, or activation. It's very possible that vitamin E maintains normal gene activity and helps turn off the abnormal gene activity characteristic of tumors.

Angiogenesis
The formation of blood vessels, which tumors need to receive nourishment and grow.

Other research shows that cancerous tumors generate large numbers of their own free radicals, thereby creating endless·mutations to circumvent various types of chemotherapeutic drugs. These drugs can be target-specific, so mutated forms of cancer cells may escape the drugs' cancer-fighting effects, allowing the cancer to thrive. By quenching free radicals, vitamin E may slow down the mutation rate in cancer, enabling other treatments to fight it.

Probably the most important way vitamin E helps ward off cancer is by boosting the immune system. As mentioned earlier, cancerous cells can develop—many experts think all people have some cancer cells in their bodies—but cancerous tumors won't take hold as long as our immune systems are strong and primed to scavenge those cells.

Vitamin E supplementation has been shown to boost the immune system in a variety of ways, including increasing the activity of natural killer (NK) cells. NK cells are "Rambo"-type cells, which can recognize cells that have gone bad; they're fully armed and ready to kill cancerous cells on the spot before the cells can divide and cause harm. This means that supplemental vitamin E helps keep your immune cells in a vigorous state, ready to attack the first cancer cells they find.

Though Not a Cure, Vitamin E Can Inhibit Cancer Cell Growth

At this time, there's no research to indicate that vitamin E can reverse cancer in humans (in other words, do not try to use vitamin E as a "cure" for cancer). There is, however, one particular type of vitamin E, d-alpha-tocopheryl succinate, that has been found to inhibit the growth of cancer cells in cell cultures (dishes of cells in a laboratory) and rodent experiments. And there is another group of vitamin E molecules, called tocotrienols, that has also been found to kill human breast cancer cells grown in cell cultures. So far, the research is preliminary, but scientists are excited about the promise of both forms of vitamin E against cancer.

Although one day certain types of vitamin E and other nutrients may be used routinely against existing cancer, the best approach is to begin taking vitamin E now to help prevent cancer. Prevention is always the best policy, especially for cancer, which can be a devastating, deadly, and emotionally wrenching disease. To put all this a slightly different way: If either of us were diagnosed with cancer, we would take supplements of the d-alpha-tocopheryl succinate form of vitamin E in addition to pursuing other types of therapies. We would not rely on vitamin E alone, and neither should you.

Vitamin E Reduces the Risk of Prostate Cancer

Vitamin E supplementation significantly lowers the risk of prostate cancer, according to recent findings reported in the *Journal of the National Cancer Institute*. In the study, Ollie P. Heinonen, M.D., D.Sc., and his colleagues at the University of Helsinki tracked the health of 29,000 men for six years. The men taking vitamin E were found to be 32 percent less likely to develop prostate cancer and 41 percent less likely to die from the disease if they did develop it. And these beneficial effects were seen within two years of starting the supplementation.

The results of this study are especially significant because the men were smokers at above-average risk of cancer. The researchers acknowledged that the simple intervention of taking a vitamin E supplement might help prevent prostate cancer, the most frequently diagnosed cancer in men, but even they were surprised by how strong the benefits were. This study used a relatively low dose—50 IU—of vitamin E, but a higher dose—400 IU—has greater overall benefits to the heart and, likely, to the prostate.

Prostate Gland
The doughnut-shaped gland below the bladder in men that surrounds the upper part of the urethra and secretes a solution that aids in sperm movement and health.

Cell studies point to a role for vitamin E in prostate cancer protection, too. In a recent study published in the journal *Nutrition and Cancer* in 2000, natural vitamin-E succinate (d-alpha-tocopheryl succinate) stopped the growth of two types of prostate cancer cells and actually caused these cells to self-destruct. Vitamin E didn't hurt normal prostate cells, though.

Vitamin E May Offer Protection against Breast Cancer

Vitamin E may protect against breast cancer as well. Research with animals suggests that vitamin E can compensate somewhat for a genetic defect that increases the risk of breast cancer. Some people have a genetic defect that results in low production of catalase, an antioxidant enzyme the body produces. Without sufficient catalase, cells have trouble neutralizing the free radicals that can cause breast cancer.

Japanese researchers at the Okayama University Medical School studied mice that did not produce enough catalase. They found that catalase-deficient mice were more likely than normal mice to develop breast cancer. But when the researchers added vitamin E to the mice's diet, the mice were far less likely to develop breast cancer.

Could vitamin E benefit people in the same way? According to the researchers, who published their findings in the *Japanese Journal of Cancer Research*, "vitamin E intrinsically has a protective effect against the development of mammary tumor, and this may apply . . . to humans." Most of us don't know whether we're producing insufficient catalase or not. However, this research suggests that taking vitamin E over a lifetime may reduce the risk of breast cancer in those individuals who unknowingly produce low amounts of catalase.

Vitamin E Protects the Skin

Vitamin E protects the skin from free radical damage, too. The skin is regularly exposed to ultraviolet (UV) radiation from sunlight that generates large numbers of free radicals, which age the skin and greatly increase the risk of skin cancer. Skin cancer is of great concern because it is the most prevalent type of cancer, and its incidence among Americans is steadily increasing.

Research in rodents has found that both internal and external use of vitamin E protects the skin from the initial damage that can occur from excessive exposure to UV radiation. It also raises the levels of protective antioxidants in the skin and reduces suppression of the immune system, which often occurs as a result of too much exposure to sunlight. Via these mechanisms, it makes the body better able to protect itself against skin cancer.

Vitamin E Protects against Mouth, Throat, and Colorectal Cancer

What's more, vitamin E helps protect against precancerous growths in the mouth and throat. These growths are predominantly found in people who smoke tobacco or drink excessive amounts of alcohol—activities that generate large numbers of free radicals. In a study conducted by Steven Benner, M.D., of the University of Texas Anderson Cancer Center, Houston, patients with these growths were given 400 IU of vitamin E twice daily for twenty-four weeks. About a quarter of the patients had a greater than 50 percent decrease in the size of their precancerous lesions and another quarter had a complete disappearance of the growths.

Another study—this one with 29,000 male cigarette smokers—found that 50 IU per day of vitamin E for five to eight years led to a slightly reduced risk of developing colorectal cancer. Larger doses might have decreased their risk of disease even more. Smokers taking beta-carotene or a placebo didn't experience this protective effect. These are some good examples of how vitamin E can quench free radicals from a variety of sources and thus protect against many different forms of cancer.

Supplementing with Vitamin E for Cancer Protection

Vitamin E is recognized as the key antioxidant for protecting cellular membranes (walls) against free radical damage, so your health will certainly benefit from taking vitamin E. As with coronary artery disease, 400 IU of natural vitamin E seems to be an effective and safe dose. But research indicates that a diverse selection of antioxidants may be more important for protecting the body against free radical damage than high doses of a single antioxidant.

Antioxidants other than vitamin E include vitamin C, alpha-lipoic acid, beta-carotene and other carotenoids (such as lutein and lycopene), coenzyme Q_{10}, selenium, and zinc. Different antioxidants scavenge different types of free radicals, so a combination of antioxidants forms a stronger antioxidant shield to protect the body against cancer and other degenerative diseases.

Antioxidants also work synergistically with each other. Vitamin C, for example, recycles vitamin E that has been used up; selenium works in concert with vitamin E; and zinc is needed to maintain normal blood concentrations of vitamin E. Taking a combination of antioxidants, therefore, better ensures that you'll get the most mileage out of the vitamin E you take.

BOOSTING IMMUNITY AND QUENCHING INFLAMMATION

Vitamin E's ability to protect against heart disease and cancer has been the focus of much research. However, its ability to boost the immune system has gone largely unnoticed until recent years. Your immune system bolsters your defenses against colds and other infections. This chapter will cover the ways in which vitamin E enhances immunity and helps protect you against everyday minor illnesses and more serious infections, while also providing safe anti-inflammatory benefits.

Vitamin E Enhances Immunity

Several studies show that vitamin E boosts the immune system and can enhance resistance to infection. This is particularly important for older people, because the immune system declines with age and this leads to an increased susceptibility to illness.

In one study, Simin N. Meydani, D.V.M., Ph.D., of Tufts University, gave vitamin E to a group of men and women sixty-five years of age and older. Subjects taking 200 IU each day for about four months showed significant improvements on various tests that assess the immune system's ability to ward off diseases. The subjects' immune responses actually behaved more like those of forty-year-olds than sixty-five- or seventy-year-olds. Furthermore, the incidence of self-reported illnesses, such as colds, declined by about 30 percent.

In other studies, vitamin E has been found to boost the

immune responses of young people. Therefore, vitamin E might keep you from being sick as often, though the effect will likely be subtle and long term instead of quick and dramatic.

The Health Consequences of Vitamin E Deficiency

A deficiency of vitamin E can make you not only more susceptible to illness, but also more prone to virus mutations that can lead to serious disease. It's well known that nutritional deficiencies reduce the ability of the immune system to fight infections.

Vitamin E deficiencies are associated with decreased immune function and decreased differentiation of immature T cells, which fight off foreign invaders like bacteria, cancer cells, viruses, and others. Basically, deficiencies of vitamin E prevent your immune system from mounting an effective counterattack against bacteria and viruses. But there has been a recent, significant twist in this field.

T Cells
Immune cells that fight off foreign invaders in the body, including bacteria, cancer cells, viruses, and more.

In groundbreaking studies, Melinda Beck, Ph.D., of the University of North Carolina at Chapel Hill, and Orville Levander, Ph.D., of the U.S. Department of Agriculture, discovered that deficiencies of vitamin E or the mineral selenium in a person or animal could turn a common virus into a deadly, rapidly producing strain.

Beck and Levander studied the Coxsackie virus, which infects about 20 million Americans annually and usually causes no more than coldlike symptoms, diarrhea, or a sore throat. However, when a person or animal is deficient in vitamin E or selenium (a mineral that works in tandem with vitamin E), the virus can mutate into a strain that inflames the heart muscle, leading to cardiomyopathy and heart failure.

Adequate levels of both nutrients, though, prevent mutations of the virus. This research provides one more convincing reason to take supplemental vitamin E, as well as selenium. But there may be more reasons in the future: Beck and Levander are currently looking into how deficiencies of vitamin E and selenium might cause other viruses, such as cold and flu viruses, to mutate.

How Vitamin E Improves Immunity

The immune system mounts an amazingly complex defense against invaders, and vitamin E stimulates many parts of this defense. Specifically, vitamin E has been found to:

- Improve the function of phagocytes (cells that act as biological "Pac-Men" against a broad range of microorganisms);

- Stimulate activity of natural killer cells (which destroy cancer and virus-infected cells);

- Enhance the body's ability to produce antibodies (which tag or damage viruses); and

- Lower levels of prostaglandin E2, an inflammation-causing substance.

Through all these mechanisms, vitamin E acts as a powerful, broad-spectrum, immune enhancer. And, in addition to stimulating immunity, vitamin E protects the immune system from the wear and tear of constantly defending the body from unwanted invaders. Although it's surprising to many people, immune cells like phagocytes generate enormous quantities of free radicals to kill bacteria, yet these immune cells are highly susceptible to damage from free radicals themselves. Vitamin E, of course, quenches free radicals, protecting healthy cells—including immune cells—from damage.

If you're wondering about the best dose for boosting your immunity, that depends on your state of health. Doses of 200–400 IU of vitamin E daily are beneficial for most people. Higher doses of vitamin E (as well as other nutrients) may be beneficial for those with severe immunity problems.

Vitamin E's Benefits for Those with AIDS

Vitamin E can help those infected with AIDS (acquired immune deficiency syndrome). Here's why: Free radicals are known to promote the replication of the HIV virus, which causes AIDS. In animal studies, vitamin E has been shown to indirectly inhibit replication of the HIV virus by quenching free radicals and by stimulating various parts of the immune system.

A number of studies have found that people infected with HIV have low levels of vitamin E and other nutrients in addition to high amounts of free radicals. One recent study, conducted in Toronto, found that supplements of vitamins E and C reduced virus levels in people infected with HIV. All of this research suggests that vitamin E may be beneficial for treating HIV infection, but more studies in humans are needed to confirm this.

It's important to recognize that people with HIV and AIDS may need far more than the standard, low RDA levels of vitamins. There are many reasons for this, not the least being that many patients with AIDS suffer from diarrhea, which promotes nutrient loss. Researchers have found that patients with HIV and AIDS have low blood levels of most vitamins and minerals, and that very high supplemental amounts are usually needed to achieve normal blood levels of these nutrients.

Does Vitamin E Exacerbate Autoimmune Diseases?

Since vitamin E boosts immunity, it's only natural to wonder whether vitamin E might exacerbate autoimmune diseases—conditions in which the immune system interprets the body's normal cells as invaders and attacks them. There are theories about what makes the immune system attack the body's own cells, but much about autoimmunity remains a mystery.

Autoimmune Disease
A condition in which the immune system attacks the body's own cells, as if they were foreign invaders.

The simple answer is that vitamin E is not likely to overstimulate the immune system and aggravate autoimmune diseases. Autoimmune diseases always involve inflammation in the body. Vitamin E enhances certain types of immune cells and dampens others that are involved in inflammation. Any time you have inflammation in the body, in fact, large numbers of free radicals accompany the inflammation, and vitamin E can serve as an antidote against these damaging molecules.

Vitamin E Helps in Lupus and Rheumatoid Arthritis

Vitamin E actually improves the symptoms of individuals with autoimmune conditions like lupus or rheumatoid arthritis, as long as it is taken in high enough doses. For example, in one study, people with lupus receiving 900–1,600 IU of vitamin E per day showed complete or almost complete clearing of symptoms. Lower dosages of 300 IU, however, had no effect. People with rheumatoid arthritis, another chronic inflammatory disease, have also benefited from supplementation, experiencing a lessening of pain and stiffness, with doses ranging from 400–1,200 IU per day.

Vitamin E seems to work well in conjunction with standard arthritis treatments, too. One example is a recent study in which thirty patients with rheumatoid disease were given either a standard drug-treatment regimen, a standard drug treatment plus a combination of low-potency antioxidants, or a high dose of vitamin E (400 IU three times a day) in combination with standard drug treatment.

Patients who took the antioxidant combination or vitamin E with the standard treatment had better control of arthritis symptoms from the first month of treatment than those who received only standard treatment. Patients who took vitamin E also had more significant improvements in disease severity, inflammation, and morning stiffness than those taking only standard drug treatment.

Vitamin E Counters Inflammation

As an antioxidant, vitamin E does a lot to counter inflammation, which is involved not only in autoimmune diseases, but also in injuries. We've already described the damage that free radicals can cause to genes, fats, proteins, and more. As if that weren't devastating enough to the body, free radicals also stimulate and intensify inflammation. They do this by turning on genes that promote inflammation.

As an antioxidant, vitamin E can quench free radicals before they have a chance to induce inflammation. This powerful vitamin also reduces important promoters of inflammation, including C-reactive protein (CRP), adhesion molecules (which help white blood cells adhere to normal cells), and interleukin-6 (IL-6). C-reactive protein is such an important marker of impending health problems that it requires a bit more explanation.

C-Reactive Protein Indicates Inflammation

CRP is a key marker of inflammation throughout the body, and high levels have been linked to a dramatically increased risk of heart attack, physical trauma, and serious infections.

High cholesterol and high homocysteine levels are associated with increased heart disease and heart-attack risk, and many people worry about these risk factors. But high levels of CRP are now considered even more predictive of a heart attack. CRP is found in atherosclerotic lesions and is related to the lesion's rupture, which can lead to blood vessel clots and, in turn, to blood-flow blockage and heart attacks.

Other conditions linked to high CRP levels are blood-sugar problems, including diabetes, insulin resistance, and Syndrome X (which you'll learn about later). Overweight people and smokers, as well as those with Alzheimer's disease, arthritis, and cancer, tend to have higher-than-normal CRP levels, too. Some of the latest research suggests that supplementing with vitamin E can lower CRP a great deal. If you wish, you can ask your physician to measure your CRP levels.

How Vitamin E Quells Inflammation

Vitamin E's benefit in preventing LDL cholesterol from being oxidized is important in how it helps quell inflammation. As we described more generally earlier, white blood cells go after oxidized LDL in the inflammation process, using an arsenal of free radicals themselves as poison to destroy the oxidized LDL.

But free radicals that leak out of the white blood cells cause more inflammation and can even penetrate artery walls where they gobble up more LDL, stick there, and grow into lesions. Smooth muscle cells try to block off the problem area by covering it, but this leads to even worse blockage. And there's more bad news: Sometimes part of a lesion will break off, leading to a potentially dangerous clot that blocks the flow of blood.

But preventing LDL from being oxidized can keep the process described above from happening. Vitamin E, as you've learned, also keeps inflammation under control by inhibiting a variety of other pro-inflammatory substances, including CRP and IL-6.

Vitamin E supplementation appears to be the best natural method of lowering CRP levels. In one study, the effects of various antioxidants on fifty-seven people with type II diabetes were investigated. As reported in *Diabetes Care*, 800 IU of natural vitamin E daily for four weeks cut CRP levels by 50 percent. Neither 500 mg of vitamin C daily nor tomato juice (rich in lycopene) daily for four weeks could match this result.

In another study, people with diabetes, healthy people, and women with heart disease took 1,200 IU of natural vitamin E daily for three months. All of these groups averaged 30 percent drops in CRP, and their levels of interleukin-6 fell by 50 percent.

Vitamin E, therefore, not only acts as an immune booster but also as an anti-inflammatory agent. Through these two mechanisms, it can protect us from minor illnesses and chronic diseases.

PRESERVING THE MIND

Vitamin E is critical for proper brain and nerve function, and supplements of it have been found to have beneficial effects against such brain and nervous system disorders as Alzheimer's disease, Parkinson's disease, and tardive dyskinesia. This section will cover the important roles of vitamin E in brain and nerve health and how vitamin E is believed to protect against these devastating diseases.

Vitamin E Is Important for Brain Health

The brain contains large amounts of polyunsaturated fatty acids (PUFAs), the types of fats most prone to free radical damage. When the fatty acids in one brain cell become damaged, they can trigger a chain reaction in which many fatty acids throughout the brain become damaged.

Vitamin E, though, can halt this wildfire reaction before it begins: It's the most important fat-soluble antioxidant to shield fatty tissues, like those in the brain, from damage. Taking supplemental vitamin E, therefore, helps promote optimal brain health and should lower the risk of Alzheimer's and other degenerative diseases associated with free radical damage.

Vitamin E Can Slow the Progression of Alzheimer's Disease

Vitamin E isn't a cure for Alzheimer's disease, but it can slow the progression of this disease more than a leading drug used for this purpose. In a recent study reported in *The New England Journal of Medicine*, Mary Sano, Ph.D., of Columbia University's College of Physicians and Surgeons, New York, and her colleagues gave patients with severe Alzheimer's disease a large dose of either vitamin E (2,000 IU), selegiline (a drug used to treat Parkinson's disease), a combination of the two, or a placebo daily for two years.

Vitamin E delayed the progression of end-stage Alzheimer's by almost eight months compared with the placebo, or slightly longer than with the selegiline. Patients who took vitamin E showed 25 percent less decline in their ability to perform daily tasks like cooking, dressing, and eating. These kinds of abilities keep those with Alzheimer's at home rather than in a nursing facility and improve the quality of life for them. For a disease that has no known cure, these results are impressive.

> **Alzheimer's Disease**
> *A degenerative brain disease caused by neuron dysfunction and death that causes problems with behavior, feelings, memory, and thinking.*

Right after this study was published, the American Psychiatric Association gave its seal of approval to vitamin E, recommending it as a normal and appropriate part of the treatment for Alzheimer's. Both the American Academy of Neurology and the Alzheimer's Association have also approved the recommendation of 1,000 IU of vitamin E twice daily to slow the progression of Alzheimer's. Another study is under way to see if vitamin E will be even more effective for those with early-stage Alzheimer's disease.

The authors of a placebo-controlled, clinical trial conducted by the Alzheimer's Disease Cooperative Study, published in the *American Journal of Clinical Nutrition*, concluded that vitamin E "may slow functional deterioration leading to nursing home placement." In the study, patients with moderately advanced Alzheimer's disease were treated with 2,000 IU of vitamin E per day. The results of additional trials should help determine whether vitamin E can delay or prevent Alzheimer's disease in older people with mild cognitive problems.

How Vitamin E Helps in Alzheimer's Disease

Here's why vitamin E may slow Alzheimer's disease and possibly even prevent or delay its onset. Vitamin E seems to prevent oxidative damage from beta-amyloid, a substance found in high amounts in the brains of Alzheimer's disease patients. Vitamin E maintains cell-membrane flexibility, and brain cells that have flexible membranes function more efficiently.

Cell membranes act like the walls and doors of cells. As long as they are flexible, they allow other important nutrients into cells and waste products out. If the membranes of brain cells start to get rigid, important nutrients can't get in and cellular waste products just keep accumulating inside these brain cells, causing poor function and, eventually, their destruction, which can lead to Alzheimer's disease.

Supplementing with Vitamin E for Protection of Brain Health

You should take vitamin E to protect your overall health, and doing this should reduce your risk of developing Alzheimer's disease over the long term. It's likely that the longer you take vitamin E, the more protected you will be against Alzheimer's disease. Although some Alzheimer's studies have used 2,000 IU of vitamin E daily, much less is probably needed for long-term prevention. Again, an ideal preventive dose would seem to be about 400 IU daily.

Beta-amyloid is the abnormal protein that accumulates in the brains of Alzheimer's patients. In lab and rodent experiments, researchers have found that nerve cells die when they are exposed to beta-amyloid. But when vitamin E is added, the cells stay healthy. Many researchers in the field believe vitamin E can act preventively against Alzheimer's disease and they take vitamin E for this reason.

If you're young, taking steps to prevent Alzheimer's disease may be the furthest thing from your mind. It shouldn't be, though. Alzheimer's disease is the fourth leading cause of death in the United States. More than 4 million older Americans have the disease, and that number is expected to skyrocket as more of us live into our eighties and nineties.

Vitamin E's Effects on Other Brain and Nerve Conditions

Tardive dyskinesia is another condition that vitamin E might help. This is a condition characterized by involuntary muscle movements. It often affects long-term alcoholics and people who have been treated with antipsychotic drugs.

Like Alzheimer's disease, tardive dyskinesia is believed to be caused by free radical damage. Several studies have found vitamin E effective in treating tardive dyskinesia, especially in those who have had the disease for five years or less. In one scientifically controlled study of twenty-eight patients, a daily intake of 1,600 IU of vitamin E for two to three months was found to reduce involuntary muscle movements by one-third.

Parkinson's Disease
A disease that involves progressive degeneration of nerve cells in the brain and causes loss of balance, rigidity, and tremors.

Parkinson's disease involves progressive degeneration of nerve cells in the brain. Symptoms include incapacitating tremors, rigidity, and loss of balance. There's some conflicting evidence on the effectiveness of vitamin E against Parkinson's, perhaps because several studies used synthetic vitamin E, which is not well assimilated. However, vitamin E still appears to be helpful. In a large-scale study of 5,342 people in the Netherlands, researchers found the risk of Parkinson's disease went up as the consumption of vitamin E went down.

Since free radicals are believed to be at work in Parkinson's disease, researchers at the Columbia University Department of Neurology gave high doses of vitamin E (3,200 IU), coupled with 3 grams of vitamin C, to Parkinson's patients. The researchers found that those on the antioxidant therapy went 2.5 years longer before requiring drug therapy to treat their symptoms than those who received no

antioxidants. The doctors conducting this trial concluded that, "the progression of Parkinson's disease may be slowed by administration of these antioxidants."

Can Vitamin E Improve Memory?

There's no direct evidence to prove that vitamin E enhances memory, but it does promote healthy brain function, and healthy brain function is needed for normal memory recall. If vitamin E is taken regularly, it's logical to think that it might help memory slightly. Researchers recently found a correlation between the amount of vitamin E per unit of blood cholesterol and memory performance among a multiethnic sample of 4,809 older people, based on data from the Third National Health and Nutrition Examination Survey.

In addition, brain function naturally declines as we age, but vitamin E can slow this aging process. In an experiment involving mice, supplemental vitamin E (in amounts equivalent to a human dose of 400 IU per day) was found to prolong the life of brain cells by preventing or delaying free radical damage to a crucial strand of proteins called band-3 proteins. This research suggests that the cells that perform thinking and memory functions are among those that receive the most protection from vitamin E supplementation.

Taking vitamin E is a good, long-term strategy to support brain health and keep you mentally sharp. If your memory has faltered some and you're actively trying to improve it, though, try taking acetyl-L-carnitine and phosphatidyl serine (other nutrients that appear to be significant memory enhancers) in addition to vitamin E.

IMPROVING SEXUAL HEALTH

In the 1920s, researchers discovered that vitamin E was necessary for reproduction in rats, and people started referring to vitamin E as the sex vitamin. Although vitamin E isn't an aphrodisiac, it turns out that it does help a wide variety of conditions related to the reproductive system— everything from impotence and infertility in men to menopausal hot flashes, premenstrual syndrome, and sore breasts in women. In this section, we'll sort through the truths and misconceptions about vitamin E as a sex vitamin.

Vitamin E May Help Impotence

Impotence, called erectile dysfunction in the medical field, affects millions of men worldwide. In one study, 52 percent of male subjects forty to seventy years old were affected. Vitamin E can help some men with erectile dysfunction, but not in the same way as the prescription drug Viagra. Viagra can improve sexual performance immediately, but it can also be dangerous and should be avoided by those with heart or eye disease. Vitamin E works in a more subtle way to improve sexual performance and, of course, heart health.

Many factors, including aging, alcohol consumption, chronic illness, diabetes, high blood pressure, medication, and smoking, can have a negative effect on the ability to have erections. However, many cases of impotence are actually related to cardiovascular disease. Basically, the blood vessels of the penis can become damaged and narrowed from a buildup of arterial plaque just like the blood vessels that surround the heart. So anything that improves cardiovascular disease—such as vitamin E—may help impotency. Vitamin E also improves circulation or blood flow to all tissues, including those in the penis. Every condition improves with better blood flow.

Some scientists think that changes in protein kinase C and free radical production in diabetes could be part of the cause of erectile dysfunction among diabetic men. In an animal-cell study, vitamin E (the alpha-tocopherol form) reduced free radical production and protein kinase C in smooth muscle cells from the penis. Future human studies should shed light on the potential of vitamin E to help men with erectile dysfunction.

Vitamin E's Effects on Improving Fertility

Vitamin E shows promise in improving fertility as well. Several studies, published in *Fertility and Sterility*, have reported that infertile men have low levels of antioxidants in their semen and high levels of free radicals, which can deform sperm and prevent fertilization of the egg.

Vitamin E strengthens and protects the cell membranes of sperm and apparently helps them go that extra inch to father a child. In one study, Ami Amit, M.D., of Israel, gave men with normal sperm counts but low fertilization rates 200 IU of vitamin E daily for three months. The vitamin E lowered free radical levels in the men's semen and boosted their fertilization rate by 30 percent.

It takes at least three months for vitamins to have an effect in fertility, mainly because it takes that long for sperm to mature. Infertile couples should supplement with both vitamin E and a high-potency multivitamin for several months before trying to conceive. If you smoke, try to stop because tobacco smoke inflicts free radical damage on sperm.

Natural Vitamin E—Important for a Healthy Pregnancy

Vitamin E not only seems to help women conceive, it also is important for a healthy pregnancy. You can and should take vitamin E while pregnant for the health of you and your baby. Vitamin E can help protect against complications that sometimes occur during pregnancy and against those that can occur in babies who are born prematurely. It's important, though, to ask your doctor for prenatal supplements that contain natural vitamin E instead of synthetic.

Synthetic vitamin E is the type found in most prenatal supplements, but a recent study reported in the *American Journal of Clinical Nutrition* found that the human placenta can deliver natural vitamin E to the fetus 3.5 times more efficiently than it can the synthetic supplement. Pregnancy is the most important time in life to ensure optimal nutrition. Give you and your baby the best by asking your doctor specifically for a prenatal supplement that contains natural vitamin E.

Vitamin E Can Ease Fibrocystic Breast Pain and PMS

Vitamin E is important for protecting the health of women who aren't pregnant, too. First, vitamin E offers relief in fibrocystic breast disease, which is not really a disease but a group of benign conditions affecting the breast. The condition, which is very common in premenopausal women, usually involves cysts, lumps, pain, or tenderness in the breasts.

Several studies show that, for many women with fibrocystic breast disease symptoms, vitamin E appears to be quite effective in relieving the condition. In one study of twenty-six women with fibrocystic breast disease, 85 percent (twenty-two women) of those who received 600 IU of vitamin E daily for eight weeks responded to treatment.

Fibrocystic Breasts *Describes a group of benign conditions of the breast, including cysts, lumps, pain and tenderness.*

In a study of twelve women taking vitamin E, benign cysts decreased in number and size and, in ten of the women, there was a total disappearance of breast tenderness and cysts. In addition to taking vitamin E, an important strategy for alleviating symptoms of fibrocystic breast disease is to strictly avoid caffeine (found in coffee, tea, cola, and chocolate). This alone can totally eradicate the symptoms of this disease in many women.

Vitamin E appears to work well for some women with premenstrual syndrome (PMS), but not for everyone. Most of the research on vitamin E and PMS has focused primarily on breast tenderness, but at least one study suggests that vitamin E may help lessen other PMS symptoms including depression, fatigue, headache, insomnia, and nervous tension.

Whether or not vitamin E by itself relieves premenstrual tension, you should take supplemental vitamin E as good preventive medicine to protect yourself against heart disease, the leading killer of women. The best strategy to overcome PMS is a comprehensive one: Take vitamin E, but try adding supplements of B-complex vitamins, chromium, magnesium, and zinc, which have proven to be of value for some women. And try avoiding all forms of sugar in your diet, as this is also effective for alleviating PMS symptoms in many women.

Vitamin E Can Reduce Hot Flashes

Finally, vitamin E offers relief for menopausal women who experience hot flashes and other uncomfortable symptoms. Most of the research regarding vitamin E for hot flashes was actually conducted in the 1940s. Several studies found vitamin E effective in relieving hot flashes (as well as menopausal vaginal complaints) when compared with a dummy pill. Since then, many health-minded women have used vitamin E for these purposes, though no follow-up tests had been done.

Recently, however, researchers at the Mayo Clinic found that women can experience a reduction of hot flashes in as little as a month of supplementing with 800 IU of vitamin E. The study was interesting because it involved 120 breast cancer survivors who couldn't take estrogen replacement therapy (ERT). Although ERT is the most common treatment for such menopausal symptoms as hot flashes, breast cancer survivors can't use it because it often stimulates the growth of breast cancer cells.

The breast cancer survivors who took vitamin E experienced a small but statistically significant decrease in hot-flash activity after just four weeks, with no risk of side effects. Taking vitamin E for longer periods of time probably would provide even more beneficial effects.

For women who cannot use estrogen replacement therapy—or for those who simply prefer not to—vitamin E appears to be a mild, natural substitute to ease hot flashes. It doesn't, however, address all menopausal health concerns, so work with a nutritionally minded health professional to devise a complete nutrition strategy if you experience difficulties during and after menopause.

SLOWING THE AGING PROCESS AND MORE

Throughout this book, you've read about vitamin E's ability to prevent free radical damage and protect against everything from heart disease to Alzheimer's disease. This section will cover a wide assortment of other health benefits from vitamin E—including its ability to slow the aging process, reduce the risk of cataracts, lessen exercise-induced fatigue, help heal burns, and possibly even protect against wrinkles.

Vitamin E Slows down the Aging Process

Vitamin E is one of a number of nutrients that seem to slow the aging process. The basic idea is that free radicals damage cells and, in effect, age them. As an antioxidant, vitamin E slows down this damage, as do other antioxidants like vitamin C and coenzyme Q_{10}. Your body is essentially composed of around 100 billion cells, and it stands to reason that slowing the aging of these individual cells will slow the aging of your entire body.

Another way to look at this is in terms of reducing your risk for some of the top age-related disease killers such as heart disease, cancer, and Alzheimer's disease. Scientific studies have shown pretty clearly that vitamin E reduces the risk of developing these diseases. It might not completely eliminate the risk—but for the sake of discussion, let's assume that vitamin E only delays the onset of these diseases. This means you might not develop heart disease until you're eighty years old, instead of sixty. If vitamin E delays the onset of these serious diseases by ten, twenty, or thirty years, you're going to live longer and more healthfully.

Realistically, then, vitamin E can slow the aging process—that is, the speed at which your body's cells age. It is not an "antiaging" vitamin in the technical sense, because aging is an inevitable process. Vitamin E will not turn a forty-year-old man into a teenager. However, it may help restore the heart function of a seventy-year-old to that of someone ten or twenty years younger. But remember that eating a good diet, exercising, and minimizing stresses in your life also retards the aging process.

Vitamin E Protects against Cataracts

Cataracts are an age-related condition that vitamin E can help you avoid. Vitamin E has been found to significantly reduce the risk of cataracts, which account for 42 percent of all vision loss and are the leading cause of blindness worldwide.

Free radicals from pollution and ultraviolet radiation damage the proteins that form the lens of the eye and cause cataracts, so it isn't surprising that vitamin E can delay the onset and slow the progression of cataracts. In a recent study, 744 older people who took vitamin E supplements lowered their risk of developing cataracts by 57 percent.

Cataract
Clouding of the normally transparent eye lens, impairing vision; often associated with aging and diabetes.

Vitamin E appears to benefit people with cortical cataracts (an opacity, or cloudy area, toward the outside of the eye lens) more than those with nuclear cataracts (an opacity in the center of the lens). In an eye-opening study, Simmi Kharb, Ph.D., of the Postgraduate Institute of Medical Sciences in Rohtak, India, found that patients with cortical cataracts had an almost 40 percent decrease in lens opacity after taking vitamin E supplements twice daily for a month. Patients with nuclear cataracts had a decrease of only 14 percent.

Similarly, vitamin E benefited cortical lens tissue more significantly in other ways—decreased free radical activity, increased antioxidant production, and increased vitamin E levels—than it benefited nuclear lens tissue. Even so, vitamin E did improve both kinds of cataracts among those studied, just to different degrees.

Vitamin E Is Helpful for Diabetics and Those with Syndrome X

Vitamin E also helps protect against two increasingly common diseases of aging—type II diabetes and Syndrome X. Type II diabetes is characterized by high blood sugar (glucose) levels and numerous symptoms, including fatigue, frequent thirst, frequent urination, and poor concentration. Syndrome X is the combination of abdominal obesity, elevated blood cholesterol or triglycerides, and high blood pressure.

Both diseases involve insulin resistance—a condition in which the glucose-lowering hormone insulin does not work efficiently—and high insulin levels at their core. Both conditions also accelerate aging and carry a greatly increased risk of diseases associated with aging, including cardiovascular disease, mental deterioration, and some types of cancer.

Part of the disease process in type II diabetes is the result of free radicals spinning off from high glucose levels. Blood glucose increases free radical damage to cells, interferes with normal cell replication and actually kills cells. Anything you can do to reduce free radicals can hold off this health-damaging process. That's what vitamin E does.

By quenching free radicals, vitamin E also limits the formation of advanced glycation endproducts—AGEs, for short. AGEs quite literally age cells. One AGE that's found in the blood is called glycated hemoglobin. This is the standard marker that people with diabetes measure to see that their condition is being controlled. High levels of glycated hemoglobin signify high glucose levels. Vitamin E can help those with diabetes manage their glucose levels and can therefore reduce the formation of AGEs that lead to many diabetic complications.

Vitamin E can also lower glucose levels and help insulin work more normally, both in people with insulin resistance and in healthy people. In a recent Italian study, a regimen of 600 IU of vitamin E daily for two weeks lowered glucose levels and free radical formation among diabetic subjects. In a study conducted by Giuseppe Paolisso, M.D., of the University of Naples, Italy, vitamin E improved glucose tolerance and insulin action in healthy people. But high levels of insulin deplete vitamin E levels in the body, so people with Syndrome X or type II diabetes have higher needs for vitamin E.

New Research on Vitamin E and Diabetes

Over the last few years, a great deal of exciting research has focused on the positive effects of vitamin E in people with diabetes. One such study found that four weeks of supplementation with vitamin E (400 IU per day) decreased oxidative stress—an excess of free radicals—in both type I and type II diabetes.

To clarify, type I diabetes, known as insulin-dependent diabetes, is characterized by inefficient production of blood-sugar-lowering insulin. Type II (non–insulin-dependent) diabetes, on the other hand, involves adequate amounts of insulin (at least in the initial stages of the disease) but the insulin that's produced doesn't work efficiently. So, vitamin E protects against complications in both types.

Another study, reported in the *American Journal of Clinical Nutrition*, found that 250 IU of natural vitamin E (d-alpha-tocopherol) taken three times a day by patients with type I diabetes decreased the oxidation of blood fats, including LDL cholesterol, after only three months of supplementation. The benefits ended after the subjects stopped taking vitamin E, leading the researchers to recommend considering lifelong supplementation with vitamin E in patients with type I diabetes. Still other studies have found that taking vitamin E might help reduce the risk of developing diabetic retinopathy (damage to blood vessels of the retina) as well as the severe kidney problems associated with diabetes in type I patients.

Patients with type II diabetes can also benefit from taking vitamin E. As you will recall, limiting oxidation of LDL cholesterol is important for decreasing the risk of heart disease, and a study published in the journal *Diabetes Care* in 2000 found that 800 IU per day of vitamin E taken for four weeks decreased LDL oxidation, as well as another risk factor for heart attack, in patients with type II diabetes. These findings are very encouraging because people with diabetes have a higher-than-average risk of heart disease.

While vitamin E is extremely safe, some caution is required in diabetics. If you are taking insulin or hypoglycemic drugs, you may have to reduce the dosages of these drugs. This is because vitamin E will improve your health so you will need less of these drugs, and if you do not reduce the dosage, you could end up overdosing. However, it is very important that you adjust the dosage of vitamin E and the drugs in cooperation with your physician.

In addition, people with "leaky" blood vessels, found in some types of diabetic retinopathy (eye disease), could develop problems with vitamin E supplements, due to the nutrient's mild anticoagulant properties. While such problems are not common, caution is warranted.

Vitamin E Protects the Skin

Wrinkles are an age-related condition that develops over time, like Alzheimer's disease and heart disease. Vitamin E slows down the aging process, so it probably can help delay the appearance of wrinkles, especially when used as part of a comprehensive program to maintain youthful skin.

Many factors contribute to the formation and deepening of wrinkles, including exposure to environmental pollutants, poor nutrition, smoking, and, especially, too much time in the sun. The damaging effects of sunlight on the skin are cumulative, but they may not be obvious until years later.

A recent cell-culture study found that natural vitamin E protects skin by blocking the activity of protein kinase C. This enzyme promotes the breakdown of collagen, one of the main structural proteins of the skin. Aging and air pollution increase collagen breakdown, but it seems that vitamin E can protect against this.

The best approach to prevent wrinkles is to avoid exposure to cigarette smoke and pollutants, eat well, limit your time in the sun, and take antioxidants—such as vitamin E and vitamin C—that help protect against the damage from sunlight, which ages the skin.

Vitamins E and C Protect against Sunburn

A recent study in the *Journal of the American Academy of Dermatology* found that taking vitamins C and E can help protect against sunburn. The vitamins do not accomplish this by acting as a sunscreen, but instead by enhancing the body's ability to withstand burning.

In the study, Bernadette Eberlein-Konig, M.D., and her colleagues from the dermatology clinic at the Technical University of Munich exposed twenty men and women to ultraviolet (UV) light. Then Eberlein-Konig gave half of the subjects either a placebo or supplements containing 2,000 mg of vitamin C and 1,000 IU of natural vitamin E daily for eight days, after which portions of the subjects' skin were again exposed to UV light. People taking vitamins C and E showed an increased resistance to sunburn while those taking the placebo showed an increased sensitivity to UV light.

"This study shows for the first time that systemic administration of vitamins C and E reduces the sunburn reaction in humans. . . Systemic photoprotection is convenient and could provide a desirable basic UV shield for the entire body surface," Eberlein-Konig wrote in the study.

In a study published in the *American Journal of Clinical Nutrition* in 2000, researchers reported that oral carotenoids and vitamin E protected against free radical damage to the skin from ultraviolet light. Benefits were greatest with the combination of carotenoids (25 mg total carotenoids per day) and natural vitamin E (335 mg, or 500 IU), as opposed to carotenoids alone.

Previous research has shown that topical applications of vitamins C and E have a weak sun-blocking effect, so using vitamin E internally and externally (both as an oral supplement and as an ingredient in topical lotions) appears to be the best way to protect yourself from damaging UV rays when you do spend time in the sun.

Vitamin E's Benefits for Minor Cuts and More Serious Burns

Vitamin E might help heal minor cuts and burns, which are a lot like sunburns. In burns and cuts, free radicals flood the site of injury, causing inflammation and redness. These free radicals are supposed to prevent infection, but sometimes the body doesn't know when to turn them off. An ointment containing vitamin E should help the healing process and restore normal vitamin E levels in the skin. You can also pop vitamin E capsules with a needle and dab the oil on minor household burns and cuts after a scab has formed.

More severe burns generate very large quantities of free radicals, which can slow the healing process. It's easy to imagine the free radical generation that takes place on the damaged skin's surface in burn victims. But the damage doesn't end on the surface.

Free radicals can wreak havoc deeper in the body as a result of burns, damaging red blood cells, oxidizing fats, and impairing the function of white blood cells called neutrophils. Neutrophils normally act as phagocytes, meaning they surround and engulf bacteria and other foreign invaders in the body, thereby protecting us from disease.

When neutrophils are impaired by free radicals (as in serious burns), our defenses against dangerous invaders are compromised. Vitamin E acts as a free radical scavenger to protect neutrophil function among human burn victims. In one recent study, oral vitamin E was also found to protect the heart in test animals suffering from burns by reducing heart inflammation that typically follows burn trauma.

Neutrophils *White blood cells that surround and engulf bacteria and other foreign invaders in the body, protecting us from disease.*

Clearly, vitamin E can quench many of the free radicals that result from burns. However, if you're talking about topical use, the problem is more pragmatic: How do you apply vitamin E to a serious burn, when the burned person is likely to scream in pain? Carlson Laboratories (1-800-323-4141), which has the broadest and perhaps most reputable selection of natural vitamin E products, sells a vitamin E spray that can be helpful in such cases.

Evan Shute, M.D., who pioneered the clinical use of vitamin E in heart disease, felt that his lasting contribution to medicine would be the use of vitamin E in treating burns. Shute treated many burn victims with vitamin E, and it consistently promoted healing and minimized scarring. If you have a burn, you're likely to get benefits by both taking the vitamin orally and applying it topically.

Vitamin E Protects against Damage from Exercise

Few people realize it, but aerobic activity, including aerobics, cross-country skiing, running, and more, increases the production of free radicals, which can damage muscle tissue and result in inflammation, aching muscles, and a feeling of being wiped out. But vitamin E acts like a sponge, soaking up those free radicals before they damage tissues.

In a study by German researchers, regular exercise increased the levels of DNA damage in human subjects. However, when these subjects took vitamin E supplements, the exercise-induced DNA damage was virtually eliminated. According to Lester Packer, Ph.D., a researcher at the University of California, Berkeley, and one of the foremost authorities on antioxidants, vitamin E can probably reduce exercise-induced fatigue. Quicker recovery from fatigue should, in turn, improve exercise performance.

Also, research published in the journal *Nutrition* in 1999 reported that marathon runners who took 1,000 IU of vitamin E daily for two weeks before a race had fewer cases of abdominal pain and less occurrence of blood in their stools (which indicates gastrointestinal bleeding) than runners in the placebo group. This type of pain and bleeding is common in marathon runners, so vitamin E might help this group in a major way.

It may seem counterintuitive that exercise—something so good for your health—actually increases the production of nasty free radicals. This doesn't mean you should become a couch potato; instead, simply add vitamin E supplements to your workout regimen.

The List of Benefits Goes on

Vitamin E protects against still more health hazards—for example, secondhand smoke. Cigarette smoke—like other forms of air pollution—increases a person's free radical burden. Even if you don't smoke, it could be a problem. Nonsmoking spouses of smokers are 3.5 times more likely to develop lung cancer, compared with people living in smoke-free houses. Breathing cigarette smoke passively is comparable to smoking anywhere from one to ten cigarettes yourself daily.

When a nonsmoker breathes in smoke from a spouse, friend, or coworker, the many pollutants and cancer-causing chemicals in tobacco smoke attack the membranes and DNA of his or her body's cells. If you live or work with a smoker, you are, in effect, a smoker. Vitamin E can help reduce the damage. So can opening the window.

Vitamin E also protects lung function. In a study of 178 men and women, it was found that those who consumed the most vitamin E had significantly better lung function than those who consumed the least amount. And vitamin E protects red blood cells from damage. Without enough vitamin E, red blood cells die sooner than they should. Adequate vitamin E, therefore, is needed to prevent hemolytic anemia and the depression and lethargy that usually accompany this condition.

Vitamin E is not a panacea (or cure-all), but it plays numerous roles in health, so it's not entirely surprising that vitamin E benefits a wide range of different conditions. Every cell in the body requires vitamin E, which is why the nutrient benefits cells as different as heart and brain cells.

Vitamin E also plays important roles in promoting the normal behavior of genes, and genes contain the most basic biological instructions for the body. When Drs. Evan and Wilfrid Shute were using vitamin E in the 1940s and 1950s, many of their critics said the vitamin seemed like a panacea. What they were lacking was an explanation of why vitamin E works. Today, we have that explanation, and time has largely proved the Shutes right about vitamin E and its many benefits.

WHAT YOU SHOULD KNOW ABOUT TOCOTRIENOLS

Vitamin E comes in eight forms and two groups: four of them are tocopherols and four are tocotrienols. Among the tocopherols are alpha-tocopherol, beta-tocopherol, delta-tocopherol and gamma-tocopherol. Likewise, the tocotrienols include alpha-, beta-, delta- and gamma-tocotrienol. All eight forms are still vitamin E, but they each have slightly different chemical structures and actions in the body.

This chapter will fill you in on the tocotrienol forms of vitamin E. As you'll discover, they have some impressive benefits that scientists are just beginning to understand. The next chapter will help you decide what types of vitamin E supplements to buy.

Tocotrienols Offer Antioxidant Activity and Heart-Protective Benefits

Tocotrienols are relatively new on the scene, but some research has shown they have impressive antioxidant activity. Tocotrienols are not as bioavailable (well absorbed) by the body after oral supplementation as tocopherols are. They do, however, penetrate the skin quickly and efficiently, fighting excessive free radicals produced from ultraviolet rays or ozone.

Tocotrienols
A group of four forms of vitamin E that differ slightly from tocopherols in their structure and function in the body.

Like alpha-tocopherol, tocotrienols may be beneficial in protecting against heart disease. One way they do this is by inhibiting LDL oxidation. Tocotrienols are also noted for their ability to lower cholesterol and reduce inflammation, according to a study published in the *Journal of Nutrition* in 2001. These actions might interfere with the formation of atherosclerotic plaque—or might reduce the size of existing lesions—which, you'll remember, can block blood flow and lead to heart attacks.

In the study cited above, mice with atherosclerotic lesions that were fed the tocotrienol-rich fraction of rice bran had a 42 percent decrease in the size of their lesions, whereas mice supplemented with alpha-tocopherol experienced only an 11 percent reduction in lesions. The toco-

Lesion
An abnormal growth of cells, such as those involved in forming "cholesterol deposits."

trienols did decrease levels of cholesterol and triglyceride (another blood lipid), but the greater improvement in lesions led the researchers to conclude that tocotrienols were superior to alpha-tocopherol in minimizing such lesions. The tocotrienol content of rice bran oil—which has cholesterol-lowering activity in humans—might help explain the purported heart benefits of this oil over other vegetable oils.

Encouraging Early Research for Fighting Breast Cancer

In recent research, tocotrienols have shown promise in fighting breast cancer cells. When the mammary cancer cells of mice were studied in culture, tocotrienols were more effective than tocopherols at inducing apoptosis, or cell death, of the cancer cells. Results with human breast cancer cells have also been promising.

In a study reported in the journal *Nutrition and Cancer*, alpha-, gamma-, and delta-tocotrienols caused cell death in human breast cancer cells in culture. Of the four tocopherols, only delta-tocopherol induced cell death in the cancer cells. The researchers concluded that naturally occuring tocotrienols and natural delta-tocopherol are effective at inducing cell death in human breast cancer cells. A recent animal study found that tocotrienols even increased the benefits of drugs, such as tamoxifen, which fight breast cancer.

Relative to the research on alpha-tocopherol, the research on tocotrienols is still in its infancy, and the research on tocotrienols does not mean they are a treatment or a cure for breast cancer. More human studies are needed to find out how, and in what amounts, tocotrienols can benefit cancer, heart health, and perhaps other conditions. However, the future looks bright for these previously underestimated forms of vitamin E.

Weighing Supplementation with Tocotrienols and Tocopherols

It's important to remember that all eight forms of vitamin E—not just alpha-tocopherol and not just the tocotrienols—are likely important to good health. The intriguing new research on tocotrienols doesn't prove that these types of vitamin E are preferable to alpha-tocopherol for all purposes. Rather, it points out the importance of the full spectrum of benefits from the whole family of vitamin E forms.

There are probably other advantages to taking both tocopherols and tocotrienols that have not yet been researched in depth. As we learn more about them, we may discover new benefits of the tocotrienols, not just as a group, but as four individual kinds of tocotrienols. In the meantime, look for "mixed tocotrienols" and "mixed toco-

pherols" on vitamin labels if you want to take advantage of the whole range of vitamin E benefits. More and more companies are incorporating a broader array of vitamin E forms into multivitamins.

Unlike alpha-tocopherol, tocotrienols (and the other three tocopherols) are only available from natural sources. That means, when comparing labels on supplement bottles, you don't have to worry about trying to tell the difference between the superior natural forms and the inferior synthetic vitamin E that you want to avoid. Whatever products you choose, be sure to check the expiration dates and to store your vitamin E in a cool, dry place away from any light, instead of in the often warm and humid bathroom medicine cabinet. In the next chapter, we'll explain everything you need to know about buying natural vitamin E products.

SHOPPING FOR AND TAKING VITAMIN E

By now, you should appreciate the health benefits of vitamin E. One of the best things you can do for your health is to begin taking vitamin E supplements, if you aren't already. While doing so might seem as simple as buying a bottle of vitamin E, finding a quality product can often be difficult and confusing. In this section, we explain the important differences between natural and synthetic vitamin E and the many different forms of this vitamin. We also offer a number of tips to help you choose among the many different types of vitamin E supplements.

Vitamin E—A Fat-Soluble Vitamin We Need

Vitamin E is an essential nutrient. It is a fat-soluble vitamin (in contrast to water-soluble nutrients like vitamin C), which means that it functions primarily in the fatty portions of cells. It also means that vitamin E supplements are best taken with a little fat or oil (as is usually found in a regular meal) for optimal absorption.

Fat-Soluble Vitamin
A vitamin that dissolves only in oil and is found in the fatty parts of food. Fat-soluble vitamins like vitamin E are best absorbed when consumed with a small amount of fat.

The Recommended Dietary Allowance is 15 mg or 22 IU daily for an adult. However, the average American gets only about 8 IU from his diet. Furthermore, vitamin E requirements increase with a higher intake of polyunsaturated fatty acids (PUFAs)—the types of fats used in fried foods and salad dressings. Americans generally eat so many PUFAs that they need to compensate for the damaging effects of these fats.

Vegetable oils are high in PUFAs, and vitamin E requirements increase when a person consumes a lot of PUFAs.

Vitamin E is needed to prevent PUFAs from oxidizing, or turning rancid. For example, anyone eating fried chicken and French fries several times a week is consuming a huge quantity of PUFAs and will need a lot more vitamin E than would, say, someone who chooses not to eat any fried foods. In fact, researchers have found that 120 IU of vitamin E supplementation daily greatly reduced DNA damage among men eating a diet high in PUFAs. Of course, it's better to avoid or strictly limit your intake of these oils and fried foods, instead of simply taking extra vitamin E.

There's also a misconception that common vegetable oils, such as peanut or soybean oil, are good dietary sources of vitamin E. Such oils tend to be very high in the gamma-tocopherol form of vitamin E, not the alpha-tocopherol form. (Tocopherol is the chemical term to describe one form of vitamin E, and the alpha-tocopherol fraction of the vitamin E molecule is the most active one in the human body.) Although gamma-tocopherol has some antioxidant properties, the body primarily needs the alpha-tocopherol form of vitamin E. It's possible that consuming of a lot of vegetable oils containing gamma-tocopherol interferes with the body's use of alpha-tocopherol.

Once again, it's important to understand that you should avoid vegetable oils (including corn, cottonseed, safflower, soybean, and sunflower oils and products made with these oils) *and* take vitamin E supplements. Doing both are critical steps for dramatically improving your health. The vitamin E protects the good oils (such as omega-3 fish oils) that should be part of your diet, and it also reduces lung damage from air pollution, a sad fact of modern life.

Eight Is Enough

Many vitamins have only one form, but—as we explained in the last chapter—vitamin E actually has eight. While keeping them straight can be a little confusing, it's important to realize that all of the various forms of vitamin E are probably important for health.

As we've mentioned throughout this book, alpha-tocopherol is the most common form of vitamin E, both in our bodies and in vitamin supplements. And, as you'll recall from earlier sections, vitamin E was first recognized for its importance in reproduction. Alpha-tocopherol is the form of vitamin E most strongly associated with that function and so it has garnered the most attention over the years.

But the other seven other forms of vitamin E are important, too. You'll recall that the eight forms of vitamin E are divided into four tocotrienols and four tocopherols. These two groups have slightly different chemical structures and functions in the body.

Choose Natural Vitamin E over Synthetic

The most important thing to know is that natural forms of vitamin E are far better than synthetic forms. For years,

researchers believed that natural vitamin E was 1.36 times more potent than synthetic vitamin E when measured in milligrams (mg). This difference was found in animal studies, and because of it, the international unit (IU) standard was developed to equalize natural and synthetic vitamin E. However, there are still major differences between natural and synthetic.

In recent human studies, Graham Burton, Ph.D., and Robert Acuff, Ph.D., found that natural vitamin E was absorbed and retained twice as well as synthetic vitamin E. Basically, when people were given equal amounts of natural and synthetic vitamin E, the levels of natural vitamin E rose twice as high in the bloodstream and in tissues. The reason, according to a number of researchers, is that the human body opts for the natural molecule over the synthetic replicas. This means that, even using the IU standard, the natural vitamin E is better absorbed—and the synthetic falls way short. Buying natural vitamin E, therefore, gives you much more value for your money.

International Unit (IU)
A measure of weight usually used for fat-soluble vitamins.

It's easy to distinguish synthetic from natural vitamin E, but you have to read the fine print on the label. Natural vitamin E is identified as "d-alpha-" tocopherol, whereas the synthetic is "dl-alpha-" tocopherol. A good way to remember the difference is that your body *doesn't like* the synthetic form (dl-alpha-tocopherol) as much as the natural form. Conversely, the natural form, or d-alpha-tocopherol, is *delicious* to your body.

d-alpha-tocopherol
The most abundant form of vitamin E in our bodies and in vitamin supplements.

Fortunately, you only have to worry about looking for the "d" when it comes to alpha-tocopherol. That's because the other seven forms of vitamin E are only available in natural forms. Unfortunately, not all labels specify whether the alpha-tocopherol is from natural or synthetic sources. If it doesn't say it's natural (that is, there's no "d"), assume it's synthetic. Natural vitamin E will be more expensive than synthetic, but you get what you pay for. And, relatively speaking, purchasing natural vitamin E is a wise investment in your health.

Natural Forms and Esterification

When choosing a vitamin E supplement that's best for you, it's important to understand the various types of vitamin E typically found in supplements. As explained above, d-alpha-tocopherol is the most biologically active among the different types of vitamin E. It is a natural and highly absorbable form of vitamin E. Its only drawback is a relatively limited shelf life, though it is stable for at least three years, provided it is stored in a cool, dry environment.

Another natural form of vitamin E, d-alpha-tocopheryl acetate, is more stable in terms of shelf life. The acetate

Natural Vitamin E
Forms of vitamin E that are derived from natural sources (such as soybeans) and are absorbed and retained best by the body.

means it has been esterified—essentially combined with an acid—to improve stability and shelf life. Without esterification, alpha-tocopherol is prone to oxidation. Once it is oxidized, vitamin E doesn't do us much good. D-alpha tocopheryl acetate is probably the best form for people actively trying to prevent heart disease, because it has been used in many medical studies.

Esterification is especially important in multivitamins and cosmetic products containing forms of vitamin E, since exposure to air and interacting with other ingredients can oxidize the vitamin E. Combining alpha-tocopherol with these acids is safe and it protects the vitamin E from damage.

Esterification
The process of combining an acid with an alcohol (as with alpha-tocopheryl-acetate) to increase stability and decrease oxidation.

Another esterified form of vitamin E, d-alpha-tocopheryl succinate, is also a stable form of natural vitamin E. The most promising studies on vitamin E's anticancer properties have tended to use this particular form.

A more "naturelike" approach to taking vitamin E is to seek out a "mixed tocopherol" product. This type of product contains a specific amount of natural d-alpha-tocopherol (usually 400 IU), plus a small amount of natural beta-, gamma-, and delta-tocopherols. Although alpha-tocopherol is considered the most biologically active form of vitamin E, the other fractions also have antioxidant properties and are believed to be of some benefit.

Finding the Best Form for You

The best form of vitamin E varies according to the individual. Each of the natural forms of vitamin E is good, though they have slightly different properties. After understanding the merits and drawbacks of each type (as we explained above), you should evaluate which type is best for you based on what diseases you're most at risk for and what you eat.

It's important to know that all four types of tocopherols are found in natural foods, but d-alpha-tocopherol is the one that gets stripped away the most in processed vegetable oils. If you eat a lot of "fast" and convenience foods, supplementing your diet with d-alpha-tocopherol can partly compensate for some of what you're missing in your diet. But again, it would be far better to avoid processed vegetable oils and convenience and "fast" foods in the first place.

If you eat a lot of unprocessed, nutrient-dense, natural foods (which you should strive to do for better health), a mixed natural tocopherol supplement is probably a better choice because it more closely reproduces how vitamin E occurs in nature, with all four tocopherols. For disease prevention, our personal preference is a "mixed natural toco-

pherol" vitamin E supplement. Most natural vitamin E supplements, by the way, are produced from soybeans.

400 IU—The Standard Dose for Most People

In general, most adults would do well taking 400 IU daily of natural vitamin E. This dosage reduces the oxidation of cholesterol and, based on human studies, leads to dramatic reductions in the incidence of coronary artery disease. Higher doses can further reduce the oxidation of cholesterol, but it might be better to take a combination of antioxidants than to take very high doses of vitamin E.

Mixed Natural Tocopherols
The four tocopherol forms of vitamin E that occur naturally in foods, including d-alpha-, d-beta-, d-gamma- and d-delta-tocopherol.

Antioxidants work as a team of synergistic nutrients. So as good as vitamin E is, a combination of antioxidants is preferable. Consider taking 400 IU of vitamin E, 1,000 mg or more of vitamin C, 15,000–25,000 IU of mixed carotenoids, 30 mg of coenzyme Q_{10}, and 50 mg of alpha-lipoic acid. Many "antioxidant formulas" contain these and other antioxidants and enable you to simplify the number of tablets or capsules you take.

Every adult should probably be taking vitamin E supplements. People who live in very polluted cities, or those who eat large amounts of fried foods or vegetable oils, exercise strenuously, or live in high altitudes should probably take at least 400 IU daily, even if they are currently healthy. Children should also take vitamin E, but the dosage should be adjusted to their weight.

The Safety of Vitamin E

In general, vitamin E is exceptionally safe. Clinical trials of vitamin E supplementation at daily doses as high as 3,200 IU in a wide variety of people for up to two years have not shown any unfavorable side effects.

There are some risks you should be aware of, however. Although vitamin E reduces the risk of heart disease and thrombotic stroke (caused by blood clots), it slightly increases the risk of hemorrhagic stroke (caused by leaky blood vessels). The risk, in general, is insignificant because the vast majority of strokes are caused by blood clots, which vitamin E can help prevent.

Along this line, some research has shown that vitamin E supplements might amplify the effects of prescription anticoagulant (or blood-thinning) drugs. However, other research has shown that vitamin E does not have this effect. We suspect the varying effects may be dose-related. If you're taking aspirin *and* a prescription anticoagulant *and* vitamin E, all these anticoagulants may be a bit too much. If you are taking an anticoagulant drug, discuss your desire to take vitamin E with your physician.

People with diabetes who take vitamin E may have to

adjust their dosage of insulin or hypoglycemic drugs—this is a good sign, indicating a lessening of diabetic symptoms. And people with rheumatic heart disease, in which half the heart is damaged, should start taking only 50–100 IU of vitamin E under a physician's supervision. The reason is, the stronger part of the heart may respond to vitamin E much faster than the weaker part.

Vitamin E Works Slowly but Surely

Occasionally people will experience quick relief from something like sore breasts by taking vitamin E—or they'll see evidence of cuts and burns healing faster. But most often vitamin E just works subtly and preventively, helping to slow the aging process and prevent degenerative diseases. On a day-to-day basis, you probably won't notice that your body has fewer damaging free radicals but your risk of disease will lessen over the long term because of this benefit. The longer you take vitamin E, the more you'll probably find you're in better health than other people your age who don't take vitamin E.

Taking vitamin E supplements can significantly lower your risk of heart disease, enhance the functioning of your immune system, and likely reduce your risk of developing Alzheimer's disease. Vitamin E, however, is not a magic bullet or panacea. You can't simply take a pill and expect to gain perfect health. The other components of a lifestyle that promotes health include eating a diet rich in protein and fruits and vegetables, exercising moderately (at least going for a walk several times a week), and managing psychological stresses. Vitamin E supplements, in combination with a general antioxidant formula or multivitamin, can provide many health benefits—and increase your likelihood of having a long, functional, and satisfying life.

CONCLUSION

Vitamin E is the main antioxidant that protects all cells from damage, so it's one of the most important nutrient supplements you can take to keep your whole body healthy and avoid disease. As you've learned, vitamin E helps protect against leading killers, including Alzheimer's disease, cancer, and heart disease. It enhances the immune system, bolstering the body's defenses against colds and other infections. Vitamin E also slows the aging process, probably delaying the onset of such conditions as cataracts and wrinkles. And it helps heal or alleviate many minor health complaints—including everything from burns to menopausal hot flashes.

If you didn't pay much attention to vitamin E until reading this book, you're probably amazed at just how much of a health protector vitamin E really is. Research on the many benefits of vitamin E continues to pile up at a furious pace and these benefits impress virtually everyone, from once-skeptical doctors to questioning health reporters.

To tap the potential of all vitamin E's benefits, though, you must take supplements of the nutrient. You simply can't get enough vitamin E for therapeutic effects from foods alone.

Numerous supplements receive a lot of hype these days and many deliver on their promises. Vitamin E, though, is one that has stood the test of time in both scientific research and clinical practice. It's a tried-and-true nutritional supplement that should be a part of everyone's supplement regimen for better health.

In sum, do as we do: Weigh the evidence, and be sure to take vitamin E supplements.

PART THREE

VITAMIN C

HYLA CASS, M.D., & JIM ENGLISH

Today, vitamin C is one of the most widely used and highly valued vitamins in the world—and for good reason. Its popularity began in 1970, when Linus Pauling published his groundbreaking book *Vitamin C and the Common Cold.* Sales of vitamin C immediately skyrocketed, with some amazing results, such as the number of deaths attributed to heart disease plummeting by a staggering 40 percent in the next decade. Scientist now estimate that more than 250,000 lives are saved every year because of the efforts of Linus Pauling and other dedicated researchers to educate the public about the benefits of vitamin C. Based on these statistics, it has been estimated that if everyone in the United States took several hundred milligrams of vitamin C a day, more than 100,000 lives and $100 billion in healthcare costs would be saved each year.

In this part of *The Users Guide to Nutritional Supplements*, we will show you how vitamin C reduces heart disease, cancer, and many of the common diseases that plague the world today. We will also look at how a genetic accident that occurred untold millions of years ago robbed our ancestors of the ability to manufacture this vital nutrient. This problem has continued to trouble humankind throughout history, and even today, it contributes to the vast majority of human diseases, such as arthritis, cardiovascular disease, strokes, and cancer. We will see that these conditions, which are so common in humans, rarely occur in animals that still possess the ability to manufacture vitamin C—often in amounts thousands of times greater than those many health authorities consider to be essential to human health.

Not only can vitamin C help us to feel better and live longer, but it also has been proven to support numerous functions that can help us attain optimal health, including:

- Antioxidant Protection. This premier antioxidant nutrient protects us from the ravages of free radicals that, if left to destroy cell membranes and damage DNA, lead to the development of degenerative diseases and accelerated aging.

- Collagen Production. Vitamin C helps manufacture collagen, the basic cellular "cement" that keeps muscles, tendons, bones, teeth, and skin healthy and strong, and aids in the repair of blood vessels and broken bones.

- Cardiovascular Support. Vitamin C benefits heart conditions of all kinds, normalizes blood pressure, reduces cholesterol levels, and aids in the removal of cholesterol deposits from arterial walls.

In the following sections, you will also see how a nutrient that is so abundant in nature—and so necessary for all life—is constantly under attack from those who argue that all good nutrition begins and ends with a fork. Can we get all the vitamin C we need from food alone? It has been shown that even the best diet cannot begin to provide the higher levels of vitamin C (500–1,000 mg per day) that research has proven can help us fend off illness, degenerative diseases, and premature aging.

We will also address the safety of vitamin C—an issue that is often at the center of seemingly biased media reporting that ignores the overwhelming body of clinical and scientific research that attests to the safety and effectiveness of this natural nutrient.

So we invite you to sit back, pour yourself a glass of orange juice (or take a good multivitamin), and come along to discover how this essential antiaging, anticancer, and antistress nutrient can help you live a longer, healthier, and more fulfilling life.

THE HISTORY OF VITAMIN C AND SCURVY

Vitamin C, also called ascorbic acid, is a powerful water-soluble antioxidant that is vital for the growth and maintenance of all body tissues. Though easily absorbed by the intestines, vitamin C cannot be stored in the body and is excreted in the urine within two to four hours of ingestion. Human history has been deeply influenced by vitamin C—or more accurately, by a frequent and disastrous lack of this vital nutrient. In his book *The Healing Factor: Vitamin C*

Against Disease, the late biochemist Irwin Stone stated: ". . . the lack of this molecule [vitamin C] in humans has contributed to more deaths, sickness, and just plain misery than any other single factor in man's long history."

Ascorbic Acid
Another name for vitamin C that derives from the Latin word ascorbic, which means "without scurvy."

Written records dating back to ancient Egypt contain the earliest reports of scurvy, a dreaded human disease caused by vitamin C deficiency. In 450 B.C., Aristotle carefully described the symptoms of scurvy, which include muscle weakness, lethargy, extreme fatigue, depression, joint pains, swollen and bleeding gums, foul breath, loss of teeth, bleeding under the skin and orifices (hemorrhages), and, eventually, death.

Scurvy has remained a constant threat to humans, causing death and misery whenever dietary sources of vitamin C became scarce. Outbreaks have been particularly devastating in times of extreme famine, such as during the Irish potato famine. And throughout history, scurvy often has been more dangerous than man-made weapons, decimating entire armies cut off from supplies of fresh fruits and vegetables. During the Crusades (A.D. 1200), untold thousands perished from scurvy, as did hundreds of thousands of soldiers fighting in the Crimean, Napoleonic, and American civil wars.

Outbreaks of scurvy have not been restricted just to the land. In the sixteenth century, the Renaissance saw the introduction of modern seafaring and a subsequent rush for global exploration. During this period, scurvy became the dreaded scourge of the sea, as sailors embarked on epic voyages that often lasted for two years or more. Frequently, captains would return from a voyage with barely a third of their crews still desperately clinging to life. Such appalling losses of life (and money) were unacceptable to European ambitions, and led to a desperate search for a cure for scurvy.

Dr. James Lind and the Birth of the "Limey"

In 1739, England was entering into a war with Spain. In a daring tactical move, the British Navy dispatched a fleet of ships to the Philippines to attack the famed Manila galleons that plied riches, men, and supplies between Manila, Mexico, and South America in support of the Spanish colonial empire. In 1740, under the command of British Admiral Anson, six ships and 1,100 men departed England. After circumnavigating the world, Admiral Anson returned four years later with thirty-two wagons of Spanish treasure, but at a terrible cost of life. He had lost almost 90 percent of his men to scurvy and, in the end, could barely muster enough men to help sail the last surviving ship back to England.

One of the survivors of Anson's epic voyage was a Scottish naval surgeon named James Lind, who returned from the trip a deeply shaken man. Appalled by the pain, suffering, and loss of life he witnessed on the ships, he was dedicated to finding a cure for scurvy. In 1746, Lind began to study the disease, taking pains to monitor the diet and health of sailors, while carefully tracking the progression of symptoms. In his book *A Treatise on Scurvy*, Lind described his observations aboard the *H.M.S. Salisbury:* "Scurvy began to rage after being a month or six weeks at sea . . . the water on board . . . was uncommonly sweet and good [and] provisions such as could afford no suspicion . . . yet, at the expiration of ten weeks, we brought into Plymouth 80 men, out of a complement of 350, more or less afflicted with the diseases."

Since the ships of Lind's time lacked modern refrigeration, sailors on long voyages lived on a diet composed of nonperishable foods, such as grains, beans, and dried bread. Lind suspected that the cause of scurvy was related to the absence of some dietary factor, other than carbohydrates, fat, and protein. To test his theory, Lind conducted an experiment during a ten-week sea voyage.

Lind first selected twelve sailors showing signs of scurvy, and divided them into six groups of two men each. During the course of the voyage, Lind gave each pair an experimental substance in addition to their basic shipboard diet. Every day each pair received either a quart of cider, an elixir containing sulfuric acid, seawater, a combination of mustard and horseradish, a spoonful of vinegar, or two oranges and one lemon.

Four of the groups showed no improvement, while the pair receiving the cider reported slight improvement of their symptoms. Most impressive was the response of the two men who were given oranges and lemons: they completely recovered from all of their symptoms. In this manner, Lind is credited with establishing that the addition of citrus fruits would effectively prevent scurvy.

He published his findings in his 1753 landmark *A Treatise on Scurvy*. Unfortunately, his discovery was largely ignored for another forty years, during which time another 100,000 British sailors died from scurvy. Eventually, the British Navy issued orders for all ships to carry lemons and limes for the sailors to consume on a daily basis. Among citrus fruits, limes from the British West Indies were especially abundant, and their frequent appearance on British ships earned English sailors the lasting, if not appreciated, nickname "limeys."

The Discovery of Vitamin C (Ascorbic Acid)

Even though Lind had proven that the missing nutrient that led to scurvy was contained in citrus fruits (as well as potatoes, sauerkraut, rose hips, and other plants), the exact nature of this vital nutrient continued to puzzle scientists for the next two centuries.

The first breakthrough in vitamin C research occurred in 1926, when the Hungarian scientist Albert Szent-Györgyi,

M.D., Ph.D., traveled to Cambridge University to conduct research on the chemical processes that caused fruits and vegetables to turn brown. Szent-Györgyi first succeeded in isolating a white crystalline substance from the adrenal gland of cows, which he referred to as Cx11.

Later, in 1928, Szent-Györgyi isolated these same crystals from the juice of potatoes and cabbages, and renamed the substance hexuronic acid. Szent-Györgyi later collaborated with the famed English chemist W. Haworth, and together they finally determined the chemical structure of hexuronic acid ($C_6H_8O_6$). Finally, in 1932, after producing the first pure crystals of vitamin C, Szent-Györgyi and Haworth once again renamed the substance, and, in recognition of its role in preventing scurvy, called it ascorbic acid, from the Latin word *ascorbic*, which means "without scurvy."

Five years later, in 1937, Szent-Györgyi was awarded the Nobel Prize in Medicine "for his discoveries in connection with the biological combustion processes, with special reference to vitamin C and the catalysis of fumaric acid."

The Missing Link—Unraveling the Secrets of Vitamin C

Following the groundbreaking work of Szent-Györgyi, researchers began to slowly unravel the structure and chemistry of vitamin C. They discovered that vitamin C is a carbohydrate closely related to glucose, the simple sugar that is used by most living organisms as a fuel for cellular energy. They also learned that most plants and animals possess an enzyme called gluconolactone oxidase (or GLO for short) that allows them to readily convert glucose into vitamin C.

Next, researchers made one of the most startling findings of all—that somehow humans had lost the ability to do what virtually every other form of life on earth can do with ease—to manufacture vitamin C. This inability, which is shared with only a few other mammals, such as apes and guinea pigs, set the stage for more research as scientists struggled to understand how humans could have lost the ability to manufacture something that is so necessary for life and so easily produced by all other living organisms. What happened, why did it happen, and what did it mean in terms of human health?

From Sugar to Vitamin C

In order to understand the importance of vitamin C and its vital role in virtually every life form, we need to momentarily gaze back through time to the earliest moments of life on earth. Scientists now know that the ability to synthesize vitamin C was a trait acquired early in the development of life. Billions of years ago, the earth's atmosphere was rich in carbon dioxide and contained only minute amounts of oxygen. In order to survive in such a hostile environment, the earliest living organisms eventually learned to "cap-

ture" or scavenge rare oxygen electrons from the environment. This new adaptation not only aided the survival of these early life forms, it also contributed to another giant leap in early evolution—the development of plant photosynthesis.

Photosynthesis, in turn, removed carbon dioxide and increased oxygen levels in the atmosphere over a period of billions of years. By radically altering the atmosphere, this process also led to the evolution of complex multicellular life forms that were totally dependent on oxygen. Interestingly, one type of life that did not acquire the ability to synthesize vitamin C was primitive, single-celled organisms that are still alive today—bacteria. This is an important point that explains why vitamin C is so effective against certain forms of bacteria. The result of this early reliance on vitamin C for scavenging electrons is that every form of life on earth today (except for anaerobic bacteria) needs vitamin C, whether they can synthesize it or not.

The "Lost" Enzyme

All life on earth was originally endowed with the ability to manufacture vitamin C from the simple sugar, glucose. Today, almost all plants produce vitamin C. Some, such as strawberries, rose hips, green peppers, and citrus fruit, produce it in relatively large amounts. Almost all animals have retained their ability to generate vitamin C in the liver, usually in amounts much higher than those that could be obtained from dietary sources. For example, a goat, weighing as much as an average man, produces 13 g of vitamin C each day—more than two hundred times the current human recommended daily allowance (RDA) of 90 mg per day. And other animals, including dogs, mice, and even elephants, also produce vitamin C in amounts that, relative to their body weight, would be the equivalent of a human taking 10 g of vitamin C every day!

At some point in the early development of life, our ancestors lost the ability to synthesize vitamin C. Scientists believe this change occurred between 45 and 60 million years ago. Some believe that early members of the primate family somehow lost the use of a gene that the body needs to produce vitamin C. The loss of this functioning gene may have been caused by random genetic mutation. Another theory proposes that the gene was actually damaged by free radicals or by an attack by a virus.

Some scientists now believe that the loss of this functioning gene was actually a beneficial change that helped our species adapt and evolve. One proposed advantage was that by getting their vitamin C from food, our early ancestors were able to use more glucose for energy production, giving them an adaptive advantage over other species. Additionally, it has been proposed that the increased production of free radicals that resulted from the loss of this gene contributed to a greater number of genetic mutations that played a role in the evolution of higher primates, including humans.

It was only when our early humanoid ancestors began to leave the vitamin C–rich habitats, such as the jungles and rainforests, that the true nature of the loss became apparent in the form of new chronic health problems, such as high cholesterol, heart disease, arthritis, colds, cancer, and in cases of severe shortage, fatal scurvy.

What Does Vitamin C Do?

As we've seen, vitamin C has played an essential role in the development of life on earth. This is apparent when one realizes that vitamin C is utilized by virtually every part of the human body. In fact, there are few, if any, biological functions that do not require vitamin C.

- Vitamin C is a water-soluble antioxidant that protects cells from free radicals. Vitamin C also prevents oxidative damage that leads to the development of atherosclerosis.

- Vitamin C is vital to the immune system, aiding white blood cells that attack and destroy cancer cells, viruses, bacteria, parasites, and other pathogens. Vitamin C also promotes wound healing and acts to control the release of histamine.

- Vitamin C is used by the body to produce collagen, which is used by connective tissues to give strength and shape to our tissues, such as muscles, blood vessels, bones, and teeth.

- Vitamin C helps the body utilize folic acid (required for maintaining DNA) and regulates the uptake of iron (needed for production of hemoglobin, the oxygen-carrying part of blood cells).

- Vitamin C is important for the synthesis of brain neurotransmitters, molecules used as chemical messengers in the body, such as noradrenaline (for energy and mood) and serotonin (for sleep, well-being, and pain control).

The Many Faces of Vitamin C

As we've seen, the history of human evolution is intimately linked with the development of vitamin C as a vital nutrient that promotes and sustains life on earth. In the following sections, we'll see how vitamin C promotes oxidation—necessary for life-giving energy—while protecting us from the dangerous byproducts of oxidation, free radicals. And we'll learn how vitamin C helps to form collagen, the basic tissues that hold our bodies together and help shape and strengthen every tissue, from bones and blood vessels to eyes and skin.

Together these and other properties form the underlying basis for the numerous health benefits attributed to vitamin

Oxidation
Refers to the loss of electrons in a chemical reaction. In the body, oxidation is used to "burn" fuel to provide energy for all life processes.

C in more than 10,000 published scientific papers. To quote from *The Vitamin Connection* by Drs. Cheraskin, Ringsdorf, and Sisley, "There is not one body process (such as what goes on inside cells or tissues) and not one disease or syndrome (from the common cold to leprosy) that is not influenced—directly or indirectly—by vitamin C."

THE ULTIMATE ANTIOXIDANT

Probably the most well known of all of vitamin C's benefits are its powerful antioxidant properties that protect us from the damaging effects of oxidation. Oxidation is the chemical process in which oxygen molecules combine with other molecules to release energy. In addition to producing energy, oxidation produces byproducts. A common, everyday example of an oxygen byproduct is rust, the result of oxygen oxidizing iron. Another example is water, the product of oxygen combining with hydrogen. In the body, cells oxidize sugar (glucose) to produce the energy they need to function.

Antioxidant
A molecule that donates electrons to stabilize damaging free radicals and render them harmless.

Even as it produces energy to make life possible, oxidation also has a negative side. When oxygen combines with other molecules, the chemical reaction often results in the production of unstable molecules that contain unpaired electrons. Since electrons are normally paired with other electrons, these unpaired fragments—called free radicals—seek out new electrons in order to return to a state of balance (a landmark discovery by Linus Pauling that led to his first Nobel Prize in 1954).

In the process of stealing electrons, free radicals cause immense damage to tissues, tearing up cell membranes and damaging DNA. Free radicals can also damage the genes in a cell and impair the cell (and any of its descendants) from performing its normal functions. Ironically, this is the very process that may have caused the loss of our gene for making vitamin C in the first place. Additionally, when stealing electrons from other sources, free radicals can set off a chain reaction, or cascade, of continuous reactions that create even more free radicals. These then contribute to even greater damage and set the stage for a number of health problems.

Free radical damage to cells throughout the body is thought to be a primary factor in the diseases of aging, and maybe of aging itself. The Free Radical Theory of Aging suggests that if we can take steps to minimize this damage, we can slow the aging process. As our knowledge of free-radical chemistry has expanded in the last half of the twentieth century, so too has our appreciation for antioxidants that can prevent or slow the devastating effects of oxidation and the production of free radicals.

Internal Production of Free Radicals

Free radicals come from several sources. Most are produced in our bodies from normal cellular processes. These endogenous (within the body) free radicals are produced from a number of normal metabolic functions. First, every cell in our bodies produces free radicals as a byproduct of oxidizing (burning) fuel and oxygen to make the energy that is essential for life. This process is a major source of free radicals—each cell in your body produces about 20 billion free radicals every day!

Free radicals are also produced by white blood cells. When the body is under attack, the immune system directs white blood cells, called phagocytes, to release huge amounts of free radicals in a process called phagocytosis. These free radicals act like molecular "bullets" that tear into, and rip apart, invading bacteria, viruses, and parasites. When the body is fighting a chronic infection, this defense mechanism can go out of control and generate massive amounts of free radicals that spill over and damage healthy cells. This problem is associated with a number of degenerative and inflammatory conditions, including arthritis, heart disease, and cancer.

Other causes of rampant free-radical production are burns, surgery, exposure to toxins, infectious and autoimmune diseases, allergies, and severe trauma. All of these conditions promote inflammation, which injures cells, causing further release of even more free radicals.

Free radicals are also produced from normal bodily functions that involve 1) the burning (oxidation) of polyunsaturated fats, 2) the breakdown and elimination of toxic chemicals, drugs, and pesticides, and 3) the increased production of hormones in response to stress.

External Sources of Free Radicals

When free radicals assault us from external sources, they are referred to as exogenous (outside the body) free radicals. External sources of free radicals include high heat, ultraviolet light, cigarette smoke, air pollution, x-rays, electromagnetic emissions, and other forms of low-level radiation. Exposure to trace metals, such as lead, mercury, iron, and copper, can also promote the production of free radicals.

Free radicals generated from internal and external sources can have a tremendous, and dangerous, impact on human health. In 1954, Dr. Denham Harman proposed that a lifetime of exposure to free radicals is a major cause of aging. Harmon also believed that free radicals contribute to the development of diseases such as heart disease, diabetes, arthritis, and cancer. In his groundbreaking paper,

"The Free Radical Theory of Aging," Dr. Harman also proposed that antioxidants, such as vitamin C, could be used to control free radicals, protect DNA, and reduce the incidence of diseases and human aging.

Antioxidants Quench Free Radicals

Just as the human body bristles with free radicals produced by internal energy production and detoxification processes, it is also equipped with a sophisticated defense system of specialized antioxidants that protect us from free radical damage. These include lipoic acid and antioxidant enzymes, such as superoxide dismutase (SOD). We also get antioxidants from our diets. Chief among the dietary antioxidants are the vitamins A, B_6, C, and E. Other nutrients, such as carotenoids, the amino acids cysteine and taurine, and the mineral selenium, have been proven to provide substantial antioxidant protection when consumed from either foods or supplements.

Enzymes *Specialized proteins that act as catalysts to promote the billions of biochemical reactions necessary for virtually all life processes.*

Vitamin C—The Ultimate Antioxidant

Remember, early life forms adapted in an environment that was very low in oxygen. As we know, oxygen is an essential ingredient for life, required for energy production and other vital metabolic functions. In order to compete for this scarce resource, early organisms learned to manufacture vitamin C, which then allowed cells to latch on to and capture oxygen molecules. Just as vitamin C aided early life forms by scavenging scarce oxygen from the atmosphere, all life today depends on vitamin C. It acts as a water-soluble antioxidant to control free radical damage, a byproduct of oxidation.

In the body, vitamin C works in concert with a number of other antioxidants, including vitamin E, lipoic acid, and glutathione. These antioxidants interact in a complex recycling process that resembles an old-fashioned fireman's bucket brigade, where buckets of water are passed, hand over hand, down a line to quench a burning fire. In this case, the body passes a dangerous free radical from one antioxidant to another, reducing its energy (and its potential to damage tissues) with each passing.

The process starts when vitamin E donates an electron to reduce a free radical back to a nonthreatening compound. But in doing this, vitamin E turns into a free radical, though one that is far less damaging than the original one. At this point, vitamin C steps in to donate an electron, and vitamin E reverts back to being an antioxidant. The newly regenerated vitamin E molecule goes back to work fighting free radicals, leaving behind another new free radical in the form of an unstable form of vitamin C called dehydroascorbate. Dehydroascorbate is normally regenerated by electrons generated by the *mitochondria*, tiny structures in

Dehydro-ascorbate
Vitamin C that has donated its electrons and is no longer able to act as an anti-oxidant.

every cell that act as powerhouses to provide energy. The process is repeated until all of the free radicals are eventually quenched. Dehydroascorbate has a half-life in the body of only a few minutes, so if it does not regain its electrons within a few minutes, it is irreversibly lost and eventually passes out of the body in the urine.

As we'll see later in this book, large doses, or megadoses, of vitamin C are frequently used to treat very serious diseases, infections, and cancer. In such large doses, vitamin C is not used for any of its proven metabolic or biochemical actions. Megadoses of vitamin C are employed strictly as a "delivery vehicle" to donate electrons to be used in the battle against the free radicals that are generated by disease processes. When used in this manner, vitamin C is "sacrificed" for its electrons, and then eliminated by the body as dehydroascorbate.

Vitamin C Supports Healthy Skin, Joints, and Vision

One of vitamin C's most vital roles in human health is in the production and maintenance of collagen. Collagen is a protein that makes up the connective tissues found throughout the body, especially in the skin, ligaments, cartilage, bones, and teeth. The most abundant protein in the body, it accounts for more mass than all the other proteins put together.

Collagen acts as a kind of intracellular "glue" that gives support, shape, and bulk to blood vessels, bones, and organs such as the heart, kidneys, and liver. Collagen fibers keep bones and blood vessels strong, and help to anchor our teeth to our gums. Collagen is also required for the repair of blood vessels, bruises, and broken bones.

Vitamin C is essential for the formation of collagen. While many vitamins and minerals act as catalysts to support the manufacture of proteins, in the case of collagen, vitamin C is actually used up as it combines with amino acids, such as lysine, glycine, and proline, to form procollagen. Procollagen is then used to manufacture one of several types of collagen that can be used for different tissues throughout the body. There are at least fourteen different types of collagen in the body, but the most common ones are:

Type I. Makes up the fibers found in connective tissues of the skin, bone, teeth, tendons, and ligaments.

Type II. Round fibers found in cartilage.

Type III. Forms connective tissues that give shape and strength to organs, such as the liver, heart, and kidneys.

Type IV. Forms sheets that lie between layers of cells in the blood vessels, muscles, and eyes.

Vitamin C Deficiency Equals Collagen Deficiency

Our bodies are continually manufacturing collagen to maintain and repair connective tissues lost to daily wear and tear. Without vitamin C, collagen formation is disrupted, resulting in a wide variety of problems throughout the body. Scurvy, the disease caused by vitamin C deficiency, is really a process that disrupts the body's ability to manufacture collagen and connective tissues. When a person is suffering from scurvy, his or her body literally falls apart as collagen is broken down and not replaced. The joints begin to wear down as tendons shrivel and weaken. The blood vessels crumble and begin to fall apart, leading to bruising and bleeding as vessels rupture (hemorrhage) throughout the body. Teeth loosen and fall out as the gums and the connective tissues holding teeth also begin to erode. Organs, once held firmly together by connective tissues, also lose structural strength and begin to fail. In time, the various body tissues weaken, and the immune system and heart give out, leading to death.

Arthritis

Arthritis is a localized degeneration of joint cartilage, mainly affecting the weight-bearing joints. More common in the elderly and in those who are overweight, osteoarthritis is also caused by the mechanical stresses and major trauma that result from sports injuries. Arthritis causes aching in the joints, limitation of movement and range of motion, and a loss of dexterity. A "wear-and-tear disease of aging," arthritis generally begins in middle age, and by age sixty, most people have some degree of osteoarthritis.

Arthritis is caused by a breakdown in cellular processes that produce, maintain, and repair cartilage. Physical stress on joints causes destruction of collagen and may also inhibit its production. When the body is unable to make enough collagen, or when there is an excessive amount of destruction of the collagen matrix, the joints start to erode.

Conventional Treatment for Arthritis

Modern medicine utilizes several classes of drugs to treat arthritis, including analgesics, corticosteroids, uric acid–lowering drugs, immunosuppressive drugs, non-steroidal anti-inflammatory drugs (NSAIDs), and disease-modifying anti-rheumatic drugs (DMARDs), such as antimalarial drugs, gold compounds, penicillamine, and sulfasalazine.

While many of these drugs provide temporary relief of pain and inflammation, they have little or no effect on the underlying disease processes. In fact, many drugs, such as the NSAIDs, actually worsen the condition by suppressing the normal tissue-building processes. Additionally, long-term toxicity and side effects associated with many approved arthritis drugs frequently require that patients be carefully monitored and reevaluated by their physicians.

Nutritional Approaches for Arthritis

Alternative nutritional approaches for arthritis have become popular over the last decade. The most popular supplements include joint-building substances, such as chondroitin sulfate, glucosamine, and SAMe (S-adenosyl methionine). Other supplements include anti-inflammatory substances, such as *Boswellia serrata*, turmeric, and essential fatty acids (EFAs).

Vitamin C for Arthritis

As we have seen, one of vitamin C's most vital functions is the production and maintenance of collagen, the tough protein that makes up the connective tissues found in our joints. The type I collagen that lines our joints is composed of a combination of vitamin C and amino acids, such as lycine, glycine, and proline. When vitamin C levels are low or become depleted, our ability to produce collagen may not be able to keep up with the constant loss of connective tissues lining our joints.

Research has shown that vitamin C can aid in reducing the pain, inflammation, and swelling of arthritis. Vitamin C can also support healthy joint functions and keep joints, particularly the knees, flexible and comfortable. Recent studies have found that vitamin C can help to reduce the progression of arthritis. After looking at the records of 640 individuals enrolled in a large study, researchers found that people taking 420 mg of vitamin C per day had a 300 percent reduction in the progression of their arthritis compared with those taking only minimal RDA levels.

This favorable effect of vitamin C was found to be due to a reduction in the loss of joint cartilage. This effect was believed to be due to vitamin C's role in making new cartilage. An additional benefit seen with higher doses of vitamin C was a significant reduction in knee pain.

In addition to the joint degeneration and loss of connective tissue that are seen in osteoarthritis, rheumatoid arthritis also involves alterations in the inflammatory response of the body. One characteristic of rheumatoid arthritis is excessive immune-system activity caused by the body's efforts to clear out the cellular debris being shed by degrading joint tissues. This results in a huge amount of free radical activity within the joint and leads to further inflammation of the tissues. Researchers have recently found that blood levels of vitamin C are extremely low in people with rheumatoid arthritis. This suggests that vitamin C may also protect against further damage to inflamed joints.

Vitamin C Reduces Risk of Cataracts

A recent study suggests that vitamin C can help to reduce the formation of cataracts. In a study published in the *American Journal of Clinical Nutrition*, researchers investigated the link between vitamin C and the incidence of age-related cataracts. At the beginning of the study, the researchers enrolled 492 women, aged fifty-three to seventy-three, who were free of cataracts. They then carefully measured how much vitamin C the women consumed over the next fifteen years.

For women younger than sixty years old, vitamin C consumption greater than 362 mg per day was found to reduce the risk of developing cataracts by 57 percent when compared with women who took less than 140 mg per day. And women who used vitamin C supplements for at least ten years reduced their risk of developing cataracts by 60 percent when compared with women who didn't consume any supplemental vitamin C.

Cataract
A clouding of the normally transparent eye lens, impairing vision.

Beauty is in the eye of the beholder, and so is the knowledge that something as simple as four or five daily servings of orange juice (or a vitamin C capsule) will help people preserve vision far into the golden years.

VITAMIN C PROTECTS AGAINST HEART DISEASE AND STROKE

In this section, we will see how vitamin C saves lives, prevents atherosclerosis, aids in the removal of cholesterol deposits from arterial walls, and regulates high blood pressure. A recent large study found that men who take vitamin C supplements live, on average, six years longer than men who get their vitamin C only from dietary sources. This very significant increase in life span seems to be due to a sharp reduction in deaths from heart disease. Based on this study, it has been estimated that if everyone took several hundred milligrams of vitamin C a day, more than 100,000 lives and $100 billion in healthcare costs would be saved each year in just the United States alone.

Cardiovascular Disease and Stroke

Cardiovascular disease, especially heart attacks and strokes, kill at least 12 million people across the globe each year. And in the United States, heart attacks and strokes remain the primary cause of mortality, accounting for a full 50 percent of all deaths.

Strokes occur when a blood clot (thrombosis) blocks a blood vessel or artery (cerebral infarction), or when a blood vessel breaks, interrupting blood flow to an area of the brain (hemorrhagic stroke). These processes cause the immediate death of brain cells in the affected area. Additionally, as brain cells die, they rupture and release a number of dangerous chemicals in a chain reaction called the "ischemic cascade." These chemicals then spread out and cause even more damage to the *penumbra,* which means "the cells surrounding the area."

Research published in the medical journal *Stroke* reports that people with high blood levels of vitamin C have a significantly lower risk of having a stroke. The findings were based on measurements of vitamin C blood levels in more than 2,120 men and women living in rural Japan. From 1977 to 1997, researchers logged a total of 196 strokes in the volunteers. After comparing vitamin C levels, the scientists discovered that people with the lowest levels of vitamin C faced a 70 percent increased risk of stroke than those with the highest levels of vitamin C in their blood. Of the 196 strokes, 109 were caused by a blockage of blood flow (infarction), 54 were caused by hemorrhagic stroke, and 33 were of undetermined types. The researchers commented on the importance of the study, stating, "This is the first prospective study to make the correlation between vitamin C in the bloodstream and incidence of stroke."

Stroke
The third leading cause of death in the U.S. It occurs when a region of the brain loses blood flow, usually from an obstructed blood vessel. Each year about 400,000 cases of stroke and approximately 150,000 deaths from it are reported in the U.S.

Because both types of stroke were reduced, researchers speculated that the protective effect of vitamin C went well beyond its well-known antioxidant actions. Cerebral infarctions are caused by atherosclerosis (blocked arteries), which can be prevented by the antioxidant effects of vitamin C. Hemorrhagic strokes, on the other hand, result from ruptured blood vessels. Therefore, the proven role of vitamin C in building collagen and strengthening connective tissues in the blood vessels seems to explain this significant reduction in hemorrhagic strokes.

Atherosclerosis

Atherosclerosis, or "hardening of the arteries," is a primary cause of heart disease. It often starts early in life as a mass of sticky fatty compounds that gradually builds up on the inner lining of arteries to form a thick "plaque." This process usually develops over a period of years or decades, until deposits become so thick that they begin to block the coronary arteries and restrict blood flow. Atherosclerosis can suddenly appear as chest pains (angina), but sometimes the first (and last) warning is a sudden—and often, fatal—heart attack. Early symptoms of atherosclerosis can include:

1. Chest pains with physical exertion (angina) caused by a blockage of the coronary arteries. If an artery is completely blocked, the result can be a heart attack.

2. Memory loss or temporary disorientation or sensory loss (transient ischemic attacks, temporary "mini-strokes") can be a sign of a blockage of arteries leading to the brain. Complete blockage often results in a stroke.

3. Pain felt in the calves after walking relatively short distances (intermittent claudication) is a sign of a blockage of the arteries in the leg.

All of these symptoms are serious signs of significant arterial narrowing in the affected areas, as well as elsewhere in the body.

Risk Factors for Atherosclerosis

Some of the risk factors known to increase the likelihood of developing atherosclerosis and heart disease include:

- Smoking.
- Hypertension (high blood pressure).
- Diabetes.
- Elevated cholesterol.
- Sedentary lifestyle.
- Obesity.
- Family history of heart disease.
- Stress.

Medical Treatment of Atherosclerosis

Over the last two decades, nutritionist and doctors have recommended various lifestyle modifications to reduce atherosclerosis. These include quitting smoking, losing weight, cutting back on dietary intake of cholesterol and fatty foods, and regular, moderate exercise. In some cases, doctors will prescribe drugs, such as ACE inhibitors, beta-blockers, and lipid-lowering statin drugs. Yet, even when following all the current guidelines and therapies, many people will still develop coronary artery disease, carotid artery disease, or other vascular illness.

Atherosclerosis
A disorder characterized by the buildup of blood fats on the damaged lining of artery walls, leading to plaques that block bloodflow.

When traditional therapies fail, surgery is often the last resort. Surgeons operate to replace, or "bypass," blocked arteries by grafting veins harvested from the legs in an attempt to restore blood flow to the heart. Alternately, balloon angioplasty attempts to restore blood flow in constricted arteries by literally smashing the plaque against the arterial walls to increase the diameter of the arteries. As impressive as these surgical advances are, they also present a number of serious side effects, including death, and even when successful, the results are often temporary and blockages can reappear within months.

Vitamin C Improves Blood Flow

The ability of blood vessels to relax and open up to blood flow (dilate) is severely reduced in people with atherosclerosis. Much of the damage to the heart during a heart attack, and to the brain during a stroke, is caused by the inability of blood vessels to open enough to allow blood to flow to the affected areas. The chest pains of angina are also caused by the inability of the coronary arteries to dilate. Doses of as little as 500 mg of vitamin C per day have consistently been proven to improve dilation of blood vessels in people with atherosclerosis, angina pectoris, congestive heart failure, and high blood pressure.

Vitamin C Lowers Cholesterol

Scientists have known for decades that dangerously high levels of cholesterol, known as hypercholesterolemia, are accompanied by very low blood levels of vitamin C. In 1981, researchers discovered that vitamin C plays a vital role in reducing cholesterol levels, by enhancing the conversion of cholesterol to bile salts that can be easily eliminated by the body. This has been supported by several large studies that proved that vitamin C can reduce the incidence of cardiovascular diseases, lower cholesterol levels, and increase the ratio of the so-called "good" cholesterol, high-density lipoprotein (HDL). When researchers gave volunteers 1 gram of vitamin C per day for three months, cholesterol levels declined by 10 percent and triglyceride levels dropped by 40 percent. A second study also found that 3 g of vitamin C every day dropped cholesterol levels an impressive 18 percent, and triglycerides by 12 percent in only three weeks.

In 1994, researchers from the USDA and National Institute on Aging conducted a trial on participants in the Baltimore Longitudinal Study of Aging to investigate the effect of vitamin C on total cholesterol levels. The researchers found that vitamin C intake that greatly exceeded the RDA of 60 mg per day resulted in a significant rise in levels of the desirable form of HDL cholesterol. The researchers stated that, in order to see positive changes in cholesterol profiles, people had to increase their intake of vitamin C to between four and five times the recommended daily dose (between 215 and 345 mg per day).

Triglycerides
Molecules formed when three fatty acids are linked together by a single molecule of a type of alcohol called glycerol.

Linus Pauling Challenges Cholesterol Theories

In 1989, the eminent American scientist and two-time Nobel Prize winner Linus Pauling announced a breakthrough in how we view and treat heart disease. In "A Unified Theory of Human Cardiovascular Disease," Linus Pauling announced that the deposits of plaque seen in atherosclerosis were not the *cause* of heart disease, but were actually the *result* of our bodies trying to repair the damage caused by long-term vitamin C deficiency. In essence, Pauling believed that heart disease is a form of scurvy, and plaque is the body's attempt to reinforce and patch weakened blood vessels and arteries that would otherwise rupture. Pauling also showed that heart disease can be easily prevented or treated by taking vitamin C and other supplements.

Plaque Deposits

Pauling based his revolutionary theory on a number of important scientific findings. First was the discovery that plaque deposits found in human aortas are made up of a special form of cholesterol called lipoprotein (a) or Lp(a), not from ordinary LDL cholesterol, as mainstream science had once believed. Lp(a) is a special form of LDL cholesterol that we now know binds to form the thick sheets of plaque that obstruct arteries.

Aorta
The largest artery in the body. It carries blood from the heart through the chest and into the abdomen where it divides and goes to each leg.

Another finding central to Pauling's theory was the observation that plaque deposits are not formed randomly throughout the circulatory system. This was first reported in the early 1950s when a Canadian doctor, G. C. Willis, M.D., observed that plaque always forms nearest the heart, where blood vessels and arteries are constantly being stretched and bent, rather than being spread evenly throughout the entire cardiovascular system. Willis also noted that damage to vessels that triggers plaque deposits always occurs in regions that are exposed to the highest blood pressures, such as the aorta, where blood is forcefully ejected from the heart.

In 1985, a team of researchers verified that plaque forms only in areas of the artery that become damaged. Just as cracks form in a garden hose that has become weak and worn from constant bending and high pressure, cracks form in the lining of the arterial wall. As these tiny cracks open up, they expose strands of the amino acid lysine (one of the primary components of collagen) to the bloodstream. It is these strands that initially attract Lp(a). Lp(a) is an especially "sticky" form of cholesterol that is attracted to lysine. Drawn to the break, Lp(a) begins to collect and attach to the exposed strands. As Lp(a) covers the lysine strands, free lysine in the blood is drawn to the growing deposit. This process continues as lysine and Lp(a) are both drawn from the blood to build ever-larger deposits of plaque. Over time, this process gradually reduces the inner diameter of the vessels and restricts its capacity to carry the blood.

Heart Disease as Low-Level Scurvy

Observing the newly described process of plaque formation, Pauling recognized a similarity to the underlying processes seen in scurvy. He also saw similarities between human and animal models of atherosclerosis that pointed to a connection with scurvy. First, cardiovascular disease does not occur in any of the animals that are able to manufacture their own vitamin C. As pointed out earlier, many animals produce large amounts of vitamin C that are equivalent to human doses ranging from 10–20 g per day. Second, the *only* animals that produce Lp(a) are those who, like humans, have also lost the ability to produce their own vitamin C.

Putting all the pieces of the puzzle together, Pauling recognized that the ability to form plaque is really the body's attempt to repair damage caused by a long-term deficiency of vitamin C. He knew that early in humanity's evolution, our ancestors lived in tropical regions where the diet consisted primarily of fruits and vegetables. With a daily intake estimated to be in the range of several hundred milligrams to several grams per day, our ancestors easily survived the loss of the gene required to manufacture vitamin C. Almost unnoticed, this mutation was passed on to successive generations, and only became a problem when early humans began to spread to other regions of the world. In effect, when humankind left the "garden," the lack of a reliable and adequate supply of dietary vitamin C led to scurvy.

Pauling thought that scurvy was one of the greatest threats to humankind's early survival, and believed that the loss of blood during times of vitamin C deficiency, particularly during the ice ages, likely brought humans close to the point of extinction.

Plaque as a Lifesaver

Evolution works by a process of trial and error that, over the course of millions of years, favors the selection of traits that increase the survival of a species. The core of Pauling's theory is that, over time, evolutionary pressures forced the body to develop a repair mechanism that would allow it to cope with the damage caused by chronic vitamin C deficiency. The repair mechanism is as elegant as it is simple. When arteries became weak and began to rupture, the body responded by "gluing" the damaged areas together with Lp(a) to prevent a slow death from internal bleeding. In essence, plaque is the body's attempt to patch blood vessels damaged by low-level scurvy. Accordingly, Pauling believed that conventional "triggers" of plaque formation, such as homocysteine and oxidized cholesterol, are actually just additional symptoms of scurvy.

Scientific Support for Pauling's Unified Theory

Pauling's theory was unique in that it addressed a fact never explained by older, mainstream theories. Specifically, Pauling finally explained why plaque isn't randomly distributed throughout the body, but restricted to areas of high mechanical stress. A surprising number of animal studies have been found to support Pauling's theory. Research conducted with animals that cannot make their own vitamin C found that when vitamin C levels are reduced, collagen production drops and blood vessels become thinner and weaker. Additional studies also confirm that when animals are deprived of vitamin C, their bodies respond by increasing blood levels of Lp(a) and forming plaque deposits to strengthen arteries and prevent vessel ruptures.

Collagen Melts Plaque, Keeps Arteries Open

In addition to taking vitamin C to prevent atherosclerosis, Pauling recommended a combination of vitamin C and the amino acids lysine and proline to help remove existing plaque while strengthening weak and damaged arteries. Since the body produces collagen from lysine and proline, Pauling reasoned that by increasing concentrations of lysine and proline in the blood, Lp(a) molecules would bind with the free lysine, rather than with the lysine strands exposed by the cracks in blood vessels.

How Much Vitamin C Prevents Atherosclerosis?

While acute scurvy can be prevented by a mere 10 mg of vitamin C per day, there is no current research showing how much vitamin C might be required to prevent the atherosclerotic plaques of chronic scurvy. In his Unified Theory, Linus Pauling often recommended 3,000 mg per day as an effective dose. Anecdotal reports from patients using the Pauling Therapy indicate that rapid recovery is frequently the rule, not the exception, allowing many people to avoid open heart surgery and angioplasty.

Vitamin C and High Blood Pressure

Blood pressure is defined as the pressure exerted by the blood against the walls of the blood vessels, especially the arteries. It varies with the strength of the heartbeat, the elasticity of the arterial walls, the volume and viscosity of the blood, and a person's health, age, and physical condition. A normal level is 120/80 where the first number is the systolic pressure and the second is the diastolic pressure.

High blood pressure, or hypertension, is a serious health problem and a major risk factor for heart disease and strokes. An estimated 25 percent of Americans suffer from the effects of hypertension. Hypertension is associated with atherosclerosis, hypertensive renal failure, stroke, congestive heart failure, and "myocardial infarction," or heart attacks. Although hypertension has been extensively studied, more than 90 percent of all cases are referred to as "essential hypertension," meaning the cause of the elevated blood pressure is unknown. Regardless of the cause, a large body of research from population studies has established that vitamin C can significantly reduce the high blood pressure of hypertensive patients.

In a recent study conducted by researchers at the Boston University School of Medicine and the Linus Pauling Institute at Oregon State University, forty-five patients were given either 500 mg of vitamin C or a placebo, daily. At the beginning of the study, average systolic pressure was 155, and diastolic pressure was 87. After a month, there was no significant change in those receiving the placebo, while those taking vitamin C had a drop in total blood pressure measurements of 9 percent. Specifically, average systolic readings dropped from 155 to 142, and diastolic readings dropped from 87 to 79. Significantly, the research showed that taking vitamin C had no effect on people with normal blood pressure levels.

> **Placebo**
> *An inactive substance that is used as a control in clinical studies instead of a drug or a nutrient.*

Vitamin C Relaxes Blood Vessels

In a series of related studies, scientists have shown that 500 mg of vitamin C daily can improve blood pressure by allowing blood vessels to relax. The research also shows that by increasing the endothelial function of blood vessels, vitamin C can help to control or prevent angina (chest pains) and reduce the risk of a heart attack or stroke.

The researchers speculate that vitamin C helps to control blood pressure by acting as an antioxidant to help protect the body's level of nitric oxide (NO). Nitric oxide is a natural compound that is manufactured in the body to act as a neurotransmitter, or "messenger molecule." In the cardiovascular system, nitric oxide acts by relaxing blood vessels to help the body maintain normal, healthy blood pressure.

> **Endothelial**
> *Refers to the cells that line and protect the inside portion of the arteries and vessels that are exposed to the bloodstream.*

When antioxidant levels are low, or when we encounter chronic stress in our lives, oxidative stresses can inhibit, and actually inactivate, nitric oxide in our bodies, leading to high blood pressure. Vitamin C helps to protect nitric oxide so it can perform its normal function of regulating blood pressure. Additionally, vitamin C is far safer, not to mention less expensive, than the prescription drugs currently used to reduce high blood pressure.

VITAMIN C FIGHTS COLDS AND PROVIDES IMMUNE SUPPORT

Vitamin C is required for the proper functioning of the immune system. Following the publication of Linus Pauling's book *Vitamin C and the Common Cold* in 1970, use of large doses of vitamin C (greater than 1 gram per day) to prevent colds and other infections increased dramatically. Vitamin C is required for the production of the white blood cells, T cells, and macrophages that defend us against viruses, bacteria, parasites, and cancer.

Vitamin C also increases the production of antibodies, boosts production of interferon, and helps to coordinate the cellular immune response. In short, vitamin C supports the immune system as it responds to constant threats from bacterial, viral, and fungal diseases. When vitamin C levels are low or become depleted, the body cannot mount an effective response to defend our health.

Vitamin C and the Common Cold

Large doses of vitamin C (2 g or more per day) can dramatically shorten both the duration and severity of a cold if taken at first sign of symptoms. Most studies show that vitamin C therapy can result in milder symptoms while reducing the duration by about a third.

More than twenty studies have found that taking vitamin C preventively reduces the annual number of colds in children. One study of more than 600 children, between the ages of eight and nine, found that 1,000 mg of vitamin C a day for three months reduced the severity and duration of colds, but not the number of colds. To understand how vitamin C can help us recover from colds, flu, and other forms of infection, we need to understand that vitamin C takes on a new role when the body is under attack.

Common Cold as "Acute Induced Scurvy"

Often, we may begin to notice that we are starting to feel ill, only to have the symptoms quickly disappear within a day or so. This is what is supposed to happen when the immune system is healthy and well supported. At the first sign of an attack, all of the components of the immune complex move quickly to identify, target, and kill the invading pathogens.

> **Immune System**
> *A complex system of responses that fight invaders such as bacteria and viruses.*

Just as often, we don't get better and our symptoms worsen as we are caught up in a cold or flu that can last for days or weeks. The invading viruses have slipped past our first lines of defense, damaging the energy-producing mitochondria in our cells. This damage results in a flood of free radicals that quickly use up all the vitamin C in the affected area, such as the nose and throat. Dr. Robert Cathcart, a pioneer in the field of orthomolecular medicine, refers to this condition as "acute induced scurvy."

> **Orthomolecular**
> *Refers to the eradication of disease by giving the body the "right molecules" it needs to stay healthy.*

When vitamin C is depleted in the affected area, the body can no longer mount an effective response until it has produced enough antibodies to attack and destroy the virus. In the meantime, the condition has time to spread to the sinuses, to the ears, and even to the lungs. This also allows bacteria to take advantage of the situation, potentially causing secondary infections, such as bronchitis, pneumonia, or worse.

Cathcart believes that taking moderate doses of vitamin C (that is, 200–2,000 mg per day) in such conditions may prevent the spread of the infection to other area of the body, but will do little to shorten the course of the illness. On the other hand, Cathcart argues that taking megadoses of vitamin C can force enough electrons into the affected tissues to neutralize all the free radicals and support the white cells that "come out fighting mad and destroy all the viruses." "It does not matter that the disease is moderately advanced," states Cathcart. If sufficient C is used, "the cold will be shortly terminated."

The Power of Megadose Vitamin C

Building on the groundbreaking work of Linus Pauling, Irwin Stone, and other orthomolecular physicians, Cathcart has helped to shape our understanding of megadose vitamin therapy, which uses vitamin C in doses higher than those required for normal cellular functions. When taken in very high doses (10–100 g or more per day, depending upon the person and the illness), vitamin C works in a uniquely different way to fight off serious illness.

We've seen that vitamin C is required to help protect the body from the ravages of free radicals and for the constant repair of our connective tissues. And, except for losses due to collagen formation, most of the time vitamin C is recycled by the body's antioxidant system. But when the body is challenged by cancer, colds, or other diseases, vitamin C takes on a new role. Dr. Cathcart and other proponents of megadose therapy contend that when we become seriously ill, the body is overwhelmed by a flood of free radicals that quickly use up all of the available stores of vitamin C. This impairs the immune response, which depends on vitamin C to mount an effective defense against the invading organisms (or tumor, in the case of cancer).

By ingesting or infusing large amounts of vitamin C, the aim is to saturate the body with enough electrons to destroy all of the free radicals being generated in the tissues affected by the disease. In short, the body is using the electrons donated by vitamin C, and then tossing away the dehydroascorbate.

The Controversy Surrounding Megadose Therapy

Megadose vitamin C therapy continues to be a highly controversial topic. Traditional medicine tends to view vitamin C as a nutrient that is useful only for preventing scurvy. In "The Third Face of Vitamin C," published in *The Journal of Orthomolecular Medicine* in 1993, Dr. Cathcart detailed his clinical experience treating more than 20,000 patients with high doses of vitamin C over a twenty-three-year period. Cathcart found that doses of up to 200 or more grams per day were effective in treating all diseases involving free radicals. These include infections, cardiovascular diseases, can-

cer, trauma, burns (both thermal and radiation), surgeries, allergies, autoimmune diseases, and aging.

Megadose therapy has caught the interest and fired the imagination of many eminent researchers. The late Irwin Stone pioneered the early use of high dose vitamin C in the treatment of disease. His close friend Dr. Frederick Klenner conducted much of the original clinical research on vitamin C megadose therapy, reporting that most viral diseases could be cured when patients were treated with intravenous sodium ascorbate in amounts up to 200 g per day.

Intravenous (IV)
Refers to the administration of a drug or nutrient with a steel needle or plastic catheter inserted into a vein.

Klenner is credited with bringing megadose therapy to the attention of Linus Pauling. Pauling went on to conduct research with the Scottish surgeon Ewan Cameron showing that high-dose vitamin C therapy doubled the life span of cancer patients. (See "Vitamin C Extends the Life Spans of People with Cancer" on page 66.)

Based on their work, a large number of physicians now routinely use massive doses of vitamin C in their clinical practice for the treatment of a wide variety of diseases. Nevertheless, most physicians still remain critical of these treatments, convinced that the usefulness of vitamin C is limited to the prevention of scurvy.

VITAMIN C AND CANCER

In the 1940s, scientists and medical researchers began to notice a strong connection between low blood levels of vitamin C and an increase in the incidence of several forms of cancer. Studies conducted over the last several decades have confirmed this link, consistently showing that eating a diet of fresh fruits and vegetables high in vitamin C can result in a significant reduction of many types of cancer. This profound anticancer benefit forms the basis for dietary guidelines issued by the National Cancer Institute recommending the consumption of at least five servings of fruits and vegetables per day. In addition to vitamin C, fruits and vegetables are also a significant source of fiber and a variety of vitamins and minerals.

Vitamin C Prevents Cancer

Vitamin C helps the body prevent cancer in a number of ways. First, research shows that vitamin C exerts anticancer effects by acting as a powerful antioxidant to prevent the oxidation of fats that can form powerful cancer-promoting compounds. When scientists gave elderly patients 400 mg of vitamin C per day for as little as one year, they noted a significant reduction in the blood serum levels of these dangerous compounds.

Second, vitamin C works inside of our cells to reduce the

effects of free radicals. Free radicals attack cellular targets, such as cell membranes, proteins, and nucleic acids, and cause structural damage to DNA. These genetic alterations appear as mutations and chromosomal alterations in certain genes that are known to cause various forms of cancer and increase the risk of developing cancer later in life.

Third, vitamin C aids the body's detoxifying systems by stimulating the production of liver enzymes that break down and eliminate dangerous environmental pollutants and toxins that are known to have powerful mutagenic or carcinogenic effects.

Carcinogen
Chemical substance or mixtures of chemical substances that are known to induce cancer or increase its incidence.

Additionally, vitamin C reduces the risk of developing cancer by preventing the formation of cancer-causing chemicals called nitro-samines. These are formed when bacteria in the stomach metabolize nitrate, a nitrogen compound found in fish and leafy green and root vegetables, such as spinach and carrots. Nitrosamines are also added to processed and cured meats, such as ham, bacon, and sausages, to prevent bacterial growth.

Researchers believe that the relatively high consumption of orange juice by people living in citrus-producing regions of the United States may explain the lower number of reported cases of cancers of the large bowel in those areas. Researchers have found that vitamin C significantly reduces urinary levels of nitrosamines in humans. Animal studies also show that vitamin C protects against nitrosamine-induced cancer by inhibiting and reducing the formation of tumors in treated animals.

Vitamin C Fights Tumor Growth

Even as cancer cells begin to spread, vitamin C plays an important role in fighting tumor growth. Dr. Ewan Cameron theorized that as cancer cells grow, they must first invade other cells to open up space for tumor expansion. In order to invade these adjoining cells, tumors must first break through the tough cell walls that are held together with "intercellular cement," as Pauling referred to the connective tissues and chains of collagen that hold cells together.

In order to break down these connective tissues and invade the tissues, cancer cells release an enzyme called hyaluronidase that weakens and breaks down connective tissues. Cancer cells also produce a second enzyme, called collagenase, which works to dissolve collagen. Under the fierce attack of these two powerful enzymes, cell walls eventually dissolve and collapse, allowing cancer cells to move in and expand.

Vitamin C is required for the maintenance of the collagen and fibrous materials that make up healthy cells. When vitamin C levels are too low to adequately maintain strong cellular walls, the damage caused by cancer enzymes is allowed to proceed unchecked. In addition to helping slow the progression of cell invasion, vitamin C has also been found to produce a substance that inhibits hyaluronidase. The more vitamin C in the system, the more this inhibitor is released.

New Mechanism of Action

A letter published in the January 12, 2002, issue of the British medical journal *Lancet* revealed a new mechanism that helps to explain why vitamin C is helpful in protecting the body against cancer. In their paper, the researchers report that vitamin C inhibits the cancer-causing effects of hydrogen peroxide. Cells must communicate with one another to stay healthy and to promote normal cell growth. Hydrogen peroxide is a known tumor promoter that works, in part, by inhibiting the normal processes of cell-to-cell communication. What the researchers discovered from animal studies is that vitamin C works to inhibit this tumor-promoting property of hydrogen peroxide.

Hydrogen Peroxide (H_2O_2)
A known tumor promoter that is produced when the body breaks down amino acids and fats for cellular energy.

Studies Show Vitamin C Reduces Incidence of Cancer

In a comprehensive review of studies on vitamin C's protective effects against various types of cancer, the *American Journal of Clinical Nutrition* reported that thirty-three studies showed a significant link between vitamin C intake (defined as 160 mg or more per day) and a lower incidence of cancer. Ongoing research continues to find a protective (as opposed to curative) effect for a number of cancers.

The most significant finding came from a published study involving 11,348 adults over a ten-year period. This study showed that males taking the highest amount of vitamin C had a 45 percent reduction in all causes of mortality, a 22 percent reduction in cancer incidence, and a 42 percent reduction in heart attacks.

Breast Cancer

Two recent studies have found that higher intake of vitamin C can protect against breast cancer in certain groups of women. The Nurses' Health Study—one of the largest investigations into the risk factors for major chronic diseases in women—found that premenopausal women with a family history of breast cancer who consumed an average of 205 mg of vitamin C per day were 63 percent less likely to develop breast cancer than similar women who consumed only 70 mg of vitamin C per day.

Another study, the Swedish Mammography Cohort, found that overweight women who consumed an average of 110 mg of vitamin C per day had a 39 percent lower risk of breast cancer when compared with overweight women who consumed only 30 mg (or less than half the RDA) of vitamin C per day.

Researchers have also shown that the spread of breast cancer, or metastasis, may be reduced by taking large amounts of vitamin C.

Mouth, Larynx, and Esophageal Cancer

In Asia, cancer of the mouth, larynx, and esophagus is the leading form of cancer in men, and the third most frequent form of cancer in women. Approximately 30,000 new cases of oral cancer are diagnosed in the United States each year, and about 9,000 people die from oral cancer each year. Research shows that a low intake of vitamin C index is associated with a significantly greater number of cancers of the mouth, larynx, and esophagus.

Lung Cancer

Researchers reviewed the intake of a group of 870 men over a period of twenty-five years. They found that men who consumed 83 mg or more of vitamin C per day were 64 percent less likely to develop lung cancer, compared with men who consumed less than 63 mg of vitamin C per day.

Pancreatic Cancer

In one study, high intake of vitamin C was shown to cut the risk of developing pancreatic cancer in half. Other studies also show that eating fruits and vegetables high in vitamin C offers significant protection against pancreatic cancer, which is the fifth leading cause of cancer deaths.

Digestive Tract Cancers

A number of studies have proven that increased intake of dietary vitamin C reduces stomach cancer. Scientists believe that vitamin C protects the stomach by inhibiting the formation of carcinogenic compounds, such as nitrosamines, in the stomach. Additionally, people infected with the common bacteria *Helicobacter pylori* (*H. pylori*) have a much higher incidence of stomach cancer. Studies have shown that supplemental vitamin C—in addition to standard *H. pylori* eradication therapies—may be effective in reducing the risk of stomach cancer.

Vitamin C–rich foods have been shown to have a significant effect in reducing both colon and rectal cancer. Supplementation with 3 g of vitamin C per day has been found to effectively prevent further polyp growth in colon cancer, and intake of more than 157 mg of vitamin C per day has been found to reduce the risk of developing colon cancer by 50 percent.

Prostate and Bladder Cancers

In a study presented at the American Institute for Cancer Research 10th Annual Research Conference in September 2001, researchers revealed that vitamin C showed potent activity against two forms of prostate cancer cells, and seven other forms of urinary tract cancers. While vitamin C didn't kill the cancer cells outright, it was found to trigger the breakdown of the malignant DNA in the cells, as well as to block the growth of the tumors.

Research has also shown that people taking 500 mg of vitamin C per day for ten years or more cut their risk of developing bladder cancer by 60 percent.

Skin Cancer

Applying vitamin C to the skin can inhibit tumor promotion in mouse skin, according to a recent study. Moreover, ascorbyl palmitate, the fat-soluble form of vitamin C, was found to be at least thirty times more effective than water-soluble vitamin C in tumor reduction. Vitamin C has also been found to reduce the number of malignant skin lesions in mice exposed to high levels of ultraviolet light (UV). Researchers have found similar results in human studies, showing that vitamin C inhibits the formation of cancer-causing compounds in skin exposed to UV radiation.

Vitamin C Extends the Life Spans of People with Cancer

While a growing number of studies show that a higher intake of vitamin C is associated with significant reductions in many forms of cancer, in general, most findings support a preventative, rather than curative, role for vitamin C and cancer.

In 1976, Dr. Linus Pauling reported on the results of cancer research he conducted in collaboration with Ewan Cameron. Pauling and Cameron treated 100 terminally ill cancer patients at the Vale of Leven Hospital in Scotland with very large doses of vitamin C (10 g per day intravenously for ten days followed by at least 10 g per day orally indefinitely). The results of their trial showed that vitamin C therapy was effective in increasing both the survival time and the quality of life of terminal cancer patients. Patients receiving vitamin C lived more than four times longer than 1,000 control subjects who received no vitamin C. Only 3 of these 1,000 patients survived for more than a year, while 16 of the 100 patients taking vitamin C lived a year or longer.

More recently, Cameron has reported similar results from a study he conducted in Alexandria, Scotland, between 1978 and 1982. Cameron created a database containing the records of every cancer patient attending three hospitals in Scotland during a four-year period. The study found that those cancer patients treated with vitamin C survived for an average of 343 days, versus only 180 days for patients not receiving vitamin C.

Abram Hoffer, M.D., Ph.D., is an internationally respected Canadian doctor who has devoted the last four decades to the field of orthomolecular medicine and the use of niacin (vitamin B$_3$) for treating schizophrenia. Dr. Hoffer has also pioneered the use of vitamin C as a primary agent in his treatment of cancer patients. A paper reporting on Hoffer's work with cancer patients detailed the results of his work between 1990 and 1994. Of the 500 patients who followed Hoffer's nutritional plan, 70 percent were still alive at the end of 1994. By contrast, of the group of 100 patients who did not follow the Hoffer vitamin C plan, only 15 were still alive after four years.

The Infamous Mayo Study

A study conducted by the Mayo clinic in 1985 made headlines across the world when this prestigious institution announced that their clinical trial, based on the methods of Cameron and Pauling, had failed to find any benefit for vitamin C in cancer patients. Even today, this study, which was led by C. G. Moertel, forms the basis for much of the resistance people encounter when asking their physicians about vitamin C therapy.

For years, vitamin C enthusiasts have pointed out that the Mayo study was seriously flawed and was based on significantly different methods from those described by Pauling and Cameron. These differences prompted researchers from the National Institutes of Health to suggest that the route of administration (intravenous versus oral) may have been the cause of the radically different results.

Intravenous (IV) administration has been shown to result in much higher blood levels of vitamin C than oral administration, and levels that are toxic to certain types of cancer cells in culture can be achieved only with intravenous administration. Part of the problem with understanding what had led to such different outcomes was that Moertel refused to release any information about the study, other than what was in the published paper.

In *Vitamin C & Cancer*, Abram Hoffer revealed the primary reason for the failure of the Mayo study to improve the survival time of cancer patients. In the Mayo therapy, researchers gave 10 g of oral vitamin C per day to a group of fifty patients suffering from advanced colorectal cancer. The significant difference was that, whereas Pauling and Cameron treated patients indefinitely, the Mayo team treated patients only for an average of seventy-five days, and then stopped treatment completely. The result was that as soon as treatment stopped, the patients began to die rapidly. Whereas only one patient died during the seventy-five days of vitamin C therapy, more than half the patients died within seventy-five days of discontinuing vitamin C.

Moertel versus Pauling?

The following are some interesting statistics that frequently appear in papers discussing the different viewpoints of Linus Pauling and C. G. Moertel:

1. Albert Szent-Györgyi took 1 gram of vitamin C every day and lived to age eighty-nine.

2. Linus Pauling consumed 18 g of vitamin C every day and died of prostate cancer at age ninety-four.

3. C. G. Moertel of the Mayo Clinic, hostile critic of vitamin C, died of cancer at age sixty-six.

Antinutrient Bias Exposed

The Mayo study is one of the most blatant examples of the antivitamin bias encountered frequently in medicine and medical research, leading one observer to note that the Mayo study was designed with the "clear intention of blowing the vitamin C and cancer controversy off the medical map." If this is true, it seems to have worked, because every physician has heard about the Mayo study, and based on the published paper, most have formed the opinion that vitamin C is useless in cases of cancer.

Is Vitamin C Toxic to Cancer Cells?

Preliminary research has recently demonstrated that very high concentrations of vitamin C, in combination with alpha-lipoic acid and other natural substances, kills cancer cells outright in laboratory tests. This cytotoxic effect is described as being similar to standard chemotherapy, but with the added benefit of leaving healthy cells undamaged. One of the pioneers in this application of vitamin C is Dr. Hugh Riordan. He has completed a ten-year research project on high-dose intravenous vitamin C and cancer, and his method passed phase I clinical trials at the University of Nebraska Medical School Hospital. These trials established that high-dose vitamin C treatment is nontoxic, and cleared the way for a phase II clinical trial under the auspices of the National Institutes of Health (NIH) for treating renal adenoma (kidney cancer). Dr Riordan has also published several successful case histories, including the results of vitamin C treatment on a late-stage lung cancer patient who remained cancer-free for five years following treatment. This is the generally accepted standard in cancer statistics for a "cure."

Vitamin C Aids Conventional Cancer Treatment

There has been some question concerning vitamin C's potential to interfere with traditional cancer therapies, including chemotherapy and radiation treatments. Abram Hoffer addressed this issue, stating, "This [vitamin treatment] would enhance the therapeutic effect of the chemotherapy and decrease its toxicity." Also, "If they [cancer patients] needed chemotherapy the program [vitamin therapy] would make it more tolerable and less painful and if they needed radiation the program would decrease the intensity of the side-effects of the radiation and increase its efficacy."

Proponents of vitamin C therapy recommend that vitamin C should not be used in place of any conventional therapy that has been demonstrated to be effective in the treatment of a particular type of cancer such as chemotherapy or radiation therapy. If an individual with cancer chooses to take vitamin supplements, it is important that the clinician coordinating his or her treatment is aware of the type and dose of each supplement. There is no clinical evidence to suggest that vitamin C has any adverse effect on the survival of cancer patients. However, there is some evidence that the vitamin C treatments should be staggered with the conventional treatments for best results.

SAFETY AND POLITICS OF VITAMIN C

Vitamin C has consistently been proven to be an extraordinarily safe nutrient. While a number of possible problems have been raised, most were based on test tube experiments. These concerns include genetic mutations, birth defects, cancer, atherosclerosis, kidney stones, rebound scurvy, increased oxidative stress, excess iron absorption, impaired copper utilization, vitamin B_{12} deficiency, and erosion of dental enamel. In reality, virtually no adverse effects (aside from the laxative effect that can cause loose stools) have been found.

Kidney Stone Formation

Fears that very high intake of vitamin C could lead to the formation of kidney stones were based on a concern that the production of oxalate, a component of stones that occurs during vitamin C metabolism, would increase stone formation. Research has shown that the oxalate produced from vitamin C is only a fraction of that derived from dietary sources, and there is no safety issue regarding kidney stones.

Rebound Scurvy

The fear that symptoms of vitamin C deficiency would suddenly appear if large doses of vitamin C were stopped (rebound scurvy) appears to be unfounded in humans, and animal studies with guinea pigs have either shown no such effect, or have been inconclusive.

Depletion of Vitamin B_{12} and Impaired Copper Absorption

Concerns that large amounts of vitamin C might destroy vitamin B_{12} were found to be the result of errors in experimental testing. Also, controlled studies have found no evidence to support the claim that vitamin C impairs copper absorption.

Diarrhea

Diarrhea is the only recognized "side effect" that may occur when taking large doses of vitamin C. Unlike diarrhea caused by illness or infection, the loose stools caused by large doses of vitamin C are the first sign that the body's tissue fluids have been saturated with ascorbic acid. This effect is due to the laxative action of vitamin C. Most people will not experience this effect unless they are taking more than 10 g of vitamin C per day. Symptoms are not serious and stop when one either discontinues or reduces the dosage of vitamin C. For more information, see "Dosing to Bowel Tolerance" on page 71.

Drug Interactions

A number of drugs are known to lower vitamin C levels and may require increased intake of vitamin C. Estrogen-containing contraceptives (birth control pills) are known to lower vitamin C levels in plasma and white blood cells. Aspirin can also lead to lower vitamin C levels if taken frequently. For example, two aspirin tablets taken every six hours for a week have been shown to reduce white blood cell content of vitamin C by 50 percent, primarily by increasing urinary excretion of vitamin C.

The Politics of Vitamin C

Vitamin C is one of the safest substances known to us. Thousands of studies and research papers support both the clinical effectiveness and exemplary safety record of vitamin C. Yet whenever vitamin C is shown to be useful for any purpose other than simply for preventing scurvy, the anti–vitamin-C lobby can be counted on to quickly produce an "expert" who immediately 1) attacks the findings, 2) questions the methods and/or qualifications of the researchers behind the study, 3) issues warnings against taking any doses greater than the sanctioned RDAs, and 4) calls for further study.

Recommended Daily Allowance (RDA) *The designated amount of a nutrient needed to prevent overt deficiency disease in most people. RDAs are not enough to promote optimal health or to prevent the incidence of many diseases in all people.*

This pattern of doubt and outright hostility is not new—vitamin C and its proponents have been under constant attack for the last several decades. Indeed, hostility to vitamin C goes all the way back to 1746, the year that James Lind proved that scurvy could be prevented with small servings of citrus fruit. The British Navy resisted Lind's findings for forty years in a show of bureaucratic obstinacy that resulted in the deaths of more than 100,000 British sailors.

Part of the hostility toward vitamin C is due to its status as a natural nutrient. Since vitamin C cannot be turned into a patented drug, pharmaceutical companies have no financial incentive to perform the double-blind studies that most of the scientific community need to be convinced of a substance's effectiveness.

Additionally, because of the seriousness of cancer and the political environment within the medical system, the use of vitamin C to prevent or treat cancer is a highly charged and controversial issue with conventional physicians.

The Attack on Vitamin C

In one recent attack, a letter published in the April 9, 1998, issue of *Nature* outlined claims by a group of British researchers who suggested that 500 mg of vitamin C per day could cause damage to human DNA. The media responded to what was essentially a press release with a flood of alarming reports stating that vitamin C caused cancer. Subsequent research found these conclusions to be entirely wrong, concluding that supplementing with 500 mg of vitamin C per day and 400 IU of vitamin E had "no significant main effect or interaction effect on oxidative DNA damage." Unfortunately, when this report was published, the mainstream press failed to share the information with the public.

The letter published in *Nature* was followed two years later by a report published in the journal *Science,* which stated that lipid hydroperoxides (rancid fat molecules) can react with vitamin C in a test tube to form products that are potentially harmful to DNA. Although the reaction of these products with DNA was not demonstrated in the study, it was suggested that vitamin C might enhance mutations and increase the risk of cancer. That this conclusion was unwarranted and contradicted countless studies showing vitamin C's benefits did little to stop the media from churning out a new rash of alarming headlines implying that vitamin C caused cancer.

Flawed Science

One of the biggest problems with the study reported in *Science* was that it tested conditions that simply do not exist in the real world. In living cells, vitamin C acts as the first line of antioxidant defense, directly preventing the formation of lipid hydroperoxides. In fact, lipid hydroperoxides can form only when vitamin C levels have been depleted. Vitamin C also works in conjunction with vitamin E—both antioxidants recycle each other to quench free radicals. Vitamin E also provides additional defense by directly preventing the conversion of unsaturated fats to lipid hydroperoxides. When (and if) lipid hydroperoxides do occur in the body, a number of cellular enzymes go to work to instantly reduce these compounds into harmless alcohols. In the study in question, researchers incubated vitamin C in concentrations of lipid hydroperoxides at least 10,000 times higher than could possibly exist in human plasma, for time periods of up to two hours—far longer than the frac-

tion of a second it would take before enzymes rendered them harmless.

Consumer Awareness

Vitamin C supplements are often singled out as potential troublemakers, though the body does not distinguish between dietary vitamin C and supplemental vitamin C. Thus, if vitamin C indeed caused cancer, as some antinutrient doctors have suggested, the only advice one could follow would be to stop taking vitamin supplements while also eliminating vitamin C–rich fruits and vegetables from the diet! In reality, we know that vitamin C–rich foods lower the risk of cancer, heart disease, stroke, and other diseases, so the more fruits and vegetables you eat, the better.

Media Bias versus Scientific Fact

While the findings reported in *Science* turned out to have little relevance to the actual processes that occur in human beings, the manner in which the story was handled revealed much about the media bias against supplements. Contemporary media is a competitive business that is driven by immediacy and sensationalism. And American media often reveals an "antisupplement" tendency in its uncritical acceptance of any report touting the potential dangers of nutrients. To support their more sensational headlines, news outlets tend to interview conventional doctors and scientist who remain steadfast in their unwillingness to accept that vitamins and minerals might have health benefits, while refusing to include opposing viewpoints.

In 1999, Dr. Hoffer summed up the problem nicely when, writing about the reluctance of orthodox physicians to accept the scientific evidence on the safety of vitamin C, he stated: "They will still promote their old ideas and will bolster them by manufacturing toxicities. As a rule, when there are no toxicities, it is simple to invent them, such as vitamin C causes kidney stones, or damages the liver, or interferes with the treatment of diabetes and so on. Every month I hear about new toxicities which totally surprise and delight me because they indicate how imaginative my colleagues can be."

HOW MUCH VITAMIN C SHOULD YOU TAKE?

Following publication of Linus Pauling's *Vitamin C and the Common Cold* in 1970, consumption of vitamin C in the United States shot up by more than 300 percent. Average intake of vitamin C continues to grow each year, and for good reason. A recent study determined that vitamin C blood levels are a good predictor of mortality risk. Higher blood levels of vitamin C have been shown to indicate a lower risk for developing cardiovascular diseases and certain types of cancer and degenerative diseases. In this section, we'll review the most common standards and recommendations for vitamin C dosages.

Recommended Daily Allowance of Vitamin C

Many people still base their vitamin C intake on the Recommended Daily Allowance (RDA). This is unfortunate because, while these amounts certainly protect against outright scurvy in most people, they fall far below the minimal levels currently shown to prevent many chronic and age-related degenerative conditions associated with long-term, low-level vitamin C deficiency. Despite evidence that higher vitamin C intake will enhance health and decrease the incidence of disease, political considerations have delayed attempts to raise the RDA for decades.

Recently, the RDA for vitamin C has been revised upward from 60 mg daily to 75 mg per day for women, and 90 mg per day for men. The recommended intake for smokers is 35 mg per day higher than for nonsmokers, because smokers are under increased oxidative stress from the toxins in cigarette smoke and generally have lower blood levels of vitamin C.

The Problem with RDAs

Today, many researchers and scientists recommend raising the RDA even higher, to a minimum of 200 mg per day, based on the current understanding of the vital role vitamin C plays in promoting health. Furthermore, even a dosage of 200 mg per day would not be enough to address the higher vitamin C requirements of women, children, middle aged and elderly adults, and individuals dealing with special circumstances (special diets, tobacco smoking, sickness, infections, trauma, metabolic and genetic disorders, or degenerative diseases).

TABLE 3.1. Recommended Daily Allowance (RDA) for Vitamin C

Life Stage	Age	Men (mg/day)	Women (mg/day)
Children	1–3	15	15
Children	4–8	25	25
Children	9–13	45	45
Adolescents	14–18	75	65
Adults	19 and over	90	75
Smokers	19 and over	125	110
Pregnancy	18 and under	—	80
Pregnancy	19 and over	—	85
Breastfeeding	18 and under	—	115
Breastfeeding	19 and over	—	120

Vitamin C for Optimal Health

Based on the overwhelmingly positive reports on the benefits of higher levels of vitamin C, many nutritionally based physicians now recommend that people base their intake of vitamin C on how much they need to promote *optimal health*, not just to prevent scurvy.

Taking a cue from animals still able to produce their own vitamin C, researchers have examined the levels produced by various species, seeking clues to help determine just how much vitamin C humans might need to maintain optimal health.

Remember that all animals, apart from primates and guinea pigs, are able to manufacture vitamin C in their livers. And while the amount produced is different in each species, every single animal produces vitamin C in levels that are hundreds, if not thousands, of times higher than those required to simply prevent scurvy. This is puzzling when one considers that glucose, which is used to make vitamin C, is absolutely vital for energy production.

Nature does not design for waste, and depleting glucose levels—and potentially running out of energy at a crucial point—can mean the difference between life and death in the constant battle for survival. The reasonable answer for these extraordinarily high levels of vitamin C, produced at the cost of life-giving glucose, is that they are essential for the health and survival of these animals.

Table 3.2 lists the average amount of vitamin C produced by each animal in the left column. In the right column, we see the equivalent amount of vitamin C, as extrapolated to the body weight of a 154-pound human. As you can see, if humans had not lost their ability to manufacture vitamin C—a loss that many now view as a genetic disease—our daily production of vitamin C would likely be between 3,000 and 15,000 mg per day, or an average of 5,400 mg per day under normal (healthy) circumstances. Research has also shown that some animals, when their health is under stress, are not always able to produce enough vitamin C. Cats and dogs, for example, are relatively low vitamin C producers, and are susceptible to stress-related vitamin C deficiency.

Optimal Doses for Humans

So what does this mean for you, and what can be considered a safe dose of vitamin C for optimal health? Recommendations differ widely, depending on the source. While many traditional doctors might feel uncomfortable about openly recommending vitamin C in doses higher than the RDAs, a recent survey in the United States found that those doctors who are the healthiest report that they consume on average at least 250 mg of vitamin C per day. Many health professionals admit to taking even higher doses.

Many holistic and alternative medical researchers suggest that, based on countless medical studies, a more rea-

TABLE 3.2.
Average Amount of Vitamin C Produced by Animals and the Human Equivalent

Animal	Vitamin C	Vitamin C equivalent produced per day for 154-pound human
Cat	336 mg	2,800 mg
Cow	1,099 mg	1,281 mg
Goat	2,280 mg	13,300 mg
Mouse	2,352 mg	19,250 mg
Rabbit	1,547 mg	15,820 mg
Rat	2,737 mg	13,902 mg

sonable therapeutic intake of vitamin C would range from 500–4,000 mg per day. This water-soluble vitamin is completely excreted from the body within four hours under normal circumstances. To maintain stable serum levels, the desired total daily dose should be divided into three separate doses taken throughout the day.

Dosing to Bowel Tolerance

Ask a vitamin C expert like Dr. Robert Cathcart how much vitamin C to take, and the answer is likely to be "a lot." Dr. Cathcart has long recommended the "bowel tolerance" method of determining one's need. This is determined by taking increasingly large amounts of vitamin C each day until your body reaches the saturation point. Any amount beyond that level and vitamin C becomes a laxative. Based on his experience with more than 20,000 patients, Dr. Cathcart believes that the bowel tolerance level for most healthy people is between 10–15 g of vitamin C per day. When fighting a cold or flu, bowel tolerance rises to between 30–60 g, and for those with a serious infectious illness, the need to induce tolerance can jump to 200 g per day or more. During an infectious illness, the best clinical results have been achieved by maintaining high vitamin C levels in the blood by taking 3 g or more of vitamin C every four hours.

When Dr. Cathcart treated patients for mononucleosis, most were functioning normally after a few days of receiving 200 g of vitamin C per day, given orally and intravenously. This was in sharp contrast to other patients in the same community, who were often hospitalized for several weeks during a mononucleosis outbreak.

Is Vitamin C "Expensive Urine"?

One of the most frequent charges made against taking vitamin C in high doses is that since much of the vitamin is excreted within a matter of hours, all one is doing is making "expensive urine." Researchers investigated this by giving increasingly larger daily doses and measuring excretion in the urine to see how much was needed to saturate tissue levels. They found that only a quarter of the subjects reached their vitamin C maximum at 1,500 mg a day. More than half of those in the study required more than 2,500 mg a day to reach a level where their bodies could use no more. In several cases, test subjects did not reach their maximum even at 5,000 mg per day!

Another consideration, pointed out by Dr. Michael Colgan, an internationally renowned nutritional research scientist, is that vitamin C protects the bowel, kidneys, and bladder as it exits the body. This is an added bonus, since the average victim of bowel or bladder cancer, aside from their pain and suffering, spends $26,000 for treatment—mostly to no avail.

Another way to look at vitamin C excretion is by thinking of what it takes to put out a house fire. The only solution is to pour as much water on the flames, as fast as possible, to put out the fire and save the house. There is little concern about "saving" the water used in this process, and no one cares that, after quenching the flames, the excess water just evaporates or drains away. The value of water in this case is not the water itself, but what the water can do to contribute to putting out the flames and saving lives. In much the same way, optimal health is not about "losing value" when vitamin C is eventually excreted, but in "getting value" by using it in high enough doses, and maintaining serum levels long enough, to quench the free radical fires damaging our bodies.

Dr. Cathcart uses a similar analogy when describing how megadose vitamin C therapy works. "Suppose you owned a farm and on one end of the property there was a barn and on the other end of the property there was a water well. One day the barn catches fire and neighbors come with buckets to set up a bucket brigade between the water well and the barn and are putting out the fire when the well goes dry.

My use of vitamin C is like thousands of neighbors coming from miles around, each with a bucketful of their own water, throwing their own water on your fire once, and then leaving."

Vitamin C for Disease Prevention

As we've seen, the amount of vitamin C required for chronic diseases is much higher than that required simply to prevent scurvy. Much of the information regarding vitamin C and the prevention of chronic disease is based on studies that measure vitamin C intake in large groups of people, over periods of years or decades, to determine a protective effect against chronic diseases. The following list describes vitamin C doses discussed in research studies conducted across the globe over the last thirty years. While not recommendations, the amounts described may serve as guidance in researching and determining your own need for vitamin C.

Age-Related Memory Impairment

Antioxidant blood levels have been shown to improve memory performance in the elderly. Higher vitamin C blood levels are associated with significant improvements in recognition, vocabulary, and memory recall. Doses of 500–1,000 mg per day have been used for this condition.

Allergies (Hay Fever)

Vitamin C is a natural antihistamine that has been shown to help suppress allergic reactions. Doses of 2,000–12,000 mg per day have been used for this condition.

Alzheimer's Disease

Researchers have shown that people with Alzheimer's disease have lower blood levels of vitamin C. When given 1,000 mg of vitamin C per day, blood levels increased significantly in people with Alzheimer's disease. In a study of vitamin C intake, out of 633 people aged sixty-five and older, 91 developed Alzheimer's disease over a period of four and a quarter years, but none of the 23 vitamin C supplement users developed the condition. Doses of 1,000–2,000 mg per day have been used for this condition.

Angina Pectoris

Vitamin C has been shown to improve blood vessel dilation that is often compromised in people with atherosclerosis. The pain of angina pectoris is also related to impaired dilation of the coronary arteries. Treatment with 500 mg per day of vitamin C has been proven to improve dilation of blood vessels in individuals with angina pectoris and congestive heart failure. Doses of 500–1,000 mg per day have been used for this condition.

Osteoarthritis and Rheumatoid Arthritis

Vitamin C has been shown effective in helping to reduce the progression of arthritis. A dosage of 420 mg of vitamin C per day resulted in a 300 percent reduction in the progression of the disease and reduced joint pain, particularly in the knees. Researchers have also shown that blood levels of vitamin C are extremely low in patients with rheumatoid arthritis, suggesting that vitamin C may offer antioxidant protection to reduce damage to inflamed joints. Doses of 420–2,000 mg per day have been used for these conditions.

Asthma

Vitamin C is helpful in the treatment of asthma, particularly in patients with food allergies. Histamine is a major factor in asthmatic attacks, and vitamin C is proven to speed up the natural clearing of excess histamine in the serum. Asthmatics can take 2 g or more of vitamin C to help break down mucus involved in attacks. Taken at bedtime, 500–1000 mg of vitamin C has been shown to reduce or prevent asthma attacks that occur in the middle of the night. Doses of 2,000–5,000 mg per day have been used for this condition.

Diabetes

Diabetes Epidemic
Diabetes has increased 49 percent from 1990 to 2000, and NIH projections indicate a 165 percent increase by the year 2050!

Numerous studies have shown that vitamin C plasma levels are about 30 percent lower in people with diabetes, as compared with people who do not have diabetes. In one study, researchers found that high doses of vitamin C markedly improved blood-sugar regulation in people with non–insulin-dependent diabetes mellitus (NIDDM). Vitamin C has also been shown to improve blood vessel dilation, which is often impaired in people with diabetes.

Also, complications of diabetes are linked to increased oxidative stresses, supporting a role for vitamin C in preventing some of the complications of diabetes. Vitamin C helps to reduce the abnormal attachment of sugars to proteins (glycosylation). Doses of between 100 and 600 mg of vitamin C per day have been shown to normalize cellular sorbitol levels, which may have implications for decreasing some of the long-term complications of diabetes. Doses of 500–1,000 mg per day have been used for this condition.

Glycosylation
A process that binds sugars (glucose) with proteins in the body to form dangerous compounds that complicate aging and diabetes.

Cancer

Vitamin C has been proven to protect against a number of types of cancer in doses as low as 100–500 mg per day. Additionally, Pauling and Cameron found that dosages of 10 g per day improved both the survival time and the quality of life of terminal cancer patients. Research has shown that high blood levels of vitamin C are toxic to certain types of cancers, and such levels can be achieved only by IV administration, as was initially used in the Pauling/Cameron study. Doses of 10,000–100,000 mg per day have been used for this condition.

Cataracts

Decreased vitamin C levels in the lens of the eye are linked to cataracts in humans. Several studies have shown that increased intake of vitamin C may decrease the incidence of cataracts. Researchers have shown that a daily dose of 300 mg of vitamin C has a protective effect against the development of cataracts when taken for a number of years. Doses of 300–500 mg per day have been used for this condition.

Gingivitis

Low levels of vitamin C are often associated with gingivitis. Doses of 500–4,000 mg of vitamin C per day have been shown to improve gum conditions.

Glaucoma

Vitamin C reduces elevated intraocular pressure (IOP) in the eye by helping fluid exit the eye and flow into the blood. Vitamin C also diminishes the production of eye fluid and improves fluid outflow. Vitamin C must be taken in large doses—between 20 and 35 g per day. Vitamin C therapy is not a cure, and if intake is reduced or stopped, glaucoma will continue to develop at its previous pace. Doses of 5,000–35,000 mg per day have been used for this condition.

Hepatitis

Reports from German literature show that high doses of vitamin C are beneficial in treating epidemic hepatitis in children. Doses of 2 g of vitamin C per day have been shown to stimulate the immune response and help to fight infection. Beneficial effects were also observed in sixty-three cases of epidemic hepatitis treated with 10 g of vitamin C daily for an average of five days. The patients' hospital stays and symptoms were reduced by 50 percent. Doses of 5,000–10,000 mg per day have been used for this condition.

HIV

Vitamin C acts as an antiviral agent, elevating the body's interferon levels. Vitamin C has also been found to inhibit HIV replication in laboratory tests. Bowel tolerance with vitamin C is recommended for its antioxidant and immunity-enhancing abilities and to increase disease resistance and improve well-being in patients with HIV. Doses of 5,000–20,000 mg per day have been used for this condition.

Hypertension (High Blood Pressure)

Several studies have shown that supplemental vitamin C can have a blood–pressure-lowering effect. In a recent study, as little as 500 mg of vitamin C per day resulted in an average drop in systolic blood pressure of 9 percent after four weeks. Doses of 6,000 mg per day have been used for this condition.

Influenza

Vitamin C has been shown to help prevent flu infection, and when taken in high doses, it speeds recovery from influenza. Doses of 2,000–6,000 mg per day have been used for this condition.

Lead Poisoning

Lead poisoning continues to be a significant health problem in the United States, especially for children living in urban areas. Children exposed to lead are more likely to develop learning disabilities and behavioral problems and to have low IQs. Abnormal growth and development have also been observed in children born to women exposed to lead during pregnancy. Several studies have shown that low intake of vitamin C is associated with higher blood levels of lead. Research suggests that vitamin C protects against lead poisoning by inhibiting intestinal absorption while enhancing urinary excretion of lead, significantly lowering blood lead levels in as little as four weeks. Doses of 1,000–2,000 mg per day have been used for this condition.

Macular Degeneration

Antioxidants have been shown to prevent the oxidative damage that causes macular degeneration. People with high blood levels of vitamin C and other antioxidants, such as vitamin E and selenium, have a 70 percent lower risk of developing macular degeneration. Doses of 500–1,000 mg per day have been used for this condition.

Male Infertility

Vitamin C protects sperm from oxidative damage, and improves sperm quality, particularly in smokers. Taking 1 g of vitamin C per day has also been found effective in treating sperm agglutination, a condition that causes sperm to clump together. Doses of 1,000–2,000 mg per day have been used for this condition.

Retinopathy

Antioxidants have been shown to prevent the oxidative damage that causes retinopathy. Vitamin C also strengthens the capillaries that supply blood to the retina. Vitamin C and other antioxidants, such as vitamin E and selenium, have been shown to reduce the damaging effects of retinopathy. Doses of 500–2,000 mg per day have been used for this condition.

Schizophrenia

In 1966, researchers showed that adult men with schizophrenia required 36–48 g of vitamin C per day to reach the vitamin C saturation level that normal men reach with only 4 g of vitamin C per day. While the patients were by no means cured, the high doses of vitamin C brought about marked improvement in the socialization of the patients. Those who were shy, reclusive, and withdrawn began to participate in ward activities and in conversation with other patients and ward personnel. Doses of 36,000–48,000 mg per day have been used for this condition.

FORMS OF VITAMIN C

When deciding which form of vitamin C is best, keep in mind that, as Linus Pauling pointed out, all forms of vitamin C are identical. The body doesn't care if the C is "natural" or synthesized, just as long as it gets enough of it. True, there are some benefits to natural food sources of C, such as fruits and vegetables. They can provide other nutrients, such as bioflavonoids. On the other hand, supplements have the advantage of packing a lot of vitamin C into a very small serving. You would have to drink eight glasses of orange juice, eat sixteen oranges, or consume fifty cups of blueberries to equal the vitamin C found in one 1,000-mg capsule. In short, when choosing your vitamin C, the most important point is choosing a form that agrees with your lifestyle and your budget.

Getting Vitamin C from Foods

Vitamin C can be obtained in various amounts from food sources, primarily from fruits and vegetables. As shown in Table 3.3, fruits and vegetables vary in their vitamin C content, but five servings should average out to at least 200 mg of vitamin C. Vitamin C is easily destroyed by heat, and because it is water-soluble, this vitamin can be drained off in liquids used in food preparation. To assure full potency of vitamin C value, it is best to consume foods raw or minimally processed.

Getting Your Vitamin C from Supplements

Vitamin C supplements are available in many forms, but according to the Linus Pauling Institute, there is little scientific evidence to show that any one form is better absorbed or more effective than another.

Natural and synthetic forms of vitamin C are chemically identical, and there are no known differences in their biological activity. The possibility that vitamin C from natural sources might be more bioavailable than synthetic vitamin C has been investigated in at least two human studies and no significant differences were found.

Mineral salts of vitamin C are buffered and are, therefore, less acidic than ascorbic acid. Some people find them less irritating to the gastrointestinal tract than ascorbic acid. Sodium ascorbate and calcium ascorbate are the most common forms, although a number of other mineral ascorbates are available. Sodium ascorbate generally provides 131 mg of sodium per 1,000 mg of ascorbic acid, and pure calcium ascorbate provides 114 mg of calcium per 1,000 mg of ascorbic acid.

Buffered vitamin C powder is prepared from beets (virtually all other forms are derived from corn). Because

TABLE 3.3	
Good Food Sources of Vitamin C	
Food/ Serving Size	Vitamin C Content
Fresh Orange Juice, 1 cup	124 mg
Green Pepper, $1/2$ cup	96 mg
Grapefruit Juice, 1 cup	93 mg
Papaya, $1/2$ medium	85 mg
Brussels Sprouts, 4 medium	73 mg
Broccoli, Raw, $1/2$ cup	70 mg
Orange, 1 medium	66 mg
Cantaloupe, $1/4$ medium	45 mg
Cauliflower, $1/2$ cup	45 mg
Strawberries, $1/2$ cup	44 mg
Tomato Juice, 1 cup	39 mg
Cabbage, $1/2$ cup	21 mg
Blackberries, $1/2$ cup	15 mg
Spinach, Raw, $1/2$ cup	14 mg
Blueberries, $1/2$ cup	10 mg
Cherries, $1/2$ cup	8 mg

Note: *Values given are estimates derived from the USDA Nutrient Values database.*

buffered vitamin C has an acid-alkaline buffering action, it can help control the increased acidity often associated with allergic reactions. Many of the most severely ill, allergic, or hypersensitive people can tolerate buffered C, even when unable to tolerate other vitamin C products.

Bioflavonoids are water-soluble plant pigments that are often found in vitamin C–rich fruits and vegetables, especially citrus fruit. Vitamin C activity is enhanced when taken with natural bioflavonoids, such as hesperidin and rutin.

Ascorbyl palmitate is a fat-soluble form of vitamin C that protects fats from peroxidation. Ascorbyl palmitate can be stored in the body in small amounts. It has been added to a number of skin creams due to its antioxidant properties and the role of vitamin C in collagen synthesis.

CONCLUSION

Millions of years ago, a genetic accident impaired our ability to produce vitamin C, a basic requirement for life. If not for this ancient genetic accident, humans today would normally produce vitamin C in levels measured in tens of grams per day. Evidence suggests that restoring vitamin C to higher levels would benefit modern human health and reduce the incidence of degenerative and infectious diseases, fend off the effects of old age, and endow all with longer lives.

Today, vitamin C is becoming one of the most widely used and valued vitamins due to its ability to help humans correct our inherited genetic defect. In addition to being the safest vitamin known to us, we have seen how the vast array of important health benefits of vitamin C improve health and prolong life by:

1. Acting as a powerful, water-soluble antioxidant to protect us against free radicals. Vitamin C has also been proven to save lives by reducing the oxidative damage that causes atherosclerosis.

2. Producing healthy collagen and strong connective tissues to keep muscles, blood vessels, bones, and teeth young and healthy.

3. Helping the body use other vital nutrients, such as folic acid (for maintaining healthy DNA) and iron (for hemoglobin, the oxygen-carrying part of blood cells).

4. Aiding the synthesis of neurotransmitters that energize us, help us sleep, control aches and pains, and maintain a positive mood.

5. Supporting the immune system in the constant battle against cancer, infections, and the degenerative diseases common to aging.

6. Increasing formation of liver bile to aid in the removal of cholesterol and potentially toxic substances, such as lead.

7. Helping to transport and burn fats and carbohydrates in the mitochondria for energy.

8. Keeping blood vessels and arteries open and dilated to prevent arterial spasms and heart attacks.

9. Maintaining antioxidant levels in the eyes to prevent macular degeneration and cataracts.

10. Protecting people with diabetes from the damage caused by increased levels of sorbitol in the bloodstream.

We hope that this brief overview of vitamin C has conveyed some of the power and importance of this essential antiaging, anticancer, and antistress nutrient. Hopefully we have conveyed the very real message, that—whether you get your vitamin C from fruits and vegetables, or high-potency vitamins—the evidence proves that you can expect to live a longer, healthier, and more fulfilling life.

PART FOUR

Coenzyme Q$_{10}$

Marty Zucker

You are the sum of your cellular parts—all several hundred trillion cells. And how you feel and function depends on how they feel and function. And how they feel and function has a lot to do with coenzyme Q$_{10}$, better known as CoQ$_{10}$, a vitaminlike substance produced throughout your body. Without this substance, your cells—and thus, you—couldn't survive.

For starters, CoQ$_{10}$ is a fundamental ingredient in the energy production that keeps those trillions of cells running smoothly. A shortage of CoQ$_{10}$ translates into an energy crunch, with you and your cells running on weak batteries.

Unfortunately, that situation describes a lot of people, many of whom are outright deficient. Low levels of CoQ$_{10}$ generate a negative impact on health and, very likely, the aging process itself.

Besides generating energy, CoQ$_{10}$ is one of the body's most powerful antioxidants. It protects you against free radicals, the destructive molecular fragments that cause accelerated aging and degenerative diseases. And, according to exciting new research, CoQ$_{10}$ also activates certain genes in a way that appears to strengthen you against disease and rejuvenate your body.

Sadly, most doctors either haven't heard of CoQ$_{10}$ or just ignore its importance. That's a tragedy because simply increasing the level of CoQ$_{10}$ in the body pays off with big health, energy, and therapeutic dividends.

Fortunately, CoQ$_{10}$ is available as a nutritional supplement. It's a natural copy of what your body makes, and it's wonderfully safe to take. Unlike pharmaceutical drugs, you don't develop bad side effects from taking it. Moreover, you don't need a prescription. You can buy it in health food stores just as you would vitamin C, ginkgo biloba, or any other supplement.

Since the 1960s, scientists in Japan, Europe, Australia, India, and the United States have been studying the healing impact of CoQ$_{10}$, primarily on cardiovascular conditions. But during the last decade, research has expanded dynamically into many age-related diseases, including baffling brain disorders, as well as the aging process itself.

To date, there have been more than four thousand scientific studies and eleven international conferences dedicated to CoQ$_{10}$. Yet researchers feel they have only scratched the surface in their understanding of CoQ$_{10}$'s formidable functions and how supplementation may contribute to better health. What's known to date distinguishes CoQ$_{10}$ as a healing superstar and lifesaver.

Continuing research promises much more good news. In laboratories and clinics worldwide, researchers and doctors are discovering major therapeutic and preventive uses for CoQ$_{10}$. In Part Four, you'll learn about the benefits and promise of CoQ$_{10}$, including:

- Disease prevention and slowing down the aging process in the body.

- Significant help for patients with heart disease.

- Reduction of mild to moderate hypertension.

- More energy, strength, and vitality, even for older people.

- Fortification of the immune system against illness, including cancer.

- Counteracting the adverse effects of cholesterol-lowering drugs.

- Improvement of nervous system and brain disorders.

- Protection against gum disease, a condition affecting most adults.

These are all major considerations for individuals interested in optimum health and optimum lifespan. As you read on, you will learn how CoQ$_{10}$ contributes to both.

THE "BIRTH" OF AN AMAZING MOLECULE

Back in 1957, Fred Crane, Ph.D., was a young research biochemist and assistant professor working at the University of Wisconsin's Enzyme Institute. He and his colleagues were investigating the biochemical sequence involved in cellular energy production.

Crane, now seventy-six years old and retired, recalls, "we could partly put the sequence together, but something was missing in our understanding of these molecular events. I was assigned the job to find the missing link."

The researchers were working with beef heart mitochondria. Mitochondria are where energy is produced inside cells. You will be hearing a lot about them in this book.

Mitochondria
Organelles—microscopic organs—within cells where oxygen and the derivatives of the food you eat are mixed to produce energy.

Mitochondria, present in both animal and plant cells, are center stage for the activity of CoQ_{10}. But Crane and his team didn't know it at the time. In fact, no scientist had ever heard of CoQ_{10}.

Extracurricular Research Pays Off

On weekends, Crane liked to return to the laboratory and continue his scientific sleuthing. At one point he began examining cauliflower mitochondria.

"This wasn't part of the program, but I always enjoyed variety, doing something different," he says. "So I chopped up the cauliflower, centrifuged the mush, and separated out the mitochondria. On Monday mornings, when my colleagues returned to the lab, they would complain that I was stinking up the place with cauliflower."

Smell aside, Crane's extracurricular research led to pay dirt. He first discovered carotenes (pigments) in the cauliflower mitochondria. He thought these could be the sought-after missing link. Turning back to beef hearts, he found a small amount of carotenes, but a large mass of yellowish substance that had different properties. He collected the material and put it aside in the lab's refrigerator while he continued studying the carotenes.

"One day I looked back in the fridge," he recalls, "and there was this tube full of the other stuff which had formed big yellow crystals. I thought maybe it might be good for something."

From Beef Hearts to the Nobel Prize

Measuring the material with a technique called light-absorption spectrum, Crane determined that it was a quinone—a family of organic compounds that he knew to have properties related to energy conversion.

Looking for confirmation, he sent off a sample of the yellow stuff to Karl Folkers, Ph.D., a leading biochemist at Merck, Sharpe, and Dohme Laboratories in New Jersey. Folkers' analysis showed that the substance was indeed a quinone, and just in case you are interested, he identified its chemical structure as 2,3, dimethoxy-5-methyl-6-decaprenyl-1, 4-benzoquinone. It was a relatively large, worm-shaped molecule. Other biochemists would call it ubiquinone because the molecule was found to be ubiquitous—widespread in living organisms.

Indeed, it turned out to be the missing link, and a major link at that.

Some years later, in 1978, British biochemist Peter Mitchell, Ph.D., would earn the Nobel Prize in chemistry for describing the complicated and exquisite process of cellular power production. And there, smack in the middle of that process, would be CoQ_{10}.

Birth of a CoQ_{10} Champion

But back in 1958, Crane's shipment of yellow stuff set off a flurry of scientific investigation at the Merck lab. Folkers and his colleagues dug into it with relish. They soon learned how to synthesize the compound, which they named coenzyme Q_{10} (CoQ_{10} for short). A coenzyme is a substance, like a vitamin, that contributes to essential chemical reactions, and in the case of CoQ_{10}, it contributes to "bioenergetics," the process of cellular energy production.

Folkers left Merck in 1963 to become president of Stanford Research Institute, a position he held for five years. Then, for the next thirty years, he served as research professor of chemistry, and later as director of the Institute for Biomedical Research at the University of Texas in Austin.

Folkers had been smitten by CoQ_{10}. And until his death in 1997 at age ninety-one, he ardently conducted and encouraged research on the basic biochemistry and clinical applications of CoQ_{10}.

Absolutely Essential for Life

In 1972, along with Italian researcher Gian Paolo Littarru, M.D., Folkers first determined there was a deficiency of CoQ_{10} in heart disease. This original research led to numerous studies showing major therapeutic benefits for heart patients supplemented with CoQ_{10}. (Later you can read more about the great connection to heart health.)

For years, much of the research and the clinical uses of CoQ_{10} centered on the heart and cardiovascular system. But more recently, scientists have looked beyond the heart and found promising uses for it against cancer, muscle, and brain disorders, as well as its intriguing potential as an "antiaging" factor.

The mounting reports from researchers worldwide validate Folkers' belief that medical science would come to recognize many important benefits for CoQ_{10}. He repeatedly told interviewers that "every life function requires biochemical energy and CoQ_{10} is a major mechanism in the process. It is absolutely essential for life."

For his years of outstanding research, Folkers received many honors, including presidential science awards from Harry Truman in 1948 and George Bush in 1990.

Your Body Makes CoQ_{10}, but . . .

Almost every cell in the body produces CoQ_{10}, yet many people are deficient in CoQ_{10}. Here are five reasons why:

Reason No. 1: Diet

It takes a number of key ingredients for your body to synthesize, or make, CoQ$_{10}$. The recipe calls for the amino acid tyrosine and at least seven vitamins (B$_2$, B$_3$, B$_6$, folic acid, B$_{12}$, pantothenic acid, and C).

According to Folkers, "The problem is that people in general eat poorly, and don't get an adequate level of good nutrients, so they often fail to produce enough."

This assessment fits right in with current nutritional surveys, which consistently find a large percentage of people deficient in essential vitamins and minerals.

Take vitamin B$_6$, for example, one of the critical ingredients in the CoQ$_{10}$ recipe. If you look at any list of common deficiencies, you'll find B$_6$ a regular entry. The vitamin is particularly low among older people and those eating a diet high in refined carbohydrates and low in vegetables and fruits. One study specifically designed to look at this connection did indeed determine that the customary intake of vitamin B$_6$ doesn't support an optimum production of CoQ$_{10}$.

You can extract some CoQ$_{10}$ directly from the food you eat. But that depends on what you eat. CoQ$_{10}$ is naturally present in small quantities in many foods. The best sources are organ meats such as heart, kidney, and liver, as well as mackerel, peanuts, salmon, sardines, and soy oil—foods we tend not to eat a lot.

Just to obtain the equivalent of a 30-mg supplement, you would have to eat one pound of sardines, two pounds of beef, or two and one-half pounds of peanuts. Thirty milligrams may be fine for general health maintenance, but it isn't nearly enough to produce therapeutic benefits against disease.

Cardiologist Peter Langsjoen, M.D., of Tyler, Texas, has used CoQ$_{10}$ for his patients longer than any other physician in the country. He says that even by eating a lot of fish you can probably consume only the equivalent of 5–10 mg a day.

"That's what the average Dane gets in a diet high in fish," he says. "But without the fish it is likely you will only get 3 to 5 mg. The key is fish. It's loaded with CoQ$_{10}$. Also beef, chicken, and pork hearts . . . but nobody eats them."

Langsjoen says his new patients are typically deficient. That's also the experience of Stephen T. Sinatra, M.D., a cardiologist in Manchester, Connecticut, who became so impressed with CoQ$_{10}$ that he wrote a book about it: *The Coenzyme Q$_{10}$ Phenomenon* (Keats Publishing, 1998).

"I regularly do blood levels of CoQ$_{10}$ and find that new patients are low," he says. "I believe there are significant deficiencies in the population."

Reason No. 2: The Aging Factor

The body's production of CoQ$_{10}$ slows down with age. Sci-entists say it starts happening after the age of twenty, with a more accelerated drop after forty.

"Production kind of poops out," says CoQ$_{10}$ discoverer Fred Crane. "And the most obvious place where CoQ$_{10}$ works is in the mitochondria. So, if you don't have enough, then you might not produce energy as well in your cells. This may help to explain why older people slow down."

Reason No. 3: Cholesterol Drugs

The pharmaceutical industry is vigorously promoting cholesterol-lowering drugs (statins), even among healthy people as a preventive agent, yet this class of pharmaceuticals has a dark side that few people know about. Research shows these drugs interfere with CoQ$_{10}$ production in the body. This is a major problem that will be discussed in detail later.

Reason No. 4: Extreme Physical Exertion

Regular moderate exercise is thought to stimulate the body's production of CoQ$_{10}$. However, experts say that exhaustive and prolonged exercise depletes CoQ$_{10}$. That's because the body needs more of it to fuel the increased activity.

At risk are high performance athletes as well as weekend-warrior types who go out and cycle 100 miles or run 20 miles on a weekend.

"They burn up a tremendous amount of CoQ$_{10}$, and other nutrients necessary for CoQ$_{10}$ production," says Langsjoen. "And if they are not replacing these factors in their diet, they may be hurting themselves."

The cardiologist cites the case of a patient fresh from Navy Seal training who had heart muscle weakness. "These are very tough and fit people who go through incredibly exhausting training," Langsjoen says. "They have a grinding schedule, and then to top it off, go days without rest.

"I have seen heart muscle weakness in many obsessive, compulsive joggers who essentially run themselves down. I wonder if that is what happened with the Navy Seal. It's not proven, but I think a deficiency state is created. The end result is a dilated heart."

Reason No. 5: Hyperthyroidism

An overactive thyroid gland—hyperthyroidism—raises the level of thyroid hormone in the body. This can cause such typical signs as anxiety, bulging of the eyes, fast or irregular heart rhythms, irritability, muscle weakness, and weight loss.

Too much thyroid hormone accelerates metabolism. One of the less recognized consequences of this is the drain put on the body's CoQ$_{10}$ supply, which can, in turn, deplete CoQ$_{10}$ and cause additional problems.

"The heart is usually a primary target," says Sinatra. "Not only arrhythmias, but even heart failure may result. I have seen the connection to heart failure in patients who were not previously diagnosed with overactive thyroid and who didn't have the usual hyperthyroid symptoms."

Sinatra suggests that patients with thyroid irregularities, and particularly with excess thyroid hormone, should be on supplemental CoQ_{10}.

THE GREAT ENERGIZER

You probably know somebody like one of my relatives (who shall remain anonymous). After a typical workday, he would sit back in his living room easy chair and do the typical couch-potato thing: watch TV for a couple of hours and then doze off. That was his pattern before he began taking CoQ_{10}.

"Now," he says, "I go out more with my wife, have gotten involved in more activities, and don't feel as bone tired as I used to. My energy level has really improved. I feel a whole lot younger."

At fifty-two, my relative had become concerned about learning new tasks at his job and about what he felt was increasing forgetfulness. He thought he might be developing Alzheimer's disease.

"But since taking CoQ_{10}, I have found that I can again concentrate and learn as well as when I was younger," he confided. "I really believe this CoQ_{10} stuff has given me a lot of physical and mental energy back."

Such comments are typical of CoQ_{10} users and even of physicians who recommend CoQ_{10} supplementation to patients.

Your Energy Level Depends on Your Cells

You eat, drink, and breathe. Deep down in the mitochondria of your cells, the ingredients of those fundamental actions are converted into the energy to unleash countless thoughts, secretions, nerve impulses, and muscle contractions.

The mitochondria, as you will remember from the beginning of Part Four, are the microscopic "power plants" in your cells where the wondrous biochemical process called "bioenergetics" goes on endlessly during a lifetime.

Inside these rod- or round-shaped dynamos is an inner sanctum of membrane folds projecting inward from the outer membrane. An extremely complex sequence of chemical reactions takes place in these membranes involving enzymes, protons, electrons, and electrical charges.

Enzymes
Specialized proteins that act as catalysts to promote the billions of biochemical reactions necessary for virtually all life processes.

For the sake of simplicity, think of a cell gathering in oxygen, along with sugars and fatty acids from food, and dispatching them to the mitochondria. There, the raw materials are processed by enzymes to produce a substance called adenosine triphosphate, or ATP for short. ATP acts like a high-octane fuel to stoke virtually all the cells in the body.

Electrons extracted from the food are utilized to make ATP. CoQ_{10} molecules carry out a starring role in this process by shuttling electrons back and forth between enzymes. This, according to Karl Folkers, is the primary function of CoQ_{10} in the body.

The arrangement inside the mitochondria is like a precision assembly line. Raw materials come in at one end. ATP molecules come out the other.

Works Like a Car Engine

You can also think of this process in terms of a car engine. It takes oxygen, gasoline, and a spark to create the energy to drive the pistons to turn the crankshaft to move the wheels.

Just as engine problems can cause a car to malfunction or operate feebly, problems with mitochondria can cause similar trouble in the body.

The cells in the body each contain between 500 and 2,000 mitochondria. When they don't function properly, an "energy crisis" develops. Faltering energy production in individual cells initiates a cascade of disorder and inefficiency throughout the body. Over time, the damage from energy shortfall spreads to tissues and organ systems.

Brain, heart, and muscle cells, the heaviest consumers of energy, start to struggle. They stop performing well. They fail to carry out their basic functions. If enough vitality and function is lost, affected cells commit suicide. Tissues begin to degenerate.

CoQ_{10} Deficiency Spells Trouble

Think about it. Cells need energy to perform all the specialized things they do for the body, such as producing enzymes, hormones, muscle contractions, and nerve impulses; fighting off bacteria and viruses; or breaking down food with acids. Cells also have to carry out basic household chores, such as nourishing themselves and getting rid of waste products. And cells also have to reproduce—we started, after all, from one fertilized egg cell. All this requires energy.

Cardiologist Stephen Sinatra sums it up this way: "Without adequate energy the cells become inefficient, lackluster, and vulnerable to disease and toxic buildup. When a deficiency of CoQ_{10} exists, the cellular 'engines' misfire and, over time, they may eventually fail or even die. The bioenergetics of a failing heart or a failing immune system will inevitably lead to the weakening of all the natural defenses against disease and premature aging."

That's how vital CoQ_{10} is to your cells and, ultimately, to you. And that's why supplementation can make a big difference in energy for so many people. Remember, we lose some of our ability to produce CoQ_{10} as we get older, so don't be caught short.

THE GREAT ANTIOXIDANT

When a nuclear bomb explodes, the blast of powerful radiation triggers a firestorm of "free radicals" that virtually wipes out everything in its path. Free radicals are not showers of shrapnel. Rather, they are runaway electrons that create chain reactions of destruction at the atomic level.

There are no atomic bombs in the cells of our body, but chain reactions instigated by electrons go on everywhere and all the time.

As we have seen, our cells utilize oxygen atoms to produce energy in the mitochondria. One byproduct of this normal process is the constant creation of a huge number of free radicals. This poses a threat not only to the mitochondria but also to the rest of the cell.

Free radicals are simply "free" electrons that have broken loose from their attachments to the nuclei of oxygen atoms during the energy process. Electrons like company, so they seek other electrons to pair up with. This activity, repeated countless times in countless cells, sets off a chain reaction of damage that starts with adjacent atoms and molecules. Over time, it engulfs tissues and eventually organ systems.

This domino effect, first theorized more than thirty years ago by Denham Harman, M.D., Ph.D., a University of Nebraska researcher, is the most widely accepted scientific explanation for aging. His free radical theory of aging holds that free radicals are causal factors in nearly every known disease, as well as the aging process itself.

Terrorists inside Our Bodies

Free radicals are like terrorists inside our bodies. They attack DNA, leading to dysfunction, mutation, and cancer. They attack enzymes and proteins, causing mayhem in normal cell activities. They attack cell membranes.

In the cells that line our blood vessels, this can lead to hardening and thickening of the arteries and eventually to heart attacks and strokes. Free radical damage to the protein in connective tissue can cause stiffness in the body.

The "oxidative stress" inflicted by free radicals on tissues is similar to the oxidation of metal that leads to rusting; or the oxidation of a fat, such as butter, that turns it rancid.

Besides the natural processes inside the body that generate damaging oxidative stress, free radical activity can also be increased and raised to dangerous overload level by lifestyle and environmental factors. They include alcohol; air pollution; chemical contaminants; chemotherapy; certain pharmaceutical drugs; excess exposure to sunlight; pesticides; physical and emotional stress; processed, smoked, or barbecued foods; and smoking.

The body fights back with antioxidants, compounds that counteract free radicals. Your cells make antioxidants, and you can also get antioxidants from food, notably fruits and vegetables, and supplements. It's when free radicals are not contained at a tolerable level by antioxidants that they set off their destructive blitz of oxidation.

Many years ago, Denham Harman, M.D., Ph.D., theorized that vitamins such as E and C could counteract free radical activity in the body and thereby slow the aging process because these nutrients were found to have antioxidant properties. Harman's subsequent research demonstrated for the first time that feeding a variety of antioxidants to mammals could extend their lifespans.

Antioxidant
A molecule that donates electrons to stabilize damaging free radicals.

There is now a massive volume of scientific evidence demonstrating that people who eat a diet high in antioxidants and who take antioxidant supplements will live longer, healthier lives.

"You can halt and even reverse many of the age-related problems that can arise (and make life so miserable) when our bodies suffer from an overabundance of free radicals and a deficit of antioxidants," says Lester Packer, Ph.D., of the University of California at Berkeley, and a renowned authority on antioxidants.

Super Antioxidants

Hundreds of antioxidants have been identified, and until recently, these compounds were thought to work independently of one another. However, at Packer's world-famous laboratory, scientists have discovered that a few of them have a unique and dynamic interplay that greatly strengthens their individual effectiveness.

The members of this select super group are CoQ₁₀, glutathione, lipoic acid, and vitamins C and E. Packer calls them *network antioxidants*.

"Network antioxidants have special powers that set them apart from other antioxidants," says Packer in his book *The Antioxidant Miracle* (John Wiley & Sons, 1999). "They are particularly effective in slowing down the aging process and boosting the body's ability to fight disease. The antioxidant network is a shield that protects the body against the forces that age us before our time and rob years from our lives."

Vitamins C and E must be obtained in food. They are not produced by the body. However, to obtain an optimum antioxidant level of these vitamins through food is virtually impossible. And while we make our own CoQ₁₀, glutathione, and lipoic acid, the levels decrease as we age.

"That is why we need to supplement all of them," says Packer. "More than 70 percent of Americans will die prematurely from diseases caused by, or compounded by deficiencies of the antioxidant network," he contends.

Why CoQ$_{10}$ Is So Special

Across the ocean from Packer's antioxidant laboratory in California, a group of Australian scientists at the Heart Research Institute in Sydney have brought to light some of the qualities of CoQ$_{10}$ that make it so special.

Under the direction of Roland Stocker, Ph.D., they made the fascinating discovery that vitamin E itself can become a highly energized and reactive compound when it "scavenges" free radicals.

"Vitamin E can become a 'hot coal,' potentially damaging other molecules, unless it is brought back to a stable condition by a further partner in a chain which eventually terminates the process," says Stocker. Such partners are CoQ$_{10}$ and vitamin C.

Researchers at the Australian institute have also demonstrated that CoQ$_{10}$ is a primary antioxidant protector of low-density lipoproteins (known as LDL, or so-called harmful cholesterol). In one 1992 study on healthy young adults, they found that CoQ$_{10}$ generated a "remarkable resistance" of LDL to oxidative damage. Too much oxidized LDL is damaging to the body because it leads to the formation of artery-narrowing plaque, a contributing condition for heart attacks and strokes.

A later study, conducted in Italy and published in the *Proceedings of the National Academy of Sciences USA*, suggested that CoQ$_{10}$ may, in fact, be far more effective than any other antioxidant in blocking LDL oxidation.

The Super Mitochondria Protector

Over the years, many laboratory and clinical studies have yielded mounting evidence that supplemental CoQ$_{10}$ offers a broad spectrum of protection against free radical activity. Research has shown it can protect, not just the arteries, but the brain, liver, muscles, nerves, and other systems in the body.

Much of this ability has to do with CoQ$_{10}$'s most critical antioxidant performance: inside the mitochondrial membranes where bioenergetics takes place.

Years ago, as Denham Harman evolved his free radical theory of aging, he introduced the idea that free radicals generated in the mitochondria "have the power to kill us." For that reason, he emphasized the importance of getting antioxidants into the mitochondria.

Today, a great deal of research has confirmed this concept. In fact, mitochondrial disease has become a booming segment of medical research and is being seen as a major cause of many degenerative conditions.

Along with this increased scientific interest has emerged a parallel interest in CoQ$_{10}$ research because of its central contributions to mitochondrial "business." In the next section, we will see yet another contribution.

THE GREAT ANTIAGING "SECRET"

So far we've seen that you need CoQ$_{10}$ to keep you energized. Just like the spark in the engine of a car. We've also seen that it's a super antioxidant snuffing out damaging free radicals throughout the body and notably the torrent unleashed by energy production in trillions of cells.

So, CoQ$_{10}$ sparks your engine and prevents it from oxidizing and "rusting." Using the automotive analogy one more time, now we'll see how CoQ$_{10}$ also puts the brakes on the aging process.

Turning Around Ailing, Aging Patients

Peter Langsjoen, M.D., has been prescribing CoQ$_{10}$ to patients since the mid-1980s. "A large number of my patients are elderly and are doing great just on CoQ$_{10}$ alone," he says. "You can't believe how active, healthy, and happy they are on virtually no medicine.

Aging
A complex biological process over time marked by a progressive decline in the performance of individual tissues and organs, and leading to age-associated disease and senility.

"When I see new patients in their 80s, coming in on walkers, I try to simplify their drugs if they are on a bunch of things, and I put them on CoQ$_{10}$. These are individuals who have been declining gradually and feeling poorly for a very long time. Typically, when I see them back again in six or eight weeks, they are different people. They can't believe how much better they feel, and how fast it has happened. It makes the practice of medicine very gratifying."

Half a world away from Texas, down under in Australia, a distinguished molecular biologist named Anthony W. Linnane, Ph.D., has repeatedly shown in scientific studies how CoQ$_{10}$ can turn aging and ailing patients like this around so dramatically.

Linnane is director of the Center for Molecular Biology and Medicine in Melbourne, a non-profit medical research institution. Interestingly, he started his career studying mitochondria in the very same University of Wisconsin laboratory where Fred Crane discovered CoQ$_{10}$ . . . and at around the same time.

In 1989, Linnane published a theory in the prestigious medical journal *Lancet* that elaborated on Denham Harman's earlier proposal that the aging process actually begins in the mitochondria. He called his theory, "the universality of bioenergetic disease."

If you happened to skip over the last two sections, I suggest you go back and read about the mitochondria, and the process of bioenergetics and free radical mayhem that goes on there. The information is key to understanding how

CoQ$_{10}$ works and also provides a background for what follows here.

The DNA Connection

The nucleus of cells, as we also know, contains the DNA that gives us our genetic heritage. For years, most scientists thought this was where aging originated.

Nuclear DNA can defend itself pretty well against free radical damage. It has good repair mechanisms. Mitochondria also have a genetic system of their own. This system, in concert with nuclear DNA, is required to maintain functional mitochondria. But unlike nuclear DNA, the genetic material inside mitochondria is much less efficient in repelling the flood of free radicals generated by the energy process.

Moreover, random mutations in mitochondrial DNA occur throughout a life of ongoing replication and increase with advancing age.

Where Aging Really Takes Place

Free radical damage increases with age as new generations of defective mitochondria replicate. Less and less energy is produced as a result. "Progressive depletion of energy production . . . is associated with the gradual decline of the physiological and biochemical performance of organs, significantly contributing to the aging process and ultimately to death," says Linnane.

In his research, the Australian molecular scientist repeatedly observed mutated mitochondria in yeast organisms, and then in the cells of laboratory animals and humans. "If you take a culture of yeast and grow them overnight, the next morning you have some mutants among them," he says. "Most of the cells will be normal, but a percentage won't be normal.

Mitochondrial Mutations: An Important Aspect of Aging

"We are basically no different. We are just an aggregation of cells, like a bacteria or yeast culture, but we are specialized, a collection of liver cells, muscle cells, or brain cells, but fundamentally the processes are the same.

"As our cells divide, more mutation occurs. The mutations add up over time. Energy degrades. We progressively lose power. And not only power, like in muscle power, but our metabolism begins to degrade as well. So, one important feature of aging, in my concept, is that we bioenergetically degrade because of mitochondrial mutation."

In other words, Linnane believes that the progressive accumulation of ongoing mitochondrial DNA mutation with age leads to a decline in cellular/ tissue bioenergy which, in turn, contributes to pathology. And in particular, he has in mind degenerative diseases of the blood vessels, brain, heart, and muscles.

CoQ$_{10}$ to the Rescue

Researchers, including Linnane, have experimented with CoQ$_{10}$ supplementation and find it inhibits the degradation and generates a partial re-energization of aging cells. This can help minimize the effects of aging and age-related diseases, they believe.

In one experiment with a long-lived breed of laboratory mice, researchers at UCLA found that the rodents supplemented with CoQ$_{10}$ after birth demonstrated a far greater level of activity as older animals than a non-supplemented group, and lived, on average, 20 percent longer.

Linnane has worked with Franklin Rosenfeldt, M.D., an Australian cardiology researcher, in both animal and human studies that have dramatically demonstrated the CoQ$_{10}$ relationship to mitochondrial stress, decline, and aging.

In one study, they experimented with specimens of heart tissue taken from patients of different ages who had been through heart surgery. In the laboratory, the specimens were exposed to oxygen deprivation and simulated ischemia, that is, interruption of blood flow. Later, the specimens were examined to determine how well they recovered from the ordeal.

It is well recognized that younger patients recover faster from a heart attack or cardiac surgery than elderly patients, so it came as no surprise that the tissues taken from older patients demonstrated inferior recovery. In addition, the researchers found a strong connection between the integrity of the mitochondrial DNA in the tissue and the recovery rate.

Differences between Old and Young Tissue Eliminated

In a subsequent study, they then exposed heart tissue to CoQ$_{10}$ and subjected the specimens to the stress of simulated ischemia. Now, they reported, the difference in recovery between the tissue of older and younger patients was "abolished."

In yet another dramatic demonstration of CoQ$_{10}$ power, they supplemented one group of old rats for six weeks and then put the animals through simulated aerobic exercise. Afterward, they compared the CoQ$_{10}$ rodents to non-supplemented rats, both older and younger, who also went through the exercise trial.

The researchers found that the supplemented older rats performed and recovered just as well as the young rats. Moreover, these older rats on CoQ$_{10}$ exhibited four times as much work capacity as the non-supplemented older rats. "We were astounded by the results," says Linnane.

In continuing studies, Linnane, Rosenfeldt, and their Australian colleagues have worked with human patients and further demonstrated the remarkable ability of CoQ$_{10}$ to rekindle mitochondrial firepower and recovery. You will read more about their amazing findings in the next chapter.

CoQ$_{10}$ and Antiaging Genes

In Anthony Linnane's latest research, he has opened an entirely new chapter on CoQ$_{10}$'s antiaging potential. Not only does CoQ$_{10}$ function as an energizer and antioxidant in the mitochondria, but Linnane now believes it also activates the genes in the nuclear DNA to combat disease and essentially "turn back the clock" in cells.

Genes
A unit of DNA, the biochemical information database carrying the complete instructions for making all the proteins in a cell. Each gene contains specific instructions to make a particular protein.

CoQ$_{10}$ does this by sending a chemical messenger to the nucleus. The process is far too complicated to explain here, but the messenger, it turns out, is actually a free radical called a peroxide that switches on certain strategic genes. The result is to fortify cellular systems in places where they have degraded, for instance, through the aging process. Thus, CoQ$_{10}$ acts as a general regulator of cell metabolism to help maintain vital cellular functions.

"A powerful reaction sweeps across the whole of cellular metabolism, and weakened cells suddenly develop renewed strength and vitality," says Linnane. He believes this is how CoQ$_{10}$ additionally benefits people suffering from a wide variety of conditions, from cancer to chronic fatigue and heart disease.

"People have never been able to understand how CoQ$_{10}$ can do so many things that are reported in the anecdotal medical literature," he says. "This particular action could be the missing component that explains CoQ$_{10}$'s impact on so many healing fronts."

Making Muscles Younger

His latest study, published in the journal *Free-Radical Research* in 2002, offers a first-ever glimpse into how CoQ$_{10}$ can regulate genes. The study made use of excised thigh-muscle tissue routinely removed from patients during hip replacement surgery. Such tissue is normally discarded.

But Linnane and his colleagues had a better use for the discards. First, they selected a group of older patients scheduled for this type of surgery at a Melbourne hospital. The patients were then randomly assigned to take either 300 mg of CoQ$_{10}$ or an inert pill called a placebo. They were to follow this routine daily for the month before surgery.

After each surgery, the researchers collected the removed muscle tissue and put the specimens through a comprehensive series of analyses. They then compared the tissue taken from supplemented and non-supplement patients.

"What we found was very exciting," says Linnane. "We found that CoQ$_{10}$ could change gene expression, that is, modulate gene expression in a significant way."

Specifically, they discovered that, after just one month, the muscle tissue taken from aging patients who were supplemented with CoQ$_{10}$ was beginning to change toward a more youthful profile.

The First-Ever Physiological Change from CoQ$_{10}$ Supplementation

In general, the quadriceps and other muscles are made up of different fiber types, like ropes, that slide across each other. The types are called slow- and fast-twitch fibers. As we age, we lose muscle tissue, but the fast type, associated with explosive strength, is progressively lost at a faster rate than slow-twitch muscles, which are associated with endurance.

"As we looked at the fibers in these specimens we could clearly see they were different from the fiber profile of a young person," says Linnane. "But when we compared the fibers of the elderly patients who were supplemented and those who were not, we found that the supplementation produced a dramatic change toward a younger profile.

"Mind you, the supplemented tissue didn't go back to a state you could say was a young profile, and we didn't make elderly people young again, but the CoQ$_{10}$ generated degrees of change in that direction," he adds. "Along with that, the supplemented people told us they began to feel better, stronger, and more energized."

The study, Linnane says, is the first demonstration of an actual physiological change from CoQ$_{10}$ supplementation.

"Huge" Antiaging Potential

"In order to do that, you would have to switch on a number of genes," Linnane explains. "You can't change muscle fiber otherwise. Hundreds of genes are required to make a muscle fiber. So, we found that CoQ$_{10}$ modulated the genes relevant to muscle biochemistry and function, switching them back toward the re-creation of a somewhat younger profile. This is a striking result that clearly warrants more research and more funding."

Linnane says that such changes wouldn't continue indefinitely and would likely reach a plateau. Still, he was delighted that a change of this nature was seen in only one month.

"CoQ$_{10}$ makes cells stronger, more energized, and more competent to combat a wide range of diseases, and perhaps even prevent degenerative diseases that develop over long periods of time," he says.

"The research suggests that CoQ$_{10}$ may dynamically support and strengthen the remaining physiological assets in an aging person. It can't put back what's gone, but hopefully it may slow the whole process. We need further research to clarify this.

"The key to all these marvelous functions of CoQ$_{10}$ is that the substance be present in enough quantity. We know that as the body ages, there is less and less of it, so that's where supplementation comes in."

When asked about the importance of CoQ$_{10}$ as an anti-aging factor, Linnane answers unequivocally: "It has a huge potential. Supplementation is clearly indicated to improve the quality of life of older people and to provide protection against many age-related conditions."

From a clinical standpoint, doctors who use CoQ$_{10}$ in their practice, believe strongly that CoQ$_{10}$ indeed protects and rejuvenates.

"I see people with heart conditions and many other additional problems and they tell me that they have their life back, that they have renewed spark and energy," says Connecticut cardiologist Stephen Sinatra. "Their quality of life as a result of taking CoQ$_{10}$, whether they have heart disease or not, or whether they have chronic fatigue, or are just elderly and moving slower, will improve with CoQ$_{10}$."

KEEPING YOUR HEART HEALTHY LONGER

It should not come as a surprise that the cells of the heart muscle are packed with mitochondria. In fact, they make up about a quarter of the volume in heart cells, more than anywhere else in the body.

That's obviously Nature's way of generating the power necessary to drive the heart's non-stop pumping action over a lifetime. Talk about a work schedule!

Your heart pushes blood (with its essential cargo of oxygen and nutrients) through a 60,000-mile network of blood vessels to nourish your brain, your feet, and everything in between. Every day, the heart muscle expands and contracts about 100,000 times, recycling 2,000 gallons of blood through your body. In a year, it contracts 36 million times.

That takes a lot of energy, and, yes, a lot of CoQ$_{10}$.

Mitochondrial Mutations and the Aging Heart

In the last chapter, we have seen how mutations of mitochondrial DNA cause a loss of energy in cells, and contribute to weakness, disease, and aging. In one Japanese study published in the *Molecular and Cellular Biochemistry Journal*, researchers found an accelerated rate of mitochondrial mutation in aging human hearts, and markedly so over the age of eighty. They concluded that such mutations play an important role in ebbing cardiac function among older people, and particularly in heart failure.

Protection of mitochondrial DNA against oxidative damage is of "primary importance in preventing the age-associated decline in cardiac performance," they emphasized.

CoQ$_{10}$, we have learned in the last chapter, protects mitochondrial DNA and the energy process from damage. It's a major mover, shaker, and protector in the mitochondr-

ial scheme of things, so it is rather sobering to realize that the heart's natural CoQ$_{10}$ content at age eighty is less than half of what it is at twenty.

CoQ$_{10}$ Deficiency Imperils the Heart

Starting in the 1970s, researchers discovered that people with heart diseases were usually deficient in CoQ$_{10}$. One study found deficiencies in three-fourths of 132 patients undergoing heart surgery.

The most extreme examples of deficiencies occur among patients with weak hearts, suffering from conditions such as cardiomyopathy or heart failure.

And it isn't just an age thing. A deficiency of CoQ$_{10}$ imperils the performance of the heart at any age. Indeed, clinicians and researchers rescue ailing hearts (young and old alike) by overcoming a deficiency with CoQ$_{10}$ supplementation. It works for teenagers with cardiomyopathy, baby boomers with blocked arteries, and octogenarians with failing hearts.

To date, more than thirty-five controlled clinical trials in Japan, Australia, Europe, and the United States have demonstrated significant benefit for angina, cardiomyopathy, congestive heart failure, coronary artery disease, heart attacks, and recovery from heart surgery. These studies involve thousands of patients. They indicate that CoQ$_{10}$ supplementation has a significant role both for early and advanced cases of heart disease, which kills 2,000 Americans daily.

Cardiomyopathy
In cardiomyopathy, the heart muscle becomes inflamed, dilated, or thicker and doesn't pump well. If the specific cause is not known, the condition is called primary cardiomyopathy. If the cause is related to a disease involving other organs or the heart, the condition is secondary cardiomyopathy.

Research in recent years has also uncovered an alarming connection between the use of common heart drugs to lower cholesterol levels and a CoQ$_{10}$ deficiency. Experts warn that the deficiency created by these drugs poses a dangerous risk to health and heart that is virtually unrecognized. We'll cover this important issue later in the chapter.

Using CoQ$_{10}$ Is Like Watering a Dry Plant

Texas cardiologist Peter Langsjoen, M.D., has participated in CoQ$_{10}$ studies since the early 1980s, when the initial clinical trials were conducted in this country. First with his cardiologist father Per, who passed away in 1993, and subsequently on his own in private practice, Langsjoen has logged more clinical usage of CoQ$_{10}$ than any other American doctor.

"CoQ$_{10}$ is the backbone of my cardiac practice," he says. "Frankly it's unthinkable for me to practice medicine without it. Based on my experience with some 10,000 patients, I can unequivocally say it's a powerful substance that can do a great deal of good for many people, and without any side effects.

"Using CoQ$_{10}$ is like watering a dry plant," he adds. "It's that remarkable. And it's that powerful. The sicker the patient, the more striking the results."

"In 80 percent of my patients, I see a clinical improvement in four weeks, with maximum improvement in six to twelve months, when they reach a plateau and have no further cardiovascular benefits. As their heart function improves, we have to decrease other medicines."

Langsjoen says that CoQ$_{10}$'s "most powerful therapeutic application is for any impairment in heart muscle function because the heart uses such a huge amount of energy. That's where you see the very dramatic lifesaving changes.

"This includes ischemic (lack of oxygen) conditions, such as coronary artery disease, because the CoQ$_{10}$ energizes the viable cells left in the heart muscle.

"We really see across-the-board benefits. CoQ$_{10}$ can help a big part of the population. This is a huge heart supplement."

A Boon for Heart Failure and Cardiomyopathy Patients

When the heart can't pump enough blood to the body, the condition is called congestive heart failure, or simply heart failure. This life-threatening situation can result from narrowed arteries, a past heart attack that causes scarring and diminished efficiency of the heart muscle, high blood pressure, a congenital heart defect (present at birth), or cardiomyopathy.

Swelling (edema) often results, typically in the legs and ankles. Fluid can build up in the lungs and interfere with breathing, causing shortness of breath. The condition also impairs the kidneys' ability to dispose of sodium and water, leading to increased edema.

Drugs, including diuretics, are the standard treatment. When that fails, a patient may become a candidate for a heart transplant.

In the early 1980s, Karl Folkers, the biochemist who first identified the chemical structure of CoQ$_{10}$, collaborated with Per Langsjoen, who at the time was associated with The Scott and White Clinic in Temple, Texas. Together, they conducted the first well-controlled medical study of CoQ$_{10}$ in the treatment of cardiomyopathy.

The effect of CoQ$_{10}$ supplementation on the nineteen patients in the study was astounding. All were expected to die from heart failure, but they rebounded with an "extraordinary clinical improvement," the researchers declared. Hearts decreased in size, became more efficient, and pumped more blood. Heart failure, including all forms of cardiomyopathy, seem to respond to CoQ$_{10}$, Per Langsjoen observed.

"CoQ$_{10}$ is not specific to any type of heart failure," he added. "All forms of cardiomyopathy seem to respond to CoQ$_{10}$, including idiopathic (unknown cause), dilated

(enlarged heart) or ischemic (reduced blood flow) cardiomyopathy."

Improved Quality of Life and Long-Term Survival

Subsequent research has confirmed the foregoing conclusion. Results include significantly improved quality of life and long-term survival from therapeutic supplementation.

One study analyzed the data compiled in eight previous controlled studies and found that patients supplemented with CoQ$_{10}$ had better scores in five key measurements of heart performance than the vast majority of non-supplemented patients. Moreover, CoQ$_{10}$ was found to be remarkably safe.

In 1994, the largest study with CoQ$_{10}$ and heart-failure patients was reported in the journal *Molecular Aspects of Medicine*. In this trial, researchers at different Italian medical centers gave more than 2,500 patients CoQ$_{10}$ in the amount of 50 to 150 mg daily for three months. The majority took 100 mg.

Improved quality of life was reported by 78 percent of the patients. Fifty-four percent attained significant improvement in at least three clinical signs that included general fluid retention, pulmonary fluid retention, heart palpitations, liver enlargement, and shortness of breath.

Such positive outcomes, along with many documented clinical reports, prompted Folkers to issue a strong appeal for the use of CoQ$_{10}$ among individuals considering heart transplants.

Writing in the journal *Biochemical and Biophysical Research Communications*, Folkers argued that research has clearly "established the efficacy and safety of CoQ$_{10}$ to treat patients in heart failure. In the United States, about 20,000 patients under sixty-five years are eligible for transplants, but donors number less than 1/10th of those eligible, and there are many more such patients over sixty-five, both eligible and ineligible."

CoQ$_{10}$ Deficiency: The Dominant Cause of Heart Failure?

In his report, Folkers, along with both Per and Peter Langsjoen, described the results of eleven transplant candidates treated with CoQ$_{10}$. "After CoQ$_{10}$, all improved," they said. "Some patients required no conventional drugs and had no limitation in lifestyle."

One of the case histories they reported was a sixty-four-year-old African-American male with a failing heart and inoperable coronary disease. After six months, he had improved to the point where there was "no limitation whatsoever on his activities."

Many such dramatically positive cases like this, combined with the absence of side effects, "justify treating patients in failure . . . with CoQ$_{10}$," the researchers said.

Heart failure has been strongly correlated with low blood and tissue levels of CoQ$_{10}$. The more severe the disease, the greater the CoQ$_{10}$ deficiency. This evidence led Folkers to theorize that the actual molecular cause of cardiac failure may be a "dominant deficiency" of CoQ$_{10}$.

"Even if you treat a patient with a conventional drug, the CoQ$_{10}$ deficiency still remains," he said. "There is no cardiovascular drug that can do for the human body what CoQ$_{10}$ can do."

The Most Dramatic Results

Peter Langsjoen agrees: "Among really complicated, critically ill cardiac patients who have been through one, two, or maybe three bypass procedures, you know that nothing really works. They are on a handful of drugs. But they feel terrible all the time.

"In this group we find the most dramatic results. These are the people who are the most severely deficient. The CoQ$_{10}$ deficiency may well indeed be a primary causal factor in some types of heart muscle dysfunction while in others it may be a secondary phenomenon.

"No matter which, the deficiency appears to be a major treatable element in the otherwise relentless decline of heart failure."

Can Supplementation Minimize the Urgency for Heart Transplants?

It's astounding to think that a simple nutritional supplement can restore to normal a patient who is in line for a heart transplant. Yet it can, for young and old patients alike.

Langsjoen recalls the case several years ago of a New Jersey man who called on behalf of his ailing teenage son. The youngster had dilated cardiomyopathy, had been placed on medication, and had been told he would require a heart transplant within a year or so. His ejection fraction was 8 percent.

"The father had done his homework and knew about CoQ$_{10}$," Langsjoen says. "He contacted me to find out if it could help his son. We sent him reprints of CoQ$_{10}$ studies on this type of condition. The father went ahead, with the agreement of his son's physician, and had the boy take 300 mg daily.

"Several months later, I heard again from the father. He was quite excited. His son's ejection fraction had gone to 24 percent. The last I heard, it was 34 percent, and the boy was beginning to do light jogging. This is obviously a striking change."

In this particular case, the youngster had just been diagnosed. Can CoQ$_{10}$ help with very advanced disease?

Ejection Fraction

The amount of blood your heart squeezes out into the bloodstream with each beat. Generally speaking, an ejection fraction reading of 50 percent or more is regarded as healthy.

"When you catch people early, the heart muscle hasn't yet deteriorated with fibrous tissue and scarring," says Langsjoen. "If someone has had a large, weak heart for years, it is unusual to get those hearts back to normal. You gradually lose heart muscle cells and you don't regrow them. A scarred heart is a tough situation.

"If the cells are weak, but alive, you then have the potential to improve them. You can gradually improve heart function for a year or two. That means decreasing heart size and increasing ejection fraction. Normally, after a year there is a leveling off."

And do patients have to continue the CoQ$_{10}$ once they have improved?

"They should not stop taking it," Langsjoen answers. "I have had patients who were doing well and decided they didn't need the supplement anymore. Usually within a month's time there is measurable decline. This has been the observation of other experts as well. I haven't seen them worse than when they started, but subjectively there is a decline and if you look at their CoQ$_{10}$ blood levels, there is a matching drop as well."

Coronary Artery Disease

Heart attacks usually result from coronary artery disease, also known as coronary or ischemic (*is-kem-ik*) heart disease. This condition is the single largest killer of American men and women, causing more than 450,000 deaths a year.

A heart attack occurs when the blood supply to part of the heart muscle is severely reduced or blocked off. This happens when one or more of the four coronary arteries feeding blood to the heart become blocked. The common cause is a buildup of plaque on the arterial walls that is called atherosclerosis. These deposits narrow the arteries, gradually choke the flow of blood, and increase the prospect for clots to block circulation.

The consequences include sudden cardiac arrest (a heart attack) or angina, where tightness and pain are felt in the chest with physical activity, emotional disturbance, or even intense elation.

CoQ$_{10}$'s "Magic"

CoQ$_{10}$ won't unclog arteries, bring back to life dead heart muscle cells, or replace lifesaving heart drugs. But it does offer impressive benefits against atherosclerosis and coronary artery disease.

First of all, it re-energizes the heart cells, including those on the edge, cells in trouble that may either die or struggle to live on. "This is CoQ$_{10}$'s magic," says Connecticut cardiologist Stephen Sinatra, M.D. "It can rejuvenate those cells."

Let's say the heart muscle is getting poor blood flow, just enough to keep it pumping. With CoQ$_{10}$, it will function better with whatever limited flow it does have. A patient will definitely have less chest pain, in fact, quite a bit less. This is not because the arteries are being opened but rather because of better energy production in the functioning areas that are poorly supplied.

CoQ_{10}, as we've seen, is also a powerful antioxidant operating in the mitochondria where tremendous amounts of free radicals are produced.

In addition, CoQ_{10} is present in the bloodstream, where it circulates with other antioxidants. As it circulates, it combines with vitamin E, another antioxidant, to help prevent lipid peroxidation. It also protects vitamin E itself from free radical destruction, a protective relationship that has been discovered only recently.

> **Lipid Peroxidation**
> A scientific term for the damaging oxidation by free radicals on fatty substances in the body.

It turns out that CoQ_{10} molecules in the bloodstream are actually transported by the LDL cholesterol. CoQ_{10} protects the LDL from oxidation, something in the Wild West tradition of "riding shotgun" on the stagecoach.

Animal studies have demonstrated that CoQ_{10} supplementation significantly protects against dangerous arterial plaque, even when animals are fed diets designed to raise the level of cholesterol and other fats in their bodies.

Thus, CoQ_{10}'s antioxidant power benefits the heart itself and the blood vessels that supply it.

CoQ_{10} Reduces Angina Episodes

A number of controlled studies have shown that CoQ_{10} generates major improvements in exercise tolerance, and reduces the frequency of angina episodes and the need for medication as well.

Dosages in these studies range from 150 to 600 mg daily.

One study also showed that when CoQ_{10} is given to patients after a heart attack, it works quickly to lower the risk of complications and additional cardiac events. In this study, patients received 120 mg of CoQ_{10} within a few days of their heart attack.

After four weeks on CoQ_{10}, they had far less experience of angina, arrhythmias, and every other measure studied, when compared with a second group of heart attack patients who were not supplemented. The CoQ_{10} group had about half as many subsequent heart attacks during this time.

The Amazing Recovery of a Three-Bypass Patient

Texas cardiologist and CoQ_{10} expert Peter Langsjoen says that these types of patients do "so well" with CoQ_{10}. As an example, he cited a female patient in her seventies who previously had three bypass surgeries. "Even after surgeries, she was having chest pain many times a day and was

> **Coronary Artery Bypass Surgery**
> A common cardiac procedure, in which a surgeon reroutes, or bypasses, blood around clogged coronary arteries to improve the supply of blood and oxygen to the heart. A blood vessel is taken from another part of the body and grafted above and below the blocked part of the affected coronary artery.

bedridden," he recalls. "Just to get up and get dressed she would have to take three or four nitroglycerine pills. She would get chest pain just sitting and watching TV.

"We started her on CoQ_{10}. Now, years later, she manages her own affairs and is quite active. She still has angina, but only from time to time. CoQ_{10} made a clear difference.

"This is somebody with extremely poor plumbing. Her arteries are a mess. Her grafts are a mess. There is nothing more to do surgically. You couldn't bypass her another time. I was amazed she even survived the third operation. Her heart is about as ischemic as you can get. We could never really improve someone in that shape without something like CoQ_{10}. She takes 120 mg twice a day along with other anti-angina medications."

Boosts Recovery after Cardiac Surgery

Supplementation with CoQ_{10} prior to heart surgery appears also to significantly help the recovery process.

"If a surgeon would like his heart patients to recover better and have a stronger heart muscle, CoQ_{10} supplementation should be a real option to use," says Franklin Rosenfeldt, M.D., of the Alfred Hospital Cardiac Surgical Research Unit in Melbourne.

Rosenfeldt has conducted multiple studies proving CoQ_{10} improves surgical outcomes. In the latest study, 122 patients scheduled for elective coronary artery bypass graft (CABG) surgery were randomly selected to take either CoQ_{10} or an inert placebo pill for one week before their operation. The amount of CoQ_{10} used in the study was 300 mg a day.

After the surgery, the researchers found that CoQ_{10} generated impressive results, including improved mitochondrial energy production, better heart muscle contraction, less heart muscle damage, and less recovery time in the hospital.

Major Implications for Life and Cost-Saving

"This is very promising and very effective in many cases," says Rosenfeldt, who reported his findings at a scientific conference of the American Heart Association in 2001.

Langsjoen emphatically agrees. "This is a great result," he points out, "obtained after just seven days. From my own experience of using CoQ_{10} for several months or so before bypass surgery, I feel that the post-operative benefits can be even more substantial."

More than a half million bypass surgeries are performed

in the United States each year. They involve increasingly older patients and an increasing percentage of repeat operations. As a result, the injury, death, and cost burden have risen substantially.

A number of studies have shown that pretreatment with CoQ_{10} improves the postoperative status of patients not just after bypass surgery, but also after heart valve replacement as well. Hopefully, cardiologists will recognize the value that CoQ_{10} can contribute to surgical outcomes and heart health in general. Up to now, however, they haven't paid much attention.

The Danger of Cholesterol-Lowering Drugs

These days the advertisements for cholesterol-lowering drugs are totally in your face. They pop up everywhere. In magazines, newspapers, and TV. And the message coming out of the pharmaceutical industry is that even healthy people should take these drugs, known technically as statins. They are, in fact, being touted as the "new aspirin."

Statins
Cholesterol-lowering drugs that were introduced in 1987 and have become blockbuster drugs with total annual sales now over $14 billion. Leading products include Pfizer's Lipitor, Merck's Zocor, and Bristol-Myers Squibb's Pravachol.

Beyond the smoke of marketing hype, a threatening fire smolders. In 2001, major headlines and news reports warned users of these drugs about the potential for deadly muscle damage. One leading statin brand, *Baycol*, was voluntarily pulled off the market by its manufacturer in the summer of 2001 after thirty-one deaths were linked to its usage. Public Citizen, a well-known consumer advocacy group, also petitioned the U.S. Food and Drug Administration (FDA) to require manufacturers to warn patients to quit the pills at the first sign of muscle pain or weakness.

What the Media Hasn't Reported

What has not been brought to public attention is that these drugs also interfere with the body's production of CoQ_{10}. They block the same enzyme system (known as HMG-CoA) that produces both cholesterol *and* CoQ_{10}.

"It is almost criminal, in my opinion, not to supplement a person who is taking statin drugs," says cardiologist Stephen Sinatra. "The drugs are creating CoQ_{10} deficiencies. The *Baycol* problem is just the tip of the iceberg. Animal studies show that statins can lead to cancer."

In his medical practice, Sinatra will only prescribe a statin drug to a very sick cardiac patient who cannot otherwise reduce his or her cholesterol by natural means.

An Impending Medical Disaster?

"But I always prescribe CoQ_{10} along with it," Sinatra adds.

"Any person taking a statin *must* take CoQ_{10}. The problem is that these drugs are big business and promoted to healthy people all over the place, and doctors aren't telling their patients about the CoQ_{10} connection. A lot of people are taking the drugs preventively but could be literally awakening a tiger inside the body that could come alive later on in life."

Says cardiologist Peter Langsjoen: "This could be the biggest impending medical disaster ever."

Experts commonly see the signs of CoQ_{10} deficiency in new patients who have been taking statin drugs for a year or more.

Warning Signs Are Deceiving

Typical signs include aches and pains, fatigue, malaise, sore muscles, weakness, difficulty getting in and out of a car, the feeling of a low-grade flu, and shorter breath with exertion. There could be mental changes as well.

The signs are deceiving and people may not link them to the cholesterol drug. With statins, the experts say, you don't have any immediate side effects. You get the immediate gratification that cholesterol is coming down, but over time you start feeling less well and just don't attribute it to something you started a year or two before.

Echo-cardiography
Ultrasound imaging technology used by cardiologists to help assess heart function, heart wall thickness, and the severity of disorders.

Moreover, adds Langsjoen, echocardiograph imaging of the heart will show an abnormality of the heart muscle function in these people, specifically a stiffening of the heart muscle.

"This is the very first thing you see with CoQ_{10} depletion," he says. "It is very common in people on statins for any length of time. It is reversible, and goes back to normal if you stop the drug."

FDA Informed about the Danger

Mounting studies proving that statin drugs seriously deplete CoQ_{10} prompted The International Coenzyme Q_{10} Association to bring the issue to the attention of the FDA in September of 2001.

In a letter to the FDA signed by fourteen scientists and clinicians in seven countries, the group pointed out that muscle destruction and fatigue linked to the drugs may in fact be a direct result of depletion. The scientists also noted that although statin therapy has benefits, its long-term benefits against heart disease may be "blunted" due to the depletion of CoQ_{10}.

Finally, the association urged the FDA to study "whether the clinical use of statins can be made safer and possibly more effective by the addition of CoQ_{10}. We should make every effort to investigate the reasons for, and to prevent further developments of what have already been serious medical consequences."

If It's So Good, Why Aren't Cardiologists Using It?

In October of 1996, Connecticut cardiologist Stephen Sinatra received an urgent call from a man who pleaded with him to take his mother in transfer from another hospital. The woman was seventy-nine years old at the time and had been admitted to a community hospital with heart failure complicated by pneumonia.

The son said she had been on a ventilator for several weeks, was getting powerful steroids and high concentrations of oxygen, but was still failing. She went into kidney failure and her doctors said there was nothing more to do.

The son, who placed the S-O-S call to Sinatra, was a biochemist and knowledgeable about CoQ_{10}. He had asked the doctors at the hospital to place his mother on CoQ_{10}. They refused. CoQ_{10} was not on their list of approved formulas.

The son brought in stacks of medical literature showing how CoQ_{10} could help patients with heart failure. The doctors would not review the information. Instead, they asked the family to end life support. The family refused.

The son went to the hospital administrators. When he insisted on the CoQ_{10}, they told him he was "interfering." The situation turned ugly, and lawyers became involved.

A Happy Ending

The story, however, had a happy ending. Sinatra told the son that if his mother could be transferred to a hospital where he could attend to her, he would see to it that she received CoQ_{10}. CoQ_{10} was approved for use at the Connecticut hospital Manchester Memorial.

Still, he warned, the transfer was risky in her weakened state. She would have to be transported in an ambulance for the forty-or-so-minute journey and be "bag-breathed" the whole way. This meant that a skilled medical technician would have to "breathe" her mechanically by hand the entire time.

The son was quick to respond. "At least with you she will have a fighting chance because, where she is, she's certainly going to die," he said.

The transfer was carried out. The elderly woman arrived, semi-comatose, and respiratory-dependent. She was placed on conventional pulmonary care similar to that received at the previous hospital.

Conventional Treatment *Plus* Supplements

The only change in her therapy was nutritional: 450 mg of CoQ_{10} daily, given through a feeding tube, along with a multivitamin/mineral preparation, and one gram of magnesium, intravenously administered.

"Although I had some hope for her, the other critical care doctors were extremely skeptical of using CoQ_{10} in this life-threatening case," Sinatra says.

On the third day, she started to "wake up." After ten days, she was weaned off the ventilator. At two weeks, she was discharged to an extended care facility, sitting up in a wheelchair with only supplemental oxygen.

Sinatra has seen Louise on a number of occasions since then. She is now eighty-three and enjoying a good quality of life. She requires routine medical therapy but also takes 500 mg of CoQ_{10} daily.

In Sinatra's words, what happened was "truly a medical resurrection" and represents the great lifesaving potential of CoQ_{10}.

But the story is not unusual, he says: "I have personally treated and heard of many cases of people seemingly 'left for dead' who have been similarly resurrected by this remarkable compound called CoQ_{10}."

Only a Small Minority of Cardiologists Use CoQ_{10}

In Japan, CoQ_{10} is the fifth most commonly prescribed heart "drug." Japanese cardiologists know its value. Up until recently it was available only through prescription there, but as of 2001 it can be bought as an over-the-counter supplement just as in the United States. Here, however, most cardiologists ignore CoQ_{10}.

"Probably less than 1 percent of cardiologists know it and use it," guesses Sinatra. "The rest are simply missing a great therapeutic tool."

How can this be, given the proven success of CoQ_{10} in scientific studies, and the excitement and gratification it generates among patients?

Why They Are Missing the Boat

One major reason is that CoQ_{10} is "only" a nutritional supplement and not a patented drug. In Western medicine, the pharmaceutical companies dominate medical practice. They research and develop drugs, patent them, and market them to practitioners, who prescribe them to patients.

Health professionals, and particularly specialists, tend to treat patients according to the accepted protocols of their specialty. The protocols emphasize medical technology and pharmaceutical drugs, not nutritional supplements.

The official position of the American Heart Association is that "the safety and effectiveness of CoQ_{10} need to be further evaluated. This requires conducting well-designed clinical trials involving large numbers of patients over a long time. Until that happens, the American Heart Association cannot recommend taking coenzyme Q_{10} regularly."

Dozens of heart-related studies from around the world overwhelmingly show that CoQ_{10} is very safe and effective. For very sick people, however, it needs to be used in high enough doses to achieve healing blood levels. But obviously, in the current medical environment, nutritional supplements, no matter how vital or how essential, typically get short shrift. They are ignored or relegated to minor importance even though medical drugs often cause nutrient deficiencies in the body. CoQ$_{10}$ is a prime "victim" of this approach.

Opposition from the Status Quo

Langsjoen adds this perspective: "While the pharmaceutical industry does a good job at physician and patient education on their new products, distributors of CoQ$_{10}$ are not as effective at this. This education is very costly and can be done only with the reasonable expectation of patent-protected profit. CoQ$_{10}$ is not patentable.

"Although this is not the first time that a fundamental and clinically important discovery has come about without the backing of a pharmaceutical company, it is the first such discovery to so radically alter how we as physicians must view disease. CoQ$_{10}$ is not revolutionary in the fields of chemistry and biochemistry, but it is revolutionary in medical practice and as such there is inherent opposition from the status quo."

Until now, CoQ$_{10}$ is best known outside of mainstream medicine—in alternative health circles. And a December 2000 report on *ABC World News Tonight* lamented that fact, citing the significant benefits to patients.

"Come on cardiologists!" chided ABC commentator Nicholas Regush. "Crack open the medical literature on coenzyme Q$_{10}$. Start reading up on how this powerful substance may be able to help patients with heart problems." Hopefully somebody was listening.

HIGH BLOOD PRESSURE, STROKE, AND DIABETES

In addition to directly helping the heart, CoQ$_{10}$ also benefits the cardiovascular system as a whole. That means the circulatory system as well. And in doing so, CoQ$_{10}$ further adds to its value as both a natural preventive and therapeutic agent.

In this section, we will discuss CoQ$_{10}$'s potential for three major conditions: high blood pressure (hypertension), stroke, and diabetes.

CoQ$_{10}$ and High Blood Pressure

You are about to read some great news if you are among the approximately one in four adult Americans with high blood pressure. What you will learn is something your doctor likely doesn't know about . . . so show this to your physician.

First, the facts. Hypertension, or high blood pressure as it is popularly called, is not really a disease. It is a byproduct of other, often more serious, underlying problems.

High blood pressure means that the force of blood pressing against the walls of the arteries is too great. Fully one-third of the individuals with high blood pressure have no symptoms and don't even know they have it.

But symptoms or no symptoms, if not controlled, high blood pressure can lead to brain damage, heart attacks, heart failure, kidney disease, and stroke.

Causes Mostly Unknown and Treatments Largely Unsuccessful

In 90 percent of cases, the cause is not precisely known and is referred to as essential hypertension. Among the causal factors are age, body weight, diet, heredity (high blood pressure is more common and severe among blacks than whites), kidney infection, and stress.

Only about 18 percent of those with high blood pressure are successfully treated. Moreover, many people fear the side effects of medication or improper prescribing by physicians.

What Determines High Blood Pressure

A person is considered to have high blood pressure when he or she has a systolic pressure of 140 mmHg or greater, and/or a diastolic pressure of 90 mmHg or greater, or is taking antihypertensive medication. *Systolic* means the pressure when the heart is beating. *Diastolic* means pressure between heartbeats. Eighty percent of people fall in the borderline-to-moderate range (120–180 over 90–114) and require no drug therapy at all. A normal blood pressure is 120 over 80.

Now that you have the facts, here is the exciting CoQ$_{10}$ connection: As far back as 1976, researchers noted that CoQ$_{10}$ could decrease blood pressure in patients with established hypertension. Over the years, the evidence has continued to grow, and now points to a possible CoQ$_{10}$ deficiency as a *cause* of high blood pressure.

Based on years of using CoQ$_{10}$ in their cardiology practices, Peter Langsjoen and his late father, Per, theorized that, with CoQ$_{10}$ supplementation, improved heart functioning precedes lowered blood pressure.

Is Hypertension the Result of a CoQ$_{10}$ Deficiency?

Here are the details: The heart muscle is packed with mitochondria and CoQ$_{10}$. In any disease that affects heart muscle function, whether it is coronary artery disease, diabetes, mitral valve disease, or the result of chemotherapy toxicity, the first change that occurs is a stiffening and thickening of the heart muscle. This phenomenon may very well be the result of a CoQ$_{10}$ deficiency.

A deficiency is seen, for instance, as a result of the regular use of cholesterol-lowering drugs, which deplete the body of CoQ$_{10}$. A depletion could also occur from polluted air, poor diet, and stress, which cause shortages in important vitamins, such as B complex, necessary for the body to produce CoQ_{10}.

We know that CoQ_{10} production declines with age. And we also know that a stiffening of the heart muscle is considered a normal aspect of aging (a senile heart).

The Heart Has to Work Harder

The stiffening means the heart has to work harder in order to fill its chambers with blood and then pump it out again. In response, the body produces adrenaline, the stress hormone. It makes the heart rate higher and improves the filling and pumping action. However, on a continual basis, the increased adrenaline causes a general constriction of the blood vessels, which means that higher (more) blood pressure is required to push the blood through narrowed arteries.

Adrenaline
Heightened secretion of this important adrenal hormone is often related to fear or anger, and results in an increasedheart rate and the conversion of stored glycogen to glucose.

"We've always looked at essential hypertension as a disease that causes thickening of the heart muscle," says Langsjoen. "That's what the textbooks say. But the experts have never looked seriously at CoQ_{10}.

"From my clinical experience, it is the CoQ_{10} deficiency that is causing the stiffening of the heart muscle, which, in turn, causes the body to respond with adrenaline. The end result is hypertension."

The concept is revolutionary and certainly warrants major clinical trials with large numbers of patients.

Hundreds of Patients Normalized with CoQ_{10}

To date there have been about ten studies, most of them small. All have shown improvement in heart muscle function and gradual lowering of blood pressure.

At the Langsjoen clinic, hundreds of patients with mild to moderate hypertension have been normalized within three to six months on CoQ_{10} *alone*. The stiffness, the increased heart rate, and the blood pressure, "all go to normal," Langsjoen says.

The CoQ_{10} results are very powerful with younger people, aged twenty to forty, says Langsjoen. "In older people, there are usually more complications involved. Nevertheless, I would say that this concept applies to a fair amount of my patients with hypertension, and maybe even a majority."

In Connecticut, Stephen Sinatra has also achieved striking results. "Since using CoQ_{10} for more than ten years, I have been able to slowly reduce at least half their cardiac medications," he says.

As blood pressure gradually normalizes, patients are often able to start reducing the amount of medication they take. They report improvement in their quality of life and vigor. Obviously, CoQ_{10} is having an energizing effect, but improvement also occurs as a result of taking less medication.

In a 1994 report published in the journal *Molecular Aspects of Medicine*, Langsjoen described a clinical study with 109 symptomatic patients. These were advanced cases where the patients had had the condition an average of nine years.

Here, about 25 percent of those studied were eventually controlled on CoQ_{10} alone, 100 mg twice daily.

"People with severe hypertension are going to need drugs," he points out. "But you can always add some CoQ_{10} in their daily routine and often be able to reduce the drugs."

Think of CoQ_{10} as a Primary Therapeutic Resource

In an informal experiment in his clinic, Langsjoen took echocardiograms of sixteen older patients with elevated blood pressure who were not initially taking CoQ_{10}. The images all showed stiffening of the heart muscle, typical for their age. All of them normalized with CoQ_{10}. "If we can reverse the stiffening with CoQ_{10}, then hypertension may not be such an unavoidable phenomenon in older people," he says.

Langsjoen suggests that patients with hypertension should bring CoQ_{10} to the attention of their physician. Because of its safety, effectiveness, and multiple benefits, he believes strongly that it should be considered prior to an escalating course of drugs.

"Consider CoQ_{10} in situations of mild or moderate hypertension, particularly when it is mild enough not to be symptomatic," he says. "You can expect to see a gradual improvement of 10 to 15 mmHg."

This promise of CoQ_{10} for hypertension takes on even greater importance in the light of new research findings showing that even slightly elevated blood pressure (in the range physicians call high normal) significantly raises the risk of heart disease. The findings, published in the *New England Journal of Medicine* in 2001, indicated the risk was 2.5 times higher than in individuals with lower normal readings, and increased with age.

"Even if blood pressure is quite high, symptoms are present, and medication is necessary, CoQ_{10} should be considered as a way of gradually decreasing the level of medicine," says Langsjoen.

"Keep in mind, however, that CoQ_{10} doesn't address all the multiple lifestyle factors that may have contributed to a person getting into the high-blood-pressure predicament to begin with. The stresses and other causal elements are still ongoing."

CoQ_{10} and Stroke

Stroke is the third leading killer disease, after coronary

artery disease and cancer. It occurs when arteries to, or inside, the head become blocked, choking off circulation to a portion of the brain. A minor stroke may cause temporary loss of sensory or organ function. But a major stroke can cause permanent paralysis, or even death.

Research into CoQ$_{10}$ and stroke has been limited to animal studies. In these experiments, animals who were supplemented for a period prior to an induced stroke were much less injured than non-supplemented animals. A similar effect has been observed in humans but has not been formally studied.

Impressive Recoveries

Peter Langsjoen describes a better-than-expected recovery among his heart patients who were taking CoQ$_{10}$ and happened to have a stroke.

"I have seen patients completely paralyzed on one side, and unable to speak, after a devastating stroke, and then after several months they get back to being pretty much normal," he says. "There might be some remaining clumsiness of the hand, or one leg not quite tracking as well, or some slight thing.

"I have seen impressive recoveries in dozens of patients, recoveries that have not only impressed me, but the physical therapy people as well."

Langsjoen says he usually increases the amount of CoQ$_{10}$ after a stroke to about 180 mg twice daily.

"I don't have any experience with people who have not been on CoQ$_{10}$ prior to a stroke, and then are put on it afterwards. At that point, it may be too late. Most of my patients take CoQ$_{10}$."

Along these same lines, John Ely, Ph.D., a research physics scientist at the University of Washington, reported the case of a remarkable recovery from a severe stroke by a sixty-nine-year-old female who had been taking 400 mg of CoQ$_{10}$ for a month prior to having a stroke.

Ely, writing about the case in a 1998 issue of the *Journal of Orthomolecular Medicine*, said the patient recovered "almost completely" in two weeks despite the "vegetative prognosis foreseen by the very experienced stroke unit specialists" at the hospital.

CoQ$_{10}$ and Diabetes

Remember Fred Crane? He's the retired researcher who first discovered CoQ$_{10}$ in 1957. Many years later, Crane developed diabetes and required oral medication to control his blood sugar. But with time the medication wasn't working well. His blood sugar level began to rise again.

As Crane tells it, "I thought that maybe CoQ$_{10}$ might help. I had been taking 30 mg a day, but then I stepped up to 180 mg. In a period of about six months, my insulin level normalized, and my blood sugar dropped down to about where it should be. I've been on this approach for seven years, taking my oral medication and the additional CoQ$_{10}$. And it's been working."

An Alarming Rise in Diabetes

The rising incidence of diabetes has health officials deeply concerned. Like Crane's case, the most common form of the disease develops slowly, usually among people over age forty-five.

The latest statistics from the Centers for Disease Control indicate that nearly 16 million Americans—6 percent of the population—have diabetes, the highest level ever recorded. Moreover, the disease is developing at the staggering rate of 798,000 new cases a year.

Although diabetes is not a cardiovascular disease per se, it has a harmful impact on the cardiovascular system. It contributes to free radical activity and a systemic deterioration of blood vessels.

Diabetics Deficient in CoQ$_{10}$

Medical studies reveal a deficiency of CoQ$_{10}$ in diabetic patients. In one study, 120 mg per day of CoQ$_{10}$ was given to thirty-nine patients with diabetes, resulting in a reduction of blood-sugar levels by 20 to 30 percent.

At his Texas cardiology clinic, Peter Langsjoen has found that CoQ$_{10}$ has improved the blood-sugar-related problems of some of his heart patients who also have diabetes. He has not done a formal study, but during one stretch of time, he carefully reviewed the progress of about 140 patients with adult-onset diabetes.

"About one-third of them were clearly doing better," he says. "By that I mean better blood-sugar control and a reduced need for medication. Among this group, patients went from insulin injections to pills, or from pills to control with diet alone." The diabetic symptoms of the other patients did not change significantly.

The CoQ$_{10}$ Connection Not Widely Known

The fact that CoQ$_{10}$ appears to help normalize blood sugar in a substantial number of cases is not well known. And clearly, much research is needed to clarify a potential role for CoQ$_{10}$.

"It appears to happen enough of the time that I inform patients they may need to substantially lower their level of insulin or oral medication," says Langsjoen.

The action of CoQ$_{10}$ is probably related to improving the bioenergetics and, as a result, the production of the so-called beta cells in the pancreas where insulin is made.

"With CoQ$_{10}$, you change the fundamental cellular chemistry of everything," he says. "So you see many improvements in the body. There are so many aspects of health that improve simply because you are energizing everything."

The Diabetes Supplement "Cocktail"

Connecticut cardiologist Stephen Sinatra uses CoQ_{10} as part of an overall supplement approach to help patients with a family history of diabetes prevent the disease. He recommends a daily "cocktail" of the following:

- Alpha-lipoic acid, an antioxidant: 100–300 mg
- CoQ_{10}: 200–400 mg
- L-carnitine, an amino acid: 1–2 grams
- Magnesium: 400 mg
- Vitamin E: 200–400 IU

"These nutrients will help prevent oxidative stress in the pancreas and also help control blood sugar," says Sinatra.

KEEPING YOUR IMMUNE SYSTEM STRONG

Energizer, antioxidant, and mitochondria protector par excellence. That's CoQ_{10}. It shouldn't come as a surprise, then, that these remarkable properties of CoQ_{10} extend to the immune system, the body's wondrous defense mechanism.

Physicians say CoQ_{10} boosts resistance to disease. People get sick less often. They get fewer colds, flu, and respiratory infections. They are not as sickly. If they come down with a viral illness, it is much milder. CoQ_{10} may also represent a front-line natural agent against more serious disorders, such as AIDS and cancer.

Although the CoQ_{10} research in the area of immunology doesn't approach the volume of scientific work done in cellular bioenergetics and heart disease, the findings nevertheless suggest a good deal of promise for CoQ_{10}.

Fortified Antibodies and Immune Cells

Antibodies
Specialized molecules made of proteins produced by immune system cells called lymphocytes that circulate in the blood and lymph fluid where they bind to "foreign invaders" (bacteria, toxic substances, or viruses) that enter the body, inactivating them or identifying them for destruction by other immune cells.

Studies show, for instance, that CoQ_{10} can improve antibody levels. In one Italian study, a group of volunteers took either 90 or 180 mg of CoQ_{10} for two weeks prior to vaccination against the hepatitis-B virus. After vaccination, they continued taking the supplement for another ninety days.

Researchers then measured the antibody levels and compared them with another group of vaccinated volunteers that was not supplemented. Both dosages of CoQ_{10} effectively improved the antibody response and the higher supplementation level increased the response by up to 57 percent.

In another human study, involving eight chronically ill patients, supplementation with 60 mg of CoQ_{10} for up to three months significantly improved their levels of IgG, the body's most common antibody.

Other studies, done with laboratory animals, show that CoQ_{10} contributes to a greater killing ability for macrophages, immune cells that devour bacteria and viruses. These studies also show that an age-related decline in immune system function can be partially reversed with CoQ_{10} supplementation. Moreover, supplemented older animals become healthier and more energetic.

People and animals alike lose energy and resistance to illness as they age. Thus, older people should consider adding CoQ_{10} to their supplement arsenal of such illness-fighters as vitamins A and C.

CoQ_{10} and Cancer

Research on the CoQ_{10}-cancer connection is limited. There have been no controlled studies. But the medical observations made to date clearly call for the therapeutic benefits of CoQ_{10} to be vigorously studied.

Karl Folkers, Ph.D., one of the original scientists involved with CoQ_{10}, believed that CoQ_{10} should be aggressively explored for its cancer-protective effects. Since it is not a patented drug, however, funding for large-scale research has not materialized.

In Europe, studies have shown a low level of CoQ_{10} in the blood and affected tissues of cancer patients.

Protective Effect for Breast Tissue

In one study, Turkish researchers noted the involvement of free radical damage to cell membranes, mitochondria, and DNA in the cancer process. Increased free radical activity, they pointed out, could cause an excess consumption of CoQ_{10} by the body.

Analyzing cancerous breast tissue removed from twenty-one mastectomy patients, the researchers found a significantly decreased level of CoQ_{10}. They concluded that supplementation of CoQ_{10} "may induce a protective effect on breast tissue."

A small-scale 1994 Scandinavian study involving CoQ_{10} and "high-risk" breast cancer was reported in the journal *Biochemical and Biophysical Research Communication*. In that study, thirty-two patients were given an array of vitamins, antioxidants, fatty acids and 90 mg of CoQ_{10}, along with conventional cancer treatment.

An Amazing Tumor Regression

Six of the cases showed partial tumor regression. One of the six women, whose tumor had stabilized in size to 1.5 centimeters over a year, was then given an increased dosage of 390 mg of CoQ_{10}. According to the researchers, after one month the tumor was no longer palpable. In another month, mammography confirmed the absence of tumor.

One of the authors commented that in treating almost 7,000 cases of breast cancer over a thirty-five year practice, he had "never seen a spontaneous complete regression" of a breast tumor that size, and had "never seen a comparable regression on any conventional anti-tumor therapy."

Another woman in the study underwent non-radical surgery for a breast tumor, but her physicians determined the presence of residual cancer. She was then given 300 mg of CoQ_{10} daily. After three months, she was described as being in excellent clinical condition with no evidence of any remaining malignant tissue.

The authors concluded their report with an appeal for more research on the effects of high-dosage CoQ_{10} for cancer patients.

Five Reasons to Consider CoQ_{10} in Cancer Therapy

It makes sense to consider the use of CoQ_{10} supplementation as part of an overall anticancer strategy for five principal reasons:

1. It is a major antioxidant, that is, it combats the free radical activity that is involved in the development of degenerative diseases, including cancer.

2. Chemotherapy increases free radical activity and impairs the immune system. For instance, *Adriamycin*, one widely used chemotherapy drug, apparently contributes to cardiac toxicity by generating overwhelming oxidative stress in the heart muscle cells, as well as inhibiting CoQ_{10}-dependent enzymes. A series of small studies have shown that CoQ_{10} supplementation can help prevent the poisoning of the heart without interfering with the antitumor effects of the drug.

3. Studies indicate that CoQ_{10} can increase the immune system's "firepower" against disease.

4. The body's natural CoQ_{10} level decreases with age, and animal studies show that the immune system's effectiveness also decreases in the presence of lower CoQ_{10}.

5. Most malignancies occur in the elderly, who have lowered immune response.

Gian Paolo Littarru, M.D., a leading CoQ_{10} researcher for thirty years, is presently directing medical investigations on the cancer–CoQ_{10} connection in Italy, where he is professor of medical chemistry at the University of Ancona.

"Our research has a two-fold purpose," he says. "First, we want a better understanding of CoQ_{10}'s anti-cancer potential and to see if it strengthens the effect of conventional therapy. And second, we want to know if administration of CoQ_{10} minimizes the side effects of the potent anti-cancer drugs."

In recent years, the medical profession has become increasingly open to alternative treatments. Given the central role that CoQ_{10} plays in the body, it seems like too important a compound to ignore in the fight against a devastating disease such as cancer where conventional therapies have a poor track record for success.

CoQ_{10} and AIDS

HIV patients often have nutritional deficiencies, points out Littarru, and as a result "probably produce less CoQ_{10} because their bodies lack certain nutrient factors essential to make CoQ_{10}."

Indeed, very low levels have been found in AIDS patients. This was first determined in 1988 by Karl Folkers and colleagues at the Institute of Biomedical Research in Austin. Individuals with ARC (AIDS-related complex), where the HIV virus is present but no symptoms are in evidence, were deficient in CoQ_{10}, too, but not to the same degree as in AIDS patients.

Acquired Immune Deficiency Syndrome (AIDS)
A contagious viral condition (attributed to the HIV virus) that weakens the immune system, leaving the body vulnerable to different kinds of infections.

Protects against AZT

In one informal case report, CoQ_{10} alone was used to treat two individuals with ARC. "These patients were doing well five and six years after they started," reported Folkers in 1991. "This is extremely encouraging. They are healthy, working, and leading normal lives. The basis of this response, we feel, is that CoQ_{10} also benefits the immune system very positively."

More recent laboratory research in Europe has shown that CoQ_{10} protects disease-fighting lymphocyte cells from the lethal effects of the AIDS drug AZT.

To date, however, not enough research has been done to determine the extent of CoQ_{10}'s value against AIDS. Still, high-dosage CoQ_{10} supplementation (keeping close attention to blood levels to make sure the compound is being absorbed well) may benefit patients at any stage of the disease.

Chronic Fatigue

From a medical standpoint, supplementation with CoQ_{10} often generates considerable energy increases in patients who for some reason are energy depleted. Clinicians who routinely use CoQ_{10} in their practice say that it is well worth trying.

One such physician is Martin P. Gallagher, M.S., D.C., a nutritional therapy expert practicing in Jeannette, Pennsylvania. He consistently finds that CoQ_{10} elevates the energy of patients. "I see many patients with chronic fatigue syndrome who reach a certain plateau of improvement on a comprehensive healing program," he says.

"The program includes detoxification, a more nutritious diet, and supplementation with a broad array of important vitamins, minerals, and herbs. I usually reserve the CoQ_{10} for when a patient hits the plateau, and then, within two-to-six weeks of starting it, there is usually a discernible improvement in energy and strength."

Chronic fatigue syndrome typically has many causes. But physicians say that CoQ_{10} almost always helps reduce the fatigue level to some degree for as long as it is taken. Any energy gains will be lost if it is discontinued.

Prominent nutritional researcher Melvyn R. Werbach, M.D., writing in *Alternative Medicine Review*, includes a low level of CoQ_{10} among a list of key deficiencies that probably contribute to the syndrome and also stymie the healing process. Other pivotal deficiencies cited include the B vitamins, essential fatty acids, L-carnitine, magnesium, vitamin C, and zinc. Because of their therapeutic benefits, Werbach suggests supplementing chronic fatigue patients with these nutrients, along with a general high-potency vitamin and mineral formula.

COMBATING NERVOUS SYSTEM DISORDERS

After starting CoQ_{10} supplementation, an eight-year-old boy confined to a wheelchair was able to walk independently, and a twenty-year-old woman was able to work outside the home for the first time.

These dramatic stories of recovery were recounted by Salvatore DiMauro, M.D., a neurologist and researcher at Columbia University in New York, in a 2001 issue of the journal *Neurology*.

DiMauro described two patients with hereditary ataxia, a rare incurable disorder that causes deterioration of the cerebellum, the part of the brain controlling coordination. Patients have difficulty with balance, coordination of arms and legs, and speech, and may develop seizures. DiMauro had discovered that the two patients, and four others with this condition he treated, had CoQ_{10} levels 70 percent lower than normal. He then began prescribing CoQ_{10} at daily dosages ranging from 300–3,000 mg.

Ataxia Patients Improved

"All of the patients improved," he reported. "They got stronger, their ataxia improved, and their seizures either stopped or happened less often." Five of the patients had been unable to walk before using CoQ_{10}. One year later, all were able to walk with some assistance, such as a rolling walker.

"Our findings suggest that CoQ_{10} deficiency is a potentially important cause of some forms of familial ataxia and it should be considered when diagnosing this condition," DiMauro said. "Where low levels are found, treatment to replace the missing CoQ_{10} should be aggressive and begin early."

DiMauro's research is part of a recent surge of medical interest in CoQ_{10}'s potential against brain and neuromuscular disorders. In the last five years, scientific investigations in this area have skyrocketed.

A Growing Field of CoQ_{10} Research

Leading CoQ_{10} researchers like Karl Folkers and Gian Paolo Littarru began studying the compound's effect on muscular dystrophy (MD) more than twenty years ago. Brought to public attention by the telethons of comedian Jerry Lewis, MD is an umbrella term for a group of genetic diseases that progressively weaken and destroy muscles controlling movement. Some forms of the disease also affect the heart and other involuntary muscles.

The early research with CoQ_{10} demonstrated that it could help improve heart function in these patients. More recently, the potential of CoQ_{10} has expanded dynamically to include Alzheimer's disease, ataxia, Huntington's disease, Parkinson's disease, and certain conditions known as mitochondrial myopathies. The latter are disorders of the muscles caused by abnormalities in the mitochondria.

How CoQ_{10} Protects Neurons

Neurons are cells in the brain and the nervous system. Like other cells in the body, they get their energy from the mitochondria. Researchers think that the combination of oxidative damage and mutations in the mitochondria, and the resulting drop in energy output, contribute to so-called neurodegenerative disorders. In English, that means conditions that disturb and kill nerve tissue.

"Even subtle functional alterations in these essential cellular dynamos can lead to insidious pathological changes in neurons," one researcher wrote. No wonder, then, that researchers have begun looking seriously at CoQ_{10}.

Just how much potential does it have? The most dramatic results so far have occurred among patients who, because of a genetic defect, have a reduced level of CoQ_{10}, a situation referred to as primary CoQ_{10} deficiency.

But even results where a primary deficiency is not involved are quite promising and have encouraged scientists to keep digging. Bioenergetic therapies, they say, may benefit the course of neurologic diseases in which mitochondrial function is impaired and oxidative stress and damage are present.

Huntington's Disease

Huntington's disease (HD) is a devastating, degenerative brain disorder without an effective treatment or cure. HD slowly diminishes the ability to reason, talk, think, and walk, and eventually causes total dependence on others for personal care. This condition is one of the more common genetic diseases. More than a quarter of a million Americans have it or are at risk of inheriting the disease.

In a major multi–medical-center study, a group of 347 patients with early-stage disease were randomly chosen to receive either CoQ_{10} (300 mg twice a day), an experimental drug, a combination of CoQ_{10} and the drug, or an inert placebo pill.

The results, published in 2001 in the journal *Neurology*, indicated that none of the treatment strategies significantly stopped the decline in functional capacity over a thirty-month period. However, the researchers did report "a trend toward slowing" the decline among the CoQ_{10} takers. There were also beneficial trends in secondary measures.

CoQ_{10} reportedly promoted a longer ability to handle daily responsibilities such as domestic chores and finances, a better ability to focus, and less depression and irritability.

"The First Real Lead"

The changes were not sufficient enough to allow the researchers to recommend CoQ_{10} for treatment of HD. Still, Karl Kieburtz, M.D., professor of neurology at the University of Rochester Medical Center, described the results as an "interesting lead" against a disease where there is currently no way to slow the progression. A bigger study was warranted, he said.

"This is the first real lead we've gotten from more than a dozen Huntington's disease patient trials," said Kieburtz. "We can't ignore it. We've got something to chase."

Mitochondrial Myopathies

Hundreds of varieties of Mitochondrial Myopathies have been identified. Symptoms include various degrees of deafness, diabetes, heart problems, learning disabilities, muscle weakness and cramps, paralysis of eye muscles, seizures, and strokelike episodes.

CoQ_{10} supplementation appears beneficial for myopathy patients who have few options. There is no cure, but research shows that CoQ_{10} helps reduce defective bioenergetics inside of cells, and helps improve muscle movement.

"In these patients, even what can be considered a small improvement by healthy peoples' standards actually represents a considerable achievement," says CoQ_{10} researcher Gian Paolo Littarru. "I have personally witnessed the heart-warming progress of some patients who are able to walk better or to climb three flights of stairs where they were barely able to make one flight before."

Brain Toxicity

Studies conducted by M. Flint Beal, M.D., a neurologist at Massachusetts General Hospital, show that CoQ_{10} helps protects brain tissue from a variety of nerve toxins. In laboratory experiments, such toxins create significantly less injury in animals who are supplemented.

Beal, along with Italian researchers, has also demonstrated that CoQ_{10} protects against "excitoxicity." This condition occurs when the energy level of nerve cells falls, leading to cell damage and death.

Parkinson's Disease

Who hasn't seen those heart-wrenching pictures of the former heavyweight champion Muhammad Ali, his hands shaking and his speech slurred. The great boxer, and more than a million other Americans, suffer from Parkinson's disease, a disorder that progressively destroys the central nervous system. The disease also causes rigidity of muscles and slowness of movement.

Parkinson's is believed to be caused by a combination of biochemical defects, including free radical damage and mitochondrial-DNA mutation, that destroy cells in the substantia nigra. This part of the brain produces dopamine, a chemical substance that enables people to move normally and smoothly. In Parkinson's, there is a severe shortage of dopamine.

Researchers know that brain tissue is highly susceptible to free radical damage. They also know that the substantia nigra has the highest level of mitochondrial-DNA mutation in the brain. These events conspire to harm cellular energy production. Researchers now believe that energy consumption plays a large role in the progression of the disease.

CoQ_{10} Studies Promising

Beal and his research colleagues at Massachusetts General Hospital have conducted a fascinating series of revealing studies on CoQ_{10} and Parkinson's. They found that the bioenergetic reduction in patients is strongly associated with the patients' blood levels of CoQ_{10}.

They also determined that CoQ_{10} supplementation could significantly reduce the amount of damage in the dopamine system of mice treated with a neurotoxin causing symptoms similar to Parkinson's.

And, in both human patients and mice, they found that supplementation helps restore sluggish energy production in the mitochondria. For humans, they found that 600 mg was an effective dose.

In a follow-up study sponsored by the National Institute of Neurological Disorders and Stroke, researchers compared daily dosages of 300, 600, and 1,200 mg on patients with early Parkinson's who as yet did not require medication. The results of this study are due in 2002 and will further clarify the extent of effectiveness and dose tolerance of CoQ_{10} supplementation.

Alzheimer's Disease

Alzheimer's Disease

A degenerative brain disease caused by neuron dysfunction and death that causes problems with memory, feelings, thinking, and behavior.

Even when the health of former president Ronald Reagan is involved, the big guns of mainstream medicine have woefully little firepower to use against the relentless loss of mental faculties and function caused by Alzheimer's disease (AD).

There is no definitive cure. No definitive treatment. No definitive explanation of causes. AD affects about 10 percent of Americans over age sixty-five and nearly 50 percent of those over age eighty-five. Four million or more Americans now have AD. Within decades, as the baby boomer generation ages, the numbers are expected to soar to about 14 million.

No one knows if AD has one underlying cause or many. Scientists have investigated biochemical deficiencies; bioenergetic deficits; free radical damage; genetic abnormalities; malfunctions in the body's defenses; toxicity from metals such as aluminum, lead, and mercury; and viruses. Some researchers talk in terms of a "deleterious network" of events that causes AD to develop and progress.

More CoQ_{10} Research Needed

There is no direct research on supplementation with CoQ_{10} for Alzheimer's disease, except for one small Japanese study reported in a 1992 issue of the medical journal *Lancet*. In that study, 60 mg of CoQ_{10} daily, along with vitamin B_6 and iron, was shown to slow down the progression of the disease.

Recent studies have linked the degree of disability in patients with a decline of energy production and mitochondrial efficiency in brain cells. This suggests a possible CoQ_{10} role.

Scientists have cited the complicity of certain toxic proteins and free radicals in the damage and death of brain cells that occurs in AD. A byproduct of this activity is a toxin called HNE, which is found in excess amounts throughout the AD-affected brain. CoQ_{10} and vitamin E, both antioxidants, have been shown to reduce HNE formation in the bloodstream.

Research Should Include Other Supplements

At this point, little can be said about CoQ_{10} and Alzheimer's except that research is certainly warranted, and probably should include both CoQ_{10} and vitamin E. Vitamin E has also been found to slow down progression of the disease.

It is worth mentioning that studies continually find the aging population suffering from malnutrition, failing to get proper amounts of nutrients because of altered gastrointestinal function, imbalances in food or diet, malabsorption, or multiple drug use. And patients with dementia and AD are more likely to be nutritionally deficient than healthy older people.

Thus, a comprehensive nutritional-supplement package should be investigated for effectiveness against Alzheimer's disease. Included in it should be therapeutic dosages of CoQ_{10} and vitamin E, along with fatty acids, the B-complex vitamins, and other cellular "energizers," such as the amino acid L-carnitine. And, ideally, such a nutritional "cocktail" should be administered at the very earliest stage of the disease in an effort to slow down its progression.

Amyotrophic Lateral Sclerosis (ALS)— "Lou Gehrig's Disease"

This devastating disease, which cut short the baseball career and life of famed New York Yankee great Lou Gehrig, attacks the nerves cells responsible for muscle control, causing loss of muscle function and paralysis. The cause of ALS is not completely understood and there is no cure. Some 5,000 Americans are diagnosed with this condition each year.

Researchers at Columbia-Presbyterian Medical Center's Eleanor and Lou Gehrig ALS Center in New York have begun investigating a possible therapeutic role for CoQ_{10}.

Promising Pilot Study on ALS

In a small pilot study completed in 2001, the center announced that high-dose CoQ_{10} supplementation had resulted in "positive trends." This development encouraged the center to set up a larger trial, which is underway.

In the pilot study, lasting nine months, six patients took 600 mg of CoQ_{10} daily. At the end of that period, researchers determined that the supplement could be beneficial for preserving motor units. A motor unit consists of a muscle-controlling nerve cell and the muscle cells it controls. A patient with ALS typically loses about 50 percent of existing motor units over a six-month period. With CoQ_{10}, three patients actually showed minimal *gains* in motor-unit numbers, while the other three had losses of 16, 23, and 38 percent.

Due to the small number of patients, the researchers were reluctant to draw conclusions from the pilot study, but felt the positive trend strongly justified a follow-up study. Enrollment for the bigger study began in October 2001.

KEEPING YOUR GUMS HEALTHY

Most people develop gum disease at some point in their adult life, and unless they take care of the problem, it's bye-bye teeth. Gum disease (also called periodontal disease or periodontitis) is the leading cause of tooth loss.

Gum disease is usually treated by specialists who perform gum surgery or extract loose teeth. These specialists are known as periodontists. Some dentists also use non-surgical methods to treat periodontal disease, including a wide variety of nutritional supplements. High on their list of supplements is CoQ$_{10}$.

Gum Disease

Problems start with gingivitis, an inflammation of the gums resulting from bacterial plaque formation. The bacteria eat away the supportive gum tissue of the teeth. Untreated gingivitis becomes periodontitis, with progressive infection, inflammation, deepening pockets between the gums and teeth, and the development of bone recession and loose teeth.

The dental use of CoQ$_{10}$ dates back to the 1970s when researchers in Europe and Japan found a common deficiency among many patients with diseased gums. Further research showed that supplementation had a beneficial therapeutic effect.

In one double-blind clinical experiment over a three-week period, a group of patients were given either a placebo or a pill with 50 mg of CoQ$_{10}$. All eight patients on CoQ$_{10}$ improved significantly. The placebo group showed no improvement.

The CoQ$_{10}$ patients had less pain, swelling, bleeding, and looseness of teeth, and reduced gingival pocket depth. CoQ$_{10}$ also helped accelerate healing. The researchers said the results seen after three weeks of supplementation would normally take six months of treatment.

In Miami, Steven Green, D.D.S., has used CoQ$_{10}$ for years. He regards it as a remarkable agent to counteract "fatigued" gum tissue. "At the most basic level there is no disease, including gum disease, that strikes anyone unless there is fatigue," he says. "CoQ$_{10}$ is great for fatigue, because it enhances energy inside the mitochondria."

In the early 1980s, Green started using a 1-mg capsule (the only potency that was commercially available at the time), but did not see any clinical benefits. The dosage simply wasn't high enough. In time, CoQ$_{10}$ capsules in 10-mg strength became available. He then recommended two capsules a day to ten patients on two-month recall. That means their periodontal disease was very advanced and they needed to be seen every other month.

"Their situations were so precarious that we would discuss at each visit whether it was time for them to bite the bullet and go for surgery," Green recalls. "They had all the classical symptoms that called for more invasive treatment—deep pockets, easily bleeding gums, rapid formation of plaque, and general tenderness of the gums. But they refused to see a specialist. They preferred to stick with the non-surgical approach. And even though I had been able to help them hold their own, I hadn't been able to make any headway."

Dramatic Improvement

"As these CoQ$_{10}$ patients started returning, I checked for results. In six out of the ten cases, improvement was dramatic: two- and three-millimeter shrinkage of pockets. I had never seen anything work like that, and so fast. There was also significantly less bleeding."

Except for adding CoQ$_{10}$, the six patients had made no other changes. The other four patients who took CoQ$_{10}$ showed no such improvement. Still, the results encouraged Green to continue using CoQ$_{10}$ on a regular basis.

Craig Zunka, D.D.S., of Front Royal, Virginia, says he often reserves CoQ$_{10}$ as the "big cannon" in resistant cases. "Because CoQ$_{10}$ is expensive, I tend to use other supplements first," he says. "Initially, I will use antioxidants such as vitamin C and E and bring in CoQ$_{10}$ when I don't see the desired results."

Reduces Pockets and Bleeding

From Zunka's observations, CoQ$_{10}$ helps reduce bleeding and improve the texture and health of the gum tissue. Polly Hoverter, a dental hygienist in Zunka's office, describes how CoQ$_{10}$ dramatically helped to restore one patient with moderate-to-severe disease.

"This woman came in with many five- to six-millimeter pockets," says Hoverter. "Within three months, all the pockets were down to three millimeters. Within six months, most had shrunk down to two millimeters. Her gums, previously bleeding and with an unhealthy grayish tint, were now pink and healthy-looking. The CoQ$_{10}$ really seemed to have helped her gums get healthy from the inside out."

Clean Pockets First, Then Use CoQ$_{10}$

Depending on what blood chemistries and other tests reveal, holistic dentists carefully individualize the array of supplements they recommend to gum-disease patients. These supplements are pivotal in the non-surgical treatment of gum disease.

"We need first of all to clean up the deep pockets between the gum and the tooth, deep down, where your brushing and flossing can't reach," says Zunka.

"It is this deep-down clearing of the bacteria that is the critical element. We then irrigate the depths of that pocket with a wide variety of natural herbal and nutritional solutions. We train our patients how to use irrigation tools on their own at home so they can become an active part of the healing process.

"Some people don't need any supplements, or just a few," adds Zunka. "They just need all the bacteria and tartar cleaned out and then their bodies will do the rest. Others need to have their immune system and cellular energetics pushed to the max with all the supplements you can throw at them."

CoQ$_{10}$ Is Part of an Aggressive Nutritional Approach

In Manchester, Connecticut, periodontist Salvatore J. Squatrito, Jr., D.D.S., uses CoQ$_{10}$ as part of an aggressive nutritional approach to improve the gum health of patients.

"In order to get good healing, patients need to eat a better diet, with five to seven fruits and vegetables a day and twelve glasses of water, and they need to minimize their intake of sugar, carbonated drinks, and alcohol," he says. "And because of the way food is grown and processed today, supplementation is a necessity."

Squatrito has been recommending CoQ$_{10}$ for nearly ten years. "Patients who stick with it have less long-range trouble than they did in the past, before I used CoQ$_{10}$," he says. There is less bleeding and a gradual improvement in periodontal health.

Particularly Effective for Advanced Cases

CoQ$_{10}$ is particularly beneficial for patients with "refractory disease." This refers to advanced cases that do not respond well to therapy. They are characterized by major pockets, pus, and inherited genetic weakness in the gums.

"These factors are indicative of low resistance," says Squatrito. "I place these patients on CoQ$_{10}$ and a low-potency antibiotic to clear up the bacterial infections. Diet scans usually turn up nutritional deficiencies, so I recommend a whole range of other supplements as well to help build up resistance. We monitor diet very closely and do a lot of nutritional counseling with these patients in order to get results.

"The nature of their condition requires more effort, and more elbow grease on their part, to overcome it. "CoQ$_{10}$ is not a panacea. You have to limit the hostile environment. That means shrinking the pockets. You have to strengthen the patient at the same time. Then the chances of recurrence are minimized. But if you have deep pockets, and you only load up with CoQ$_{10}$ and think you will be OK, it won't happen."

The Risk of Spreading Infection

Squatrito says that a detailed periodontal charting and pocket-depth reading is necessary. Pockets deeper than four or five millimeters must be treated professionally. If not treated, they will accumulate hostile bacteria and the periodontal infection will advance.

"The risk is not just losing teeth," he says. "The infection can seep into your system, sap your energy, and even attack your heart."

Squatrito recommends that patients obtain a blood test to determine their CoQ$_{10}$ level. Such a test may or may not be covered by insurance, and will have to be done through a physician.

"From my experience, if the blood level is not over 2.5 micrograms of CoQ$_{10}$ per milliliter of blood, the likelihood of periodontal disease and recurrent infection is high," he says. "I try to have patients take enough CoQ$_{10}$ bring them up to a 2.5 or 3 microgram level. That's what can make a difference.

"I might start patients with 60 milligrams in the morning and another 60 milligrams in the evening, and see what kind of response they get. When I recheck them, and I find that the gingival fluid is cloudy, then I know they need more CoQ$_{10}$ and should probably be on an antibiotic as well.

"I am often able to get patients to the point where I only see them every six months or a year, and then I have little to do. That's a whole lot better for patients than having to return every two months, getting reamed out and having their gums drained."

The Patient Who Benefited Despite Himself

The great thing about CoQ$_{10}$ is that it also does so many other good things for the body, dentists note. As an example, Squatrito cites a patient who "doesn't give a damn about his teeth," but without CoQ$_{10}$ he can't walk up and down the steps without leg cramps. "That's why he takes it. It's the only reason. And it helps his teeth whether he's interested or not."

Dentists familiar with CoQ$_{10}$ recommend taking 30–60 mg daily for prevention.

HOW TO TAKE CoQ$_{10}$

Before we get into specifics, keep in mind that while CoQ$_{10}$ can do wonders, it is not a panacea. Don't expect it to serve as a rescue remedy for every physical ailment or for a ruinous lifestyle.

It is also important to point out that people with CoQ$_{10}$ deficiencies often have deficiencies in other key nutrients that can contribute to ill health or poor healing. This is particularly true of older individuals and those with medical conditions taking pharmaceutical drugs, but nutritional surveys consistently show that Americans of all ages are deficient in many vital nutrients.

In view of this, it is probably in the best interest of overall good health to take CoQ$_{10}$ along with a high-quality multivitamin and mineral formula, at the very least.

How Much to Take for Disease Prevention

Unlike many vitamins and minerals, CoQ$_{10}$ is not considered an essential nutrient that we must obtain in our diets or perish. That's because we make CoQ$_{10}$ in our bodies. And even though we may become deficient in CoQ$_{10}$ as a result of the aging process, certain genetic conditions, poor diet, stress, or the use of particular medications, the medical community is not yet advising supplementation for prevention.

Research on CoQ$_{10}$ is extensive and increasing all the time, but no one really knows precisely what represents an ideal "preventive" dose of CoQ$_{10}$. The research on this has not yet been done, so at this point we need to rely on the CoQ$_{10}$ experts, the researchers and clinicians most familiar with it.

Take 30 to 100 Mg for General Health

One obvious expert is Texas cardiologist Peter Langsjoen who has himself been taking CoQ$_{10}$ and recommending it to patients for twenty years. He believes that a healthy person in their forties could probably take 30 or 60 mg a day and see a variety of benefits.

"What we know is for illness," he says. "You see measurable changes in blood levels and heart function somewhere between thirty and sixty milligrams a day. It would seem reasonable to take that much for general health purposes and energy."

Langsjoen takes 100 mg twice a day. "I'm forty-seven, a very busy practitioner, and in good health," he says. "I feel it gives me great energy."

To Help Prevent Heart Attacks

Fellow cardiologist Stephen Sinatra believes that CoQ$_{10}$ can help both young and old. He recommends a preventive dose of 100 mg daily.

"If you are older and tired, double that amount," he says. As a supplement to help prevent heart attacks, he suggests 100 or 200 mg a day, along with natural vitamin E (200 IU for women and 200 to 400 IU for men).

"Be sure to use a form of vitamin E that contains not just alpha tocopherol, the most common form, but also gamma tocopherol," he adds. "This form is more expensive but it is also more protective. Take at least twenty-five international units of gamma tocopherol."

"I strongly believe CoQ$_{10}$ helps prevent cancer," says Sinatra. "There are no controlled studies, but from what we know of blood levels in patients with cancer, I don't have reservations about younger people taking CoQ$_{10}$."

Over Fifty? Take CoQ$_{10}$ for the Rest of Your Life

Australian expert on aging and CoQ$_{10}$ Anthony Linnane, age seventy, believes that "everyone over fifty should take CoQ$_{10}$ for the rest of their life."

He also recommends 100 mg a day, and takes 500 mg a day himself. "You should also take plenty of vitamins C and E for their additional antioxidant benefits," he says. "We aren't perfect machines, so there is no reason we can't give our normal processes a bit of nutritional help from the outside and improve them."

How Much to Take for Therapeutic Effect

Therapeutic doses generally range from 100–600 mg a day.

Langsjoen recommends at least 100 mg to his heart patients for general therapeutic purposes.

"If you can afford it, take 100 milligrams twice a day," he says. "And people who are very sick should take 400 milligrams. I have used even more in some cases. People may need the higher doses if they don't absorb it well, or if they have substantial heart failure and a lot of edema."

Subjectively, how can you tell if the CoQ$_{10}$ you are taking is working for you? "The most obvious thing you'll notice is improved energy and stamina," says Langsjoen.

If Possible, Have Your Blood Level Checked

Objectively, you can ask your physician to conduct a blood test that measures CoQ$_{10}$. More and more medical laboratories are offering this service as interest in CoQ$_{10}$ rises. And with this development comes more accurate and reliable tests.

A normal blood level is .8 to 1.2 micrograms per milliliter of blood. However, to obtain therapeutic benefits, the experts say the level must be driven up into the 2.5 to 3.5 range through sustained supplementation.

Cardiologist Stephen Sinatra notes that CoQ$_{10}$ has occasionally failed to show therapeutic potency in medical studies because researchers weren't getting high enough blood levels due to inadequate doses being administered to those in the study. "I find that the higher the blood level of CoQ$_{10}$ in very elderly or sicker patients, the greater the benefits," he says.

Other Key Supplements May Be Necessary

"However, about 15 percent of my cardiac patients do not experience therapeutic improvements with CoQ$_{10}$ supplementation, even when I raise their blood levels to 3.5 micrograms," he adds.

"The CoQ$_{10}$ is indeed getting into the body but is just not enough on its own to achieve the desired results. In those cases, I add other key supplements, such as L-Carnitine and NADH."

Among nutritional supplements, CoQ$_{10}$ is relatively expensive. Capsules typically come in 10, 30, 50, 60, or 100 mg. A bottle of sixty 10-mg capsules may retail for around $7; a bottle of sixty 100-mg capsules for about $45.

You May Require Less Medication

If you are under a doctor's care, please consult with your physician before starting CoQ$_{10}$. As we've seen throughout this book, CoQ$_{10}$ has the ability to improve cellular energy and thus have a positive impact on many symptoms. The effects can be very striking.

For instance, it can lower high blood pressure. And if you take a significant dose of blood-pressure medication, you may become lightheaded because your pressure drops as a result of CoQ_{10}.

It is indeed probable that some medications can be reduced or somehow adjusted after CoQ_{10} is started. This is generally desirable since drugs typically cause side effects and disturb normal processes in the body. But don't stop or reduce medication on your own. That should be done only under the guidance of a physician.

Your doctor may not know about CoQ_{10} or may dismiss it. In either case, you may want to show him or her this book and mention that there have been thousands of scientific studies proving CoQ_{10}'s effectiveness and safety. Keep in mind also that your doctor may have a bias against a simple nutritional supplement that he or she is not familiar with.

How to Take CoQ_{10}

If you slug down your vitamins with a glass of water whenever you remember, it is very probable you aren't getting a big bang for your CoQ_{10} buck. It works better if you take it with a meal, and preferably with a meal that has some fat in it. CoQ_{10} is a fat-soluble compound. That means it dissolves, and absorbs, more effectively in a fatty environment.

There is also a saturation effect with CoQ_{10}. Research shows that your body can only make use of about 180 mg maximum at a time, so if you take more in a single dose, you may not be utilizing the excess. If you take more than that amount, divide your daily dosage. "Most of my cardiac patients take it twice a day," says Langsjoen.

"To get the big heart benefits and other improvements, sick people need to take CoQ_{10} in big enough doses and with their food. Those are the two biggest mistakes when you don't see results: using Mickey-Mouse doses or not taking it with food."

Experts advise keeping CoQ_{10} away from heat and out of direct sunlight, so keep it stored in a cool, dark pantry, for instance.

How Safe Is CoQ_{10}?

CoQ_{10} is extremely safe to take. I've never heard of anything in the way of complaints in any shape, form, or fashion," says Langsjoen. "And I have prescribed CoQ_{10} to thousands of patients." The medical literature mentions 1 or 2 percent of users experiencing some upset stomach. "But I have never come across this or any other effect in nearly twenty years of using CoQ_{10}," Langsjoen adds. If an upset stomach develops, try reducing the amount of CoQ_{10} you take, or switch to a different form (see page 103 for more on forms of CoQ_{10}).

One recent Scandinavian report stated that the effec-

tiveness of Coumadin, a commonly prescribed blood thinner, was decreased in three patients who took CoQ_{10}. Langsjoen has specifically looked for this effect and has never observed it, even using amounts much greater than those used in the Scandinavian cases.

Are All Forms of CoQ_{10} Equal?

Although the original discoveries of CoQ_{10} occurred in the United States, Japan has dominated the commercial production. In the mid-1970s, the fermentation technology that produces pure CoQ_{10} from yeast was developed there. Today, two Japanese pharmaceutical companies supply most of the CoQ_{10} used in supplements and medical research. Quality is quite good, say the experts.

Supplements are commonly found in three forms: as capsules containing yellow powder, soft-gels with CoQ_{10} dissolved in a natural oil base, or tablets. If you don't see the expected results from one form of CoQ_{10}, you may want to switch to another. It could be you are not absorbing that particular supplement well.

"When you treat people with CoQ_{10} and they don't react to the compound, they are probably not absorbing it," says cardiologist Stephen Sinatra. "I have seen patients taking as much as 500 milligrams daily, yet they have an ordinary blood level that they might have from just their regular diet.

"I saw a young man with cardiomyopathy who was taking 200 milligrams a day and yet his blood level was .8 micrograms. I put him on a different form of CoQ_{10} which elevated his blood level up to 3.5 micrograms, and he had a totally different quality of life."

Langsjoen contends that "no matter what kind of CoQ_{10} you take, you can get just about a doubling of the blood level by swallowing it with a meal as opposed to taking it with water alone. That alone makes a big difference."

The Vitamin B_6 Connection

The B-complex vitamins, and particularly B_6, are key ingredients used by certain enzymes in the body to produce CoQ_{10}. Both vitamin B_6 and CoQ_{10} levels decline as we age. For that reason, researchers at the University of Texas in Austin recommended that patients receiving supplemental CoQ_{10} also be supplemented with vitamin B_6. That would enhance better synthesis of CoQ_{10} in the body to go along with the supplement, they wrote in a 1999 report in the journal *Biofactors*.

As noted, CoQ_{10} is relatively expensive. Thus, individuals who cannot afford the higher therapeutic doses may want to boost their own CoQ_{10} production with a B_6 supplement. B_6 is inexpensive.

Peter Langsjoen relates the case of a patient with very low levels of B_6 and CoQ_{10}. The patient couldn't easily afford CoQ_{10}, but was readily able to purchase the vitamin. "I suggested 100 milligrams of B_6 a day," recalls Langsjoen.

"I rechecked his CoQ_{10} level in about two months, and it had significantly increased. The level wasn't as high as the therapeutic dose of CoQ_{10} I felt he needed, but I was impressed by the increase created by B_6. And his B_6 level was now normal."

THE FUTURE OF CoQ₁₀

Modern medicine has taken the approach that a disease can be furiously and selectively attacked with the likes of antibiotics, powerful drugs, chemotherapy, and surgery, without any damage to the host body. It's a medical myth.

Someone may be cured of one condition only to suffer or die from something else caused by the treatment. In general, the time borrowed with medication and surgery does not mean that health has been restored.

Patients are demanding a change. And as our medical system matures, it will likely come to honor the need to strengthen the body with key nutritional supplements such as CoQ_{10}. This is what an integrative medical approach is all about, and today many large hospitals and major university medical centers have taken steps in this direction by opening "complementary" or "alternative" clinics.

The Changing Medical Scene

In this shifting ambiance, interested patients should have more access to savvy doctors who believe in and use many natural healing remedies. Such practitioners may recommend a certain drug and a nutritional supplement to prevent side effects and bolster the body from the onslaught of drug or surgical stress. The idea is really to use the best combination of approaches, not just one that takes away the symptom and leaves the cause of the disease still smoldering in the body.

CoQ_{10} is not a patented drug. It's a natural compound. You can't patent it. And because of this, it has no big pharmaceutical sugar daddy pushing major research, advertising in medical journals, peddling it to doctors, and staging media blitzes. This is why it has taken decades to get the word out. But CoQ_{10} is just too good for researchers and doctors to ignore.

The late Karl Folkers, the respected University of Texas researcher who studied CoQ_{10} for decades, believed that the supplement had huge medical applications, from brain disorders to cancer to heart disease. "When you favorably affect the bioenergetics of your cells, the results show up in all tissues," he said.

Even a Small Deficiency Could Be Critical

As medical science probes deeper into the mitochondrial and bioenergetic basis for disease and the aging process itself, CoQ_{10} figures to keep gaining more importance. Rolf Luft, M.D., Ph.D., of the Karolinska Hospital in Sweden, and one of the pioneers in mitochondrial medicine, has observed that even a relatively small deficiency of CoQ_{10} may be a key factor in the development of mitochondrial disorders.

Mitochondrial medicine is a dynamic frontier of current research. Some scientists refer to it as a revolution in medical and aging research. And the results of 4,000 studies already make it clear that we have a uniquely powerful healing and protective friend in CoQ_{10}.

Researchers in Europe even think that CoQ_{10} may reduce the detrimental oxidation of skin tissue that contributes to wrinkling and aging skin. Thus, you can now buy skin creams containing CoQ_{10}.

And recently, Italian researchers found that patients with macular degeneration, the leading cause of blindness in people older than fifty, have low levels of CoQ_{10}. They believe that CoQ_{10} may be able to help counteract the free radical damage thought to be the basis of this age-associated disease.

An Exciting Future

CoQ_{10} has gained increasing attention simply because it plays a very central role in the body. Can you name a single drug with so many healing benefits? And can you name any drug that does so much without any side effects?

Many practitioners of nutritional medicine have long used CoQ_{10} as part of their treatment strategies. Often, they use it as part of a multiple antioxidant combination (along with such nutrients as alpha-lipoic acid, l-carnitine, and vitamins A, C, and E) to generate a broad-spectrum healing effect.

But whether alone or in combination, CoQ_{10} clearly represents a major weapon for doctors in their battle against disease. Hopefully, they will recognize it and use it because ignoring it is a major disservice to patients.

Fred Crane, the research biochemist who started it all with his discovery of CoQ_{10} back in 1957, sums it up when he says, "what we do know about CoQ_{10} is very exciting . . . and what we still don't know figures to be even more exciting."

PART FIVE

CALCIUM & MAGNESIUM

NAN KATHRYN FUCHS, PH.D.

Calcium. It's not just a miracle mineral for strong bones. Calcium helps your heart contract, lowers your blood pressure, and nourishes your nerves. In some people, it protects against colon cancer and reduces symptoms of PMS.

But calcium doesn't work alone. Without enough magnesium, calcium can actually cause more harm than good. Calcium is better known than magnesium. But magnesium is so important to our health, and so lacking in our diets, that people who supplement with it often think they've found a miracle mineral. In many ways, they have.

Magnesium is calcium's partner in many body functions. Without enough magnesium, calcium can't get into your bones. It's simply not absorbed. And this unabsorbed calcium can lead to such health problems as arthritis and heart disease. Although a great many supplements contain both calcium and magnesium, you may need more magnesium and less calcium than they contain—especially if you also eat a high-calcium, low-magnesium diet.

A typical American diet tends to be high in calcium and low in magnesium. Most supplements contain more calcium than magnesium, as well. Calcium supplements are among the most widely taken of all nutrients. More people take extra calcium than even vitamin C! The result is that our mineral balance has become calcium heavy and magnesium deficient.

Low magnesium can contribute to high blood pressure, premenstrual mood swings and anxiety, sore muscles, depression, headaches, diabetes, and more. You need plenty of magnesium for a healthy nervous system, for energy, and to build strong bones. When you increase your magnesium, all of these conditions improve. There's no doubt that getting enough calcium is extremely important. But getting adequate magnesium is often even more important.

If you're taking a lot of calcium and not paying attention to magnesium, it's probably because that's the advice you've heard. It's information that's generally accepted as being accurate. However, the amount of calcium and magnesium you've been told to take is based on very old

research. Newer studies indicate that we need less calcium and more magnesium than previously thought.

This part of the *User's Guide to Nutritional Supplements* is designed to clear up the confusion about these two very important minerals and explain how they work together. It will answer your questions about the role of calcium and magnesium in various diseases and help you decide how much of each you need to get and stay healthy.

Each of our bodies has slightly different needs so not everyone needs the same amount of every nutrient. This is not a "one size fits all" situation. There are always variables that are not addressed in the studies that have been conducted. Your body's calcium and magnesium requirements may not only be different from someone else's, they may also change with age, stress, the medications you take, and your particular health conditions.

The amount of calcium and magnesium you need depends also on their forms. Not all of the minerals we get in our food or supplements can be well absorbed. Some forms of calcium and magnesium are well absorbed, like calcium citrate and magnesium citrate-malate. Others are not, like calcium carbonate and magnesium oxide. Since unabsorbed calcium can cause painful and life-threatening health problems, it's important to understand which forms are best absorbed and to use only them.

This part of the guide helps you understand how your particular health and age affect your body's needs for calcium and magnesium. With this information, you can decide how much of each of these important minerals your body needs, and in which forms.

UNDERSTANDING CALCIUM

You can't escape it. News about calcium is everywhere—in magazines, on TV, and in newspapers. Everybody's talking about the need for extra calcium to prevent osteoporosis. The reason for this is that 98 percent of all calcium is needed to continuously make bone. But if you think that calcium's only job is to build strong bones, you're mistaken. Calcium is essential for heart and nerve function, even though only 2 percent gets used for that purpose.

The 2 percent of calcium that stays in your blood and soft tissues is vitally important to your health and well-being. All of your muscles—including your heart—need calcium to contract. In addition, your blood needs calcium to clot. And your nervous system needs enough calcium to send messages throughout your body.

The problem is that you may be taking too much of a good thing. Taking too much calcium can be as much of a problem as getting too little. Excessive amounts of calcium can contribute to muscle cramping, heart palpitations and heart disease, fibromyalgia (nonspecific muscle pain), and some premenstrual syndrome (PMS) symptoms.

Cofactor
A substance that helps another substance perform its functions.

This is why it's important to take the amount of calcium your particular body needs, and to take it in an easy-to-absorb form. Since calcium doesn't work alone, it's essential to take it with enough of its cofactors. Calcium can't be well absorbed or be used effectively without other nutrients, such as vitamin D, potassium, iron, and magnesium.

Why Calcium Is So Important

Calcium is the most abundant mineral in your body. Almost all of it is in your bones. Don't think of bones as being dead sticks that hold your body together and keep you from collapsing. They are living tissues that are constantly breaking down and being rebuilt. The minerals that make up bone tissue need to be constantly available so that bone can be made continuously. Since some calcium is naturally excreted from your body every day, you need to get sufficient calcium in your diet and supplements every day.

In addition, your body needs calcium to help transmit nerve impulses along nerve cells to send messages across your nervous system. Calcium also helps blood to clot and is involved in many other chemical reactions throughout your body.

What do minerals do?
Minerals help build bones and connective tissues. They also help messages travel along the nerves and support enzyme production.

One of calcium's major jobs is to help all of the muscles in your body to contract. Magnesium, on the other hand, helps them to relax. Together, these minerals regulate your heartbeat by contracting and relaxing as necessary. So, calcium is vital to a healthy heart. The right amount of calcium helps maintain a regular heartbeat, but too much or too little calcium can cause an irregular heartbeat, called an arrhythmia.

Because too much calcium can contribute to health problems, it's important to take just the right amount. This can be confusing because different people look at the amount of calcium we need differently.

RDAs, DRIs, and Other Opinions

There are a lot of opinions about how much calcium we need. Most medical doctors and registered dietitians follow the recommended guidelines given by a government agency. The Food and Nutrition Board of the National Academy of Sciences/National Research Council has assessed our need for nutrient doses at various stages of our lives based on a number of studies. This government agency updates the recommended amount of vitamins and minerals as new information becomes available. However, there are always conflicting studies giving different information. The amount of any nutrient this government agency says we need is called either an RDA or a DRI.

Recommended Daily Allowances (RDA)
Recommendations by the National Academy of Sciences for the amount of nutrients an "average" healthy person's body needs.

Dietary Reference Intakes (DRI)
A combination of RDAs and other values. Presently, they're essentially the same as RDAs and may be used interchangeably.

The RDAs for calcium for adolescents and adults are between 1,000 and 1,300 mg a day.

• Males and females ages 25 to 49: 1,000 mg per day.

• Males and females over age 50: 1,200 mg per day.

• Adolescents and teens: 1,300 mg per day.

• Children ages 4 to 8: 800 mg per day.

• Pregnant and lactating women: 1,000 mg per day.

Grams and Milligrams
A gram (g) is a unit of weight. One pound equals 454 grams. A milligram (mg) is one-thousandth of a gram.

Even though these recommended amounts are based on scientific studies, numerous doctors, scientists, and nutritionists are finding that these doses don't work for all of their patients. If only it was this simple, all we would need to do is to find the RDA or DRI for calcium and take that amount. Unfortunately, it's not that cut-and-dried. Not only are many health practitioners questioning the RDA for calcium, newer studies are finding that these amounts may be too high for many people, especially if they already have health problems.

Many health practitioners are finding that 500 mg of supplemental calcium a day reduces health conditions like heart disease and fibromyalgia, and still protects bone density. If you look only at RDAs and DRIs without considering your body's individual needs, you may be overlooking important information that could impact your health greatly.

These RDAs and DRIs are based on the amount of calcium a healthy person needs, but these standards do not account for individual differences in absorption. People with serious health conditions like colon cancer and heart disease need more or less calcium. Also, many people are neither sick nor healthy, but are somewhere in between. They can have symptoms of a calcium deficiency or excess, but these symptoms may not be severe enough to be called a particular disease. To meet your particular calcium requirements, you need to look more closely at your age, health, and diet.

Calcium for Osteoporosis

The most popular reason for taking large amounts of calcium is to prevent osteoporosis. Fear motivates many women to take more than their bodies can use. Wherever we turn, we see advertisements for calcium supplements that show women's bodies bent and twisted from osteoporosis. These ads are designed to help sell more calcium supplements. And they do. In theory, taking a lot of calcium may make sense. But in practice, it doesn't always work. In fact, it can backfire.

To prevent osteoporosis, calcium has to get absorbed into your bones. David Levinson, M.D., of the Cornell University Medical Center in New York City, found that the highest amount of calcium anyone should take at one time for good absorption is just 500 mg. This makes sense. If you look at the amount of calcium in many healthy meals, it rarely tops 500 mg. Over the centuries, our bodies have learned to utilize that amount at any one time, but not a great deal more.

It's not unusual for people to take 1,000–1,500 mg of calcium supplements a day in addition to any calcium in the foods they eat. And they often take these supplements all at once, so they won't forget to take them later. The problem is that very little of these high amounts of calcium can be absorbed. Perhaps this is one reason why an article published in *The New England Journal of Medicine* reported that a two-year clinical study that gave 2,000 mg of calcium a day to participants showed little to no effect on bone density.

Other studies have had similar findings. A four-year Mayo Clinic study, also published in *The New England Journal of Medicine*, divided its participants into two groups. One group took 1,400 mg of calcium supplements a day. The other group took less than 500 mg. The rate of bone loss in both groups was the same. Clearly, there's more to bone density than taking a lot of calcium.

When you take more calcium than you can use, the extra calcium isn't automatically excreted. In fact, it can con-

Absorption
The passage of substances, such as the nutrients in food, into the blood and tissues.

Osteoporosis
A condition of reduced bone density and increased bone brittleness that can lead to bones that break easily.

tribute to uncomfortable and dangerous conditions like arthritis and heart disease. The key is to take the right amount of a well-absorbed form of calcium along with other nutrients needed to help it work.

Make Sure Your Body Can Use Calcium

Calcium doesn't work alone. In order to perform its various functions, it requires cofactors like magnesium and phosphorus, along with vitamins A, B$_6$, C, D, and E. Of all the cofactors calcium needs, magnesium is perhaps the most important. It helps carry calcium into the bones, and it allows muscles to relax, after calcium causes them to contract.

Dairy products are high in calcium, but they don't have enough magnesium to help move it into your bones. Whole grains and green leafy vegetables, on the other hand, contain calcium as well as many of its cofactors. A combination of a little dairy along with some whole grains and green vegetables may be your best approach to getting sufficient calcium in your food. However, dairy is not essential. Even vegans can get plenty of calcium if they eat a healthy diet.

Before your body can use calcium, it has to be absorbed. Some calcium supplements are poorly absorbed; others are better absorbed. Calcium seems to be best absorbed when it is in the presence of some kind of acid. This acid may be in your food, or it may be the acid secreted by your stomach to help with digestion. The form of calcium you take helps determine how much of this mineral gets into your body. Calcium carbonate, for example, is low in acid and is very poorly absorbed by people who have low stomach acid compared with the more acidic calcium citrate. (More about this later.)

Vegan
A vegetarian who does not eat eggs or dairy. Vegans can get enough calcium if their diets contain sufficient servings of beans, whole grains, nuts, and green vegetables.

How Age Affects Your Need for Calcium

You have a smart body. It knows which nutrients you need and how to conserve them. It knows that the need for calcium is highest in pregnant women, babies, young children, and young adults, when most bone tissue is forming.

Teens need a lot of calcium. This is because the teen years are the body's last chance to store away extra calcium in the bones and protect them against bone loss later in life. So at these times when we need the most calcium, our bodies absorb it best and excrete it less.

A baby whose bones are forming rapidly can absorb up to 400 mg of calcium a day and excretes only 10 to 40 mg. Calcium absorption changes dramatically after age twenty. From then on, our bodies excrete more calcium and retain less than before—except during pregnancy. An adult absorbs only 20 to 30 percent of the calcium they consume.

Postmenopausal women can often absorb no more than 7 percent. While some might interpret this to mean that post-menopausal women should be taking very high amounts of calcium, remember that whatever the body doesn't absorb and excrete can create other health problems.

Adults don't excrete all the unused calcium in their diets and supplements. This is why it's so important for all adults to make certain that the calcium they take is absorbed as well as possible. If your body can't absorb and store it as well as when you were younger, your choice of calcium sources becomes extremely important.

You need about the same amount of calcium as an older adult as you needed as a younger adult. It's just that as you age, less calcium gets absorbed and more is excreted. Again, it's not only the amount of calcium you take that's important with aging, but also calcium absorption and retention.

Other factors enter the calcium-absorption picture as you get older. Poor kidney function can affect calcium absorption. To prevent too much calcium from being excreted in your urine, your kidneys save and reuse some of it. If your kidneys are not working properly, they may not be conserving enough calcium. When this happens, calcium gets stored in soft tissues rather than in bones. This can lead to arthritis, heart disease, hypertension, and even senile dementia.

Digestion and Calcium Absorption

Poor digestion can greatly affect your calcium absorption because of the connection between calcium absorption and acid. A number of studies suggest that calcium needs some form of acid in order to be broken down into a usable form. If you don't have enough acid present with calcium, you may not be absorbing it well. While not all studies have come to this conclusion, your calcium absorption should increase if you take it with some form of acid.

Fortunately, your smart body already makes an acid. When you eat, your stomach secretes hydrochloric acid (HCl). This acid helps digest protein. It also helps break down calcium, magnesium, and other minerals. But as we get older, our bodies make less HCl.

When you chew your food, a message travels from your taste buds to your stomach, telling it to secrete HCl. One method of increasing calcium absorption is simply to chew your food better. This can help your digestion in general, as well as increase your body's ability to use calcium.

Antacids have the opposite effect. They interfere with calcium absorption. Antacids neutralize HCl, reducing that very same acid that helps your body break down and use calcium. If you don't have much HCl due to aging, or if you're taking antacids, there's another possible solution (unless you're unable to eat the following suggested foods and beverages). You can accompany foods high in calcium with small amounts of tomato, orange juice, lemon water, or a little vinegar. The acids in these foods and beverages can help break down and utilize calcium. For instance, when you add an oil-and-vinegar dressing to a salad, you absorb more of the calcium in the salad greens, as well as the calcium in any cheese that may be contained in either the salad or dressing.

The connection between calcium and HCl is not clear-cut. Robert R. Recker, M.D., is one of several authors of a study published in the journal *Calcified Tissue International*. This study found that HCl is needed to break down calcium, but it wasn't essential for calcium absorption. In a previous study, however, Dr. Recker found that people with low HCl had poor calcium absorption.

Since we don't know exactly what role acid plays in the utilization of calcium, you may want to take steps to maximize calcium absorption. First, take calcium supplements with your meals. Avoid antacids whenever possible. Take calcium with acidic foods. And chew all your food better to help your body secrete needed HCl.

Antacids and Calcium Absorption

Many doctors insist that antacids are a perfectly good source of calcium supplementation because they are inexpensive and high in calcium. If your doctor recommends that you take calcium-containing antacids instead of another form of calcium, ask why. Acid helps the body utilize calcium.

Numerous studies have concluded that antacids are not protective against osteoporosis. A six-year study of more than 6,000 women, published in the *New England Journal of Medicine*, found that women who used Tums antacid as their only source of supplemental calcium had more broken arms than women who didn't. This was a large enough study to get the attention of many people, but not enough to stop doctors from suggesting their patients continue to use this inexpensive form of calcium.

Another study of more than 9,000 women over age sixty-five studied calcium intake versus broken bones. Information on broken bones was collected every four months for more than six years. Those women who took high-calcium antacids had more broken arms than those who took other forms of calcium.

The calcium in antacids is calcium carbonate, a poorly absorbed form of calcium that needs to be in the presence of some kind of acid before your body can use it. The calcium in an antacid begins by being difficult to absorb. Then, if you take an antacid with a high-calcium meal, you will not be able to absorb much of the calcium in your food, either. Antacids may prevent heartburn, but the calcium they contain isn't your best source of absorbable calcium.

What about Prilosec or other drugs that block the production of HCl? They may also interfere with calcium absorption. However, if you have an ulcer, acid reflux, or other medical condition where HCl causes pain, you may need to continue taking these medications, even if they affect your calcium levels.

The Consequences of Too Much Calcium

If you're boosting your calcium intake both in your diet and in supplements just to be on the safe side—take another look at what you're doing. This approach is not necessarily safe, and it could even be dangerous. Extra calcium can cause as many problems as not having enough. And taking a lot of calcium doesn't guarantee that it's getting into your bones.

Guy E. Abraham, M.D., is a research gynecologist and endocrinologist who has researched the subject of calcium and magnesium for decades. He has also published dozens of studies in scientific journals. Dr. Abraham points out that when calcium isn't absorbed into your bones, it doesn't just magically disappear. It can lead to clogged arteries (atherosclerosis). Or it can collect in your joints where it contributes to arthritis, or in your kidneys where it can contribute to the formation of kidney stones.

In addition to clogging your arteries, calcium can accumulate in your aorta. This can reduce the aorta's elasticity and lead to heart disease. When too much calcium gets into muscle tissues, it can produce muscle cramps and fibromyalgia (nonspecific muscle pain). Excessive calcium can also cause irritability, while the right amount can keep you calm.

Stephen Seely, a professor of cardiology in England, wrote in the *International Journal of Cardiology* that many diseases could be avoided if calcium consumption was reduced. He found that hypertension in older age is virtually nonexistent in countries where calcium intake is low.

Too much calcium doesn't protect your bones. In fact, it can lead to the formation of brittle bones that break easily. To avoid this brittleness, you need to be getting plenty of magnesium in your diet and supplements. Magnesium makes bones more flexible and less prone to breaking. Some nutrients strengthen bones, while others, surprisingly, have the opposite effect.

Calcium, Vitamin C, and Broken Hips

You'd think that it's a good idea to take a lot of vitamin C and calcium. Many people do. But it may not be a good idea or even safe. Here's an example of when "more" may not be "better." It concerns women who take a lot of vitamin C along with high amounts of calcium. A Swedish study with 65,000 participants published in the *International Journal of Epidemiology* found that women who took high amounts of both vitamin C and calcium had the highest number of hip fractures. When they reduced their vitamin C intake, they had fewer cases of broken hips.

We don't know what would have happened if they reduced their intake of calcium and not vitamin C. But it seems clear that the combination may not be as beneficial as you thought. For now, you may want to take high quantities of vitamin C supplements as needed, and just the amount of calcium your body needs.

Take a Look at the Whole Picture

It should be clear by now that calcium doesn't work alone, that too much calcium can cause health problems, and that high amounts of calcium are not the answer to forming and maintaining healthy bones. So what's next?

First, take a closer look at magnesium, a mineral you may know little about. Once you understand what magnesium does, you'll be ready to take a look at various health conditions and the role of both calcium and magnesium in each. From there, you can decide how much calcium you need, and how much magnesium should accompany it.

UNDERSTANDING MAGNESIUM

Magnesium is at least as important as calcium. It not only affects the health of your bones, it also plays a significant role in a wide number of body functions. You need lots of magnesium for strong bones, a healthy heart, and to alleviate PMS (premenstrual syndrome) and muscle cramps.

While most calcium is stored in bones, most magnesium remains in your muscles. Calcium causes muscles to contract, while magnesium helps them to relax. Your heart is a muscle that relies on this combination of relaxing and contracting. All of your muscles contain, and need, more magnesium than calcium. It is extremely important that you get enough magnesium for all muscle-related conditions including arrhythmia (irregular heartbeat), headaches, muscle cramps, fibromyalgia, and restless leg syndrome.

But magnesium does even more. It is a natural, safe calcium-channel blocker, protecting you against heart disease. And it is just as important as calcium in preventing osteoporosis. In addition, magnesium helps reduces stress by having a calming effect.

Calcium-Channel Blocker
A substance, often a drug, that protects against heart disease by preventing excess calcium from getting into the smooth muscles of your heart.

Magnesium's Many Functions

Magnesium works both in partnership with calcium, and independently. On its own, magnesium helps "turn on" hundreds of enzymes. These enzymes allow the carbohydrates (starches and sugars) and fats in your diet to be used as energy. So getting enough magnesium is important in fighting fatigue.

Magnesium also helps regulate nerve cell function,

allowing your nervous system to relax. One sign of stress that can signal a need for more magnesium is a sensitivity to loud noises.

Magnesium helps your mood and affects how well you sleep. Serotonin is a chemical that produces a feeling of well-being. Melatonin is a hormone that helps you sleep. You can't produce enough of either of these brain chemicals without sufficient magnesium.

> **Melatonin**
> *A hormone made from serotonin that helps regulate hormone secretion, sleepiness, and wakefulness. Supplemental melatonin can help prevent jet lag.*

Our bodies make less and less melatonin as we age. In addition, many older people eat diets low in magnesium, which could boost their melatonin production. If you're depressed or have trouble sleeping, you may not need an antidepressant or a sleeping pill. You may just need more magnesium.

Magnesium and Calcium Work Together

You want your heart muscle to both contract and relax. Because calcium causes your muscles to contract while magnesium helps them to relax, you need a balance of these two minerals for a healthy heart. If you have too many contractions and not enough relaxing, you can have an irregular heartbeat or a heart attack.

Magnesium can prevent and reverse constipation. Your colon is a long muscle that requires calcium and magnesium to contract and relax, allowing waste products to be eliminated. If you have too much calcium or not enough magnesium, you may have spasms in your colon. Or you could become constipated. After ruling out more serious problems, many health practitioners now look at constipation as a possible sign of a magnesium deficiency.

RDAs for Magnesium

Of all the RDAs, the ones for magnesium may be the most misleading. With diets already low in magnesium, and increased magnesium excretion from stress and other health conditions, your need for this mineral may be greater than the RDAs suggest. Author and physician Alan R. Gaby, M.D., is just one of a growing number of medical doctors with a practice that focuses on nutrition. He has found that most of his patients are magnesium-deficient.

The RDAs for magnesium are between 320 and 420 mg a day for adolescents and adults. Interestingly, although there are more signs of magnesium deficiency symptoms in women than in men, magnesium RDAs are higher for men than for women.

- Males ages 25 to 49: 420 mg per day.
- Females ages 25 to 49: 320 mg per day.
- Children ages 4 to 8: 130 mg per day.
- Pregnant and lactating women: 310–360 mg per day.

How to Know if You Need More Magnesium

If your diet is low in magnesium-rich foods like whole grains, nuts, seeds, and beans, chances are you need more magnesium. This is especially true if you eat a lot of dairy products, which are high in calcium with almost no magnesium.

Most dietary supplements contain twice as much calcium as magnesium. In theory, this may reflect the body's need for these two minerals. But practically speaking, years of stress and diets low in magnesium upset nature's balance. Many people need at least as much magnesium as calcium. If you take high calcium supplements with half as much magnesium, or less, chances are you would benefit from more magnesium.

Are you a chocoholic? It may be a sign that you have a magnesium deficiency. Chocolate is very high in magnesium. If you crave chocolate, either all the time or when you are premenstrual and your need for magnesium increases, you may need more magnesium. Constipation, irregular heartbeat, muscle cramps, and muscle pain (fibromyalgia) are all signs of a possible need for more magnesium.

Why So Many People Are Low in Magnesium

Blame it on your ancestors. Research gynecologist and endocrinologist Guy E. Abraham, M.D., looked back in history and found an interesting explanation for magnesium deficiencies. Thousands of years ago, he discovered, our ancestors ate diets high in magnesium—nuts, seeds, whole grains, and beans. In fact, the magnesium in their diets often provided them with twice as much magnesium as calcium. Dairy products were not abundant at that time, so their calcium intake was low.

Their bodies adapted to this low-calcium, high-magnesium diet by retaining and reusing calcium. Since magnesium was available on a daily basis, unused magnesium was excreted. Our bodies still function like those of our ancestors. Our kidneys still recycle some calcium, but don't retain magnesium. This is why we need to concentrate on getting enough magnesium every day.

Both calcium and magnesium are important. But Dr. Abraham is one of a growing number of health practitioners who has found that getting enough magnesium corrects a wide number of health problems. Unfortunately, you can't just get a blood test to see if you're getting enough magnesium.

The Problem with Magnesium Blood Tests

They're just not accurate, says Mildred S. Seelig, M.D., one of the world's authorities on magnesium. Magnesium is a difficult mineral to measure. When you have a yearly blood test, you can have your magnesium level tested. But this test, called serum magnesium, may not reveal low magnesium.

Some doctors, including Dr. Abraham, believe that a Red Blood Cell (RBC) magnesium test is a better indicator of magnesium levels. But not all laboratories do this particular test, and many doctors are unfamiliar with it. Studies have shown that there are no blood tests that are sensitive enough to accurately diagnose magnesium deficiencies.

So where does this leave you? Dr. Seelig suggests that taking more magnesium than the RDAs is safe unless you have kidney problems. The primary common side effect from taking too much magnesium is loose bowels. There's an easy way to tell whether or not you have a magnesium deficiency. Increase your magnesium for a few months and see if your symptoms lessen or disappear.

Some Symptoms of Low Magnesium

Sherry Rogers, M.D., of Syracuse, New York, finds that one of the most common symptoms of magnesium deficiency is pain in the back or neck. But there are many other signs as well.

Low magnesium can cause high blood pressure, irritability, nervousness, and anxiety. It can lead to muscle cramps and spasms and muscle tension, including constipation. Magnesium deficiency can cause depression, fatigue, exhaustion, learning disabilities, and an excessive sensitivity to noise and pain. If that wasn't enough, it can contribute to poor appetite—even anorexia—and irregular or rapid heartbeat.

Problems from Taking Too Much Magnesium

You can take too much of a good thing, even when it's magnesium. But for the most part, magnesium is a very safe nutrient to increase due to its self-limiting attributes. When you take more magnesium than your body can handle, you're likely to have intestinal gas or loose stools.

Some doctors suggest you take magnesium "to bowel tolerance." This means taking enough to allow you to have stools that are comfortable, but not too loose. Some practitioners begin by adding 100 mg of magnesium a day for a few days. If their patients' stools aren't too soft, they increase it gradually until the stools are comfortably soft.

If your stools are already soft and you suspect a magnesium deficiency, you have a few choices. Begin by increasing your dietary magnesium: whole grains, nuts, seeds, beans, and dark green vegetables. Then try taking magnesium glycinate, a form of magnesium that is less likely to cause loose bowels. If you can't find magnesium glycinate, try magnesium from amino acid chelate. It works almost as well.

Finally, if your need for magnesium still seems clear, talk with your doctor about a more extreme, but effective solution: getting magnesium injections. Before you do, however, make sure that your body is able to use the magnesium you're already taking.

Absorbing and Using Magnesium

If you can't absorb magnesium, your body can't use it. Several dietary factors get in the way of magnesium absorption and utilization. Both a high-fat diet and a diet high in phosphorus block magnesium absorption. So begin by looking at your diet to see if you're unknowingly getting in your own way and creating a magnesium deficiency.

The phosphoric acid in most cola drinks, along with the phosphates in baking powder, processed meats and cheeses, and other processed foods, combines with magnesium to form a substance called magnesium phosphate. The majority of the magnesium you take is able to be absorbed in your intestines. But magnesium phosphate prevents magnesium from being absorbed and causes it to be excreted in solid wastes.

A high-fat diet also reduces magnesium's availability. When fats combine with magnesium, they turn into a soapy consistency that can't get into your intestines and become absorbed. Diets high in fried foods, cheese, and fatty meats interfere with your body's ability to use magnesium.

Perhaps the least known reason for poor magnesium absorption is getting too much calcium either in your diet or in supplements. Because both calcium and magnesium are absorbed through the same parts of your intestines, when you have too much calcium, you block magnesium absorption.

The amount of available magnesium that is able to keep you healthy depends on how much you take, how much is absorbed, and how much is excreted. Some factors cause your body to excrete more magnesium than it should.

Excessive Magnesium Loss

Your body loses magnesium from diarrhea, diet, and stress. Diarrhea causes much of the magnesium in your intestines to be excreted. The diarrhea may be a result of illness or laxative abuse. It doesn't matter. The results are the same. Some of the foods you eat and the supplements you take also cause increased magnesium excretion.

Magnesium excretion is promoted by drinking too much alcohol or caffeine and by eating high amounts of animal protein or sugar. The kind of sugar that contributes to low magnesium is not limited to refined sugar. It includes fructose, the sugar found in fruits and fruit juices. To prevent too much magnesium from being excreted unnecessarily, reduce your intake of these foods and beverages.

All kinds of stress contribute to excessive magnesium loss. The reason for this is simple. Your adrenal glands make hormones that allow you to handle stressful situations. When these hormone levels get too high, magnesium spills out in the urine. Stress does not just mean a difficult emotional

Adrenal Glands
These glands sit on top of your kidneys and make hormones in response to stress that provide increased energy for emergencies.

time. It includes mental, physical, thermal (being too hot or too cold), and other kinds of stress. Very loud noises, like fireworks or music played at many rock concerts, can cause this stress response and contribute to magnesium excretion, as well.

How Magnesium Influences Calcium Absorption

Parathyroid Gland
A small gland that secretes hormones used to regulate calcium and phosphorus metabolism.

Calcium absorption is governed by the parathyroid gland, a tiny gland that sits behind the thyroid (a gland in your neck). But magnesium is part of the equation. Your body can't use the calcium in either your diet or supplements without enough magnesium. Here's how it works.

Your parathyroid makes hormones called PTH (parathyroid hormones). PTH controls calcium absorption. But your parathyroid needs enough magnesium to make sufficient PTH for calcium absorption.

An interesting study in the *American Journal of Clinical Medicine* reported that taking one gram (1,000 mg) of magnesium a day increases the absorption of *both* calcium and magnesium. When you take extra magnesium, your calcium levels can go up even higher than your magnesium levels. If you're concerned about getting enough usable calcium, you have to first get enough magnesium.

Evaluate Your Mineral Needs

The amount of calcium and magnesium you need depends to a great extent on a number of factors that differ from person to person. You may be someone who can take the RDA of each and be fine. But to best use these minerals to support your health, it's a good idea to look more closely at each condition that is dependent on both calcium and magnesium, and evaluate your body's particular needs.

In the following sections, you will find information on calcium and magnesium that can help reduce your risk for heart disease, osteoporosis, headaches, muscle cramps, fibromyalgia, and PMS. You will find out how to use these minerals to support your body during pregnancy, and how they can help improve your mood and energy. Used properly, calcium and magnesium can both prevent health disorders and often reverse them.

PROTECTING YOUR HEART

A healthy heart needs both calcium and magnesium in the right amounts and balance to help it beat regularly and to keep your blood pressure regulated and stable. Magnesium is nature's calcium-channel blocker. It prevents extra calcium that your body can't use from damaging your

heart cells. It keeps calcium from clogging up and hardening your arteries. So getting enough magnesium is key to having a healthy heart.

On the other hand, some people with high blood pressure need more calcium than they're getting. So the balance between these two minerals is very important. This is why you need to look at your present health and your family's health history to help evaluate just how much of each you need.

How Calcium and Magnesium Regulate Your Heart

Your heart is a muscle that pumps by constantly contracting and relaxing. Calcium helps your heart and other muscles to contract. Magnesium helps them to relax. Together, they work as a team to keep your heart pumping day and night.

Both of these minerals also help send electrical messages to your heart, reminding it to contract regularly. Too much of either one can lead to heart problems by upsetting a delicate balance.

Magnesium also dilates (opens up) blood vessels in your heart, arms, and legs. This allows more oxygen to flow to your heart. Minerals researcher Thomas Steinmetz found that a magnesium deficiency was the cause of death from sudden heart attacks in 8 million people in this country between 1940 and 1994. Clearly, magnesium is not only important to a healthy heart function. It is also essential in preventing heart problems.

Calcium-Channel Blockers

Calcium that's not absorbed into your bones or other tissues can collect in your arteries where it can lead to atherosclerosis. When this buildup reduces the amount of blood

Atherosclerosis
A disorder characterized by the buildup of blood fats on the damaged lining of artery walls, leading to plaques that block blood flow.

from flowing through your arteries, you can have a heart attack.

The idea is to prevent calcium from building up in your arteries. This calls for something to block calcium deposits—a calcium-channel blocker. A number of pharmaceutical drugs are calcium-channel blockers. Magnesium is a natural substance that has the same effect. You can use magnesium, drugs, or both to prevent excess calcium from clogging your arteries.

Procardia and Cardizem are two medications commonly prescribed to block calcium deposits and to regulate heart arrhythmias. All drugs have side effects in some people, and calcium-channel blocking drugs are no exception. Magnesium has the same blocking activity and also regulates the heartbeat with no side effect except, occasionally, loose stools. And magnesium does more than just block calcium deposits and help regulate your heartbeat. It opens up your arteries to allow more blood to flow through, as well.

Don't think you can just stop taking your medications and use magnesium instead. You may be able to, but this is a decision that should be made with your doctor's input and with your being monitored. If you think additional magnesium could be helpful to your heart, talk with your doctor first—especially if you have a heart condition or are at risk for heart disease. If magnesium is a viable option, you may find that when you increase your magnesium you don't need to take calcium-channel blocking drugs. Some people use both magnesium and medications. Be sure to check this out with your doctor before making any changes.

Magnesium's Role in Heart Disease

Low magnesium has been seen in people with irregular or rapid heartbeat and mitral valve prolapse, a disorder of the heart valves. Magnesium is also often low in people with congestive heart failure and high blood pressure.

A review of magnesium and the heart in *The American Journal of Medicine* found that low magnesium is so common that as many as 65 percent of patients in intensive care suffer from it. What's interesting about this finding is that these low magnesium levels were determined through blood tests. That's right. The same inaccurate blood tests that frequently miss detecting low magnesium in many people. If 65 percent of this group of people were found to have low magnesium using inaccurate tests, it's likely that more accurate tests would reveal a still greater need for additional magnesium.

Surviving a Heart Attack

Magnesium can save your life if you're having a heart attack. If you or anyone you are with is having a heart attack, call 911 and ask the paramedics or emergency room doctor to administer a magnesium IV immediately. Emergency room doctors around the country are now giving intravenous magnesium to people who have heart attacks or heart spasms because it helps reduce mortality.

One study of more than 100 heart attack patients found that the survival rate increased almost ten times when patients were given additional magnesium. In a review of heart attacks and magnesium published in the journal *Circulation,* intravenous magnesium was given to 1,300 patients. There was a significant reduction in their irregular heartbeats and death.

It's worth discussing the subject of using magnesium for heart attacks with your doctor. Have this information added to your chart so that if it is ever necessary, you and your doctor will know your desire to be given additional magnesium.

Calcium and Arrhythmias

When your blood test shows high serum calcium, you're at an increased risk for irregular heartbeats, or arrhythmias. Irregular heartbeats can lead to blood clots and stroke.

Melvyn R. Werbach, M.D., explains that even when your blood magnesium level is normal, you may be able to reduce your irregular heartbeat by taking more magnesium. He also found that when magnesium is known to be low, it may be necessary to take higher than normal amounts of magnesium supplements to eliminate arrhythmias.

Calcium's Role in a Healthy Heart

Your heart needs calcium, but not too much of it. High amounts of calcium can be harmful, especially if you don't have enough magnesium to use it. But you do need enough calcium for your heart to keep contracting regularly.

As you age, a number of factors can lead to heart problems. These include getting less calcium, making less stomach acid (hydrochloric acid, or HCl), getting less vitamin D (the sunshine vitamin), and having poor calcium absorption through your intestines.

Since your heart can't function without enough calcium, if you're not getting enough in your diet and supplements to help it contract, your body will pull calcium out of your bones. This can lead to osteoporosis, or brittle bones. So for a healthy heart and strong bones, you may want to consider getting equal amounts of calcium and magnesium.

Regulating Your Blood Pressure

If you have high blood pressure (hypertension), you may need more calcium—or more magnesium. Some people need more of one; others need more of the other.

Many people with high blood pressure have diets low in calcium. They may need more calcium to reduce their blood pressure. A study in *The New England Journal of Medicine* reported that group of people with high blood pressure were given 1,000 mg of calcium a day for four months. At the end of that time, their blood pressure was reduced significantly. David A. McCarron, M.D., also found that calcium lowered blood pressure. He noticed that when people were hypertensive (had high blood pressure), they excreted more calcium in their urine than necessary. When he added calcium to their diets, their blood pressure began to drop.

But sometimes it takes more magnesium to lower blood pressure. Nutritionist Ann Louise Gittleman, M.S., C.N.S., found that some people with high blood pressure, especially those taking diuretics, have low magnesium levels. Diuretics not only lower potassium, they also cause more magnesium than usual to be excreted in the urine.

Diuretic
Something that increases the excretion of urine. Diuretics may be either herbal or pharmaceutical.

A need for magnesium to lower blood pressure is not limited to people using diuretics. A study published in the *British Medical Journal* found that nineteen out of twenty people lowered their high blood pressure using magnesium supplements. No one in the control group experienced that effect.

If you have high blood pressure, look at your diet and supplements. If your overall intake of calcium is high, you may need more magnesium. Or vice versa. Always discuss the supplements you want to take with your health-care provider if you're under a doctor's care for hypertension.

PREVENTING OSTEOPOROSIS

Osteoporosis doesn't just mean having thin bones. It also means that your bones are brittle. Unfortunately, there are no tests for bone brittleness. If you frequently break bones from relatively minor falls, you already know that your bones are brittle. Otherwise, you may have no idea. Doctors tend to rely solely on bone density tests to diagnose osteoporosis because brittleness can't be evaluated. However, your bones may be thinning but they may not be particularly brittle. It depends, to a great degree, on the balance of calcium and magnesium you're getting.

Both calcium and magnesium control the density and brittleness—or flexibility—of bones. Calcium makes bones more brittle, and magnesium makes them more flexible. A good example of this can be seen when you look at the difference between chalk and ivory. Blackboard chalk is calcium carbonate. Drop it and it breaks easily. Ivory is a combination of calcium along with good amounts of magnesium. Drop a piece of ivory and it bounces without breaking. Your bones may be more like chalk, or more like ivory.

An article in *Nutrition Reviews* explains that bones containing less magnesium have larger bone mineral crystals with more perfect shapes. Bones with more magnesium form smaller, more irregular crystals that attach more firmly to one another. The larger, more perfectly shaped crystals are more brittle than the smaller, irregularly shaped bone crystals.

Although your bones contain more calcium than magnesium, magnesium plays an essential role in bone health. It helps transport calcium into the bones and it makes bones stronger. Still, your bones need more than these two minerals. Vitamins C, D, and K, along with boron, manganese, and other trace minerals, are all necessary components of healthy, strong, and dense bone tissue.

Calcium Blood Tests and Your Bones

If a blood tests shows that your calcium is normal, it doesn't mean you have strong bones. Blood tests only test the amount of calcium in your blood, not in your bones. Less than 2 percent of the calcium in your body stays in your blood, so a blood test isn't a good indicator of bone density.

But this small amount of calcium in your blood is so essential for your heart and other functions that if its levels drop, calcium is released from your bones. So a normal calcium blood test could even mean you have less calcium in your bones—especially if your calcium intake is low. Calcium blood tests are used to evaluate parathyroid problems, some kinds of cancers, and bone diseases, but not osteoporosis.

Bone Density Tests and Osteoporosis

There are several types of tests that look at bone density. They can measure the thickness of your bones, but not how fragile or brittle they are. Often, thinner, more porous bones are fragile and break easily. But not always. Bones break when they're brittle, even if they're dense.

Bone density tests vary in their ability to evaluate density. x-rays only detect osteoporosis when 25 percent of bone has been lost. Dual x-ray absorptiometry (DEXA) can detect as little as a 3 percent bone loss. Ultrasound tests measure the bone density of your heel, which is a close match to the bone in your spine. (The bone in your heel and spine is different from the bone in your hips.) Therefore, these tests measure the type of bone found in your spine more accurately than the bone found in your hips.

Newer, better tests are constantly being developed. Check with your doctor before having a bone density test and ask what it will and will not show.

High Calcium and Osteoporosis Prevention

Studies don't agree that taking between 1,000 and 1,500 mg of calcium a day protects your bones. In fact, research has shown that large amounts of calcium don't increase bone density. Smaller amounts, it turns out, may be more than enough to prevent bone loss and fractures.

A four-year study published in the *American Journal of Clinical Nutrition* concluded that taking a lot of calcium isn't the answer to the osteoporosis question. Participants took 1,500–2,000 mg of calcium a day. They had a little less bone loss in their arms than women taking less calcium. But the density in their spines and hips didn't improve at all.

A Mayo Clinic osteoporosis study concluded that women who took 1,400 mg of calcium a day had the same amount of bone loss as those who took less than 500 mg a day. What we're seeing now is that current scientific literature suggests that a smaller amount of well-absorbed calcium may be better, along with enough magnesium for optimal calcium absorption.

Susan E. Brown, Ph.D., director of the Osteoporosis Education Project in Syracuse, New York, studied calcium and osteoporosis in women around the world. She discovered that women in underdeveloped countries who had diets with between 200 and 475 mg of calcium a day had strong bones. Women who took 800–1,000 mg a day had more osteoporosis and broken bones.

In spite of the findings that various cultures with low calcium intake have a lower rate of osteoporosis than cultures with high calcium consumption, people still think that high amounts of calcium prevent bone loss. Where did this belief originate? And what was the science behind it? The answer is surprising.

An Explanation of High Calcium Recommendations

Recommendations for taking high amounts of calcium began in 1978 when a poorly conducted, short study conducted by Robert Heaney, M.D., was published in *The Journal of Laboratory Clinical Medicine*. In this study, forty-one women in Nebraska kept a one-week food diary and gave Dr. Heaney their dietary history. Their average calcium intake was estimated from this information. Nothing was calculated.

Calcium absorption for these women was also estimated, since there wasn't any way to calculate such general information. The calcium intake for this small group of women averaged around 670 mg a day during this single week. None of the women took as much as 1,500 mg. This study concluded that all women should take more than twice the amount of calcium taken by these Nebraska women. It's not clear how this conclusion was formed.

Marketing Study Results

What happened next shouldn't surprise you. The dairy industry heard about Dr. Heaney's study and saw an opportunity to sell more high-calcium foods. With the help of the media, they took this one-week study and promoted an increased need for their products to worried women who wanted to protect themselves from osteoporosis. Drug and supplement companies saw that they could use this study to sell more calcium supplements. Today's high calcium recommendations originated from Dr. Heaney's one-week study.

Later, Dr. Heaney published a study on 200 nuns. He observed them for fifteen years and found that the nuns who were on low-calcium diets excreted more calcium each day than they took. Since then, a great many sound scientific studies have concluded just the opposite: When a person's diet is low in calcium, their body conserves and reuses more of it.

In spite of studies concluding that small amounts of calcium can protect the bones when enough magnesium and other nutrients are present, many doctors still recommend the higher amounts. You can now find good studies that say you need a lot of calcium, or just a little. Perhaps both are right and the amount you need depends on your own body's particular needs.

A Look at Individuality

It's easiest to take someone's recommendations and follow them. Especially if they come from an authority like the National Academy of Sciences/ National Research Council or your family doctor. Still, your needs may differ greatly from conclusions found in studies.

Your body theoretically needs 1,000–1,500 mg of calcium and half as much magnesium a day. This is the amount advised by most doctors and found in most supplement formulas. But this high calcium formula may work for only a small number of people. Dr. Abraham discovered that this amount of calcium may actually work against conserving bone as you age. You may need less calcium and more magnesium than you've been told.

Dr. Abraham conducted a small double-blind one-year study and found that women who took 500 mg of calcium and 600 mg of magnesium had an 11 percent increase in bone density. At the end of two years, one woman in the study had an increase in bone density of over 20 percent. This is much higher than any improvement found by taking high amounts of calcium, hormones, or osteoporosis-protective drugs.

Alan R. Gaby, M.D., recommends between 600 and 1,200 mg of calcium for his postmenopausal patients. He uses the higher amount only when he finds specific evidence of a calcium deficiency. Dr. Gaby has found that for the majority of older women who already get about 500 mg of calcium in their diets each day, no supplemental calcium is necessary.

He also recommends taking 250–600 mg of magnesium supplements each day. If your diet is very high in magnesium-rich foods, the lower amount may be enough. If your diet is low in magnesium, you may want to take the higher amount. This higher amount is the quantity that Dr. Abraham's research found to be beneficial. Some foods contain a balance of both minerals. Include them in your diet each day.

Calcium- and Magnesium-Rich Foods
Whole grains, beans, nuts, seeds, and green leafy vegetables are all high in both calcium and magnesium.

Calcium Can Contribute to Osteoporosis

Taking too much calcium can create a vicious cycle. Too much calcium keeps you from utilizing magnesium. And you need magnesium to move calcium into your bones. This means that the calcium you're taking is not preserving your bones.

Many people who take high amounts of calcium are under the mistaken impression that it is preventing osteoporosis. In fact, it may be contributing to fragile, porous bones. Without enough magnesium, bone crystals that make up your bone tissues are larger and smoother, resulting in bones that are fragile and weak.

Both magnesium and vitamin D are needed to transport calcium into bone tissues. Neither are found in large enough quantities in high-calcium foods like dairy. They also tend to be low in some supplements. In addition, dairy products contain a lot of phosphorus. Phosphorus is a mineral that blocks calcium from getting into your bones.

The answer is not to take more calcium. It may very well be to take less of a better-absorbed calcium along with more magnesium and vitamin D.

Magnesium Can Protect against Osteoporosis

Magnesium has two roles in bone health. It can make bones more flexible and less brittle. And it can help bone regain some of its lost density. Since osteoporosis is a condition where bones both lose some of their density and become brittle, adding magnesium to your program can protect your bones. Magnesium is often low in women's diets, especially as they age: They tend to eat fewer nuts, seeds, and whole grains in an effort to keep their weight down.

A study on bone density and nutrition, published in the *American Journal of Clinical Nutrition*, found that magnesium was low in the diets and supplements of many post-menopausal women. Their blood levels of magnesium were also low. This is interesting because blood magnesium levels often don't register as being low even when they are. Therefore, these low blood magnesium levels indicate a significant lack of magnesium.

The researcher on this study also noticed that women with osteoporosis who had spongy bones (that is, bones that lack density and break easily) were low in magnesium. When women took more magnesium, they had fewer broken bones, less bone loss, and an increase in bone density.

Other Bone-Strengthening Nutrients

Vitamin D is called the "sunshine vitamin." This is because your skin uses the ultraviolet rays off the sun to make vitamin D. After calcium and magnesium, this vitamin is the most important nutrient for strong healthy bones. (Vitamin D helps calcium absorption through the intestines.) Vitamin D is often lacking in people who don't spend enough time outdoors. This is particularly true of older people who often spend the majority of their time indoors.

Studies show that when you combine vitamin D with calcium, the rate of hip fracture goes down. One study of nearly 350 women over age seventy were given either 400 IU of vitamin D a day or a placebo for two years. Hipbone density increased 2 to 2.5 percent in the women who took the vitamin. You can get vitamin D by spending time outdoors every day, by taking 400–700 IU of it daily in supplement form, or by getting it from your food. Vitamin D–fortified dairy products, fish, and eggs all contain some of this sunshine vitamin.

Neither calcium nor vitamin D works as well alone as in combination.

Other trace nutrients that help form strong bones

International Unit (IU)
A measure of weight usually used for fat-soluble vitamins, like vitamins D and E.

include manganese (15–30 mg per day), boron (3–5 mg per day), zinc (15–20 mg per day), copper (1.5–3 mg per day), folic acid (400–500 mcg per day), vitamin B$_6$ (50–100 mg per day), vitamin C (500 mg per day), and vitamin K (150–500 mg per day). Many of these are available in sufficient quantities in a healthy diet. If not, they can be included in a good multivitamin/mineral supplement.

Vitamin K is the vitamin that helps blood clot. Vitamin K is also needed to produce a protein called osteocalcin that helps calcium build bones. Green leafy vegetables are high in vitamin K. But people who are taking Coumadin or other blood thinners must eliminate most vitamin K from their diets and supplements. This lack of vitamin K can contribute to osteoporosis. If you're taking a blood thinner, you'll want to take all the bone-protecting nutrients you safely can.

PMS AND PREGNANCY

Adequate calcium and magnesium are needed to reduce or eliminate premenstrual syndrome (PMS), and are needed during pregnancy. Studies have linked both calcium and magnesium deficiencies to PMS. But compelling evidence from research gynecologist Guy E. Abraham, M.D., and magnesium expert Mildred S. Seelig, M.D., points to a magnesium deficiency in women with emotional premenstrual symptoms like anxiety and depression. And when Dr. Abraham examined the diets of two groups of women with emotional premenstrual symptoms, he found that they ate five times more dairy than other women. It seems that some premenstrual symptoms occur when there is too little magnesium and too much calcium.

Premenstrual Syndrome (PMS)
A number of physical or emotional symptoms that occur during the week before menstruation. They usually disappear with menstruation or after it begins.

With pregnancy comes an increased need for calcium. But pregnant women have an increased ability to absorb it. This means that the amount of calcium in a pregnant woman's diet and supplements does not have to be extremely high because of this increased absorption. Pregnant women also have a need for enough magnesium to prevent them from going into early labor. They also need enough calcium and magnesium to prevent a condition called preeclampsia.

A woman's need for various nutrients changes during different life cycles. Menstruation and pregnancy are two cycles when it is particularly important to get sufficient calcium and magnesium.

Causes of PMS

Hormone levels fluctuate before, during, and after the menstrual cycle. This causes an ever-changing need for a number of nutrients—particularly calcium and magnesium.

It appears that hormonal and nutrient excesses and deficiencies lead to premenstrual symptoms. Some are physical—like tender breasts and weight gain. Others are emotional. Each has their causes that often stem from nutrient deficiencies. Dr. Abraham has separated PMS into four categories: anxiety, depression, cravings, and hydration (water retention). The first two categories are emotional; the second two are primarily physical.

Preeclampsia
A complication of pregnancy that can include high blood pressure, water retention, and protein in the urine.

Emotional premenstrual symptoms like anxiety, depression, and mood swings are often a sign of a magnesium deficiency, calcium excess, or both. A study published in the *Journal of Orthomolecular Psychiatry* found a connection between high-dairy diets and aggressiveness in girls. High amounts of calcium interfere with the body's ability to break down sugar. Large quantities of sugar in the bloodstream, which causes magnesium excretion, can contribute to mood changes and aggressiveness. This may be one explanation for how a high-dairy diet negatively affects emotional premenstrual symptoms.

Magnesium's Role in PMS

Estrogen and progesterone are the primary hormones that regulate menstruation. Their production increases and decreases around the monthly menstrual cycle. Hormones can greatly influence your moods. In fact, estrogen contributes to premenstrual symptoms of anxiety and depression. It also increases magnesium excretion just when it is needed the most. Magnesium plays an important role in these monthly hormonal changes.

Production of estrogen and progesterone increases during a normal menstrual cycle. But to make progesterone, a hormone that has sedative effects, the body needs enough magnesium.

Low levels of progesterone appear to be responsible for premenstrual symptoms like anxiety and depression. In some women, progesterone levels remain low because there are not enough nutrients, like magnesium, present to increase them. High-magnesium foods, like whole grains and beans, contain good amounts of vitamin B$_6$. This vitamin helps the body make more progesterone.

Neurotransmitter
Molecules used as chemical messengers in the body. Serotonin and dopamine are well-known neurotransmitters.

Magnesium also plays an important role in the production of brain chemicals. Before menstruation, the body makes a number of stimulating chemicals called neurotransmitters that can lead to anxiety. Magnesium helps the brain make a calming neurotransmitter, dopamine, which counteracts the effects of the stimulating neurotransmitters.

All stress, like the hormonal fluctuations caused by the menstrual cycle, results in your body excreting magnesium faster than normal. This is another reason why women need extra magnesium before menstruation. One possible signal of a magnesium deficiency is craving chocolate. The common phenomenon of chocolate craving before menstruation may be your body's way of telling you it needs more magnesium.

Chocolate Craving and Magnesium Deficiency

There are a number of reasons why people crave chocolate, including a magnesium deficiency. The reason is simple: Chocolate contains some of the highest amounts of magnesium of any food.

But eating a lot of chocolate to raise your magnesium levels is not the answer. Foods containing chocolate are high in sugar and fat, as well as in magnesium. The sugar causes drowsiness, difficulty concentrating, nervousness, and water retention—other premenstrual symptoms. The fat binds with magnesium making it difficult to absorb. However, a chocolate craving may help you recognize that at some stressful times, your body needs more magnesium.

When Calcium Helps PMS

Some women with PMS may need more calcium, rather than more magnesium. One study had women take either 1,200 mg of calcium a day or a placebo. After three months, almost half of the women who took the calcium supplement had fewer PMS symptoms.

Placebo
An inactive substance that is used as a control in clinical studies instead of a drug or nutrient.

The same researchers had conducted a smaller study with similar results. In both studies, they used calcium carbonate, a poorly absorbed form of calcium. It is possible that smaller amounts of a better-absorbed calcium, like calcium citrate, would give similar results without risking a calcium overload that could lead to arthritis and heart disease.

Most researchers have found that increasing magnesium is more effective than increasing calcium for women with PMS. This is especially true for those who eat a lot of dairy products—foods that are high in calcium and low in magnesium.

Mildred S. Seelig, M.D., points out that since calcium impairs the absorption of magnesium, any time you take extra calcium you also need to take more magnesium. Today's emphasis on calcium has encouraged many women to eat diets that create a wider and wider gap between calcium and magnesium balance, creating a greater and greater magnesium deficiency.

Calcium Needs during Pregnancy and Nursing

Calcium requirements for women increase during pregnancy and lactation, but that's not the whole story. In fact, concentrating on calcium can be misleading. At times when more calcium is needed, like during pregnancy, the body is able to absorb more from both foods and supplements.

Nature knows that fetuses need calcium to form bones, and that mother's milk needs to provide babies with plenty of calcium for the same reason. Doctors know this, too. This is why the revised U.S.-Canadian dietary guidelines no longer recommend that pregnant or lactating women take extra calcium. The recommendation is for 1,000 mg of calcium a day. This includes all calcium in foods and supplements, not just supplements.

Calcium and magnesium are both helpful in preventing leg cramps associated with pregnancy. Once again, the idea is to get enough, but not too much, of each mineral. And in looking at calcium requirements during pregnancy, it's easy to overlook the importance of magnesium. (See the discussion "How Magnesium and Calcium Help Preeclampsia.")

Magnesium and Pregnancy

Long-term studies indicate that at least 450 mg of magnesium a day is needed to keep both mothers and their fetuses healthy. Once again, some women may need much more. Dr. Seelig reports that a woman who had a number of uncomplicated pregnancies and gave birth to healthy babies needed to take as much as 600 mg of magnesium a day during the last half of her pregnancy. When she took less than 300 mg a day, her doctor found her to be deficient in magnesium.

Magnesium is a valuable nutrient for pregnant women because it can prevent premature birth and reduce pregnancy-related constipation. In a four-month study of more than 550 pregnant women, those who took magnesium supplements had fewer premature babies. In addition, fewer mothers were hospitalized before giving birth, and fewer newborn babies needed to be in intensive care. Naturopath Tori Hudson, N.D., Professor at the National College of Naturopathic Medicine in Portland, Oregon, explains that the best time for pregnant women to increase their magnesium is during their first trimester if they want to prevent low-birth weight in their babies.

Many women now take extra magnesium to prevent constipation during pregnancy. Gynecologist Uzzi Reiss, M.D., has told some of his patients they could take magnesium to bowel tolerance during their pregnancies to avoid this pressure-related constipation. Some of his patients took as much as 1,000 mg of supplementary magnesium a day in addition to whatever amounts they got from their diets. Before increasing magnesium, pregnant women should always check with their doctors.

A number of studies have shown that a magnesium deficiency is common in both normal pregnancies and those complicated by diabetes or high blood pressure. And, as mentioned previously, sufficient magnesium can help prevent preeclampsia.

How Magnesium and Calcium Help Preeclampsia

Preeclampsia can occur during the last trimester of pregnancy when blood pressure is elevated. Among other symptoms, it may result in kidney damage and water retention. Preeclampsia can also restrict blood flow to the fetus. This limits the amount of oxygen and nourishment available to the developing baby.

Magnesium may counteract the constriction of blood vessels. These blood vessels need calcium to contract, but they also need sufficient magnesium to relax and open up. Magnesium acts as a calcium-channel blocker to help regulate blood pressure. Without high blood pressure, preeclampsia is rare.

In addition to bed rest, a high-protein diet, and at times taking medications to reduce high blood pressure, magnesium is the major treatment of choice for this complication of pregnancy. However, too little calcium can also lead to preeclampsia. So once again, the proper balance of these two minerals is of vital importance.

How Much Calcium and Magnesium Is Needed during Pregnancy?

The amount of calcium and magnesium needed by a pregnant woman depends, in part, on the absorbability of the calcium in the diet and the supplement. When you take a well-absorbed form of calcium like calcium citrate or calcium malate, you need less than when you're taking calcium carbonate or dolomite. Pregnant women who consume 500–750 mg of good quality calcium each day in their diets and supplements should have plenty for themselves and their babies. This can be achieved either with or without dairy products.

Dr. Seelig recommends that pregnant women take 450 mg of magnesium. This is slightly higher than the 350 mg suggested by the current RDAs, and less than the 1,000 mg some physicians suggest their patients take to counteract constipation.

It makes sense to take some extra magnesium, since this is a mineral that is excreted when we're under stress, and pregnancy is physiologically, as well as emotionally, stressful. There may be fewer times in a woman's life when her body is under more stress than during pregnancy.

COUNTERACTING DEPRESSION AND FATIGUE

It takes a complex series of biochemical activities to convert food into energy, and another series of actions to produce brain chemicals that give you a feeling of either well-being or depression. In both cases, you need enough specific nutrients to turn your food either into energy or into mood-elevating brain chemicals. These specific nutrients include calcium and magnesium.

One of the most important nutrients to help you feel energetic and happy is magnesium. But once again, while magnesium has been recognized as being of primary importance, some studies indicate that calcium needs must be met, as well. Although you may need to emphasize magnesium over calcium to counteract depression and fatigue, these two minerals work so closely together that you can't consider one without the other.

How Calcium Affects Depression

While calcium is not commonly known to affect moods, two preliminary studies, published in the *Journal of Orthomolecular Psychiatry*, indicate it may help reduce depression. These studies took a group of college students, both male and female, and gave them either 1,000 mg of calcium with 600 IU of vitamin D twice a day for a month, or a placebo. The students who took the calcium and vitamin D had half as much depression as those who took the placebo.

Depression
A common mood disorder that may include poor appetite, insomnia or excessive sleeping, lack of interest, fatigue, feelings of worthlessness, and an inability to concentrate.

On the other hand, too much calcium can cause depression in some people. A number of studies have associated personality changes and depression in psychiatric patients with high calcium levels. Too much calcium can contribute to depression, irritability, and a lack of initiative.

More studies on the connection between calcium and depression are needed, but calcium may play a role in your mood. Too little, or too much, can affect the way you feel. If you suffer from depression, you may want to have your calcium levels evaluated by your doctor both through blood tests and by looking at your dietary calcium intake. Take a look at how much calcium you get each day and see how your mood changes if you take less or more. Calcium's role in depression is unclear at this time. Magnesium's role is better understood.

How Magnesium Helps Reduce Depression

Magnesium, along with vitamin B_6, helps produce serotonin, an important brain neurotransmitter. Serotonin is considered to be a natural antidepressant, and a serotonin deficiency is one common cause for depression. In these cases, when a lack of serotonin contributes to depression, taking more magnesium can be helpful.

Psychiatrist Hyla Cass, M.D., explains that low serotonin production can cause a number of symptoms from depres-

sion to obsessive thinking, anxiety, violent behavior, PMS, and alcohol or drug abuse.

Many medical doctors treat a serotonin-deficiency depression with a class of drugs called SSRIs (selective serotonin reuptake inhibitors). These drugs, which include Prozac, Zoloft, and Paxil, make serotonin more available to brain cells. But certain amino acids like l-tryptophan or its derivative 5-HTP can have the same effect. However, these amino acids need to be taken along with magnesium for them to work.

Amino Acids
A group of organic compounds that are the building blocks of protein. Along with vitamins, minerals, and enzymes, they help make other needed chemicals, like neurotransmitters.

Since serotonin can't get from the bloodstream into the brain, your brain needs to constantly make this chemical. The raw ingredients needed to make a substance like serotonin are called precursors. Magnesium is a precursor to serotonin production.

Tryptophan, 5-HTP, Magnesium, and Depression

To counteract many forms of depression, you may need more serotonin. But before serotonin can be produced, your body needs to have enough tryptophan and magnesium. Here's how serotonin production works.

Tryptophan is an amino acid that gets into your brain where it is converted into serotonin. But first it needs to be changed into a chemical called 5-HTP (5-hydroxytryptophan). Then, 5-HTP needs helpers—mainly magnesium and vitamin B_6.

These three nutrients—5-HTP, magnesium, and vitamin B_6—work together to help make serotonin, a neurotransmitter that carries messages throughout your brain, which affects your mood, sleep, and other body functions.

An article in *Alternative Medicine Review* examined a Swiss study of more than 500 participants with a variety of types of depression. Some of the participants were seriously depressed while others were just a little sad. Everyone was given 5-HTP, and the study concluded that this nutrient worked even better than SSRI drugs in reducing depression.

You may not need to take 5-HTP. Since your body needs magnesium to make serotonin, you might just want to begin by taking more magnesium. If that's not enough, you can always try adding 5-HTP. Psychiatrist Priscilla Slagle, M.D., who has worked extensively with natural solutions to depression, notes that people who are depressed may need to take as much as 100–500 mg of magnesium orotate three times a day. Other forms of magnesium should work as well as the orotate.

If you decide next to take 5-HTP, which is better absorbed and easier to find than tryptophan, Dr. Slagle has found that healthy people need 100–200 mg of 5-HTP (or

1,000–2,000 mg of tryptophan) a day. Someone who is depressed, she says, may need even more. She gives her patients an average of 300–400 mg of 5-HTP a day. But don't just run out and buy this supplement. Talk with your doctor first. It could be just what you need, or just the reverse. If you sleep a lot when you're depressed, for instance, you may not need tryptophan or 5-HTP at all.

Amino acids are powerful nutrients, and the balance between all of them is important. You don't want too much of one and not enough of another. Magnesium is a bit different. It's clear that so many people are magnesium deficient; therefore, adding more magnesium to your diet and taking supplements is likely to do one of the following: help, have no effect, or cause loose stools. So, it's a pretty safe nutrient to try for depression.

Fighting Fatigue

Magnesium is also an important ingredient in creating energy. Without enough magnesium, you can feel tired and drained. You need enough magnesium for your body to turn all of the sugars in your diet into energy. This includes cookies, fruit, honey, and all starches (carbohydrates) that eventually turn into sugar.

You also need magnesium to give your muscles their strength. If you have weak muscles, it may be because you're not exercising enough. Or it could be due to a deficiency of either magnesium or its partner in energy production: potassium. Or you could need both.

Use Potassium along with Magnesium

Fatigue and muscle weakness are the most common symptoms of a chronic potassium deficiency. But potassium doesn't work alone. It needs magnesium. In fact, a magnesium deficiency may be one reason why you need more potassium. If your potassium and magnesium levels are both low, taking more potassium without also boosting your magnesium intake is often not enough. Taking potassium by itself could cause more magnesium to be excreted in your urine. If it seems like you may need more potassium, make sure you're getting enough magnesium, as well.

Dr Alan R. Gaby found that when fatigue is due to low potassium, taking a potassium/magnesium aspartate supplement often helps. Aspartic acid is an excellent chemical to transport both potassium and magnesium into cells. Dr. Gaby noticed that between 75 and 91 percent of participants in several double-blind studies who took this combined supplement had much more energy after taking it. Talk with your doctor about the advisability of using potassium/magnesium aspartate supplements for low energy. The amount suggested is 70 mg of magnesium aspartate and 99 mg of potassium aspartate three times a day.

Potassium can be found in a healthy diet. It is abundant in all vegetables, but especially dark green leafy ones. Orange juice, whole grains, sunflower seeds, and potatoes are also high in this mineral. But alcohol, caffeine, and sodium all increase the excretion of potassium.

Chronic Fatigue and Magnesium

Chronic fatigue is more than a feeling of lethargy. It is a complex syndrome that often includes muscle and/or joint pain, headaches, poor sleep, poor memory, and a sore throat. Rest doesn't help people with chronic fatigue feel better. Medical doctors are often puzzled by how to treat their chronic fatigue patients unless they are well versed in nutrition. Then, they find magnesium can frequently help.

Scientific studies on magnesium's effect on chronic fatigue have resulted in mixed results. Some say magnesium helps; others say it doesn't. When it does work, it is impressive in alleviating some of the debilitating fatigue that prevents people with this condition from accomplishing even the simplest of daily tasks.

It appears that chronic fatigue patients who have low magnesium levels respond positively to taking additional amounts of this mineral. And these are the majority of chronic fatigue patients. A lack of magnesium has been associated with fatigue, pain, weakness, muscle spasms, irritability, and numbness—all symptoms of chronic fatigue. The only people who should avoid taking extra magnesium are people with chronic kidney failure. Very few of them have chronic fatigue.

Jacob Teitelbaum, M.D., a leading researcher in the field of chronic fatigue, suggests that people who have either fatigue or chronic fatigue syndrome should take magnesium supplements. It will either do nothing or result in more energy and a reduction in other chronic fatigue symptoms within two or three weeks. But magnesium supplements are not the only answer. Dr. Teitelbaum stresses that a healthy diet, along with magnesium, is essential.

OTHER USES FOR CALCIUM AND MAGNESIUM

The amount of calcium and magnesium you get affects a wide variety of health conditions. This balance of calcium to magnesium affects stress, twitching muscles, hyperactivity, muscle pain including fibromyalgia, and headaches. While you need enough calcium to keep your bones healthy and your body functioning properly, taking additional magnesium is often even more helpful in a number of conditions that affect the muscles. This is because magnesium helps muscles to relax.

Also, magnesium has been found to be low in many people with diabetes. So anyone who has diabetes should have their magnesium intakes evaluated, and consider increasing this mineral in their diets. People with a family history of colon cancer, on the other hand, may benefit from taking extra calcium. Once again, your body's particular needs, rather than a "one size fits all" approach, help determine how much of each of these minerals you should be getting. Look at your diet and your health to see whether you need more calcium, magnesium, or both.

How Magnesium Helps Stress

Whenever you're under stress, your body excretes more magnesium than usual. This is a normal stress response. When you're under any kind of stress, your body produces particular hormones to help you handle it. These hormones contribute to a magnesium deficiency by increasing magnesium excretion.

Your brain needs plenty of energy when you're under stress to help you cope and make wise decisions, and glucose is the brain's energy source. But to turn foods into glucose, you need enough magnesium. Your nervous system also needs extra magnesium when you're under stress. You need plenty of magnesium every day, but especially whenever you're stressed and nervous. Foods high in magnesium include whole grains, beans, nuts, seeds, and green vegetables. One reason why it's important to eat very well when you're under stress is that a healthy diet is high in magnesium.

Stress
Anything that disturbs your balance. Stress can be emotional, mental, physical, thermal (too hot or too cold), or economic.

Mildred S. Seelig, M.D., explains that stress causes fatty acids to be released. These fats attach themselves to magnesium. When magnesium gets stuck to fatty acids, it isn't well absorbed.

Other nutrients besides magnesium are needed when you're under stress. They include B vitamins, zinc, and vitamin C. These vitamins and minerals can also be found in a high-magnesium diet.

Restless Legs

If your legs twitch and you can't stop them from twitching, you may have a condition called restless leg syndrome (RLS). This neurological condition can include tingling, itching, burning, and other uncomfortable sensations that are often relieved by walking. While some people have restless legs during the day, their symptoms are often worse at night. This makes it difficult to get a good night's sleep.

The cause of RLS isn't understood, but we know it involves a problem in the nervous system, a system dependent on getting enough magnesium. Both calcium and magnesium are needed to strengthen your muscle function. And both are needed by your central nervous system. But additional magnesium is often needed even more than calcium.

A number of anecdotal reports indicate that magnesium supplementation reduces RLS. This makes sense, since a deficiency of magnesium can increase muscle excitability, or twitching. If you have restless leg syndrome, you can begin by boosting your dietary and supplemental magnesium. Loose stools are a sign that you're taking more magnesium than your body can handle. If this occurs, reduce your intake to an amount that causes comfortably loose stools. If your symptoms don't improve, see if additional calcium improves or worsens your condition.

A study published in the journal *Sleep* reported a 75 to 85 percent improvement in sleeping with RLS patients who took magnesium. Previously, twitching legs awakened them or prevented them from getting to sleep. Magnesium was most helpful in people with mild to moderate restless leg syndrome.

A deficiency of folic acid has also been associated with RLS. Taking 400 mcg twice a day with a little vitamin B_{12} often helps reduce twitching. So does eliminating coffee and other sources of caffeine.

Restless Children

Hyperactivity can affect children, adolescents, and adults. It is now popularly called ADHD, or attention-deficit hyperactivity disorder. While hyperactivity may be caused by prenatal alcohol or drug abuse, a reaction to certain foods or medications, or lead poisoning, it can also be due to a need for specific nutrients. Calcium and magnesium are two of the most important nutrients to counteract hyperactivity.

Acupuncturist Janet Zand, LAc, OMD, suggests that children aged five to seven who have ADHD begin by taking one teaspoonful of a liquid calcium and magnesium supplement once a day. For children aged seven to ten, she suggests this amount twice a day. Children over ten, she says, should take one tablespoon once or twice a day. After two months, Dr. Zand reduces this supplement to five times a week for three more months. Then the supplement is stopped. Hyperactive children have an increased need for calcium since their bones are forming. Adults may find a reduction in restlessness by taking magnesium alone. Magnesium without additional calcium may work for children, also, if their diets contain dairy and other calcium sources.

In a six-month study published in *Magnesium Research Journal*, half the children with ADHD were given 200 mg of magnesium a day. The control group took nothing. The children who took magnesium had a noticeably greater reduction in their hyperactivity. There was no change in the control group.

Other nutrients besides magnesium appear to be helpful in counteracting ADHD. Hyperactive children often need a vitamin B complex to help support their nervous systems. But magnesium may be a significant part of the puzzle.

Headaches

Headaches can be triggered by a number of factors including food sensitivities, low blood sugar, and stress. But migraine headaches, including premenstrual migraines, may be caused by low magnesium.

In a study published in *Contemporary Nutrition*, 3,000 female migraine sufferers were given 100–200 mg of magnesium a day. Eighty percent of the participants had a reduction in the frequency and severity of their migraines.

Another study, published in a headache journal, *Cephalagia*, observed eighty people for one month. Then, half were given 600 mg of magnesium a day for three months while the other half were given a placebo. Within nine weeks, magnesium reduced the severity and length of migraines in more than 40 percent of the participants. While it's true that magnesium didn't provide an immediate solution, it was a considerable help to a good percentage of migraine sufferers. And it allowed them to reduce their migraine medicine, as well.

Some migraines are associated with menstruation. Dr. Abraham and his colleagues conducted a study on premenstrual syndrome (PMS) with more than two dozen women. They measured both serum magnesium and red blood cell magnesium in all participants. Women with premenstrual migraines had low red blood cell magnesium levels although their serum magnesium levels were normal. Serum magnesium is the most common way of measuring magnesium. It is not as accurate as red blood cell magnesium—a test that is rarely done because of the expense.

Tight muscles may contribute to everyday tension headaches. Because magnesium relaxes all muscles, it may be helpful for this common variety of headaches. If you have frequent tension headaches, you may want to increase your magnesium.

Fibromyalgia

No one knows what causes fibromyalgia. But this painful condition results in fatigue, along with stiffness and aching in muscles and soft tissues—areas that contain high concentrations of magnesium. In fact, there's an overlapping between fibromyalgia and chronic fatigue syndrome. In fibromyalgia, there's more pain; in chronic fatigue there's more fatigue.

Jorge D. Flechas, M.D., a physician from North Carolina, measured red blood cell magnesium in fibromyalgia patients. The results were stunning. He found low magnesium in twelve out of thirteen patients.

One theory about the relationship between magnesium and fibromyalgia is that the painful muscles may not have enough magnesium to relax them. Another concerns a connection between pain and serotonin. We know that fibromyalgia patients have low levels of serotonin. And when serotonin is chronically low, pain feels even more severe. Without enough magnesium, your brain can't make serotonin.

Magnesium is an important nutrient in the production of a compound called adenosine triphosphate (ATP). ATP furnishes energy to muscles. Both magnesium and malic acid, a substance found in apples and some other fruits, are needed to make ATP. It is very possible that fibromyalgia is a result of a deficiency of both magnesium and malic acid.

ATP
The "energy currency" for your cells. ATP is composed of one adenosine molecule and three phosphate molecules.

Dr. Flechas conducted several studies treating fibromyalgia patients with a combination of magnesium and malic acid. The patients who took 300–600 mg of magnesium, and 1,200–2,400 mg of malic acid, each day had less pain within one or two months. Other controlled studies showed a 50 percent reduction in fibromyalgia pain in two months using both supplements. Two days after the subjects stopped taking magnesium with malic acid, their pain returned. While not all studies show this degree of effectiveness, it is safe enough and inexpensive enough to try for several months to see if it works for you.

Magnesium and Diabetes

Magnesium is the most common mineral deficiency in insulin-dependent diabetes. In fact, low magnesium is more common in people with both insulin-dependent (type I) and non–insulin-dependent (type II) diabetes than in any other group of people. The reason is simple.

A balance is needed between insulin and magnesium to regulate blood sugar. Your body needs magnesium to secrete enough insulin to keep your blood sugar level, and insulin helps transport magnesium into your cells. In a seven-year study of 14,000 middle-aged people called the Atherosclerosis Risk in Communities Study (ARIC), people who had the lowest magnesium levels were twice as likely to get diabetes as those with the highest magnesium levels. To prevent or support the treatment of diabetes, getting enough magnesium is key.

Magnesium and Type II Diabetes

Type II diabetes; or non–insulin-dependent diabetes, is often a result of obesity in later years. Type II diabetes often can be controlled by diet and weight loss. But additional magnesium helps.

Maria De Lourdes Lima, M.D., and her associates conducted a study in Brazil with more than 124 people with type II diabetes. Twenty-five to 38 percent of the participants had low magnesium. Some diabetics in this study were given additional magnesium, while others were given a placebo. The magnesium was given to participants whether or not they had low magnesium levels. Magnesium helped improve blood sugar regulation, especially in people with neuropathy (damage to nerve tissue) or with heart disease.

Dr. Lima and her colleagues noticed that the participants in this study had to be given higher than usual doses of magnesium to get results. In fact, they needed 800–1,600 mg a day. If you have type II diabetes, you may want to talk with your doctor about adding more magnesium to your diet and supplement program. The amount you need may be quite a bit lower than this. Naturopath Kathi Head suggests 200–500 mg of supplemental magnesium a day.

Diabetic Neuropathy

A condition that occurs in some people who have diabetes that can cause muscle pain, tingling, and numbness, commonly found in the legs. It can also occur in the hands and arms.

Calcium's Role in Diabetes

Too much calcium is more likely to be a problem for people with diabetes than too little calcium. Several studies indicate that diabetes may accelerate the deposit of calcium in the walls of arteries. This can lead to high blood pressure and heart disease—conditions that are common in people with diabetes. Don't overdo dietary calcium by eating a lot of dairy products. Even low-fat and nonfat dairy contains high amounts of calcium. Keep your calcium supplements low, around 500 mg a day, and be sure to take enough magnesium with it.

As you've learned, magnesium is a natural calcium-channel blocker. It prevents calcium from adhering to artery walls. For this reason, it appears to be even more important for people with diabetes to concentrate on getting enough magnesium. And keep calcium intake reasonable, not high, to guard against an excess of calcium, and to prevent these calcium deposits.

Colon Cancer

Extra calcium may be important if you have a family history of colon cancer. The connection between this mineral and colon cancer is just now starting to be understood.

Both dietary fats and bile, a substance produced in the liver to help digest them, can irritate the intestines. This, in turn, causes a buildup of protective cells, like a Band-Aid. But this buildup of cells is abnormal, and in a small but significant number of people, it could lead to cancer.

A study published in *The New England Journal of Medicine* found that calcium supplements slowed down cell growth in the intestines most successfully in people with a family history of colon cancer. There seems to be a genetic tendency for this buildup in some families. When this particular subgroup of people increased their calcium from 700 mg to 1,250 mg a day, fewer "Band-Aid" cells were made. Both cancerous and precancerous cells grew faster in people with a genetic tendency for colon cancer who ate a high-fat, low-calcium diet.

A more recent study by the Calcium Polyp Prevention Study Group, also published in *The New England Journal of Medicine*, found that taking calcium supplements could be helpful to people who have had colon cancer in the past. This study took more than 900 people with a recent history of colon cancer and gave half of them 1,200 mg of calcium a day and the other half a placebo. At the end of this four-year study, those people who had taken extra calcium had fewer recurrences of colon cancer than those on the placebo. In this particular study, dietary fat and dietary calcium had no effect; only calcium supplements had an effect.

If you have a concern about colon cancer, reduce the amount of all fats in your diet. If you have a family history of this disease, or have had colon cancer yourself, consider increasing your supplemental calcium.

How to Get Enough Calcium

Calcium absorption is even more important than the amount of calcium you get. You may think that if a food contains 100 mg of calcium, then 100 mg of calcium is absorbed and available to your bones and other tissues. But this isn't true. Only a fraction of the calcium in different foods is usable. It's the same with calcium supplements. Some are well absorbed; others are not. Whatever your body can't use becomes a potential problem.

When calcium isn't absorbed into your bones and other tissues, it can contribute to heart disease, kidney stones, and arthritis. Taking high amounts of calcium to prevent bone loss does not guarantee strong bones. The key is to take enough, but not too much, calcium. And it's just as important to get enough magnesium and other cofactors to help your body use the calcium in your supplements and diet.

Many nondairy sources of dietary calcium contain these cofactors. Dairy does not. Look for foods, such as whole grains, dark green vegetables, and beans, that have both calcium and magnesium for best absorption.

To evaluate your daily intake, count all the calcium in your foods and supplements. Not just the amount in the pills you take. And be sure to include enough magnesium whenever you take calcium. This means doing more than merely taking a handful of calcium supplements or eating a lot of dairy.

Assessing Your Calcium Needs

Not everyone needs 1,000–1,500 mg of supplemental calcium a day. The total amount of calcium your body needs comes from both diet and supplements. Still many people eat dairy and other high-calcium foods while taking 1,000 mg or more of a calcium supplement. As you've learned, this can be dangerous.

To decide how much calcium you may need, first look at your personal and family health histories. Some disorders are a sign of low or poorly absorbed calcium. These include arthritis, heart disease, and osteoporosis. If you have any of these health problems, look to see whether you need to take more calcium than you've been taking, or a better-absorbed form.

Next, look for reasons why calcium may not be well absorbed. These include not getting magnesium and having low amounts of hydrochloric acid (stomach acid). Acid is needed to break down and use both calcium and magnesium. For this reason, calcium in antacids is not as well absorbed as other forms. See the discussion "Antacids and Calcium Absorption" on page 108.

There is compelling evidence to suggest that high amounts of calcium are not necessary and may even contribute to health problems. If you're taking a well-absorbed form, you may need much less than the amount most people recommend.

Look for signs of calcium excess. If you're taking too much calcium, you may have muscle cramps, fibromyalgia, irregular heartbeat (arrhythmias), restless leg syndrome, or premenstrual syndrome (PMS). In these cases, symptoms may improve by lowering supplemental calcium to 500 mg a day.

If you are determining how much calcium your child needs, remember that children and adolescents, whose bones are still forming and growing, need more calcium than adults do.

Dairy Products as a Source of Calcium

We've been taught that dairy products are a good source of dietary calcium. In fact, we've heard so much about dairy that few people realize that there are other calcium-rich foods. But dairy has limitations that you should consider when you're evaluating your calcium intake.

Dairy is rich in calcium, with very little magnesium, which is needed to help move calcium into your bones. So, a diet containing dairy should also include high-magnesium foods like nuts, seeds, whole grains, beans, and green vegetables.

Dairy is also high in phosphorus, and while you need phosphorus for strong bones, too much can interfere with calcium absorption and cause increased calcium excretion. The typical American diet contains too much phosphorus. High-phosphorus foods include animal protein and colas. You need equal amounts of calcium and phosphorus for healthy bones. While small amounts of dairy may have its place in a diet designed to help bones stay strong, high-dairy diets may not be protecting your bones as much as you think—especially if you're eating a lot of protein and drinking colas.

Limitations of Dairy

The association between eating a lot of dairy and osteoporosis is not what you think. People who live in countries with the highest dairy consumption—the United States, Great Britain, and Sweden—have the highest amount of osteoporosis. People on diets low in dairy, like Asians and many Africans, have stronger bones. Clearly, dairy is not the solution for strong bones.

In addition, not everyone can digest dairy. Lactose intolerance is another reason why dairy is not the only, or best, source of dietary calcium for many people. Yogurt is one form of dairy that is low in lactose and easier for people with lactose intolerance to digest.

Lactose Intolerance *The inability to digest milk sugar. This intolerance leads to bloating and cramping after eating milk, cheese, and other dairy products.*

Drinking milk is not natural. Michael Klaper, M.D., points out that of all the animals on earth, humans are the only species that drink the milk of other species. We're also the only species to drink milk after we're weaned. It appears that nature is trying to tell us something, but we're not listening. The voice of vested interest groups, like the American Dairy Association, are shouting in our ears, preventing us from listening to other, more logical, messages.

Scientific Studies and Dairy

There have been numerous studies that looked at dairy products and osteoporosis. One impressive twelve-year study of 78,000 women, published in the *American Journal of Public Health*, had a surprising finding. Women who drank two or more glasses of milk a day had more hip fractures than those who drank it once a week or less.

Cardiologist Kurt Oster, M.D., has published studies that found that an enzyme in cow's milk could lead to heart disease. This enzyme damages cell membranes in the arteries. Normally, digestive juices destroy this enzyme. But when the milk is homogenized, the enzyme can get into your arteries and cause considerable damage. Since most dairy products are homogenized, it might be wise to limit dairy products to protect against heart disease.

In an article published in the *International Journal of Cardiology*, Stephen Seely, M.D., points out that our need for calcium decreases as we age. He found that a diet high in calcium could lead to small amounts of the mineral getting into soft tissues, like the aorta, resulting in heart disease. He also found that high blood pressure does not exist in countries where calcium intake is low. (See "Calcium's Role in a Healthy Heart" on page 113.)

Dietary Sources of Calcium

Calcium is everywhere, and all calcium counts toward your daily dose. Beans, whole grains, green vegetables, and fish (with small edible bones, like canned salmon) all contain good amounts of calcium. Canned salmon, for instance, has 350–550 mg of calcium. Fresh salmon, without bones, has none since the calcium in fish comes from the bones.

Many common foods have good amounts of this important mineral. A cup of broccoli has 178 mg, and a cup of most any kind of beans supplies at least 130 mg. Some contain much more. Half a cup of garbanzo beans, for instance, will give you more than 200 mg of calcium. Half a cup of tofu (soybean curd) contains 100–300 mg. Even an orange has 56 mg. Of all nuts, almonds are highest in calcium content. One tablespoon of almond butter has 40 mg, while an ounce of the nuts themselves contains nearly 80 mg.

Many foods have smaller amounts of calcium. Add them up at the end of the day and you will find your calcium intake is much higher than you thought. For instance, a cup of blackberries (46 mg), a kiwi fruit (74 mg), or a single dried fig (19 mg) added to a salad, broccoli, and a few nuts gives you a good amount of usable calcium.

Absorbing Dietary Calcium

Contrary to popular belief, calcium from plant products is well absorbed. Registered dietician Vesanto Melina points out that 50 to 70 percent of the calcium found in cooked vegetables like broccoli and kale gets into tissues. Only 32 percent of calcium from dairy products, on the other hand, is used.

You can increase the absorption of calcium by soaking beans overnight, sprouting seeds (like sunflower seeds), roasting nuts, and cooking grains. And you can get more usable calcium just by chewing better.

As mentioned previously, when you chew your food well, your body secretes hydrochloric acid (HCl), the acid made in your stomach that helps you use calcium, magnesium, iron, and protein. As you've learned, it's not a good idea to take antacids when you eat calcium-rich foods or when you're taking calcium supplements. Antacids neutralize stomach acid and lower calcium absorption. Add acidic foods like lemon juice, orange juice, vinegar, or tomatoes to high-calcium foods, or when you take calcium supplements.

Limit your calcium intake to about 500 mg at any one time. This is the amount found in many healthy meals. Your body will use more calcium if you take it frequently in small quantities rather than if you take large amounts all at once. Finally, choose a calcium supplement that is easy for your body to use.

Evaluating Calcium Supplements

Some calcium supplements may contain lead, a harmful heavy metal. Lead has been found in bone meal and dolomite. Avoid these forms. Lead is lowest in supplements where calcium is attached to citrate, fumarate, succinate, or aspartate, or amino acid chelate. In addition to not containing lead, they are better absorbed than calcium carbonate, an inexpensive and frequently used calcium source.

To give you an idea of the absorbability of calcium supplements, look at calcium carbonate versus calcium citrate. About 45 percent of calcium in a citrate form can be absorbed by people with low stomach acid. Only 4 percent of calcium carbonate is available to these same people. Once again, because acid is needed to utilize calcium, antacids are not a good source of calcium.

Calcium hydroxyapatite is a popular ingredient in several bone-building formulas. But Tori Hudson, N.D., points out that this form of calcium is simply purified bone meal and may also contain lead. While claims of superior absorption have been made for calcium hydroxyapatite, Dr. Hudson finds it is even less absorbable than calcium carbonate.

The best forms of calcium supplements are calcium citrate, calcium malate, calcium fumarate, calcium succinate, calcium aspartate, and calcium amino acid chelate.

How to Get Enough Magnesium

You may not be getting enough magnesium in your diet, especially if you have signs of a magnesium deficiency. As you may recall, high-magnesium foods include nuts, seeds, whole grains, beans, and dark green vegetables. Even if you eat these foods every day, you may be losing valuable magnesium due to stress, a high-fat diet, colas, or too much vitamin D (from dairy products). Diets and supplements that emphasize calcium over magnesium contribute to many magnesium-deficiency problems. High dairy consumption also adds to this deficiency.

Alan R. Gaby, M.D., gives magnesium supplements to almost every one of his patients. He found that taking extra magnesium eliminated magnesium-deficiency symptoms and prevented calcium deposits like kidney stones and atherosclerosis.

Assessing Your Magnesium Needs

Most doctors suggest you need only the RDA of magnesium (320–420 mg) each day. But magnesium expert Mildred S. Seelig, M.D., disagrees. She says this RDA is based on an erroneous theory and that we need much more. A review on magnesium from the Yale School of Medicine supports Dr. Seelig in its finding that magnesium deficiencies are common. Today, more nutrition-oriented doctors are emphasizing the importance of additional magnesium for their patients.

The theory on which today's RDA is based stated that only half the magnesium we get in our foods and supplements is absorbed. It went on to say that since our kidneys can recirculate magnesium, like they can with calcium, there is no real magnesium deficiency. But since the RDAs were established, follow-up studies indicate that we don't absorb this much magnesium at all. What's more, unabsorbed magnesium is not recirculated, but excreted. Since your kidneys recirculate calcium, this creates an even greater need for additional magnesium.

Your diet and lifestyle may create a need for still more magnesium. A high-salt diet, drinking alcohol, taking hormones, and using diuretic medications all increase the requirement for this mineral, as do tight, painful muscles, heart disease, and osteoporosis.

Some people need equal amounts of magnesium and calcium. Others need even more magnesium than calcium. Since the side effects from taking too much magnesium are mild—loose stools, diarrhea, or stomach irritation—many health practitioners suggest taking it to bowel tolerance. They have their patients add supplemental magnesium up to 1,000 mg a day until they have comfortably loose stools. Some people can tolerate only 100 mg of magnesium a day while others can take as much as 1,000 mg.

Symptoms of Magnesium Deficiency

Constipation is one possible sign of a magnesium deficiency. Increasing magnesium relaxes the intestinal muscles and often alleviates constipation. Before taking magnesium for constipation, check with your doctor to make sure you have no underlying health problem that's causing this condition.

Craving chocolate is another possible sign of a magnesium deficiency, since chocolate contains more magnesium than any other food. When magnesium is increased, chocolate cravings can take a backseat to simply enjoying this flavor. Instead of trying to resist eating chocolate, you might want to increase your magnesium and see if you still crave it as much.

Sore muscles, headaches, tight muscles, irregular heartbeat, PMS, cramps, heart disease, and osteoporosis are other signs that you may need more magnesium. If you're taking a lot of supplemental calcium or eating a diet high in dairy, you may need less calcium, as well.

How Calcium Affects Magnesium Needs

If you're taking a calcium-magnesium supplement, you may not be getting enough magnesium because most supplements contain twice as much calcium as magnesium. In theory, this makes sense because your body contains more calcium than magnesium. But practically speaking, this ratio leaves many people with unabsorbed calcium and a need for more magnesium.

High calcium, accompanied by low magnesium, can lead to a condition called hypocalcemia. Hypocalcemia, in turn, leads to hypomagnesia, or low magnesium. Correct-

Hypocalcemia
Abnormally low levels of calcium in the blood that can lead to low magnesium and kidney problems.

ing both of these imbalances requires an increase in one mineral: magnesium.

Sometimes both calcium and magnesium levels are low. When a person with low calcium and low magnesium is given extra calcium, both levels remain low. When extra magnesium is added, both levels improve. Magnesium is one important key to calcium absorption. Since calcium and magnesium are both absorbed in the same sites in your intestines, too much calcium prevents you from absorbing magnesium.

Foods That Interfere with Magnesium

Magnesium is normally excreted in the urine. Some foods increase this excretion. They include high amounts of alcohol, caffeine, sugars of any kind (even fruits and fruit juices), colas, and animal protein. Some drugs, like diuretics, also increase urinary excretion of magnesium. Other medications, like Digoxin (used for heart problems) and Cisplatin (a chemotherapy drug), block the body's ability to absorb and retain magnesium. In addition, a high-fat diet interferes with the absorption of magnesium. This is because when fats and magnesium are combined, they form soaps that prevent magnesium from being absorbed.

Foods High in Magnesium

Magnesium is found in chlorophyll, which is why green leafy vegetables are a good source of this mineral. For example, one cup of cooked spinach contains more than 100 mg.

Magnesium is stored in the outer layer of grains. You can increase your dietary magnesium simply by eating more whole grains. A cup of wild rice contains 238 mg of magnesium, while a cup of whole-wheat flour has 136 mg. One cup of refined, enriched white flour, on the other hand, has only 34 mg of magnesium.

All beans are a good source of magnesium. Split peas and lentils contain the most: 270 mg per cup. Nuts and seeds are also high in magnesium. One-fourth of a cup of almonds, cashews, or Brazil nuts will give you between 85 and 95 mg of magnesium.

Unfortunately, few people eat nuts, beans, and whole grains daily. This leaves green vegetables as their major food source of magnesium. It's not likely that anyone can get enough magnesium eating one or two helpings of vegetables a day and only occasional servings of whole wheat bread and beans. In addition, today's foods contain less magnesium than they did in the past. It's becoming almost impossible to meet rising magnesium needs with foods that have less magnesium than ever before.

Why Our Foods Are Low in Magnesium

Foods normally high in magnesium, like green vegetables,

can only contain good amounts if the soil they grow in has enough. Unless soil is amended with magnesium, spinach, for example, will contain less magnesium than it should. Magnesium is not found in synthetic fertilizers. Unless soil has been amended naturally, your food may have less magnesium than you think. For this reason, organic foods may contain more magnesium than their conventionally grown counterparts.

Magnesium is one of the nutrients removed from grains when they are refined, and it is not replenished when these foods are "enriched." Whole-wheat flour loses 96 percent of its magnesium when it is refined into white flour.

During the refining process from sugarcane to white sugar, 99 percent of the magnesium it originally contained is lost. And up to 50 percent of the magnesium in vegetables is lost in the water in which it is cooked. For this reason, vegetables that are stir-fried will have more magnesium than those that have been boiled or steamed.

Even the water you drink helps determine how much magnesium you get. Most of our drinking water has been fluoridated. The magnesium naturally found in drinking water is lost during fluoridation. In addition, hard water has more magnesium than soft water. A number of studies have shown that people who drink soft water have more deaths from heart disease than those who drink hard water.

Since fats, meats, and dairy contain very low amounts of magnesium, it's no wonder that we have difficulty getting enough of this important mineral from our food. When dietary sources are not enough, it's time to add magnesium supplements.

Taking Magnesium Supplements

The American Diabetes Association suggests that magnesium chloride is more soluble than most other forms. But there are many well-absorbed forms including magnesium glycinate, magnesium citrate, magnesium aspartate, magnesium gluconate, magnesium lactate, and magnesium amino acid chelate.

The least absorbable forms are magnesium oxide and magnesium hydroxide. They need to be in the presence of stomach acid to be broken down and used. If you're taking antacids or have poor hydrochloric acid (HCl) production due to aging, you may want to avoid these forms of magnesium.

Guy E. Abraham, M.D., who has researched magnesium's role in PMS and osteoporosis, says that any form of magnesium is fine if there's enough hydrochloric acid present. Since your stomach makes HCl to help digest certain foods, it's best to take magnesium supplements along with, or right after, meals.

CONCLUSION

There's no doubt that calcium is an extremely important mineral to help build healthy bones. Our need for this mineral increases throughout our lives at critical times, such as during childhood when bones are forming, and during pregnancy when a fetus needs extra bone-building nutrients. It helps regulate our heart and blood pressure, protects some people against colon cancer, and, if enough can get into our bones, guards against osteoporosis.

But by emphasizing calcium in our diets and supplements, many people have created a magnesium deficiency. This deficiency can affect a wide variety of health conditions from a simple headache to arthritis or a deadly heart attack. It may not be a good idea to take high amounts of calcium supplements, especially when magnesium intake is relatively low. A lower quantity of well-absorbed calcium appears to be more appropriate.

While our need for calcium has remained constant for hundreds of years, our need for magnesium has increased with changes in lifestyle, diet, and the stresses of daily living. Dietary stressors, including too much sugar, alcohol, and caffeine, have left many people deficient in magnesium. This important mineral has been depleted from our soil and removed from foods during refining processes. Yet, as we have seen, without sufficient magnesium, the calcium we require is unable to make its way into bone and other tissues.

The answer is to reduce stress or find ways to handle it better, increase magnesium in our diets and supplements, and evaluate our particular nutritional requirements for calcium. Finally, to be most easily absorbed, these two minerals should come in contact with some form of acid, like the hydrochloric acid naturally secreted by our stomachs.

Calcium and magnesium supplements should be attached to an acid, like citric acid (citrate), aspartic acid (aspartate), or malic acid (malate), for best absorption. When it comes to calcium and magnesium, you are not what you eat. You are what you eat, digest, and absorb.

PART SIX

CHROMIUM

MELISSA DIANE SMITH

Can a trace mineral make a huge difference in health? Absolutely, especially when that mineral is chromium. Needed in minute amounts by the body, chromium promotes optimal health by protecting against the most common chronic diseases in our modern world.

Why is chromium so health promoting? Chromium helps the blood–sugar-lowering hormone, insulin, function more efficiently. This benefit may seem minor or only important for diabetics, but it's important for all of us. Insulin, the master hormone of our metabolism, regulates the body's breakdown of carbohydrates, protein, and fats for energy. Obviously, the better insulin functions, the better the body functions.

We now know that most health problems and chronic diseases that plague the Western world are brought on by uncontrolled blood sugar and disturbances of insulin function. By helping insulin work more effectively, chromium combats these problems—not only several different types of diabetes, but also obesity, prediabetes, hypoglycemia, unhealthy cholesterol levels, high blood pressure, Syndrome X, and heart disease. By keeping insulin and blood sugar levels in check, chromium can also delay the effects of aging. It is even helpful in some cases of depression, premenstrual syndrome, seasonal affective disorder, and osteoporosis. In other words, chromium is a tiny nutrient that packs a mighty therapeutic punch for its size.

Nutritionally speaking, it's usually best to get nutrients from food whenever possible. However, chromium levels have been depleted from our soil, and few foods today have high amounts of chromium. Amazingly, 90 percent of Americans don't receive adequate amounts of chromium from their diets. What's more, most Americans eat excessive amounts of sugar and refined grains, which deplete chromium levels.

With most people running on low levels of chromium, it shouldn't be surprising that the incidences of insulin-related health conditions such as type II diabetes and obesity are at all-time highs. But they don't have to be. Insulin-related health problems are nutritional diseases that can be corrected and prevented with nutrition. One of the first places to start is with chromium supplementation.

All nutrients are important, but chromium may be a little extra important in this day and age. Delve into this part of the *User's Guide to Nutritional Supplements* and find out the many reasons why.

BASICS ABOUT CHROMIUM

Chromium is an essential nutrient that's needed for optimal blood sugar function. Lack of dietary chromium is widespread in industrialized nations and is a contributing factor in the development of many common blood–sugar- and insulin-related health problems.

A Mineral Needed in Small but Regular Amounts

Chromium is a mineral, not a vitamin. Vitamins and minerals are both necessary for health, but minerals are simpler in chemical form and are tiny in comparison to vitamins.

Unlike calcium and magnesium, which are found in large amounts in the body, chromium is a trace mineral found in minute amounts. It doesn't take much chromium to fulfill our basic need for this mineral. However, if we don't get the small amount we need, our health suffers.

Minerals
Elements that cannot be broken down into simpler substances. A trace mineral is one that is needed in very tiny amounts.

Chemistry: Nutritional versus Industrial Chromium

It should be pointed out that chromium in this book refers to nutritional chromium, which is technically known as trivalent chromium because it has a net electronic charge of plus three (+3). There is another type of chromium, hexavalent chromium (Cr6+), which I'll call industrial chromium, just to keep it simple. Industrial chromium forms as a byproduct of certain industrial processes, such as the making of stainless and hard-alloy steel.

If you saw the movie *Erin Brockovich,* you may recall that industrial or hexavalent chromium has been shown to cause cancer. But don't be alarmed: industrial chromium has nothing to do with nutritional chromium—and nutritional chromium cannot change into industrial chromium inside the body. There are numerous examples of substances having vastly different properties in different forms. For example, oxygen is health promoting in some forms, while it is hazardous to health in other forms.

> **Trivalent Chromium**
> *The scientific name for nutritional chromium, the type of chromium we need for health.*

If you read about chromium in scientific terms, here's how to keep the two forms straight: When you hear about hexavalent chromium, think of "hex" as something that brings you very bad luck. However, when you hear the prefix "tri" in trivalent chromium, think "Three's a charm." As you read this book, you'll learn just what kind of magic nutritional chromium can do for people with many different kinds of blood–sugar- and insulin-related health problems.

Chromium's Essentiality Discovered in the 1970s

By the 1950s, chromium was known to help control blood sugar in animals, but it wasn't until 1977 that chromium was proven to be essential for human health. Hospitalized patients who could not take in food by mouth were given Total Parental Nutrition (TPN)—a solution of all the nutrients they needed to maintain health—directly into their veins. Some of these patients developed high blood sugar levels and other diabetic-type symptoms. Doctors tried to start insulin therapy to treat the condition, but it didn't work very well.

Physicians got the idea that the patients were showing signs of chromium deficiency. Small amounts of chromium were added to the patients' intravenous feeding solutions. With the addition of this one nutrient, the patients quickly improved: their blood sugars and other abnormalities returned to normal. The Food and Drug Administration (FDA) and the Food and Nutrition Board of the National Research Council, therefore, designated chromium an essential trace mineral for human health.

The Relationship between Chromium and Insulin

To understand what happens when we don't get enough chromium, it's important to understand more about chromium and the hormone insulin.

Insulin is the master hormone of our metabolism. It controls blood sugar levels, regulates many aspects of the breakdown and utilization of carbohydrates, fats, and protein for energy, and directly affects certain genetic proc-

esses. Keeping insulin working correctly is an important factor in health.

> **Insulin**
> *A key metabolic hormone that lowers blood sugar levels by increasing the rate at which glucose is taken up by cells throughout the body.*

Here's where chromium comes in: the trace mineral helps insulin work more efficiently to allow blood sugar (or glucose) to move from the blood into the cells. Glucose is a fuel that cells need for energy.

Researchers still don't know exactly how chromium does its magic, but it may help insulin attach more easily to the necessary molecular docks. Also, it may be involved in enzyme reactions that lead to increased insulin sensitivity (or receptivity). Regardless of the mechanism, without chromium, the blood–sugar-lowering hormone insulin won't work properly and blood sugar, in turn, will rise to unhealthy levels.

Insulin Resistance—The Root of Many Health Problems

Before blood sugar levels rise to consistently unhealthy levels, a condition called insulin resistance usually develops. Insulin resistance sneaks up on people over years and sometimes decades, primarily from eating the wrong foods and not getting enough nutrients.

> **Insulin Resistance**
> *A condition in which the body does not respond to insulin efficiently. High insulin levels usually accompany insulin resistance.*

What happens is this: Sugary treats and a lot of white-flour products provoke a steep rise in blood sugar. The body responds by releasing insulin to lower blood sugar to healthy levels. This works fine for a while; however, the more often blood–sugar-rising foods are eaten, the more the body has to pump out extra levels of insulin to keep blood sugar in a normal range.

Eventually, the body becomes overwhelmed by so much insulin that it doesn't respond as efficiently to insulin's blood–sugar-lowering effects. (This condition—insulin resistance—is very much like taking so much of a drug that it loses its effectiveness and a person needs a larger amount of it to get the same effect.) When insulin isn't working efficiently, the body compensates by churning out even greater insulin levels to keep glucose levels in check.

Chromium Fights High Insulin and High Blood Sugar

The combination of insulin resistance and high insulin levels can go on silently for years or decades without a person knowing it. Unfortunately, all the while, the excess insulin does damage and sets disease into motion inside the body. If this continues, blood sugar levels gradually rise, either because body cells become even less responsive to the action of insulin or because the workhorse pancreas eventually tires and stops producing adequate amounts of insulin.

Later, you'll learn that both high insulin levels and high blood sugar levels are hazardous to health and contribute to premature aging. Fortunately, chromium protects against both conditions because it helps insulin work more effectively.

Chromium Needs Vary

The amount of chromium that people need varies. It depends primarily on their intake and state of health. Those who are most lacking in the nutrient need it the most.

The symptoms of chromium deficiency include elevated blood sugar, insulin, and cholesterol; elevated blood triglycerides; and decreased levels of the good HDL cholesterol. All of these conditions have been shown to respond well to chromium supplementation.

The Recommended Daily Allowance Committee recommends 50–200 mcg of chromium per day. This amount seems reasonable for the average healthy person, but higher amounts are needed for people with many conditions involving insulin resistance, such as type II diabetes and prediabetes.

50–200 mcg
The estimated safe and recommended amount of chromium the average healthy person needs on a daily basis.

Low Intakes Are Exceedingly Common

Unfortunately, most Americans don't obtain the minimum 50 mcg of chromium from their daily diets. Research from the USDA found that men average 33 mcg of chromium per day in their diets and women average 25 mcg per day—and the situation is similar in other countries. Even diets designed to be well balanced by nutritionists almost always contain less than 50 mcg of chromium.

What makes it so difficult to meet our needs for chromium? To begin with, only a few foods are rich sources of chromium. Second, our soil has been depleted of many minerals, including chromium; foods that grow in the depleted soil are therefore low in chromium and other minerals that we need.

The best sources of chromium are organ meats, oysters, broccoli, mushrooms, brewers yeast, brown rice, barley, and wheat germ. Unfortunately, the first two foods aren't widely eaten. Also, there are a large number of people who are susceptible to yeast infections or who have yeast or grain sensitivities and should therefore avoid or limit some of the other foods.

Our bodies are designed to thrive on an ample supply of chromium along with few or no foods that act as chromium depletors. Our Stone-Age ancestors regularly ate organ meats, so they likely had a higher intake of chromium than we have today. In addition, Stone-Age people ate no refined sugar or refined grains, which are very low in chromium and also promote chromium losses in the urine.

Chromium excretion also increases with infection, strenuous exercise, pregnancy, and stress, and we lose chromium as we age. The highest tissue levels of chromium are found in newborns; tissue levels decrease from then on throughout the rest of our lives. Because of all these factors—inadequate chromium intake, increased chromium losses, and decreasing chromium tissue levels as we age—virtually all of us can benefit from rebuilding the body's stockpile of chromium by taking chromium supplements.

In the sections that follow, you'll read over and over again how chromium's ability to improve faulty insulin function carries considerable therapeutic weight against a wide variety of blood–sugar- and insulin-related conditions. We'll start the discussion by covering chromium's impressive health benefits for people with the most serious of these conditions, diabetes.

NUTRITIONAL THERAPY FOR DIABETES

Diabetes can come in several different forms, but it's always characterized by abnormally high blood sugar levels. Diabetes is a serious disease that's out of sight and out of mind to many people, but it shouldn't be: it greatly increases the risk of coronary artery disease, stroke, blindness, nerve disorders, kidney disease, cancer, and impotence (in men). Moreover, the incidence of one particular type of diabetes, type II diabetes, is growing at an outstanding rate.

Improving insulin function to reduce blood sugar levels is the prime strategy for treating diabetes. Chromium improves insulin efficiency, so not surprisingly, chromium supplements have been found to be therapeutic for relieving symptoms and improving blood sugar and insulin levels in many different types of diabetes. Chromium also benefits the most common type of hypoglycemia (low blood sugar), which is often considered a precursor to type II diabetes.

The Different Types of Diabetes

Diabetes is generally classified into two main types, type I and type II. Type II is by far the most common type, accounting for 90 to 95 percent of all cases. Historically, this type of diabetes developed primarily in adults; therefore, it is often called adult-onset diabetes. Today, however, type II diabetes is developing in children at an alarming rate, including some children as young as ten years old. Primarily a disease brought on by an unhealthy diet and lifestyle, type II diabetes is insulin resistance in its worst form. Fortunately, it usually responds incredibly well to nutritional treatment.

Type I diabetes, also called insulin-dependent or juvenile-onset diabetes, is an autoimmune disease that usually develops in children or adults before age thirty. This type of diabetes isn't characterized by inefficient use of insulin but rather by a lack of insulin production. Something, perhaps a virus or a dietary factor, causes the immune system to destroy the insulin-producing cells in the pancreas.

> **Diabetes Mellitus**
> *A condition caused by undersecretion of the hormone insulin (in type I diabetes) or cell insensitivity to insulin (in type II diabetes), leading to high blood glucose levels.*

There also are a few types of diabetes that develop during stressful periods on the body. These include gestational diabetes (which develops during pregnancy) and drug-induced diabetes (which develops when people take certain drugs). The good news is that chromium has been found to be a helpful nutritional treatment for these many different types.

Chromium's Effectiveness in Type II Diabetes

Since chromium helps insulin to function better, researchers naturally suspected that supplemental chromium might help treat type II diabetes, the type in which insulin isn't used efficiently. Chromium, you'll recall, was deemed essential for human health after it was found to reverse diabetes in hospitalized patients. Research has found that chromium can do the same for large groups of type II diabetics.

Most of the studies involving supplemental chromium for type II diabetes have shown positive results of one type or another. However, when one particular form of chromium—the most bioavailable form, chromium picolinate—has been used, *all* of the studies have yielded positive results (in blood sugar, blood insulin, and/or blood lipid [cholesterol and triglyceride] readings).

One of these studies, a 1997 study involving 180 type II diabetics in China, is a classic. It documented "spectacular" results in diabetics who took 500 mcg of chromium picolinate twice daily. After four months, nearly all of the diabetics no longer had traditional signs of diabetes. Their blood sugar and insulin levels dropped to near normal—something that medications could not achieve. Even more important, the "gold standard" diagnostic measure of diabetes—blood levels of hemoglobin A1c (sugar-damaged proteins that age cells)—also dropped to normal.

A follow-up study by some of the same researchers monitored 833 type II diabetics who took 500 mcg of chromium picolinate twice daily. A significant reduction in fasting blood sugar levels and in post-meal blood sugar levels was found during the ten months of the study. No negative side effects were shown from taking the supplements. In addition, more than 85 percent of the patients reported improvements in the common diabetic symptoms of excessive thirst, frequent urination, and fatigue.

Type II Diabetics Have Higher Needs for Chromium

It's important to understand that type II diabetics have altered chromium metabolism—greater excretion of chromium, lower tissue levels of chromium, and less of an ability to convert chromium to a usable form in the body. For all of these reasons, chromium supplements are a must for diabetics.

Supplements usually work very well if taken in high enough doses and effective forms. But the dose and form really makes a big difference. Type II diabetics who have taken chromium picolinate in low doses—200 mcg per day—have had some improvements in their condition; however, they have not had the same spectacular results as type II diabetics who have taken 1,000 mcg per day.

There's one big caveat about taking chromium supplements: *If you're a diabetic who takes insulin injections or sugar-lowering drugs, you should not take chromium supplements without working with a knowledgeable doctor who can help you safely adjust the dosages of your medications.* Supplemental chromium works so well at improving insulin function that less medication usually is needed. (And, sometimes, medication can be eliminated completely over time.) This is a good thing—it indicates a reversal or lessening of insulin resistance—but it also means that you should work with your doctor to carefully monitor your condition and avoid overmedicating yourself.

Chromium picolinate is very beneficial by itself for type II diabetics, but there appears to be a nutrient combination that's even more effective. That combination is chromium picolinate plus biotin, a B vitamin. Recent research indicates that this combination of nutrients stimulates greater blood sugar usage and greater improvements in cholesterol readings compared with those seen when chromium picolinate is taken alone. You'll learn more about this synergistic combination later.

Chromium Helps Prevent Type II Diabetes in Those at Risk

Although the incidence of type II diabetes is increasing in record numbers, many people don't yet have diabetes but are at high risk for developing it. Chromium supplements can help in these cases, too.

A study directed by William Cefalu, M.D., of Wake Forest University, monitored individuals at risk—people who were moderately obese and had a family history of diabetes. Some people received a placebo; others, 1,000 mcg of chromium picolinate daily. After four months of treatment with chromium, insulin resistance was reduced by 40 percent. Insulin resistance, you'll recall, is the condition at the core of type II diabetes. Chromium supplements, therefore, help reverse the underlying disease process that leads to type II diabetes. In other words, they help both prevent and reverse type II diabetes.

Chromium Helps Type I Diabetes, Too

Many diabetics who inject insulin—both type I diabetics and type II diabetics who are in more advanced stages of the disease—respond positively to chromium picolinate supplementation. About 70 percent of both types show improved insulin responsiveness after taking 200 mcg of supplemental chromium per day. Some experience such an improvement in insulin sensitivity that they are able to reduce the amount of insulin they inject or the amount of other blood–sugar-lowering medications they take.

Chromium can't cure type I diabetes—in other words, it can't make type I diabetics produce more insulin. But chromium helps make the injected insulin taken by type I diabetics work more effectively, so less is often needed. Therefore, type I diabetics, like type II diabetics, should monitor their condition carefully and work with their physicians regarding the appropriate dosages of medications.

Chromium and Other Types of Diabetes

Chromium supplementation has been found to be helpful for still other types of diabetes. Gestational diabetes is a transitional diabetes that develops during pregnancy and can cause numerous health problems, including loss of the child. It's the most common medical complication of pregnancy today. Just eight weeks of supplementation with chromium picolinate can significantly improve glucose intolerance and reduce blood sugar and insulin levels in those with gestational diabetes, thereby reducing the risk of health problems for both the mother and her child.

The use of certain pharmaceutical drugs, such as corticosteroids or Thiazide diuretics, lead to significant chromium losses and can also sometimes induce diabetic-type conditions. Fortunately, chromium supplementation can lead to improvements in the body's handling of blood sugar in both cases. In one study, steroid-induced diabetes was ameliorated in thirty-eight of forty-one patients following supplementation with 200 mcg of chromium three times per day. This occurred even though blood–sugar-lowering drugs were reduced by 50 percent in all patients who were given chromium supplements.

A Blood Sugar Balancer That's Helpful for Hypoglycemia, Too

It is important to keep in mind that chromium is a nutrient, not a drug. Chromium helps insulin function more efficiently. It benefits people with all types of blood sugar and insulin disorders—not just people with insulin resistance and diabetes, but also people with reactive hypoglycemia (those who experience quick blood sugar highs followed by quick blood sugar lows). Reactive hypoglycemia may seem very different from diabetes, but it represents the beginning stages of blood sugar imbalance or glucose intolerance and is considered a precursor to diabetes.

In people with reactive hypoglycemia, supplemental chromium normalizes insulin function, leading to increased insulin efficiency and a return to normal glucose levels more quickly after a high-sugar intake. It also alleviates hypoglycemic symptoms, including sweating, trembling, blurred vision, and sleepiness. In people with diabetes, improved insulin efficiency leads to a more efficient removal of sugar from the blood and reduction of diabetic markers, such as hemoglobin A1c levels. It also leads to a reduction of diabetic symptoms, such as increased thirst, frequent urination, and fatigue. Chromium, therefore, can be considered a blood sugar balancer as well as a blood sugar regulator.

Reactive Hypoglycemia
A condition characterized by unstable blood sugar and symptoms such as mood and energy swings, sugar cravings, anxiety, and trembling.

Chromium is not a magic bullet, however. Diabetes and blood sugar problems can be due to many different factors. Chromium deficiency (even if it is just marginal) is one of those factors, but not the only one.

As you've learned, in many of the studies, chromium supplementation by itself is often quite effective in alleviating many different types of glucose intolerance. Sometimes, however, it is not. The best approach involves taking chromium supplements as well as taking supplements of other nutrients important for proper blood sugar and insulin function; eating a protein-rich, low-carbohydrate diet rich in vegetables; reducing stress; and being physically active. More information on these synergistic strategies will be covered later.

A PROTECTOR AGAINST CHOLESTEROL PROBLEMS, SYNDROME X, AND HEART DISEASE

Insulin resistance and high insulin levels are major risk factors for heart disease. In addition, these conditions either directly or indirectly lead to other strong risk factors for heart disease, including upper-body ("apple-shaped" or abdominal) obesity; abnormal blood fat levels (that is, high triglycerides and high cholesterol or poor ratios of high-density lipoprotein to low-density lipoprotein cholesterol); and high blood pressure. This cluster of symptoms is known as Syndrome X.

Chromium helps improve insulin function so it's a critical nutrient for preventing and treating Syndrome X and thereby protecting against heart disease.

What Is Syndrome X?

Syndrome X *Insulin resistance plus abdominal obesity, high blood pressure, high blood triglycerides, and/or unhealthy blood cholesterol levels.*

Syndrome X may sound mysterious, but millions of Americans have it and don't know it. The term refers to a group of conditions many Americans are very familiar with: abdominal obesity (a "spare tire" around the middle); high blood pressure; high blood triglycerides; and high blood cholesterol levels or poor HDL-to-LDL cholesterol ratios. These heart disease risk factors tend to occur together—that's why they're called a "syndrome." Sixty-five to 70 million Americans are estimated to have this syndrome.

Each of the components of Syndrome X increases the risk of heart disease and diabetes. A combination of two or more of these components has an additive, or cumulative, effect in increasing the risk all the more.

The Chromium Connection to Syndrome X

Insulin resistance is at the root of Syndrome X; hence, Syndrome X is sometimes called the insulin resistance syndrome. It should be thought of as a prediabetic condition.

Chromium helps insulin work properly and helps reverse insulin resistance. Therefore, it gets to the root of the problem and helps reverse Syndrome X, just as it does with type II diabetes.

The symptoms of chromium deficiency are actually the symptoms of Syndrome X—high blood sugar, high insulin, high cholesterol, high triglycerides, and low levels of the "good" HDL cholesterol. A lack of chromium can cause all these conditions, so it makes sense that supplemental chromium can help improve these conditions. You'll learn that chromium does indeed do this.

Chromium and Fat Metabolism

Chromium is important for fat metabolism as well as for carbohydrate metabolism. Numerous studies have found that chromium supplements have beneficial effects on blood fats—including decreasing high total cholesterol and high LDL cholesterol, increasing beneficial HDL cholesterol, and decreasing triglycerides.

One double-blind, placebo-controlled study found that dietary supplementation with chromium picolinate for two months lowered blood levels of triglycerides in diabetics by an average of 17.4 percent. Another study by Richard Anderson, M.D., and his colleagues at the USDA observed a 15-percent decrease in total cholesterol when type II diabetics were given 1,000 mcg of chromium picolinate per day. Since elevated triglycerides and elevated cholesterol are risk factors for heart disease, chromium's ability to favorably influence them makes the mineral important in the prevention of cardiovascular disease, especially for diabetics who are at increased risk.

Chromium Acts as a Cholesterol Normalizer

Not all studies have found that chromium supplements lower blood cholesterol. This is likely because of two reasons. One, it takes a while, sometimes several months, to improve insulin sensitivity and high blood cholesterol levels. Studies that have not found cholesterol-lowering effects from chromium supplementation have lasted fewer than six weeks.

Two, chromium seems to act as a cholesterol normalizer instead of an overall cholesterol reducer. Gilbert Kaats, Ph.D., of the Health and Medical Research Foundation in San Antonio, Texas, designed an innovative study to examine this effect. He grouped people according to their cholesterol levels; then he gave them 400 mcg of chromium picolinate daily. He found that people who already had high cholesterol levels (greater than 199 mg/dl) experienced a drop in blood cholesterol of 17 mg/dl. In people who had normal cholesterol levels (150–199 mg/dl), the levels didn't change. And in people with low cholesterol levels (less than 150 mg/dl), chromium supplementation raised blood cholesterol by 8 mg/dl.

Therefore, just as chromium acts as a normalizer of blood sugar levels (helping people with both diabetes and hypoglycemia), it also acts as a normalizer of cholesterol levels, reducing cholesterol levels if they are too high but increasing them if they are too low.

Most people are concerned about high blood cholesterol levels, but few know that there are dangers in having low blood cholesterol levels. Research has shown that cholesterol levels below 150 mg/dl are associated with an increased risk of stroke, depression, violence, and suicide. Therefore, it's beneficial to health to raise cholesterol if it is too low, reduce cholesterol if it is too high, and maintain cholesterol if it is in the normal range. That's exactly what chromium supplements do.

This section focuses on reversing Syndrome X and preventing heart disease, so lowering high cholesterol levels is the most applicable part. But it's reassuring to know that chromium doesn't lower cholesterol levels in everyone. It simply promotes healthy cholesterol levels. In addition, those who need chromium the most respond to supplemental chromium the best.

Chromium's Effect on Blood Pressure

For many decades, high blood pressure was called "essential hypertension," which meant that the cause was not known. However, research over the past few decades has changed all that, showing that most hypertension is caused by excessive insulin.

Insulin can increase blood pressure in numerous ways. The hormone can increase the retention of sodium, which can raise blood pressure. Insulin also excites the body's sympathetic nervous system, which in turn speeds up the heart rate and raises blood pressure. And it increases the secretion of the stress hormone cortisol, which constricts blood vessels and can promote high blood pressure.

Chromium's ability to augment insulin sensitivity, therefore, can fix the root cause of many cases of high blood pressure. Animal studies at Georgetown University suggest that eating sugar raises blood pressure, but chromium picolinate supplements reduce typical sugar-induced elevations in blood pressure—at least up to a point. The best strategy for correcting hypertension, of course, is to take chromium supplements *and* to avoid eating sugar.

Chromium's Effect on Overweight

Chromium's role in helping overweight and obese people slim down will be covered in detail in the next section. Right now, let's cover a few basics.

The majority of Americans are now overweight and one-quarter are obese. Upper-body, "apple-shaped" obesity (seen often as a potbelly or beer belly) is a hallmark of Syndrome X, and it greatly increases the risk of heart disease and diabetes.

Upper Body Obesity
Extra weight carried through the middle of the body, often seen as a potbelly or beer belly. It's a common indicator of Syndrome X.

Insulin is a hormone that promotes the storage of fat when in excess. The higher insulin levels are, the more your body will pack on the pounds. Lowering insulin levels will help you burn fat and lose weight because you won't have the hormone working against you.

As already mentioned, most Americans don't get adequate chromium from their diets. They also eat excessive amounts of sugar and white-flour products, which deplete chromium levels in the body and raise blood sugar levels. Over time, the typical American diet leads to insulin resistance and high insulin levels, which in turn can lead to obesity.

It makes sense that the only way to break this vicious cycle is to start a program that improves insulin efficiency and lowers high insulin levels—first, by eating a lower-carbohydrate, protein-rich, vegetable-rich diet, and second, by taking chromium supplements.

Chromium—An Integral Part of an Anti-X Plan

Chromium doesn't act as a magic weight loss pill or a cholesterol- or blood–pressure-lowering drug (which is good because it doesn't come with any side effects!). Instead, it's a nutrient that combats all of the components of Syndrome X because it corrects the underlying problem—faulty insulin function.

Chromium supplements are indispensable for the nutritional treatment—and prevention—of Syndrome X. However, they're best used together with a blood–sugar-balancing diet and supplements of other nutrients important for proper blood sugar and insulin function (which you'll learn more about later).

As the coauthor of *Syndrome X: The Complete Nutritional Program to Prevent and Reverse Insulin Resistance* (John Wiley & Sons), I have put many clients on this type of nutrition plan and have also gotten feedback from many readers. The conclusion: An Anti-X nutrition plan, including chromium supplements, is very effective at improving heart-disease risk factors—or Syndrome X—all across the board.

When insulin resistance is reversed and numerous heart-disease risk factors fall by the wayside, the risk of developing heart disease and diabetes drops dramatically. Besides that, people who conquer Syndrome X feel more energetic and mentally focused—and look better—because insulin is functioning the way it should. The next section will cover the many ways chromium can help make it easier to lose weight and firm up the body.

AN AID IN FIGHTING THE BATTLE OF THE BULGE

Sixty percent of Americans are now overweight, 25 percent are obese, and the numbers increase every year. Some experts believe that if something isn't done soon to correct this trend, nearly everyone will be overweight by the year 2020. Overweight and obesity greatly increase the risk of chronic diseases, such as type II diabetes, and are therefore public health problems.

For most people, going on a lower-carbohydrate diet is important for stimulating weight loss, but taking chromium supplements is another good bet for firming up and losing unwanted fat. Chromium can help fight the battle of the bulge on several fronts.

Better Functioning Insulin Means Better Fat Burning

Chromium's key role, again, is it helps insulin work efficiently. When insulin is working properly, the fat-burning mechanisms of the body operate optimally. Less insulin is needed to do its job, so the body produces less insulin. Important body processes—thermogenesis (the production of heat by the body through the burning of sugar or fat) and the basal metabolic rate (the rate at which the body spends energy for the maintenance activities of the body)—hum along efficiently, so there's little chance for energy to be stored as fat.

When insulin doesn't do its job properly, all of this is reversed. More fat-promoting insulin is pumped out, the body's fat-burning processes are inhibited, and it's next to impossible to lose fat and get lean and trim. This is a common occurrence today because most people aren't getting adequate chromium and are eating foods that lead to further chromium losses.

Chromium Can Increase Lean Body Mass

When most people try to lose weight, they starve themselves on low-calorie diets, which cause a loss of lean body mass and a substantial decrease in their metabolic rates. Dieters following low-calorie diets, therefore, can lose weight, but they lose more muscle than fat and often become weak. Their metabolisms also slow down so they have a tendency to easily regain weight after they go off low-calorie diets.

The name of the game in weight control is not so much what you weigh as how much muscle you have compared with how much fat. (Lean muscle tissue actually weighs more than fat.)

Chromium, fortunately, can prevent loss of lean muscle tissue when a person moderately restricts calories. Better yet, when a person doesn't restrict calories, chromium can increase a person's total lean body mass. This in turn increases metabolism and the body's ability to burn fat.

Chromium helps maintain or build muscle mass because it's a potentiator of insulin. Among the many jobs insulin has, insulin directs amino acids (protein components) into muscle cells to build muscle. It also slows the breakdown or catabolism of body protein. When you're trying to lose weight, you want to lose fat but maintain or build muscle. Chromium supplements help you do that.

Exercise also increases insulin sensitivity, so physical activity and chromium supplementation often can work together to promote a trimmer, stronger body. Working out, however, increases a person's excretion of chromium, increasing his or her need for extra supplemental chromium.

Chromium Improves Body Composition

Several double-blind, placebo-controlled studies have shown that chromium supplementation stimulates fat loss, increases lean body mass, and helps lower body weight. In college-aged male weight lifters, male football players, and male and female swimmers, increases in lean body mass and reductions in body fat have been documented in those who have taken chromium supplements.

Chromium seems to be helpful for improving body composition in obese people, too. One 1998 study—after controlling for differences in calorie intake and expenditure among subjects—found that compared with those who received a placebo, obese subjects who received 400 mcg of chromium per day lost significantly more weight and fat, and had a greater loss in their percentage of body fat, without any loss of lean body mass. Supplemental chromium, therefore, can gradually improve body composition, but it often takes several months to see significant effects.

Even more exciting, a new combination of chromium picolinate and three other natural ingredients seems to magnify and quicken positive effects in weight and fat loss. You'll learn more about this new product in the section on nutrients and other factors that enhance chromium's effects.

Chromium Reduces Sugar Cravings

By improving insulin sensitivity and keeping blood sugar levels more even, chromium also reduces cravings for sugar and refined white-flour products. This is important because carbohydrate cravings and chromium deficiency tend to form a vicious cycle.

When the body has low levels of chromium, cravings for sugars and heavily refined grain products increase. People then give in to the cravings and eat those foods, but the more sweets they eat, the more they deplete chromium stores in the body. With even lower levels of chromium, cravings for more sweets develop and the unhealthy cycle can go on and on.

Fortunately, chromium can come to the rescue and stop this process. For example, some of my clients tell me they have had a lifelong sweet tooth, but when they start taking chromium supplements, their urges to eat sweets dramatically diminish. The more they stay away from sweets, the more they can build up their chromium reserves—and the more they do this, the easier it is for them to lose weight and look great.

In sum, chromium supplements aren't magic pills that automatically make people thinner and firmer. However, they do a lot to help people lose fat and improve body composition, particularly in conjunction with a good diet (and moderate physical activity).

An Antiaging Agent

Antiaging therapy is the rage these days, but most of the information written in this area is misleading. The truth is aging is inevitable: nothing can keep us young forever. But there's a lot we can do to age slowly and gracefully and delay or avoid developing the common chronic diseases of aging.

High insulin and high blood sugar levels—two factors that develop over time from eating the typical American diet—age us faster than anything else. Chromium brings down high insulin and high blood sugar and, therefore, plays a critical role in delaying the aging process.

Type II Diabetes—A Model of Accelerated Aging

To understand how chromium helps slow the aging process, it's important to know more about diabetes and the dangers of high insulin and high blood sugar.

Researchers see type II diabetes as a model of accelerated aging. Why is this? Because diabetics develop risk factors, symptoms, and chronic diseases of aging (such as heart disease) earlier in life than nondiabetics, and they generally die of chronic diseases at younger ages. Chromium supplements help prevent and reverse type II diabetes, a prime risk factor for heart disease and many other potentially fatal health consequences. So, for this simple reason alone, they hold back the aging process.

In addition, a decline in glucose tolerance is one of the changes normally associated with aging. Chromium supplementation is indispensable for improving glucose tolerance, so it holds back the aging process in this way, too.

The Aging Effects of High Insulin

We now know that the high insulin levels and high blood sugar levels that characterize type II diabetes both accelerate the aging process. You don't have to have diabetes to have either or both of these conditions and be on the fast track to aging. If you eat a diet that causes your body to pump out high levels of insulin—say, you're overweight around the middle—you're also aging prematurely.

Insulin is a powerful mitogen—it stimulates the division of cells and the activation of genes. Prolonged exposure to high levels of insulin, therefore, actually accelerates the aging of cells or makes cells act like older (instead of younger) cells. High insulin levels, it turns out, have their hand in the development of numerous age-related, chronic conditions—not just heart disease and type II diabetes, but also cognitive disorders, impaired thinking processes, dementia, Alzheimer's disease, and liver, pancreatic, endometrial, breast, and colorectal cancers.

The Aging Effects of High Blood Sugar

High blood sugar (or high glucose) also does damage in the body. First, high blood sugar generates a lot of free radicals—destructive molecules that damage and age cells. The more free radicals there are in the body—without an equal balance of protective antioxidants, molecules that quench free radicals—the faster that cells are damaged and the body ages.

Second, high blood sugar reacts with and damages proteins in organs and tissues, forming "advanced glycation end-products." The abbreviation for these substances, AGEs, is appropriate: AGEs toughen proteins and quite literally age cells.

Blood sugar that combines with the protein hemoglobin in your blood is glycosylated hemoglobin or hemoglobin A1c. AGEs are also involved in clouding the proteins in the lens of the eye (forming cataracts), and in the development of wrinkled skin and stiff joints. Often it's the combination of lots of AGEs and lots of free radicals that leads to so many of the complications of type II diabetes.

With blood sugar, you don't just run into trouble if your fasting blood sugar levels are high enough to qualify as diabetes (above 125 mg/dl). Prediabetic blood sugar levels (above 110 but below 125) greatly increase the risk of heart disease and diabetes—two of the most common diseases of aging. In addition, fasting blood sugar levels in the upper range of normal (say, 109) substantially increase the risk of death from heart disease than in someone with blood sugar readings at the lower range of normal (say, 80). The more you can lower blood sugar readings toward optimal levels, the least likely you are to age prematurely.

Hemoglobin A1c *Sugar-damaged hemoglobin. A marker that diabetics measure in their blood to monitor control of their condition.*

Chromium Lowers High Insulin and High Blood Sugar

Through its ability to improve insulin efficiency, chromium lowers high blood sugar and insulin levels, staving off the consequences from these conditions that promote aging. Even if supplemental chromium reduces blood sugar and insulin levels just slightly, it reduces the risk of age-related disease a little. Therefore, taking chromium supplements can help delay aging.

Animal research bears this out: Rats that are deprived of chromium have shorter life spans, while rats that are supplemented with chromium picolinate live 37 percent longer than they do in their natural habitat.

The rats that have longer life spans because of chromium supplementation have lower blood sugar, lower insulin, and lower blood levels of hemoglobin A1c—the marker that indicates good diabetic control and normal aging. Once again, supplemental chromium enhances insulin sensitivity, and by doing that, it helps maintain more youthful cell performance.

Supplemental Chromium— A Bit Like Caloric Restriction

The effect of supplemental chromium is very similar to that of caloric restriction on aging. To explain, researchers have known since the 1930s that restricting an animal's lifelong caloric intake by one-third extends its life span by one-third. Eating less protects against diabetes—and it also slows the aging process.

Currently, researchers at the University of Wisconsin, Madison, are applying caloric restriction to monkeys (not just rodents). Monkeys are biologically very similar to humans. While this experiment is still in progress, the researchers have reported that the calorie-restricted monkeys are showing no signs of type II diabetes and are acting, in effect, like young monkeys. In contrast, monkeys that are allowed to eat as much as they want—as many people do—are developing the early signs of diabetes.

Now, you're probably asking, what does caloric restriction have to do with chromium? The answer is simple. If you would like to add a few years to your life, would you prefer to do it by cutting your calorie intake by one-third and always being a little hungry, or would you prefer to eat a normal calorie intake (that is, not overeat) and just take some chromium supplements?

Chromium can complement the beneficial effects of a lower-carbohydrate, lower-sugar diet to delay aging and likely add years to your life. Not only that, it will probably help you feel younger during those extra years.

Supplemental Chromium Raises DHEA Levels

Hormones have a powerful effect on body function, and chromium supplementation helps in a key way to keep our bodies hormonally younger: It helps increase the body's production of dehydroepiandrosterone (DHEA). One study found that after taking chromium supplements for a month, the DHEA levels of postmenopausal women increased to levels that would be typical of thirty- to thirty-five-year-old women.

DHEA
A key hormone in the body that promotes youthful body function. Its production is suppressed when insulin levels are high.

This is significant because DHEA levels are perhaps the most telling of all the markers for aging. People with higher DHEA levels live longer and feel better: they have a greater sense of overall well-being and a better ability to deal with emotional and physical stress.

On the other hand, the lower people's DHEA levels are, the more likely they are to develop degenerative diseases of accelerated aging, including hardening of the arteries, diabetes, cancer, osteoporosis, and lowered immunity. In addition, they're more likely to die from an age-related disease. For example, one 1986 *New England Journal of Medicine* study found that men with low DHEA levels were 3.3 times more likely to die of heart disease than those with normal levels.

Your body's levels of DHEA peak when you're in your twenties. After that, the amount of DHEA you produce declines at the rate of about 2 percent a year. By the time you're forty, you make only about half the DHEA you did at age twenty, and at age sixty-five, your level is only 10 to 20 percent of what it was at its peak.

Insulin, more than anything else, will suppress your natural DHEA production. Keeping insulin levels low—by following a lower-carbohydrate diet and taking chromium supplements—is one of the best ways to maintain a high DHEA level. If you do that, you keep the intricate network of hormones in your body functioning in a more youthful way.

The Hormone Connection to Aging

With the main exception of insulin (which can rise if we eat the wrong foods and don't take our chromium supple-

ments), levels of virtually every other hormone in our bodies decline as we age. Hormones regulate every aspect of our bodies' functions, from metabolism to body temperature to sex drive. When levels of most hormones decline, youthful body function declines, too. When levels of those same hormones stay higher, the body functions as if it were younger.

Hormones
Regulatory substances produced by the endocrine glands that control numerous functions in the body.

Made by the adrenal glands, DHEA is the precursor or source for other adrenal hormones, including the stress hormone cortisol, and all the sex hormones, such as estrogen, progesterone, and testosterone. It's often called the "mother" hormone for this very reason.

Clearly, if your body's production of DHEA declines, the cascade of hormone production that follows will be seriously disrupted, too. A steady drop in your hormone levels ushers in older body function and symptoms of aging, such as decreased resistance to infection, brittle bones, loss of muscle mass and tone, diminished libido, lower stamina, and trouble with short-term memory.

A drop in hormone production and a decline in mental and physical function are considered a natural part of aging, but you can do a lot to slow this process. If you maintain high DHEA levels—or raise DHEA levels if they're low—you automatically help your body improve its production of numerous hormones that keep it functioning more youthfully. You may feel decades younger and people may say you look and act decades younger than your chronological age.

Of course, many people today take DHEA supplements for this very reason, but DHEA supplements really shouldn't be taken without the supervision of a doctor. If too much DHEA is taken, it can throw off the whole intricate web of hormone function in the body, sometimes causing side effects, such as acne and excessive growth of facial hair in women. The far safer route to improve DHEA levels and feel better is to do it the natural way by taking chromium supplements, eating a lower-carbohydrate diet, and reducing stress.

Chromium Gets to the Roots of Aging

A lot of information has been covered in this section, but it boils down to this: an excess of free radicals and advanced glycation end-products, rising blood pressure, and diminishing levels of DHEA and other hormones all have been implicated in the aging process. Chromium positively influences all of these factors because it improves insulin sensitivity and lowers blood sugar and insulin levels.

Chromium supplementation extends the lifespan of rats, and all evidence suggests that it can do the same for us. Our modern lifestyle promotes high blood sugar and insulin levels, which are at the root of aging. Supplemental chromium can make a major dent in combating those roots. When combined with a lower-carbohydrate diet, some antioxidant supplements (which you'll learn more about later), physical activity, and stress reduction, taking chromium supplements is the closest thing we've found to a natural fountain of youth.

A Natural Remedy for Depression and Premenstrual Syndrome

Chromium normalizes blood sugar, and people with minor and major blood sugar disturbances often report increased mental focus and steadier moods from chromium supplementation. Recently, though, supplemental chromium has shown promising results in an exciting new area: the treatment of depression and premenstrual syndrome.

There are many different varieties and underlying causes of depression and premenstrual syndrome. Supplemental chromium isn't a panacea for all types of these conditions, but it has been found to be helpful for several types, both when used alone and when used with antidepressant drugs.

Basics about Depression

Depression has sometimes been described as "the common cold of mental illness." At any time, 13 to 20 percent of us have at least some degree of it.

Major depression and dysthymia—the two main classifications of depression—differ according to how chronic, severe, and long lasting they are. Major depression, which isn't too common, is characterized by a sharp contrast to usual functioning. A happy person can go along with his normal life and then, over a period of several days or weeks, can rapidly develop severe symptoms of depression. Dysthymia, on the other hand, is a chronic depression of low to moderate severity that lasts many months or years. It can hang like a pall over people's lives for years and years, eroding confidence and initiative and greatly diminishing joys and pleasures that are experienced.

Whether major or minor or some other type, depression can also be described by its features or symptoms. For example, some depressions involve biological or environmental triggers. These include premenstrual, postnatal, and menopausal depressions and seasonal affective disorder, or SAD (winter depression).

Atypical features, another classifier or subtype, involve mood reactivity and at least two of the following: increased appetite and/or weight gain, unexplained profound tiredness and exhaustion, too much sleep, and excessive sensitivity to rejection. Percentage-wise, this cluster of symptoms is the largest subtype of depression.

The Disadvantages of Antidepressant Drugs

Several different types of drugs are used in treating the various forms of depression, but each one has troublesome side effects. Tricyclic antidepressants, for example, often cause lethargy and lead to weight gain. Selective serotonin reuptake inhibitors (SSRIs), a popular group of antidepressants including Prozac and Zoloft, can cause fuzzy thinking, nausea, diarrhea, headache, and sexual side effects. Some physicians have even attributed an increased incidence of suicide or violence in people who take certain SSRIs.

Monoamine oxidase inhibitors (MAOIs) are so problematic that most psychiatrists no longer recommend them. The use of these drugs requires a number of strict dietary restrictions and special precautions (such as avoiding certain other drugs). If these precautions aren't followed, patients can develop a dangerous side effect—a severe hypertensive crisis. People who take MAOIs are instructed to carry an antidote and rush to the nearest emergency room if a severe, throbbing headache develops.

Clearly, natural treatments that work well for depression but don't have adverse side effects are desirable to many of the standard antidepressant drug treatments. Supplemental chromium appears to be one such natural treatment: It's been found to both boost the action of SSRI antidepressants and act as an antidepressant in its own right.

The Fascinating Way Chromium's Effects Were Discovered

The discovery of chromium's beneficial effects on depression began in a serendipitous way. One day, a longtime depressed patient of Malcolm McLeod, M.D., of Chapel Hill, North Carolina, told the psychiatrist that he had experienced dramatic improvements in his condition after taking a multivitamin and mineral supplement. McLeod was skeptical of supplements, so he subjected the patient's pills to scientific scrutiny.

After studying the supplement label, McLeod asked his patient to stop taking the supplement and participate in an experiment. McLeod gave the patient only one of the supplement's individual ingredients for an entire week; then he switched to a different individual ingredient the next week. The patient didn't know which of the individual supplements he was taking.

During the first, third, fourth, and fifth weeks of the experiment, the patient didn't feel any improvement and, in some cases, felt worse. During the second week, however, he felt a dramatic and immediate relief in his depression, along with other beneficial health effects, such as a decrease in appetite and an increase in energy.

At the end of the fifth week, the patient insisted on knowing what he took during the second week. He was told it was chromium picolinate. On his own initiative, the patient began to take 400 mcg of chromium daily from chromium picolinate. His sleep improved, his thinking became clearer, he lost his cravings for food and alcohol, and he became hopeful about the future. His depression cleared so completely that he eventually stopped taking the SSRI drug he had been taking.

McLeod's Discovery of Chromium's Beneficial Effects in Others

Amazed by the effects supplemental chromium had on this one patient, McLeod tried the experiment on several more patients with different symptoms. He got similar results. The difference in some of his patients after taking chromium supplements was so dramatic that McLeod had no choice but to believe he was on to something.

He applied for patents on the use of chromium for treating depression and premenstrual syndrome (PMS). He also published the results of his experiment in the April 1999 issue of the *Journal of Clinical Psychiatry*.

Then he began hearing from other psychiatrists—from around the United States and even from Australia and Sweden—who had witnessed similar positive effects from supplemental chromium in their practices. They told him that in some cases, supplemental chromium was life transforming for several of their patients.

McLeod also oversaw two more studies that found chromium supplementation helpful for many types of depression—as well as for premenstrual syndrome. And other researchers at the University of North Carolina and Duke University are now following up on his work: they're currently conducting studies of their own to try to verify his findings.

Chromium's Antidepressant Action

McLeod's first scientific paper—the write-up of his initial experiments—showed that chromium supplementation led to remission of longstanding, minor to moderate depression (dysthymia) in patients who were taking SSRI drugs. The SSRIs by themselves didn't eradicate these patients' depression, but when the patients took chromium supplements along with the SSRIs, their depression dramatically lifted and so did the side effects, such as fuzzy thinking, that they were having from taking the SSRIs.

Chromium supplementation, therefore, potentiated the action of the antidepressants and reduced the side effects of antidepressants. McLeod at first thought that's all chromium did. However, experiments with other patients confirmed that chromium supplementation all by itself acts as an antidepressant and is sometimes all that is needed to eradicate depression.

A few examples: one patient who had bipolar disorder and major depression had developed unacceptable side effects from several antidepressants. Lithium treatment caused a feeling of being slowed down and a thirty-pound weight gain. After starting to take chromium supplements,

the patient was able to stop taking lithium and continue with chromium alone. He felt increasingly relaxed and stable and gradually lost twenty-three pounds. Other patients who couldn't take antidepressant drugs because of undesirable side effects, such as loss of interest in sex, had their depression completely go away when they took chromium supplements.

How Chromium Might Work

Based on clinical evidence, McLeod and his colleagues at the University of North Carolina department of psychiatry have a few ideas about how chromium might work in the body to alleviate depression. As a potentiator of insulin, chromium allows blood sugar to enter brain cells more easily. Blood sugar is a primary fuel the brain needs to make chemical messengers that regulate mood and help us think clearly.

Chromium may also help facilitate the entry of tryptophan, an amino acid, into the brain. Tryptophan serves as an essential building block for chemical messengers, such as serotonin, which regulate mood, emotions, sleep, and appetite. Low levels of serotonin or dysfunctions of serotonin activity are associated with depression. Chromium may also enhance the release of stored chemical messengers, such as norepinephrine, that help promote normal mood functioning.

Serotonin
A neurotransmitter that regulates mood, emotions, sleep, and appetite. Disorders of serotonin activity are thought to be involved in depression.

It's interesting to note that depression is often associated with insulin resistance and poor utilization of blood sugar. Several studies show that type II diabetics are at increased risk for depression. Chromium of course improves insulin sensitivity and helps reverse type II diabetes—and many type II diabetics who take chromium supplements often report improvements in mood. By improving insulin sensitivity, chromium probably facilitates serotonin activity in the brain, thereby exerting some antidepressant effects.

The Type of Depression Chromium Seems to Help

Depression is a complex disorder; it should be emphasized that chromium isn't a cure-all for all types of depression. However, the more McLeod investigates the effect of chromium supplementation on depression, the more he suspects that it's helpful for people who have what psychiatrists call "depression with atypical features." These features, you'll recall, include cravings for sugar and carbohydrates, weight problems, lethargy, excess sleepiness, and excessive sensitivity to rejection by others.

The term "atypical" is something of a misnomer because about 40 percent of depressed people have these features. People with atypical symptoms usually don't receive effective treatment. They typically don't respond to common antidepressants, and MAIOs, which have been used as a treatment, have such dangerous side effects that most doctors don't want to use them.

The good news is chromium supplementation seems to be particularly helpful for treating people with this subtype of depression. However, some depressed people without atypical symptoms also have responded to chromium supplements. Researchers need more time and study to determine all the different types of depressed people who respond favorably to chromium supplementation.

> **Atypical Features**
>
> *A term that classifies depression with symptoms including sugar cravings, overweight, lethargy, sleepiness, and sensitivity to rejection.*

Chromium Is Also Helpful for PMS and Painful Periods

Some of McLeod's depressed female patients also suffered from premenstrual syndrome—characterized by such symptoms as mood swings, increased irritability or anxiety, carbohydrate cravings, overeating, marked lack of energy, and sleep disturbances during the last week or several days before menstrual periods. Other female patients had painful periods with menstrual cramps. Upon receiving chromium supplements, their PMS symptoms and painful periods were alleviated.

In some women with severe PMS, chromium taken in combination with standard SSRI antidepressants totally eradicated their symptoms. In other women, chromium alone was all that was needed.

Most of these experiments were done under single-blind conditions—when the doctor knows what the patient is taking but the patient does not. However, one small pilot study that involved six women was a double-blind, placebo-controlled study—in other words, neither the doctor nor the patient knew what the patient was taking. This study found similar results: chromium augments the effects of standard antidepressants when needed. Some women got such marked relief that they made comments like "Without a doubt, that's the easiest period I've had in years" and "When my period started, I was completely surprised. I had none of the usual, difficult warning symptoms."

Chromium Might Alleviate Seasonal Blues

Some of McLeod's patients with seasonal affective disorder (SAD) also have been helped by chromium supplementation. Technically, SAD can mean recurrent mood swings during a particular season. However, it most often refers to recurrent depression during the fall and winter, when the daylight hours are shorter. Symptoms of this type of SAD include depressed mood, difficulty concentrating, excess sleep, decreased energy, increased appetite, and carbohy-

drate cravings—symptoms very much like those in depression with atypical features.

Recent research has found that mood swings during the winter months are common in healthy people. These people don't technically have SAD, but they feel slightly down, sadder, more irritable, or worry more during winter than they do during other times of year.

Simple treatments—such as getting more sun exposure, increasing physical activity, and making dietary changes—have been recommended for the seasonal blues. Taking chromium supplements seems like another good strategy because it has already proven helpful for some people with SAD.

I believe another reason for the winter blues is that many people eat more chromium-depleting sugar and refined grains during the winter holidays, especially from Halloween through New Year's Day. An increase in the intake of refined carbohydrates lowers chromium levels, probably inducing chromium deficiencies and subsequent winter blues in many people, escalating their need for chromium supplements.

Common Threads in Disorders Helped by Chromium

It may seem unbelievable that chromium could be effective for so many different mood disorders—depression, premenstrual syndrome, and winter blues. But researchers have noted that these disorders often share common symptoms—such as carbohydrate cravings and lethargy.

In addition, all of these disorders have responded to antidepressant medicines that increase serotonin levels in the brain. This suggests that these disorders are closely related and are associated with low serotonin levels. Since chromium improves insulin sensitivity and probably, as a result, increases serotonin levels in the brain, supplemental chromium may prove to remedy a key factor in these mood disorders.

Chromium Is Worth Trying for Depression and PMS

Supplemental chromium is probably worth a try if a person has any of these disorders and hasn't responded to other treatments. Chromium is a very safe supplement; most people are lacking in chromium and can benefit from taking supplements.

There have been few side effects reported in studies with depressed people, and those that have occurred have been mild. Some people report having vivid dreams (but not nightmares)—an effect that usually subsides after a few weeks.

Some people also report that if chromium is taken too late in the day, it may interfere with falling asleep. This effect can be counteracted by simply taking chromium earlier in the day, at least eight hours before bedtime. When taken early in the day, chromium tends to have an energizing effect for the first six hours or so and then seems to regulate sleep and reduce insomnia, according to McLeod.

Chromium doesn't seem to negatively interact with any medications. But chromium taken with excessive amounts of caffeine may cause some people to feel wired, so this combination is best avoided. Also, for reasons that aren't understood, a few patients who have taken chromium while also taking the popular antidepressant herb, St. John's wort, found that the combination worsened their depression and PMS. Therefore, it's probably best not to take chromium and St. John's wort at the same.

Chromium can make SSRI medications more effective and reduce the side effects they cause. If you currently take an SSRI or any other psychiatric drug and want to try chromium supplements, it's best to talk with your healthcare provider.

Chromium—A Natural Antidepressant

Chromium is an essential nutrient our bodies need on a daily basis to maintain blood sugar balance and insulin sensitivity. By boosting these actions, supplemental chromium acts as a natural antidepressant.

Consider that chromium supplements act faster than antidepressants, usually showing beneficial effects within a few days, rather than at least a month for antidepressants. Chromium supplements also have no serious side effects and are 20 to 50 times less expensive than antidepressant drugs. Considering all the evidence so far, chromium supplements probably should be the first choice for the treatment of mood disorders, before antidepressant drugs.

OTHER BENEFITS AND AREAS FOR FUTURE RESEARCH

Chromium's beneficial effects on diabetes, Syndrome X, cholesterol problems, overweight, aging, depression, and PMS are very impressive. But this mineral has even more benefits, as well as potential benefits yet to be researched. For starters, supplemental chromium helps prevent osteoporosis. There's also evidence to suggest that chromium may be helpful for conditions as varied as acne, alcoholism, bulimia, nearsighted vision, and a common cause of female infertility. This section will fill you in on all the latest thinking of future areas of research for chromium supplementation.

Chromium Improves DHEA Levels and Helps Prevent Osteoporosis

In 1996, the results of an innovative study led by Gary Evans, Ph.D., was published in the *FASEB Journal*. Unfortunately,

as is often the case, health writers and researchers missed the boat on how significant this research actually was.

At the time, it was known that insulin resistance interfered with calcium absorption into bone and led to high insulin levels, which markedly reduce the production of the antiaging, feel-good hormone DHEA. Evans also learned that postmenopausal women who had high insulin levels had low levels of DHEA. He wondered if chromium supplementation would reduce insulin levels and raise DHEA levels and therefore improve bone health in these women.

To put this idea to a test, Evans had twenty-seven postmenopausal women, ages fifty-two to sixty-three, take two capsules per day that contained either a placebo or 200 mcg of chromium as chromium picolinate for two months. For three months after that, no supplement was given; then the women were given the opposite supplement. The results that occurred during the period of chromium supplementation were impressive. Blood insulin levels dropped 38 percent, blood sugar levels decreased 26 percent, and DHEA levels increased 24 percent. In addition, the amount of calcium the women excreted decreased by half, and two key indicators of bone breakdown—the urinary hydroxyproline/creatinine ratio and the urinary calcium/creatinine ratio—decreased by about 20 percent.

This study showed that supplementing with chromium picolinate can go a long way toward preventing osteoporosis, especially in people who have insulin resistance—in other words, most people who are overweight, people who have Syndrome X or type II diabetes, and one-quarter of the thin population. Essentially, efficient insulin activity builds bone; inefficient insulin activity breaks down bone.

Osteoporosis *A condition of reduced bone density and increased bone brittleness that can lead to bones that break easily.*

Chromium Boosts Postmenopausal Women's Estrogen Levels

Another key finding of this study was after taking chromium supplements for one month, the postmenopausal women's estrogen (estradiol) and DHEA (which can be converted to estrogen and other sex hormones) increased to levels resembling those of women in their thirties. Chromium supplements, therefore, can turn back the hormonal clock, perhaps delaying menopause and possibly reducing the adverse symptoms caused by the dramatic loss of hormones that typically occurs during menopause.

Osteoporosis and difficult menopauses are treated with estrogen by many doctors. However, estrogen is not an ideal treatment because it has been shown to increase the risk of certain types of cancer. This study suggested there is a natural way to increase estrogen levels in the body without actually taking estrogen: that is, to take chromium supplements. It seems that when insulin is functioning efficiently in the body, it keeps other hormones functioning more efficiently, too. Controlling insulin levels seems to be an effective way to hold back, delay, or improve age-related conditions, including osteoporosis and menopause.

The Chromium Connection to Alcoholism and Bulimia

In the last section, you learned that depression, premenstrual syndrome, and seasonal affective disorder all share a common link: low levels of serotonin or inefficient serotonin activity in the brain. Two other disorders, alcoholism and bulimia nervosa (bulimia, for short) share that same link. Chromium supplementation seems to enhance serotonin activity in the brain, and there's evidence to suggest that it may be helpful as an aid in the treatment of alcoholism and bulimia, just as it is for depression, premenstrual syndrome, and seasonal affective disorder.

Alcoholism is characterized by a tendency to drink excessively, unsuccessful attempts at stopping drinking, and continuing to drink despite adverse social, occupational, and health consequences. Bulimia is characterized by repeated episodes of binge eating (usually of sweets and grain-based foods), followed by purging (self-induced vomiting or taking laxatives or diuretics), or excessive exercise to counteract the effects of bingeing. Like alcoholics, bulimics have trouble stopping their behavior even when they understand that it is unhealthy for them.

Uncontrollable cravings (for alcohol or carbohydrates, probably stemming from disordered serotonin metabolism) seem to drive people to drink or eat excessively. Chromium supplementation diminishes cravings for sweets and carbohydrates, and it was reported to diminish cravings for alcohol in some of McLeod's depressed patients with frequent alcohol cravings. One of McLeod's patients who benefited had a family history of alcoholism.

Nutritionally oriented physicians have long believed that blood sugar imbalances lie at the core of alcoholism. Chromium, which acts as a blood sugar regulator, should therefore be helpful. My limited experience counseling people with bulimia leads me to believe that chromium is helpful for some of them, too.

A Success Story of One Woman Overcoming Bulimia

One of my clients—I'll call her Hope—had bulimia, depression, and Syndrome X (with high cholesterol, high triglycerides, and abdominal obesity). She was taking an SSRI antidepressant for the bulimia and depression, but it didn't seem to help much. Hope typically made herself vomit twice a day, even though she knew she shouldn't. She contacted me because she knew I specialized in the nutritional treatment of Syndrome X.

The standard nutrition-oriented approach would be to ignore the fact that she had Syndrome X and treat her eating disorder first. But I got the sense that disturbed blood sugar metabolism was at the crux of her problems. It seemed to cause her nearly uncontrollable cravings for carbohydrates, which prompted her to binge on carbohydrates, which in turn led her to induce vomiting because she felt so uncomfortably full.

I put her on an Anti-X program, which included a sugar-free, grain-free diet and a number of supplements, including chromium. It worked like a charm: she stopped bingeing, so she stopped purging, and conquered her longstanding battle with bulimia. She also felt brighter spirited and gradually started to lose weight and have her cholesterol and triglyceride levels come down.

It's hard to say whether it was the diet, the chromium supplements, or some of the other supplements (such as liquid zinc sulfate) that worked so effectively. I believe the whole program worked together to improve her inefficient insulin sensitivity and the numerous conditions that stemmed from that.

However, Hope is certain that chromium played an important role. A few times she forgot to take her chromium supplements and her cravings for carbohydrates came back with a vengeance, making it much more difficult for her to stay on her nutrition program.

Both bulimia and alcoholism are complex mind-body disorders with numerous factors that are probably involved. The story of Hope is not meant to indicate that chromium supplementation is effective for all cases of bulimia—only that it has proven tremendously helpful in some cases. The clinical and theoretical evidence suggesting beneficial effects from chromium supplementation for bulimia and alcoholism is so intriguing that both conditions should be future areas of research.

The Growing List of Conditions Associated with High Insulin

You've learned that insulin resistance and high insulin levels can lead to the development of type II diabetes and cardiovascular disease, two of the most common diseases of aging. You also learned that high insulin levels accelerate aging all throughout the body.

It shouldn't be surprising, then, that high insulin levels are associated with other diseases of aging. Several studies have established insulin resistance and high insulin levels as factors in cognitive disorders, impaired thinking processes, dementia, and even Alzheimer's disease. There is also substantial evidence that elevated levels of insulin increase the risk of breast, prostate, and colorectal cancers. Consider that type II diabetics have an increased risk of developing all three cancers.

The list of insulin-related disorders and disease processes keeps growing. Colorado State University health science researcher Loren Cordain, Ph.D., for example, has recently explained that the high insulin levels that go hand in hand with insulin resistance cause a cascade of hormonal shifts that favor unregulated cell growth in a variety of tissues. This unregulated cell growth may lead not only to breast, prostate, and colon cancers, but also to—believe it or not—acne, nearsightedness, and a female-specific condition called polycystic ovary syndrome. Reversing insulin resistance and reducing high insulin levels should nip these problems in the bud. Chromium supplementation, as you've learned, reverses insulin resistance and lowers insulin levels.

At first, the idea of chromium helping these varied conditions may seem farfetched. The insulin connection to these conditions is so new that, unfortunately, no research evaluating the effectiveness of chromium supplementation in these conditions has been conducted. But clinical and theoretical evidence suggests therapeutic value from supplemental chromium, so future studies are warranted.

The Chromium Connection to Acne

As early as 1940, research suggested that acne is a result of impaired sugar metabolism or insulin resistance of the skin. To measure the ability of the body to handle sugar, glucose tolerance tests have been performed on acne patients. Blood sugar levels during glucose tolerance tests seem to be normal in acne patients, but repetitive skin biopsies reveal their skin's glucose tolerance is significantly impaired. Considering this evidence, one researcher coined the term "skin diabetes" to describe the disorder of acne.

Chromium regulates blood sugar levels and improves insulin sensitivity. Insulin promotes the uptake of blood sugar by the cells, including skin cells. When insulin is functioning efficiently, improved glucose tolerance results throughout the body, including the skin.

As another line of thinking, consider that teenaged boys who eat many junk foods and drink a lot of soft drinks are the group of people most likely to develop acne. Sweets and white-flour products, such as pizza, pasta, and bread, are deficient in chromium, and soft drinks are totally void of chromium. Furthermore, sweets, white-flour products, and soft drinks promote losses of chromium from the body. It's very possible that low chromium levels are a factor in the development of acne.

In one study from nearly twenty years ago, high-chromium yeast was reported to produce rapid improvements in acne patients. Unfortunately, no one has followed up on that research yet. Nevertheless, most Americans (and teenagers in particular) are lacking chromium in their diets, so chromium supplementation, together with avoiding sugar and refined grains, seems like a worthwhile nutrition strategy.

High-chromium yeast can be problematic, so I would recommend a better-tolerated source of chromium, such as chromium picolinate. Many people have hidden yeast sensitivities or a tendency to develop yeast infections and do best avoiding daily supplements of yeast.

The Chromium Connection to Nearsightedness

The idea that chromium supplementation might help prevent or delay the development of nearsightedness may seem harder to believe than anything else discussed here. However, keep in mind that research over the last decade or so has proven that optimal levels of nutrients are critical for protecting eye health and vision.

Nearsightedness *Difficulty seeing things at a distance. Poor nutrition, including lack of chromium, plays a role in its development.*

First, some basics: Nearsightedness may be partly genetic in origin, but it is also attributed to the extra strain industrialized people put on their eyes by constantly reading or performing near-visual tasks during the growing years. Poor nutrition, especially a high intake of chromium-depleting refined carbohydrates, plays a contributing role.

Benjamin Lane, O.D., C.N.S., an optometrist, nutritionist, and researcher from Lake Hiawatha, New Jersey, discovered the chromium connection to nearsightedness in the early 1980s. He evaluated the results of 120 consecutive nutrition workups from his files and reported his results in the *Journal of the International Academy of Preventive Medicine:* Chromium deficiency is strongly tied to the development and progression of nearsightedness.

Chromium is needed for the proper function of all muscles, but the muscles that we use more today than ever before are the ciliary muscles, the muscles that help the eyes focus so we can read. If there isn't enough chromium in our bloodstream, then long, sustained eye focusing cannot be maintained.

Many children eat tremendous amounts of chromium-depleting sugar and white-flour products, but they don't develop nearsightedness until their chromium reserves run out. As soon as they lose their chromium reserves, they rapidly develop nearsightedness under that stress of eye focusing, according to Lane.

Avoiding chromium-depleting, blood–sugar-raising, refined carbohydrates is one of the best nutritional strategies to try to prevent the development or progression of nearsightedness. But many people continue to eat these foods. In addition, Lane believes some people have inborn chromium deficiency. So, chromium supplementation may be needed for extra protection against nearsightedness. With our society doing more near-visual work than ever before, this is an important area for future research.

Polycystic Ovary Syndrome— A Newly Recognized Condition

Polycystic ovary syndrome (PCOS) is a newly recognized

condition associated with insulin resistance and high insulin levels. It's characterized by symptoms such as ovarian cysts, irregular menstrual periods, elevated levels of male sex hormones such as testosterone, excess facial hair, acne, and often obesity. The most common cause of infertility among women in the United States, this disorder involves a woman's eggs maturing in the ovary but not being released.

Polycystic Ovary Syndrome
An insulin-related condition that affects females, causing ovarian cysts, irregular menstrual periods, excess facial hair, and sometimes infertility.

Studies have shown that high insulin levels stimulate the production of male sex hormones by the ovaries and may impede ovulation and contribute to infertility. High levels of insulin, as you may recall, affect the balance of other hormones in the body.

Like Syndrome X, PCOS increases the risk of other serious diseases associated with insulin resistance, such as type II diabetes. Virtually no nutritional research has been done on this condition, but improving insulin sensitivity has become established as a baseline treatment strategy in PCOS. In addition, improvements in PCOS have been reported by some women who have followed an Anti-X-type program that included chromium supplementation. Since chromium supplementation has fewer side effects than insulin-sensitizing drugs, its effectiveness in PCOS should be pursued in clinical trials.

Other Insulin-Related Conditions

There are several lines of research to suggest that sleep apnea and some types of iron overload may result from, or be aggravated by, insulin resistance and high insulin levels—and may, therefore, benefit from chromium supplementation.

Sleep apnea is a potentially fatal disorder of a breathing disruption during sleep. Loud snoring, gasping sounds, and disordered breathing during sleep are common symptoms. People who have abdominal obesity and type II diabetes are most apt to develop this problem. I have not had any clients diagnosed with sleep apnea, but I have had a number of Syndrome X clients who have reported that their snoring dramatically decreased after following an Anti-X program. McLeod has also reported that chromium supplementation can improve sleep disturbances. Since sleep apnea is such a serious disorder, investigating whether chromium supplementation could improve this condition seems like an area worth pursuing.

Iron overload is a storage of excess iron in organs such as the liver. There is hereditary iron overload (called hereditary hemachromatosis), and there is also insulin–resistance-associated iron overload. In one study, 94 percent of people with unexplained iron overload in the liver had Syndrome X. The standard treatment for both types of iron overload is to have blood drawn regularly to reduce iron levels in the body. However, chromium supplementation may also be helpful. Many people with iron overload have reduced insulin sensitivity, and iron is antagonistic to chromium. Excess iron, therefore, may be displacing chromium, causing chromium deficiency; so supplemental chromium (in addition to blood draws) may be therapeutic.

The web of diseases and abnormalities associated with insulin resistance and high insulin levels seems to be far reaching and complex. Researchers will likely be investigating all the insulin connections to various ailments for decades. In the meantime, before all the research is conducted, you should become savvy to protect your health. If you learn that poor insulin function may be involved in the development of a condition you have or are prone to, think about supplemental chromium as a possible remedy that may be helpful.

HOW TO BUY AND USE CHROMIUM

By now, you've read about the impressive health benefits of chromium and learned that taking chromium supplements is one of the best things you can do to protect yourself from the blood–sugar- and insulin-related health problems that run rampant in our society. You're probably ready to learn more about how to supplement with chromium. This section will answer what you need to know about chromium supplements, so you can make the most educated decisions about to how to use chromium for your best health.

Who Should Take Chromium Supplements?

From my experience counseling clients, virtually everyone can benefit from supplemental chromium. Most Americans have grown up on a diet containing chromium-depleting sugar and white-flour products, which gradually leads to at least marginal chromium deficiencies. This is why blood sugar highs and lows and conditions such as overweight, Syndrome X, and type II diabetes are so common today.

The best way to know if you need chromium supplements is to consult a nutritionist or nutrition-oriented health professional who can evaluate your individual intake, needs, and symptoms. The second best way is the try-it-and-see approach: Try chromium supplements for a month or two and see if you experience beneficial effects on your health. Look for improvements in energy, mood, weight control, sugar cravings, or heart disease risk factors. The more you need chromium, the more you'll respond to supplementation. Some people with depression respond within a day or two.

Even if you are healthy (not overweight and not at risk for

diabetes or heart disease), a small dose of supplemental chromium—say, 100–200 mcg—is recommended to insure that you meet your daily needs. As you'll remember, 90 percent of Americans don't meet the minimum suggested safe and adequate daily intake for chromium of 50 mcg. Over the long run, this puts people at risk for many health problems. Fortunately, a deficiency can be prevented with daily chromium supplements.

The Different Forms of Chromium Supplements

There are many different types of chromium supplements. Most people don't have any idea which one they should choose. The terms can get a bit confusing, so here are the basics:

GTF refers to glucose tolerance factor, the term originally given to an active form of chromium that researchers found affected blood sugar control. This active form of chromium was isolated from yeast and was better utilized by animals than chromium chloride, one of the earliest chromium compounds—an inorganic compound of chromium combined with chloride. The active form isolated from yeast is sometimes called yeast GTF.

Some researchers proposed a possible composition for GTF, but it was never shown that this specific composition existed. While GTF is sometimes still found in supplements, the term GTF is outdated and not used by many researchers today.

Chromium polynicotinate, a type of chromium supplement now out on the market, is a mixture of nicotinate (a form of vitamin B_3) and chromium combined with water. There's been a lot of hype about this form, but it has not proven to be absorbed well by the body.

Several organic compounds of chromium (compounds that contain carbon) are on the market. The different forms are compounds of chromium combined or chelated with various amino acids or organic acids in an effort to facilitate chromium absorption. To give you a few examples, chromium picolinate is chromium combined or chelated with picolinic acid; chromium arginate is chromium combined with arginine; chromium aspartate is chromium combined with aspartic acid; and chromium citrite is chromium combined with citric acid. Most of these forms, other than chromium picolinate, have not been extensively studied.

Chelator
A chemical or carrier protein that combines with a mineral and aids in moving it into the bloodstream and throughout the body.

Speaking a bit more scientifically, the minerals we need in our bodies are electrically charged. They have to be de-energized before they can approach and enter the body's cells. This can be done if they're attached to special chemical substances called chelators. Gary Evans, Ph.D., a USDA researcher, discovered picolinate to be a superior chelator and showed that it very effectively cloaks the charge of

chromium so it can be carried by the blood to the cells that need it. Chromium picolinate is the most researched form of chromium. Numerous studies have found it's the best absorbed and best utilized form of chromium on the market.

The Safety of Chromium Supplements

If you're concerned about the safety of taking chromium, don't be. Nutritional chromium, the form of chromium found in foods and nutritional supplements, is considered one of the safest mineral nutrients. In animal experiments, chromium has demonstrated a lack of toxicity at extremely high levels—levels several thousand times the estimated safe and adequate daily dietary intake (ESADDI) limit of 200 mcg per day. There is no evidence of toxic effects or widespread health problems related to chromium supplementation in humans or in animals.

Unfortunately, in 1995, a controversial study was conducted, and some people got the idea that chromium picolinate could cause cancer. In the study, chromium picolinate caused chromosome damage in hamster ovarian cells in test-tube experiments. This result wasn't particularly surprising: the amount of chromium that was applied directly to these cells was 3,000 times the blood level of people who take chromium picolinate supplements. Very few essential minerals tested in this way would pass.

The standard test for determining whether chemicals cause cancer is the Ames test—an experiment in which a chemical is added to five different types of bacteria that reproduce rapidly and show adverse changes in their offspring. Chromium picolinate has been independently tested using the Ames test and has passed with flying colors.

The real test is not so much what happens in test-tube experiments but what happens in human and animal experiments. Chromium picolinate has been found to be extraordinarily safe in human and animal studies, and it certainly hasn't caused cancer. Its effects have been therapeutic, not toxic. As one example, remember that rats whose diets were supplemented with chromium picolinate lived 37 percent longer than rats who didn't receive supplemental chromium. Chromium supplements are safe: The far greater risk to health is not to take chromium supplements than to take them.

Side Effects from Chromium Are Rare

Most people do not experience any side effects from taking chromium. The side effects that have been reported have been few and minor, such as slight rashes or dizziness. If you experience symptoms such as these, try switching to a different form of chromium. Several of McLeod's depressed patients experienced dizzy spells while taking chromium polynicotinate but didn't have this symptom when they took chromium picolinate.

A few other side effects that McLeod has noticed from his research are increased and vivid dreaming after beginning chromium supplementation (which usually subsides after a few weeks) and a tendency to have trouble falling asleep if chromium is taken too close to bedtime. Trouble falling asleep can easily be avoided by taking chromium early in the day.

Also, a few people have developed headaches *after* discontinuing chromium. This symptom generally is considered to be a sign of glucose tolerance problems. When these people started taking chromium supplements again, their headaches disappeared.

Choosing a High-Quality Supplement

Choosing a chromium supplement isn't as simple as walking into a store and grabbing any supplement that says chromium. To get the most value for the money you spend, there are several tricks of the trade.

First, avoid brand-name supplements sold in drugstores and supermarkets, and look instead for one of the quality brands sold in health food stores and natural food supermarkets. Commercial brands often contain artificial colors (for example, blue, red, or yellow dyes), hidden forms of sugar (for example, maltodextrin), mineral oil, and long lists of unrecognizable words that are usually unnecessary excipients, binders, and fillers. Health food brands usually don't have these ingredients: They may be slightly more expensive, but you get better value in terms of quality.

Second, when choosing between capsules and tablets, keep in mind that capsules tend to be "cleaner"—in other words, they usually have fewer undesirable fillers than tablets. I also usually recommend capsules over tablets because capsules tend to be easier for the body to break down and easier for people to swallow.

Third, read labels carefully and look for the amount of elemental, or pure, chromium a supplement supplies. Chromium comes in different forms (chromium picolinate, chromium aspartate, chromium chelate, and so on), and each one of these forms supplies a different amount of elemental chromium. The amount of chromium compound that the supplement supplies is not important, but the amount of *elemental* chromium is.

This used to be a bit confusing for consumers, but supplement labels now should list the amount of elemental chromium in a standardized way—stating, for example, "200 mcg chromium (as chromium picolinate)" or "200 mcg elemental chromium (from chromium picolinate)." Either of these two listings means that the supplement supplies 200 mcg of elemental chromium from chromium picolinate.

Another way of finding a good chromium supplement is to look for the Chromax trademark in the supplement facts label on many supplements. Chromax® chromium picolinate is the best-absorbed form, and the form that has proven most effective against insulin resistance. Therefore, it's the form that's worth seeking out.

Guidelines for How Much Chromium You Should Take

The amount of chromium a person needs depends upon age, overall health, diet, and stress and activity levels. Here are some guidelines:

- The amount of chromium considered safe and adequate for children seven years and older is 50–200 mcg. However, health conditions such as diabetes increase those needs. If you're a parent planning supplementation for a child, it's always best to discuss supplementation with a nutritionally oriented professional.

- If you're an adult, 200 mcg daily should be sufficient for the general prevention of insulin resistance and all the adverse health conditions that result from it.

- If you have reactive hypoglycemia (blood sugar lows a while after eating sweets) or if you're mildly depressed and/or slightly overweight, 400 mcg daily seems to be more therapeutic.

- If you have any one of the conditions involved in Syndrome X—obesity, hypertension, unhealthy triglyceride levels or poor cholesterol profiles—or if these conditions run in your family—try 400–800 mcg daily. It's best to split the amount you take in two to three smaller doses during the day. This amount also can be helpful if you have strong cravings for sugar.

- If you have type II diabetes, 1,000 mcg daily is recommended. This recommendation, though, comes with a caveat: if you are taking medication to control your glucose, start with 200 mcg of chromium per day for a week and monitor your glucose levels closely. Continue to increase the amount of chromium you take by 200 mcg per week until you reach 1,000 mcg, and then have your physician adjust your medication accordingly. Supplemental chromium works so well at improving insulin function that less medication to control glucose usually is needed.

Finding the Dose That's Right for You

If you have health problems, determining the dose of chromium that's best for you sometimes takes a bit of experimenting. If you have sugar cravings, for example, you'll probably find 200 mcg helpful but not near as effective at controlling your symptoms and improving your condition as 400 mcg daily. Most people can experiment with daily doses between 100–400 mcg and evaluate how they feel to determine the dose that's best for them.

If you run into trouble figuring out how much chromium

to take, or if you have a serious health problem, see a nutritionist or nutrition-oriented physician who can help you fine-tune your supplement program. A nutrition-minded health professional can evaluate your needs based on your diet, physical activity levels, symptoms, and medical history and may sometimes order hair analysis or other tests to better assess your chromium status and make recommendations of the doses that are best for you.

What Doctors Tend to Think about Chromium

Don't expect your physician to agree with your decision to take chromium or to be knowledgeable about the many ways supplemental chromium can help your health. As Nobel laureate Linus Pauling, Ph.D., once said, "If a doctor isn't 'up' on something, he's 'down' on it."

Most doctors and health educators haven't received much nutrition training and tend to dismiss nutritional treatments because they don't know much about them. Even if doctors or health educators are open to the idea of nutritional treatments, they often are so busy that they have a hard time staying up to date on the latest nutritional research.

The evidence pointing toward the use of chromium for conditions covered in this book is unmistakable (or, in the case of the conditions mentioned in the section "Other Benefits and Areas for Future Research," strongly suggestive). By reading this book, you probably know more now about chromium than your doctor does. Don't get frustrated by this. Just try to encourage your doctor to learn more. Share this book with him, pointing specifically to the scientific references in the Selected References section of this book. That way your doctor can look up the studies himself and see that the information written in this book is grounded in science. If your doctor seems unwilling to do this, switch to a doctor who is more willing to work with you or seek guidance from a nutrition-oriented health professional.

Choosing between Chromium in a Multiple and Chromium by Itself

Most multivitamin and mineral supplements contain chromium, so a natural question is whether you should take a multiple that contains chromium or a chromium supplement by itself. The answer to that question depends on your reasons for supplementing with chromium.

If you're healthy and simply want to stay healthy, taking a multivitamin/mineral that contains chromium offers good assurance that you're covering the bases of your daily needs for chromium and other essential nutrients. However, many multivitamin/ minerals that supply chromium use a form such as chromium chloride, which is the least effective type, or other types that haven't been properly researched. To get your money's worth and to make sure you're getting

chromium in its most absorbable and usable form, look for a multiple (or diabetic or sports formula) that contains chromium from chromium picolinate. To do that, you usually have to read the fine print.

If you need supplemental chromium for therapeutic reasons—say, to help reverse insulin resistance—then taking separate chromium supplements along with a multivitamin and mineral supplement or other therapeutic supplements usually works best. For the layperson who wants to keep supplements simple, I often recommend starting with something like Alpha betic once-a-day formula by Abkit. It has 200 mcg of chromium (as chromium picolinate), along with other nutrients important for insulin function, such as alpha-lipoic acid (which you'll learn about in the next section). Therefore, it's a good base supplement for people with insulin resistance, such as those who are overweight or have Syndrome X or type II diabetes. However, type II diabetics and those with Syndrome X respond best to higher doses of chromium, so they should take extra chromium supplements to reach a total of between 600 and 1,000 mcg of supplemental chromium per day.

Advantages of Having Separate Chromium Supplements

Even if you take a multiple that supplies adequate chromium, it's a good idea to have separate supplements of 200 mcg of chromium on hand to take if you occasionally indulge in a sweet or white-flour product, such as white bread or pasta. This is unconventional nutrition advice, but it works well for most of my clients (as long as it's not taken to an extreme or taken too late in the day).

As a nutritionist, I must emphasize that one of the best things you can do for your health is to steer clear of nutrient-deficient refined sugars and grains as often as possible. The more you do this, the better your health will be. However, practically speaking, many people find it difficult to avoid these foods completely (especially during special occasions). At those times, it makes sense to supplement with chromium.

When refined carbohydrates are eaten, blood sugar levels rise and the body reacts by releasing insulin into the bloodstream to stimulate the uptake of blood sugar into the tissues. What most people don't know is that the body also signals the release of an active form of chromium from sites in the liver and other areas into the bloodstream to help insulin do its job. Once chromium is done being used this way, it is lost in the urine.

Eating refined carbohydrates, therefore, is a double-whammy for maintaining optimal chromium levels: These foods are deficient in chromium, and eating these foods provokes chromium losses. For these reasons, you should try hard not to eat refined carbohydrates and should supplement with extra chromium if you do. Supplementing with chromium helps some of my clients have their cake and eat it, too, so they can enjoy special occasions without such severe nutritional consequences.

NUTRIENTS AND OTHER FACTORS THAT ENHANCE CHROMIUM'S EFFECTS

As you've learned throughout this book, supplemental chromium works well all by itself to improve many different conditions. But chromium can work even better when you combine it with other synergistic nutrients, a good diet, stress reduction, and physical activity. This section gives you a rundown of the many factors that can help you get the most effectiveness out of the chromium you take so you can enjoy better overall health.

Chromium Works Best with Other Nutrients

The health benefits of chromium are impressive, but chromium is still just one nutrient. There are more than twenty other essential nutrients we need to keep our bodies functioning optimally. We shouldn't forget about our needs for other nutrients or our health will suffer.

Nutrients always work best when they're part of a balanced or targeted program designed specifically for the individual. This section will highlight some of the other nutrients you should think about to help chromium work best for the improvement or maintenance of your health.

Vitamins C and E

As you learned earlier, high blood sugar levels generate high levels of harmful free radicals that damage and age the body. Blood–sugar-related conditions such as Syndrome X and type II diabetes are characterized by excessive levels of free radicals and low levels of protective antioxidants. That's why these conditions are associated with accelerated aging.

Chromium is a natural for improving insulin function and thereby lowering blood sugar levels. But people with Syndrome X and type II diabetes can also benefit from supplementing their diets with antioxidants to squelch the excess free radicals that are produced, which contribute to the insulin resistance disease process.

The most important antioxidants are vitamin C, the key water-soluble antioxidant in the body, and vitamin E, the key fat-soluble antioxidant. These nutrients not only work synergistically to scavenge free radicals and reduce damage and aging in the body, they also play important roles in protection against cardiovascular disease. Vitamin C and vitamin E, therefore, are important nutrients for the public at large, but they're even more important for those with Syndrome X and type II diabetes who are much more prone to developing cardiovascular disease.

Just as most people don't get adequate levels of chromium in the diet, many people also don't get adequate levels of vitamins C and E from the diet. Supplements, therefore, are recommended, particularly for people with insulin–resistance-related conditions. Individual needs vary, but 500–2,000 mg of vitamin C and 400–800 IU of natural vitamin E are prudent doses for most people.

B Vitamins

The B vitamins include B_1 (thiamine), B_2 (riboflavin), B_3 (niacin and niacinamide), pantothenic acid (vitamin B_5), B_6 (pyridoxine), B_{12}, folic acid, biotin, choline, inositol, and PABA (para-aminobenzoic acid). Each B vitamin has its own unique roles and properties, but they often work together in the body and are commonly talked about together.

As a group, B vitamins help the body burn the food we eat efficiently, thereby helping to give us energy. They're often called "the antistress vitamins," because our need for B vitamins increases dramatically during times of stress. B vitamins have a well-documented role in maintaining a healthy nervous system, which has led many practitioners to use B-complex vitamins or individual B vitamins to alleviate psychiatric symptoms such as mild depression, anxiety, and nervousness.

Multi-ingredient supplements containing chromium picolinate and specific B vitamins found synergistic in alleviating depression or anxiety may one day be developed. In the meantime, many people who are under a lot of stress can benefit from taking a B-50 or B-100 complex (which supplies 50–100 mg of most of the major B vitamins) in addition to taking chromium supplements.

Minerals

There are more than a dozen essential minerals; each has critical roles in maintaining health. After chromium, the two most important for supporting optimal insulin function are zinc and magnesium. Zinc is needed to help the pancreas produce insulin, to allow insulin to work more effectively, and to protect insulin receptors on cells. Magnesium is needed for the production and release of insulin and to maintain insulin sensitivity. Therefore, while chromium is critical for preventing and reversing insulin resistance, so are zinc and magnesium. Doses of 30–50 mg of zinc and 400 mg of magnesium are often used in therapeutic programs for combating insulin resistance.

Many people can help meet their daily needs for minerals by taking well-rounded multiminerals or multivitamins/minerals. However, caution should be taken about supplementing with iron. Excessive amounts of iron can increase free radical activity in the body and are associated with insulin–resistance-related conditions. Iron may crowd chromium out from doing its job as an insulin potentiator. Therefore, unless a legitimate iron deficiency has been diagnosed, people should choose multimineral supplements without iron.

Essential Fatty Acids

Like chromium, omega-3 essential fatty acids help improve glucose tolerance and reverse insulin resistance. They also lower high blood pressure and high blood triglycerides and protect against heart disease.

Eating coldwater fish, omega-3-enriched eggs, flaxseeds, and dark green leafy vegetables boosts omega-3 intake adequately for the promotion of good health in many people. But some people, especially those with Syndrome X or those who don't eat fish, can benefit from taking 1–3 grams of EPA- and DHA-rich fish oil supplements daily. Diabetics, however, should work with a nutrition-savvy healthcare professional before they try omega-3 supplements.

Alpha-Lipoic Acid and Silymarin (Milk Thistle)

Alpha-lipoic acid, a vitaminlike substance, and silymarin, the active ingredient in the herb milk thistle, are not essential nutrients. But both are antioxidants that bolster liver function, lower blood glucose levels, and reverse insulin resistance.

In my nutritional practice, I have found that one or both of these supplements work well with chromium supplements for countering Syndrome X and type II diabetes. Therapeutic doses range from 280–525 mg of standardized milk thistle extract daily and 100–600 mg of alpha-lipoic acid daily, depending on the severity of the condition.

A Picture of the Future— Chromium Nutrient Combinations

Right now, it's best to work with a knowledgeable health professional to take the many nutrient supplements that are available and develop a targeted nutrition program with chromium for the treatment of various conditions. But there's good news on the horizon for consumers.

Researchers are currently investigating different individual nutrients to find nutrients that help chromium work even better for the nutritional support of various systems and conditions. Areas of investigation include synergistic chromium-nutrient compounds for better blood sugar control, the normalization of cholesterol levels, maintenance of cardiovascular health, bone health support, and improved mood.

Two chromium-nutrient combinations seem especially promising right now. One is chromium picolinate plus conjugated linoleic acid (CLA), which is a fatty acid. In test-tube studies, the two ingredients together dramatically improved glucose uptake into human muscle cells, even without the presence of insulin! Researchers aren't quite sure how the ingredients are working without the action of

insulin, but this finding is dramatic. It might mean that in the near future, chromium picolinate plus CLA could be used to promote better blood sugar control in type I diabetics who no longer produce adequate insulin.

The second chromium-nutrient compound worth keeping an eye out for is chromium picolinate plus niacin (vitamin B_3). Both chromium and niacin are known independently to lower high blood cholesterol levels. But niacin is usually needed in high doses of several grams a day to produce therapeutic effects. These doses often lead to side effects such as flushing—an uncomfortable tingling of the skin. Combining chromium picolinate with niacin seems to solve this problem. It allows much lower doses of niacin to be used for therapeutic benefits without side effects.

Some supplement manufacturing companies plan to make targeted chromium compound products like these available to consumers over the next several years. These products have the potential to make supplemental chromium even more therapeutic, so keep an eye out for them.

A New Product—Chromium plus Biotin

One targeted chromium compound has just recently become available. It's a combination of chromium picolinate plus biotin. It can be found under the trademark name Diachrome—both on the supplement facts label and sometimes as the name of the product itself.

This product was developed after researchers tried to find nutrients that worked synergistically with chromium to improve sugar and fat metabolism. They investigated several different nutrients and found that biotin worked best with chromium for this purpose.

Chromium Plus Biotin Improves Blood Sugar and Cholesterol

Studies conducted at the University of Vermont College of Medicine and the Chicago Center for Clinical Research have found that this combination leads to enhanced blood sugar control and improvements in cholesterol profiles. Here's a rundown of this recent research:

- In muscle cell culture studies, supplementation with chromium picolinate plus biotin enhanced blood sugar uptake four times more than supplementation with biotin or chromium picolinate alone.

- In studies with obese rats with high insulin levels—Syndrome X animal models—supplementation with chromium picolinate plus biotin (and chromium picolinate alone) improved rates of glucose disposal compared to the rats who received no chromium supplementation.

- In studies with type II diabetics who drank a high-carbohydrate, meal–replacement-type drink twice daily, fasting blood sugar levels and glycated hemoglobin levels skyrocketed in the diabetics who did not receive any chromium supplements. However, these levels did not significantly change in diabetics who took chromium picolinate plus biotin. This means that chromium picolinate plus biotin significantly controlled some of the negative effects of sugar intake in diabetics.

Therefore, chromium picolinate plus biotin is a combination that can help maintain and control healthy blood sugar levels, promote healthy fat metabolism, improve insulin sensitivity, and promote healthy cholesterol profiles. It's an exciting new nutrient combination that should be helpful for people with Syndrome X and type II diabetes.

A Multi-Ingredient Chromium Compound to Promote Weight Loss

A multi-ingredient product that enhances chromium's ability to promote weight and fat loss also has recently been developed. The patented combination of four ingredients is found in one new product called Metabolic Makeover, which is available exclusively through the QVC home shopping television channel and its website, www.qvc.com. You should be able to find similar products by other companies on store shelves in the near future.

The combination of ingredients to look for is chromium picolinate along with three other ingredients—carnitine, hydroxycitric acid (HCA), and biotin or pyruvate. Carnitine, often called an amino acid, is a nutrient that picks up fats and drops them off where the body burns them for fuel. HCA is a natural substance extracted primarily from the dried rind of the fruit of a South Asian plant, *Garcinia cambogia*. Pyruvate is a key compound needed for the body to produce energy.

The combination of these four ingredients has been found to have a "hepatothermic effect"—in other words, they enhance metabolism in the liver, which is important for enhancing weight loss.

A short pilot study involving sixteen primarily Samoan-American, obese people who weighed between 200 and 500 pounds showed that this combination is beneficial for weight loss. Supplementation with the four ingredients, together with a high-protein diet and moderate walking, led to dramatic results in three to four weeks. The people lost an average of three pounds of weight and five pounds of fat per week. The heaviest person actually lost twenty-six pounds of weight and fifty pounds of fat in twenty-four days! What's more, lean body mass increased and the supplement takers reported increased energy.

Improving Your Diet to Help Chromium Work Better

You can take chromium or chromium combination supplements regularly, but if you consistently eat a junk-food diet, the supplements aren't going to work very well. Chromium can improve blood sugar and insulin function, but eating foods that stress blood sugar and insulin function can negate many of chromium's positive effects.

Remember: Insulin-resistance conditions such as overweight, Syndrome X, and type II diabetes are nutritional conditions. That means that diet plays an indispensable role in the reversal of these conditions.

If you're really serious about wanting to overcome insulin-related conditions, you should take chromium supplements *and* change your diet. This section will give you diet tips so you can enhance chromium's key role of improving insulin sensitivity and thereby lowering blood sugar and insulin levels.

Lower Your Carbohydrate Intake

Rule number one with diet is to avoid high-carbohydrate refined sugar and refined grains, those pesky ingredients that find their way into popular foods such as sweets, candy, bread, pasta, and snack foods, as well as soft drinks. Following this guideline can be difficult at first because refined carbohydrates are virtually everywhere in our modern society. However, when you go against the grain of social pressure to eat these foods, you go a long way toward improving blood sugar function and allowing the chromium you take to work more effectively at improving insulin function.

If you have severe blood sugar problems such as type II diabetes, it's best to avoid other high-carbohydrate foods such as whole grains, starchy vegetables like potatoes, and dried fruits. Although these foods are generally more nutritious than refined carbohydrates, they're not as good at promoting optimal blood sugar and insulin function as non-starchy vegetables—such as salad greens, spinach, broccoli, cabbage, cauliflower, green beans, and asparagus. By avoiding grains and other high-carbohydrate foods and eating non-starchy vegetables, carbohydrate intake is dramatically reduced. This helps lower blood sugar and insulin levels, giving you some of the benefits of calorie restriction that you learned about earlier. Together with chromium supplementation, a lower-carbohydrate diet works very well at reversing insulin resistance.

Get Adequate Protein and Fat

Getting adequate protein and fat also is important for eating a diet that works well with chromium supplementation. Protein stimulates the production of glucagon, a hormone that opposes insulin and is needed for the maintenance of a healthy metabolism and the building and repairing of muscles. If you take chromium but don't eat enough protein, metabolism can slow and muscle mass can be lost rather than be improved.

Getting adequate protein—and fat—also satisfies the appetite and makes it easier to stick to a lower-carbohydrate diet that can lower insulin levels. Although many people think all types of fat are unhealthy, that's simply not true. Reducing carbohydrate intake and eating more monounsaturated fats, such as olives, olive oil, avocado, and many nuts, improves insulin sensitivity. Emphasizing monounsaturated fats *and* omega-3 fats, such as those in coldwater fish, while avoiding other types of fat, is even better. Eating the right types of fat and avoiding the wrong ones adds to the effect of taking chromium supplements to improve insulin sensitivity.

Lastly, try adding a little spice to your diet. Laboratory experiments by USDA researchers have found that cinnamon, cloves, apple pie spice, bay leaves, and turmeric potentiate insulin activity more than threefold. Using these flavorful additions to your cooking is another way to keep insulin working effectively, along with the help of supplemental chromium.

The Importance of Stress Reduction, Adequate Sleep, and Exercise

Many people don't realize it, but lifestyle factors, such as excessive stress, lack of sleep, and lack of physical activity, contribute to the development of insulin resistance. Addressing these factors can only add to the effects of taking chromium supplements to improve insulin sensitivity.

Excessive stress interferes with efforts to improve insulin sensitivity. It raises levels of cortisol, and chronic elevations of cortisol lead to increased insulin levels, diminished muscle use of blood sugar for energy, and lower levels of the antiaging hormone DHEA.

Stress reduction through various means helps promote health and youthful body function because it raises DHEA levels. You learned that taking chromium picolinate supplements also raises DHEA levels (in addition to lowering insulin levels). So the combination of chromium supplementation and reducing stress is likely to be extra effective at holding back aging.

People who sleep seven and a half to eight and a half hours a night process carbohydrates more efficiently than those who sleep less. People who deprive themselves of sleep, on the other hand, are on the fast track to developing insulin resistance. Getting adequate sleep, therefore, is another effective strategy to avoid sabotaging the beneficial effects of chromium on insulin sensitivity.

Physical activity increases insulin sensitivity, helps build muscle, and reduces stress, not to mention that it significantly reduces the risk of cardiovascular disease and type II diabetes. Many people actually can reverse insulin resistance with diet and chromium and other supplements, but some people need the extra benefits of regular physical activity. If you start an exercise program, keep in mind that strenuous exercise increases chromium losses from the body, so chromium supplementation is more important than ever.

CONCLUSION

Chromium is an essential mineral that is needed in tiny amounts by the body, but one that has an incredibly important job. Its one key role is it helps insulin work more efficiently. This seemingly minor role has tremendous effects for preserving and improving health throughout the body. Unfortunately, most people don't get the tiny amounts of chromium they need from their diets.

As you've learned, supplementing the diet with chromium can offer widespread health benefits. Chromium protects against a long laundry list of common health problems, including two top killers in our society—diabetes and cardiovascular disease. Chromium slows down aging. It normalizes blood sugar function and staves off carbohydrate cravings. It regulates blood cholesterol profiles, lowering the bad types and increasing the good. It combats Syndrome X and helps improve body composition. It alleviates some types of depression and premenstrual syndrome. And it improves bone health and helps prevent osteoporosis.

Although chromium sounds like a panacea and too good to be true, it isn't. Chromium offers all these benefits because it helps insulin works more efficiently. Insulin that works efficiently does the rest.

The most common health maladies facing our society today are disorders of inefficient blood sugar and insulin function. Any nutrient that improves blood sugar and insulin function turns out to be an all-star nutrient. That's exactly what chromium is.

It's time now to weigh the evidence and use this information to your advantage. Make the decision to fortify yourself with supplemental chromium and let this mighty mineral work for you.

PART SEVEN

GLUCOSAMINE & CHONDROITIN

VICTORIA DOLBY TOEWS

If you have osteoarthritis, you've got company. Osteoarthritis, the most common form of arthritis, affects about 21 million Americans, giving this disease the dubious distinction of being more common than heart disease or diabetes. And these numbers are on the verge of ballooning as the Baby Boomers are firmly entrenched in the middle-aged years, with the achy joints to prove it. In fact, by the year 2020, the number of those with osteoarthritis is expected to hit 30 million.

The sad truth is that going to your doctor's office is unlikely to result in lasting relief from your joint complaints. In short, conventional medicine has failed many with arthritis. In fact, the side effects of doctor-prescribed medications, such as nonsteroidal anti-inflammatory drugs (NSAIDs) that are used to mask the pain of osteoarthritis, often rival the discomfort of the disease itself. To add insult to injury, NSAIDs (the most commonly prescribed drug for osteoarthritis) can, in some cases, even promote additional joint damage. And to date, conventional medicine has nothing to offer in terms of a medication that repairs or rebuilds an osteoarthritic joint.

This is where the natural dietary supplements glucosamine and chondroitin come in. Conventional medicine, at best, only addresses the symptoms of osteoarthritis. The crucial difference with glucosamine and chondroitin is that, for the first time, there is a remedy available which actually reverses the damage of osteoarthritis, getting to the source of the problem and repairing joint cartilage.

With glucosamine and chondroitin, you feel better not just because your symptoms are masked, but because your joints are growing new and healthy cartilage to cushion the space where bones meet. While neither promises to be a magic bullet, more often than not they succeed in reducing the pain and impairment of mobility in arthritis.

Perhaps you've been intrigued by natural remedies' claims for aiding health woes such as osteoarthritis, but worry that it's "too good to be true." Think again. Scientifically based clinical trials are stacking up in favor of the ability of glucosamine and chondroitin to provide real relief for aching joints.

It can be hard to get the real scoop about dietary supplements. Some things you read are just hype, overstating the value of a particular supplement with the goal to simply sell more bottles, while other sources are overly skeptical of any supplements and dismiss them all as a waste of money. It's time that the plain truth is told.

This part of the *User's Guide to Nutritional Supplements* provides straightforward information—not hype—about glucosamine and chondroitin. It starts with the basics of understanding the problem of osteoarthritis and how your joints are damaged by this condition. The next section puts this into perspective by explaining how glucosamine and chondroitin can provide symptom relief and rebuild damaged cartilage. Realistic information about how you can expect to feel while taking these joint-friendly supplements is found here, too.

Subsequent sections share the history and development of glucosamine and chondroitin, as well as the nuts and bolts of how to use glucosamine and chondroitin dietary supplements and information about a handful of additional supplements that aid in joint recovery. The role of conventional medications, such as NSAIDs will also be explored. Other health conditions, such as heart disease and migraines, that can benefit from glucosamine and chondroitin will also be discussed. Finally, this part will touch on minor safety concerns with the use of these supplements to ensure that you get the maximum benefit, with the minimum risk, from choosing these dietary supplements.

Isn't it time that you found relief for your osteoarthritis? Read on to finally find an osteoarthritis remedy that offers a long-term solution to your ailment.

JOINTS IN TROUBLE

Osteoarthritis is no fun at all. It's a thief that can take away your ability to be fully engaged in daily activities. As it progresses, you might have days you can't even get out of bed. It is one of the oldest and most common diseases suffered by humans. Arthritis can hit only one joint, which is especially common in the early stages of the disease, or it may affect many joints in the body. In addition, arthritis can vary in severity from a mild ache and stiffness to crippling pain and even joint deformity.

What, Exactly, Is Osteoarthritis?

Osteoarthritis is a medical disease name created from Greek terms, with "osteo" referring to bones, "arthro" indicating that joints are involved, and "itis" meaning inflammation. This is actually somewhat of a misnomer, since pain is the hallmark feature of this condition while inflammation is only rarely implicated, although it certainly involves the bones and joints. Osteoarthritis is a chronic disease involving the breakdown of the joints and surrounding tissues.

In osteoarthritis, the problem lies with the cartilage that protects the ends of bones. This cartilage is a necessary cushion between bones and when it wears away, the bones grinding together cause the common complaints of stiffness and pain. As such, osteoarthritis is the leading cause of disability. Osteoarthritis can have a huge impact on the quality of life. About 100,000 people in the United States alone are estimated to be unable to walk because of severe osteoarthritis in the hip or knee.

Osteoarthritis comes in two "flavors." Primary osteoarthritis is the more prevalent flavor, and it is a slow, but progressive, type of osteoarthritis that generally develops after age forty-five. With primary osteoarthritis, the knees and hips are the main target. The exact cause of primary osteoarthritis is not known, although obesity and family history of this disease do play a role.

Secondary osteoarthritis, on the other hand, can be traced to a specific cause. In many cases, this cause was a traumatic event, such as a sports injury, that left the joint vulnerable. In other cases, it can be related to joint infection, surgery of the joint, or chronic trauma. An example of chronic trauma would be a repetitive motion that damages the joint, such as a baseball pitcher repeatedly throwing a ball. Most younger people with osteoarthritis have secondary osteoarthritis.

How Joints Work

Joints, as the name implies, are the point at which two bones meet. And the human body has over 100 different joints. The joints of the body are known as the articulation system and are responsible for the body's ability to move.

There are three kinds of joints in the body, each with different movement capabilities. The three joint types are cartilaginous, fibrous, and synovial. The synovial joints, including elbows, fingers, hips, and knees, are the most complex since they allow for the greatest movement. The cartilaginous joints, such as the joints between ribs, are slightly movable. The fibrous joints, such as the bones of the skull, are generally immovable.

Synovial Joints
Synovial joints, such as those of the knee and hip, are highly movable joints and are the joints most frequently affected by osteoarthritis.

Osteoarthritis overwhelmingly favors the highly movable synovial joints (although cartilaginous joints very occasionally develop osteoarthritis). The term synovial joint reflects the fact that these joints contain synovial fluid. This clear, sticky fluid lubricates the joints for ease of movement and is produced in the synovial membrane, which lines the joint. Synovial fluid is very important for healthy joints because cartilage does not have its own blood supply. This fluid supplies the building blocks for the repair of cartilage and removes waste products.

Cartilage Is the Key to Healthy Joints

Cartilage acts as a smooth, slippery surface so the bones can move easily past one another. It's the layer of resilient tissue cushioning the ends of bones where joints meet that allows flexible movement and absorbs shock. Cartilage is

Cartilage
Cartilage is mostly water. It also contains a special type of protein called collagen that forms a mesh framework. Attached to this framework are protein-sugar compounds that trap the water to give cartilage its resiliency.

made up of three primary substances: collagen (a special kind of protein), proteoglycans (compounds made of protein and sugar), and water. You may already be familiar with collagen, since it is also the building block of bone, skin, tendon, and other connective tissues.

A mesh network of collagen fibers forms the framework of cartilage. Proteoglycans work and act like miniature sponges to trap water within the cartilage structure. This trapped water is what allows cartilage to absorb shock and spring back after being compressed during the normal movements of a joint.

Additionally, cartilage also contains cells called chondrocytes, which manufacture new collagen and proteoglycans, as well as secrete enzymes to degrade old collagen and proteoglycan molecules. In other words, chondrocytes are the birthplace of both the collagen and proteoglycans that, in turn, create cartilage. Sometimes these chondrocytes malfunction and the balance between the degrading enzymes and the rebuilding process is disturbed. In addition, the new proteoglycans that are made in the malfunctioning chondrocytes are sometimes incomplete and defective, which means they are simply not up to the important job of contributing to strong, resilient cartilage. When these things happen, the stage can be set for osteoarthritis.

The spongelike qualities of cartilage are due in large part to the fact that cartilage contains up to 80 percent water. This unique blend of collagen, proteoglycans, and water means that joints of the body are able to absorb the shock of walking, running, jumping, and all other manner of activities. In fact, for someone who weighs 200 pounds, the weight-bearing joints (knees and hips) have to sustain up to a ton of pressure during active use. Ideally, the joints can handle this load, but joints with osteoarthritis are simply not up to the challenge and regular activities can become painful.

The Osteoarthritic Joint

You've just read how the inside of a healthy joint looks. Now let's take a look inside a joint with osteoarthritis. In the early stages, the first thing that happens is an increase in the enzymes that break down proteoglycans. Unfortunately, the creation of new proteoglycans just can't keep pace with the destruction and, without them, collagen fibers become exposed. Not normally exposed, these fibers are now attacked by enzymes, degrading them further.

In the final stages of arthritis developing in the joint, the entire cartilage matrix has been dissolved, the chondrocytes are disappearing, and the ends of bones are exposed and rubbing painfully together. In addition, the area becomes inflamed as the body tries to protect the joint. However, this inflammation contributes to the breakdown of tissue and this, in turn, promotes more pain in the joint.

Who Gets Osteoarthritis?

With age comes wisdom, and also—for many of us—osteoarthritis. This joint disease generally sets in after age forty and is the most common source of physical disability in adults. With increasing age, the risk of osteoarthritis rises dramatically. On average, each year after age forty, there's a 2 percent rise in the rate of osteoarthritis. Looking at the population as a whole, 21 million Americans can be counted among those with osteoarthritis.

Joints at Risk for Osteoarthritis
Osteoarthritis could theoretically strike any of the body's joints, but it most often affects the feet, fingers, hips, knees, lower back, and neck, rarely the elbows or shoulders.

By age sixty-five, the average person getting an x-ray of a weight-bearing joint would have a 50 percent chance of learning they have osteoarthritis. Since the numbers of Americans reaching age fifty-five and beyond is increasing, so too are the numbers of people developing osteoarthritis.

Lots of people younger than forty develop this joint condition as well, but their cases can generally be traced to a specific joint injury. Both men and women have this disease. Before age forty-five, however, more men have it, while after age forty-five, osteoarthritis is far more common in women.

If you have a close family member with osteoarthritis, your chances of also getting the disease yourself are higher. In addition, being overweight places an extra load on your joints and increases your risk. The connection between obesity and osteoarthritis seems straightforward at first glance, since extra weight makes the weight-bearing joints of the knee and hip work harder. While this is true, it is not yet understood why being overweight also increases the risk of osteoarthritis in the hand. The good news is that weight loss can keep you from getting this disease if you don't yet have it, and if you already do, losing weight helps lessen symptoms.

Secondary osteoarthritis, as previously mentioned, is related to a specific cause. This can include a sports or other injury to a joint, an infection in a joint, a metabolic imbalance (such as calcium deposits), or chronic overuse of a joint from hard labor or sports. In other words, specific stresses on a joint stemming from overuse, trauma, and certain occupations that demand high use from joints, can accelerate the aging of cartilage. It is important to point out here that regular exercise does not cause osteoarthritis and, in fact, does the opposite, since being physically active can help those with osteoarthritis. But it is very important, when working a physical job or when involved in athletics, to be careful that the joints are not overburdened and put at risk for developing secondary osteoarthritis.

What Are the Symptoms?

Osteoarthritis can sneak up on you. It probably started out with one joint (most likely your knee or hip) feeling just a bit stiff in the morning. In general, the pain is asymmetrical, with only the knee or hip on one side of the body being bothered. Over time, however, this can change, with multiple joints developing problems.

What began as morning stiffness can then extend throughout the day in the form of pain, with the affected joint manifesting pain anytime it is used, especially if used actively. The joint will generally feel better with rest. Late in the disease process, however, the joint can be painful with the slightest movement, or even when at rest. Also, as the disease progresses, morning stiffness can occur anytime a joint is not used for a while (such as on a car trip), and the range of motion of the joint can be diminished.

Joint cracking, with both an audible sound and a sensation of crunching, also occurs in the joint. While this can be loud, it is not usually a painful experience.

Shooting pain down the arms or up the back of the head and down the back of the thighs may result from osteoarthritis and is called *referred pain*. Other possible symptoms are muscle spasms and bony growths (called *nodes*) in the fingers.

Inflammation occasionally occurs with osteoarthritis, but is not the primary symptom. If there is inflammation related to osteoarthritis, it is probably very late in the course of the disease. Inflammation is the hallmark of rheumatoid arthritis, a different form of the disease that is not the focus of this discussion.

Osteoarthritis is a progressive disease. This means your symptoms will tend to worsen over time. In advanced cases, bone spurs can form and bones can even become deformed.

Just Part of the Aging Process?

Some people assume that osteoarthritis is simply an inevitable part of the aging process due to wear and tear on the joint. In fact, this is why osteoarthritis used to be known as "wear and tear" arthritis. But modern understanding of this condition now shows that osteoarthritis is not just the result of joints worn out by decades of use, but instead is caused when the body's process of maintaining healthy cartilage is no longer functioning properly.

Key Signs of Osteoarthritis
1. Joint pain, either steady or intermittent.
2. Stiffness in the joint upon first getting out of bed.
3. Joint cracking.
4. Limited range of motion.

There are a few theories about what goes wrong in the cartilage repair process that leads to osteoarthritis, and several of these may be happening at the same time. In some cases, the chondrocytes that make new cartilage seem to put out the wrong mixture of cartilage ingredients. In other cases, the chondrocytes are sending out too many of the cartilage-destroying enzymes and not enough of the materials needed to build new cartilage.

It used to be assumed that this malfunctioning of chondrocytes was not reversible. Today, we know this is not necessarily true. Glucosamine and chondroitin provide the help your body needs to correct the process of creating new, healthy cartilage. You'll learn more details about this amazing breakthrough later.

Preventing Arthritis

Arthritis is not inevitable, there are ways to minimize the risk that it will develop, or at least stave off the inevitable for as long as possible. As the saying goes, an ounce of prevention is worth a pound of cure.

The most important tool for preventing most types of arthritis is exercise. The reason for this lies in the unique anatomy of the joint. Joints do not have a blood supply to nourish them, as other body tissues do. Rather, joints get oxygen and nourishment and eliminate waste as the result of joint movement. During motion, synovial fluid is squeezed into the space between joints and then squeezed out. "Use it or lose it" does seem to apply in this situation. Without joint activity and motion, joints become starved for oxygen and other nutrients which contributes to joint degeneration and arthritis.

Exercise, including stretching, strengthening, and aerobics, is a common recommendation for patients with arthritis, but the pain and mobility impairments associated with arthritis often make it difficult for an individual to comply with this advice. Still, it is important to find an exercise, even if it is only slow walking, that is comfortable for your body.

Exercise has several benefits. The bones respond to exercise by growing stronger and becoming better support structures. And improved muscle tone resulting from improved fitness assists in supporting and stabilizing the joints. Keeping active also maintains the health of cartilage, while inactivity leads to cartilage degeneration. Finally, the beneficial psychological effects of exercise help to prevent anxiety and depression. Biking, swimming, and walking are great exercises to start with, but it is very important to begin any exercise program slowly.

Avoiding injuries is another key factor in an arthritis prevention plan. Of course, the nature of injuries is that they are unplanned; nonetheless, there are ways to minimize the risk. For example, wear shoes that fit properly. Shoes that are too tight can damage the toe joints and lead to arthritis. Likewise, certain occupations can lead to joint problems. If the chair of someone who sits all day is not supportive, or if their posture is incorrect, extensive vertebral damage can develop.

The last piece of advice for reducing the risk of arthritis is already well-known to most people: maintain a healthy weight. The strain of extra weight on the weight-bearing joints (hips, knees, and ankles) can actually destroy the joint. Overweight men and women are 30 percent more likely than their normal weight counterparts to have arthritis. The situation gets worse as the pounds add up. Obese men are at 70 percent higher risk and obese women are at 50 percent higher risk of developing arthritis. But the good news is that losing the weight reduces the risk of arthritis.

Diagnosing Arthritis

Finding out whether the ache you feel in your knee, or the catch in your hip is osteoarthritis is not as easy as you would think. There's no single, clear-cut test for osteoarthritis. Instead, your doctor will use a combination of the methods described here, as well as rule out other conditions.

Osteoarthritis vs. Rheumatoid Arthritis
The joint pain and stiffness of rheumatoid arthritis can be very similar to osteoarthritis, but it is an autoimmune disorder and has a different treatment.

Your doctor will probably start by asking you to describe your symptoms, when they first developed, and how they have changed over time. This is known as a clinical history. Specifically, the doctor will want you to describe any pain, stiffness, and range-of-motion limitation in the affected joint. Next up is a physical examination of the joint to check how impeded the joint usage is.

In addition, x-rays may be taken to determine the extent of joint damage. X-rays can show if there has been any cartilage loss, bone damage, or if bone spurs are present. Disease severity as it appears in x-rays does not always closely match how much pain or disability a person with osteoarthritis experiences. Furthermore, early stages of osteoarthritis do not always appear in x-rays.

In order to confirm a diagnosis of arthritis, a physician may use a syringe to extract some fluid from the affected joint and examine it microscopically for the presence of microorganisms, uric acid, or other substances. This fluid may also be cultured in order to analyze it for infections.

Other joint disorders will be ruled out. For instance, blood tests are utilized in some cases to determine the presence of proteins typical of rheumatoid arthritis or high levels of uric acid indicative of gout. Bursitis symptoms can mimic osteoarthritis symptoms, but the treatment would be different.

Once you know you have osteoarthritis, the next natural step is trying to determine how you can regain as much of your health and quality of life as possible. This is where glucosamine and chondroitin enter the picture. The following sections will focus on how you can use these dietary supplements to reduce your symptoms, and rebuild healthy cartilage in your ailing joints at the same time.

THE CARTILAGE HEALING SOLUTION

Successful treatment of osteoarthritis has two main goals. The first is to control pain, and the second is to slow down—and ideally reverse—the progression of this disease. Conventional medicine has worked hard on this problem, but to date it has only been able to address the first part of this solution—minimizing some of the discomfort that defines osteoarthritis.

Glucosamine and chondroitin are the first well-researched compounds that are meeting both arthritis treatment goals: to control pain *and* to afford some recovery of cartilage function. These supplements don't just ease joint pain and tenderness and improve range of motion, they also promote healing of cartilage.

What Is Glucosamine?

Glucosamine (glue-KOSE-a-meen) is the fundamental building block for the key cartilage ingredient called proteoglycans. You may recall from the last section that proteoglycans act as sponges to contain the water necessary for resilient joints. As the name implies, glucose (sugar) and an amino acid (protein building block) are combined to create "glucosamine." Although the body creates its own glucosamine, in cases of osteoarthritis an extra boost in supply can make a big difference to joint health.

This is one little compound that certainly gets around. In addition to helping make cartilage in joints, glucosamine is also needed, either directly or indirectly, for the formation of blood vessels, bone, heart valves, ligaments, nails, skin, synovial fluid, tendons, and mucus secretions of the digestive tract. Glucosamine is also needed by the body to make chondroitin.

Glucosamine taken orally in a capsule is quickly and almost completely (90 percent) absorbed from the GI tract. In processing this compound, the body sends the lion's share to areas of cartilage where it can be used to build new, healthy cartilage in joints.

What Is Chondroitin?

Much like glucosamine, chondroitin (kon-DROY-tin) is also made within the body and is a necessary component of cartilage and other connective tissues. Chondroitin sulfate, its technical name, belongs to a class of compounds called glycosaminoglycans. Although chondroitin sulfate is often referred to as if it were one thing, there are actually several unique, yet structurally similar, types of this compound. The most abundant in the body are chondroitin-4-sulfate and chondroitin-6-sulfate. The number in each of the names refers to the location of the sulfate molecule along the chondroitin chain.

Chondroitin Family
Supplements of chondroitin sulfate are actually a group of compounds with very similar structures. The differences involve where the sulfate joins onto the chondroitin molecule, which affects how well the body uses each type of chondroitin.

Because there are slightly different structures of chondroitin sulfate molecules, each of the individual structures has different weights. There has been some discussion amongst chondroitin researchers about how the different weights influence the absorption and use of these compounds. Some evidence indicates that the lower weight compounds are more readily absorbed, but the ideal structure of chondroitin remains unknown.

Unlike glucosamine, chondroitin is not well absorbed when ingested orally. In fact, the absorption numbers are mirror images of each other: while 90 percent of glucosamine is absorbed, less than 10 percent of chondroitin is absorbed. This absorption issue is still being researched, since there are many factors—such as molecular weight and location of sulfate groups—that affect the absorption of chondroitin. Some experts theorize that low-molecular-mass chondroitin would be better absorbed. There are currently several products on the market that are designed as low molecular mass.

Even without the specific details of what happens to chondroitin molecules after they are swallowed in a supplement, numerous scientific studies have shown that taking chondroitin sulfate as a dietary supplement results in better joint health.

Joint Benefits of Glucosamine

Osteoarthritis causes cartilage to be worn away, but the good news is that glucosamine can help your body rebuild this cartilage. Here's how: When glucosamine is taken as a supplement, most of it ends up in joint tissues. Once in the cartilage, glucosamine enters the chondrocytes, the cartilage-building factories located within the cartilage tissue, and they utilize the glucosamine to create new proteoglycans.

This revved-up manufacture of proteoglycans helps, in turn, to restore healthy joint function. Remember, it is the proteoglycans that trap water and give joints their springy quality. Increased proteoglycan production is important since one of the hallmarks of osteoarthritis is the body's inability to create enough new proteoglycans to keep up with the loss of this cartilage component.

But that's not all. In any body tissue, new cells are constantly being manufactured to take the place of old cells, a cell-replacement process that is facilitated by enzymes that degrade the old cells. Sometimes, however, the enzymatic breakdown of proteoglycans in cartilage occurs more quickly than their replacement by new cells, which can result in fragile and inelastic cartilage. Here's where glucosamine comes in. It inhibits this misguided, too-rapid enzymatic destruction of proteoglycans, in addition to having an anti-inflammatory effect on the joint.

Joint Benefits of Chondroitin

The beneficial role of chondroitin is both similar and complementary to that of glucosamine. For starters, chondroitin also plays an important role in creating new crops of healthy water-trapping proteoglycans. Since it has a negative charge, each of its molecules is slightly pushed apart from nearby molecules to create small spaces within the cartilage matrix, which are then filled with water. Both glucosamine and chondroitin have been observed in the laboratory to stimulate the creation of proteoglycans by chondrocytes.

The absorption of water into the cartilage matrix is important, since cartilage has no blood supply of its own and depends on the movement of fluid into cartilage to bring necessary nutrients into the joint. The water that fills the spaces within the proteoglycans also acts as a shock absorber for the compression caused during joint movement.

As previously explained, there are enzymes released within the joint that destroy proteoglycans, preparing the way for new proteoglycans to take their place. In osteoarthritic joints, these enzymes are out of balance with the creation of new proteoglycans.

Chondroitin inhibits several of these degrading enzymes, thereby slowing the out-of-balance destruction of proteoglycans and collagen in cartilage. Italian researchers have documented this in a study that found that the oral use of chondroitin sulfate for five days by one group of individuals with cartilage degeneration and a second group with healthy cartilage significantly decreased the levels of cartilage-degrading enzymes in both groups.

As with glucosamine, chondroitin also has the ability to lessen joint inflammation. Although this is not the core problem in the early stages of osteoarthritis, it can become quite debilitating as the disease progresses. This anti-inflammatory effect of chondroitin (as well as glucosamine) is special because, in contrast to prescribed NSAIDs, it does not alter hormonelike substances in the body called prostaglandins, and their function is allowed to continue unharmed. (You'll learn in more detail later about how NSAIDs alter prostaglandins in order to quell inflammation, and how this, in turn, can lead to a bevy of side effects, such as stomach upset.)

Helping Cartilage Rebuild Itself

Both glucosamine and chondroitin bring the joint remodeling process back into balance by quelling the destructive enzymes and beefing up the proteoglycan-building ability of chondrocytes. What this means, specifically, is that osteoarthritis progression can be stopped in its tracks. A landmark study that brought together arthritis experts from four countries and 212 people with osteoarthritis found irrefutable proof that glucosamine does in fact prevent this disease from progressing.

Chondroprotection
The ability to protect cartilage integrity. Glucosamine and chondroitin have this ability since they stimulate the metabolism of chondrocytes, the cells that produce collagen and proteoglycans, inhibit the production of cartilage-degrading enzymes and lessen swelling.

This study, reported in the prestigious medical journal *Lancet,* adhered to the strictest scientific principles. It was double blind, which means that neither the patients nor the doctors had any idea which person was taking glucosamine and which was taking a placebo (dummy pill). Comparing the glucosamine supplements to a placebo was an important aspect of this study, since it takes away the possibility that any benefit found in this study only occurred because of wishful thinking.

All the patients had osteoarthritis of the knee. Half the people took 1,500 mg of glucosamine sulfate per day, the other half were given a placebo. This supplement regimen was continued for three years, and during that time, pain symptoms increased by 10 percent in the placebo group, but dropped by 20 to 25 percent for the glucosamine sulfate group. Similarly, the placebo group continued to experience worsening knee-joint abnormalities while the glucosamine sulfate group showed no deterioration based on x-ray examinations. This is considered landmark research since it was the first time that glucosamine was documented to stop the progression of this disease.

Another group of researchers, however, was not necessarily surprised by these exciting results, since they had already viewed cartilage that was able to rebuild itself with the help of glucosamine. When scanned electron micrographs of cartilage were examined in their study, people who had taken glucosamine showed evidence that their cartilage was actually rebuilding itself.

Chondroitin supplements share a similar success story. When 226 adults with thinning cartilage were administered oral doses of chondroitin sulfate or an inactive placebo daily for one year, the cartilage of those taking the chondroitin sulfate stopped thinning or even improved in thickness. In addition, the chondroitin sulfate group showed significant improvements in all measured parameters, including pain and joint mobility.

In an exhaustive review and reanalysis of all research related to knee and hip osteoarthritis from 1966 to 1999, researchers publishing in the *Journal of the American Medical Association* concluded that glucosamine and chondroitin do, in fact, show a "moderate to large" effect for easing osteoarthritis symptoms. Coming from such a prestigious publication, it is reassuring news that these supplements are no flash in the pan, but a serious treatment consideration for osteoarthritis.

Good Things Are Worth Waiting For

Researchers conducting studies with glucosamine and chondroitin for osteoarthritis can sometimes sound like broken records because they repeat the same recommendation over and over: Glucosamine and chondroitin should be considered as the first-choice, basic therapy for the management of osteoarthritis.

In other words, highly trained researchers recommend that glucosamine/chondroitin should be tried as an osteoarthritis treatment before aspirin, NSAIDs, or surgery. This does not mean that these supplements will completely resolve the disease in every person, but rather that it is the most sensible place to start since the potential for benefit is high and the risk of side effects is exceedingly low.

So how are you likely to feel different after using one or both of these supplements? For starters, you'll need to be prepared to not feel anything for several weeks. Numerous studies have noted that, similar to vitamin and mineral intake, there is a lag time before glucosamine and chondroitin cause noticeable changes. For instance, most people with osteoarthritis who take ibuprofen, an NSAID, notice some pain relief within a week of use, whereas it might take several weeks before glucosamine/ chondroitin approaches the pain relief afforded by an NSAID.

Hang in there, though, because in just a couple more weeks of use, the glucosamine/chondroitin users will usually have surpassed the pain relief of the ibuprofen users. Although it will likely take at least one solid month of daily use before glucosamine and chondroitin will exert their full benefit, it's a classic case of "good things being worth waiting for." This time lag is understandable once you realize that glucosamine/chondroitin are not just applying Band-Aids, they are working to root out the cause of the problem by rebuilding the joint structure, and it takes time to create new, healthy tissue.

While an escape from pain and discomfort is very welcome indeed, it is not the only change the typical user of glucosamine and/or chondroitin experiences. Taking these supplements helps to reduce the swelling of an inflamed joint and lessens the nagging sensation of stiffness in the joints, primarily in the morning, but also any time a joint hasn't been used in a while. People who take glucosamine/ chondroitin report being able to more fully move their affected joint through its normal range, while others report an improved walking speed as one more benefit of these supplements.

So that's what to expect if you take them. But what if you choose not to? The science on this is clear. Untreated osteoarthritis is a progressively worsening condition, and you will most likely feel worse as time goes by.

For example, in one study comparing glucosamine to a placebo (dummy pill), those taking glucosamine had a 24 percent decrease in their symptom scores, but the placebo group's symptom score *increased* by 10 percent. Furthermore, according to x-rays of their knees, the glucosamine group showed no further joint deterioration, but the placebo group continued to show a significant increase in abnormalities. There is definitely a risk involved if you choose to do nothing about your osteoarthritis.

Getting to the Source of the Problem

Treatments for osteoarthritis are generally divided into two categories: symptom-modifying and structure-modifying. As yet, no prescription or over-the-counter medication has been found to be in the latter category. All that doctors have in their current arsenal to mask some of the symptoms of osteoarthritis are drugs, namely NSAIDs. But that's not all. Some of the NSAIDs in common use by conventional medicine are actually known to *worsen* the progression of osteoarthritis.

Fortunately there is glucosamine and chondroitin. These supplements qualify as both symptom-modifying and structure-modifying. Not only do these natural remedies mask osteoarthritis symptoms, they are actually the only remedy yet found to favorably modify the structure of the joint. In short, it's the answer that millions of people with osteoarthritis have been waiting for: a remedy to ease discomfort and heal the joint.

Here are five key ways that glucosamine and chondroitin act as both symptom-modifying and structure-modifying agents for osteoarthritis treatment. They:

1. Reduce joint pain and swelling.

2. Increase water content of cartilage.

3. Slow down action of cartilage-eating enzymes.

4. Step up production of new cartilage components (proteoglycans and collagen).

5. Improve viscosity of synovial fluid (joint lubrication).

Putting Glucosamine/Chondroitin to the Test

The National Center for Complementary and Alternative Medicine and the National Institute of Arthritis and Musculoskeletal Disease are funding a $14-million study to examine whether glucosamine and chondroitin supplements can ease the pain of osteoarthritis.

This study—the Glucosamine/Chondroitin Arthritis Intervention Trial (GAIT)—will last for twenty-four weeks and enroll almost 1,600 patients at thirteen different clinical centers. The efficacy of glucosamine and chondroitin alone, in combination, compared to a placebo, and compared to a conventional medication (celecoxib) for relieving osteoarthritic knee pain will be measured.

The trial will continue with a subset of the participants for another eighteen months to assess how the supplements might alter the progression of the osteoarthritis. The final results of this ambitious study won't be available until 2005. You probably won't want to wait until then, however, to give these great supplements a try.

A STAR IS BORN

The United States is generally thought of as a leader in science and medicine, but in the case of alternative medicine, we are playing catch-up. Many other countries are researching and using natural therapies at a much higher rate than the United States, and glucosamine and chondroitin are a case in point.

Glucosamine Enters the Scene

You may be hearing about glucosamine for the first time, but it is by no means a "new" supplement. Glucosamine is a substance naturally made by and found in the human body. The synthesis of glucosamine sulfate was first described by a chemist back in 1898. However, it took until relatively recently to develop a more stable compound with a long shelf life. Today, supplements of glucosamine are made from chitin, a source material found in crab, shrimp, and lobster shells.

Glucosamine Could Be Considered a Nutrient
Glucosamine is made by the body, and is naturally found in meat, poultry, and fish. The body readily absorbs and uses the small amounts of glucosamine from food sources, and for this reason some experts suggest that it could legitimately be considered a nutrient.

Scientists first got an inkling that glucosamine could play a role in joint problems about half a century ago. Laboratory studies using petri dishes of cartilage cells found that the addition of glucosamine kicked the secretion of glycosaminoglycans and collagen into high gear. A few years later, in 1969, glucosamine was documented to relieve human patients with osteo-

arthritis. German researchers used an injectable form of glucosamine sulfate to bring about reductions in pain and improve mobility. These first human studies, however, were not controlled, meaning that no placebo was used and the study was not double blind, so there was always a chance that the promising results were actually a result of wishful thinking on the part of the patients or doctors.

Over the next two decades, several controlled studies were published by researchers from several countries (including Italy, Portugal, and the Philippines) that showed that glucosamine really does aid joint health. During this time, the United States virtually ignored the building body of research in favor of glucosamine, even though the results of these studies uniformly found that glucosamine reduced joint pain and improved range of motion in affected joints.

In time, an Italian pharmaceutical company developed glucosamine in an oral (pill) form much preferred by patients to the injected form. The standard dose was established as 1,500 mg. The body of research documenting the benefits of glucosamine continued to grow, and the low incidence of side effects from this supplement became irrefutable.

Chondroitin Makes Its Mark

Chondroitin was first identified as a component of cartilage in the 1940s. Supplements of chondroitin sulfate use cartilage from pigs, chicken, fish, and cows as a source material. Regarding the latter, there have been concerns raised about the risk of mad cow disease (bovine spongiform encephalopathy) contaminating chondroitin supplements. This concern is discussed in more detail later, but the bottom line is that supplement manufacturers take the same steps as companies producing beef products to ensure that this animal-based product has an extremely low risk for transmitting this disease.

The early research with chondroitin primarily used this supplement in animals to demonstrate its application for joint health. Other laboratory research on animals showed that chondroitin increases proteoglycan production. Trials involving people with osteoarthritis soon followed and, as with glucosamine, this supplement was repeatedly shown to relieve joint pain, improve mobility, lessen swelling, increase walk time, and decrease the use of NSAID medications.

Also Used by Veterinarians
Glucosamine and chondroitin are used increasingly in veterinary medicine to treat arthritis in dogs, horses, and other animals.

The Overlooked Medical Miracle

Although glucosamine is a mainstay treatment for osteoarthritis in Europe, and has been for years, glucosamine and chondroitin have only recently become commonplace in the United States. What accounts for this disparity in how osteoarthritis is treated on either side of the Atlantic? To find the answer to this question, one simply needs to "follow the money."

Pharmaceutical companies spend an enormous amount of money researching and marketing drugs to treat diseases. The way they recoup all this outflow of money is by investing in drugs they can patent. Patented medicines, such as the NSAID medications, are protected and allow the patent holder to corner the market and charge higher prices than are charged for a product produced by competitive manufacturers.

While this situation leads to the development of some very useful and life-saving medications, it does have the downfall that products like nutritional supplements that cannot be patented are often left by the wayside. Thus, the medical-pharmaceutical industry ignores these natural agents because there is no money to be made. Instead they turn out, one after another, new drugs, such as Cox-2 inhibitors that drain pocketbooks, and rack up unfortunate side effects.

There simply isn't as ready a source of research dollars to study nutritional supplements as there is for pharmaceuticals. This doesn't mean that nutritional supplements lack amazing potential for healing, it just means they lack funding.

But this has been changing. Overall, there is growing interest in natural healing modalities. With the rise of the Internet, more of the international research on glucosamine and chondroitin has gotten attention, and more physicians are becoming open to the use of dietary supplements.

For glucosamine and chondroitin, the biggest moment of change came in 1997 when a book called *The Arthritis Cure* took the morning news programs, newspapers, and the awareness of the general public by storm. The authors of this book, Dr. Jason Theodosakis, Brenda Adderly, and Dr. Barry Fox, contended that glucosamine and chondroitin could halt, reverse, and even cure osteoarthritis. It truly caused a groundswell of interest in these supplements by the average person that could no longer be ignored. Overnight, glucosamine became a household word. Since then, much more has been learned about using these supplements.

Quality Control Remains Strong

You shell out the money for a bottle of pills, but how do you really know what's in those pills? In the case of glucosamine and chondroitin, you don't have to worry. Although there has been in-fighting between supplement companies accusing each other of putting out poor-quality products, the bottom line seems to be that the average bottle of glucosamine/chondroitin really is of high quality.

A non-profit organization related to the natural products industry put twenty-eight brands of glucosamine to the test. All the supplement bottles were randomly purchased from stores, and then sent to independent laboratories for analysis of the amount and type of glucosamine. To achieve a passing score, the products needed to pass both tests within a 5 percent margin of error. Every single product passed, which indicated that it contained exactly what the label listed in terms of product type and quantity.

This should give glucosamine users peace of mind that they are getting what they paid for.

Costs of Supplementation

Consumers spend about $400 million on glucosamine and chondroitin supplements annually. That might sound like a lot, but it is really just a drop in the bucket compared to the annual $6.6 billion spent on pharmaceuticals for arthritis. Clearly, there are legions of ailing joints out in the world. The lower amount spent on glucosamine and chondroitin is partly related to their less frequent use, but primarily it reflects a more reasonable price compared to the patented pharmaceutical drugs.

The High Cost of NSAIDs *Not only are NSAID medications expensive, they also lead to costly treatment of their side effects. Each year, $2 billion is spent to treat the side effects of NSAIDs.*

In fact, the cost of these nutritional supplements has been dropping rapidly as numerous companies competing for consumer business have entered the marketplace. As an example, a one-month supply of a combination product supplying 1,500 mg of glucosamine sulfate and 1,200 mg of chondroitin sulfate is as little as $20 per month. And this is not an off-label bargain basement reject. This particular brand was independently tested for potency, as many brands have been. The monthly cost of taking glucosamine and/or chondroitin is quite reasonable in comparison to the cost of prescription osteoarthritis products. (A typical brand-name NSAID could cost up to $100 a month, or about $40 if it's a generic, but even this lower cost is double that of the natural glucosamine/chondroitin supplements.)

There's never been a better time to give glucosamine/chondroitin products a try to see if they will help your joints because product quality and cost are both the best they've ever been.

HOW TO TAKE GLUCOSAMINE AND CHONDROITIN

By now it's clear that glucosamine and chondroitin get to the root of the problem: the joint, where they repair the damage caused by osteoarthritis. You are probably anxious to find out if you'll be among the majority of those with osteoarthritis who find relief with glucosamine and chondroitin. But you'll want to make sure you use these supplements in the best way—the way that has solid scientific research as a successful treatment for osteoarthritis behind it. That's what this chapter is all about. Here is where you'll find the nuts-and-bolts information on how to incorporate these supplements into your life.

Glucosamine Comes in Different Forms

Glucosamine is commonly available in three forms: glucosamine sulfate, glucosamine HCl, and N-acetyl glucosamine. The vast majority of the scientific research has used the glucosamine sulfate form. However, this does not mean the other forms of glucosamine are not effective. There are a few studies that have focused on the glucosamine HCl and N-acetyl glucosamine forms with promising results.

Which Product Is Best? There have not yet been studies comparing the forms of glucosamine (glucosamine sulfate, glucosamine HCl, and N-acetyl glucosamine) to one another. For this reason, it is not yet known if one is more effective than another.

There are no studies comparing these glucosamine forms to each other, so it is difficult to know if one is better than another. It would be prudent, if you had to choose only one, to stick with the glucosamine sulfate form since it has been the most thoroughly researched. However, there is also something to be said for hedging your bets by taking one of the combination products on the market which contain glucosamine sulfate, glucosamine HCl, and N-acetyl glucosamine.

Lower Weight Chondroitin Preferable

Unlike glucosamine, chondroitin is generally available in only one form: chondroitin sulfate. There are, however, varying weights of chondroitin sulfate and, as previously stated, the low-molecular-mass chondroitin is theoretically better absorbed. Chondroitin sulfate compounds differ slightly in terms of where the sulfate is attached to the chondroitin molecule and this difference in location accounts for the different weights of chondroitin sulfates (the lower weight chondroitin-4-sulfate and chondroitin-6-sulfate are the most plentiful chondroitin sulfates in the body).

Researchers have noted that the lower weight compounds are more easily absorbed, and are for this reason theoretically the preferred form. Some products on the market will specify on the label that the product contains "low-weight chondroitin sulfate."

Sulfate Plays a Role

It might be a good idea to make sure that there is at least some sulfate in the product you buy. In other words, including some glucosamine sulfate or chondroitin sulfate as opposed to only glucosamine HCl or N-acetyl glucosamine could be prudent.

There is some evidence that part of the reason why both

glucosamine sulfate and chondroitin sulfate supplements aid joint health is because of the sulfate molecule they are attached to. Sulfate is a form of sulfur, and sulfur is an essential nutrient needed for the stabilization of the connective tissue matrix as well as for the manufacture of collagen. The idea that sulfur is needed for joint repair is nothing new. Back in 1934, a researcher first proposed that sulfur halts the degeneration of joints in those with arthritis.

When sulfate levels are low, the manufacture of new glycosaminoglycans (the complex compounds in the joint tissue, including chondroitin) is drastically stepped down, according to research in animals. In humans, it has been shown that a limited supply of sulfate also interferes with the production of new glycosaminoglycans.

This slowing of glycosaminoglycan production can be a big problem for those with arthritis. Joints suffering from arthritis have an increased demand for glycosaminoglycans, so at the time when the joints are calling for more of these important compounds, they might not have enough sulfate available to produce them.

Glucosamine versus Chondroitin

Glucosamine and chondroitin play slightly different roles in joint tissue, but both have the end effect of rebuilding damaged cartilage. However, it is always reassuring to have a solid foundation in scientific research, and the simple fact is that glucosamine has been scrutinized in far more studies than chondroitin. This is not to say chondroitin doesn't work. It just means that glucosamine has been put under the microscope more often and in more people so, if you had to choose just one, for this reason glucosamine would be the better bet.

But why not hedge your bets and take a combination product? There are numerous products on the market today that contain a mixture of glucosamine and chondroitin. This way you'll be able to garner the benefits of both supplements.

Synergy Gives More "Bang for the Buck" Synergy is the concept that two substances, when used together, provide more benefit than when either was used individually.

Choosing to take a combination product has another, even more valuable benefit. Glucosamine and chondroitin have been found to have a synergistic benefit to the joints, rather than a simple additive effect which means that the total benefit exceeds that expected of each taken alone. This is because glycosaminoglycan production is being stimulated by the glucosamine while, at the same time, the chondroitin is inhibiting the breakdown of glycosaminoglycans. The net effect is the production of greater quantities of healthy cartilage.

For example, supplements of glucosamine HCl, low-molecular-weight chondroitin sulfate, and manganese ascorbate (a vitamin-mineral complex) were tested separately and in combination for how well they slowed cartilage degeneration in rabbits. While each of these supplements helped the rabbits a bit, when they were given as a combination product, the rabbits had the most joint protection. In the laboratory, petri dishes of cartilage show a much greater amount of new glycosaminoglycan growth when this same combination is given than when each of the components is used separately.

Who Should Consider Taking These Supplements?

The primary use of glucosamine and chondroitin is for the healing of joints addled with osteoarthritis damage (although later I'll discuss additional health benefits of these supplements). For this reason, adult men and women who have been diagnosed with osteoarthritis by a physician are the core group of people who should consider taking these supplements.

> **Three Types Are "Right" for Taking Glucosamine/Chondroitin**
> 1. *Adults with active cases of osteoarthritis—to restore joint health.*
> 2. *Adults with osteoarthritis that is currently under control—to reduce chances of relapse.*
> 3. *Healthy older people who are at risk for this disease—to lower the chances that it will ever develop.*

Even if your osteoarthritis is under control (either with the use of conventional NSAID medications or other means), you might want to consider taking glucosamine and chondroitin in order to prevent a future flare-up. However, there is no reason you can't wait until a flare-up starts before resuming, or commencing, the use of glucosamine and chondroitin.

Even people without any signs of osteoarthritis might consider these supplements. On each birthday after age sixty-five, you have a 2 percent greater risk of developing osteoarthritis. Thus, healthy older people might want to use glucosamine and chondroitin as insurance against developing osteoarthritis. This is particularly prudent "insurance" if you have other risk factors for osteoarthritis, such as prior joint injuries, family history, or obesity.

The Right Amount

Virtually all human research has uniformly used 1,500 mg of glucosamine per day, an amount that seems appropriate for most people. However, after taking this full amount of glucosamine for six to eight weeks, you could experiment to see if taking 1,000 mg per day, or even as little as 500 mg per day as a "maintenance" dose, will keep your symptoms at bay. The standard dose of chondroitin is 1,200 mg per day.

For example, Ray, a fifty-nine-year-old man with osteoarthritis of the knee, took 1,500 mg of glucosamine sulfate daily for several years and got significant relief from his knee discomfort. When he experimented with phasing out glucosamine altogether, his symptoms returned. Today, however, he is able to maintain the same level of relief that 1,500 mg per day initially provided by taking just 1,000 mg per day as a maintenance dose.

It is probably a good idea to start out at the recommended dosage of 1,500 mg per day, rather than experimenting with lower levels. Jeff, a thirty-five-year-old with osteoarthritis of the hip and knee as a result of sports injuries, had tried taking just 500 mg of glucosamine off and on for several months without significant pain relief.

> **How much glucosamine and chondroitin should I take?**
> *According to numerous research studies, a daily intake of 1,500 mg glucosamine and 1,200 mg chondroitin is an effective amount for most people.*

After upping to the full 1,500 mg per day (along with 1,200 mg per day of chondroitin) and diligently taking it every day, he was able to start running again after having avoided that joint-jarring activity for the previous five years. He reports that his joints feel almost as good as in his younger years.

Once a Day Is All You Need

Taking glucosamine and chondroitin is more convenient than ever before. For starters, they are no longer sleepy, backwoods specialty supplements, they can now be found virtually everywhere: in natural foods stores, pharmacies, grocery stores, even warehouse discount stores.

In addition, glucosamine is easier than ever to use. The original studies with this supplement used injections of glucosamine, a drawback because a medication that only comes in injectable form means people have to spend extra time and money at a physician's office. Fortunately, glucosamine in pill form that was stable and well absorbed was developed. This original pill form was taken three times per day—500 mg each time, the standard recommendation—an improvement over injections, but still a hassle. Having to cart around your bottle of supplements all day, as well as remember to actually pop all three pills, was hard to do.

Now, research has found that taking 1,500 mg in one sitting is just as effective as the divided doses. You only have to remember once a day to take the supplement, and you can choose whichever time of day is most convenient for you.

The story is just about the same with chondroitin: It is also now known to be effective when taken once daily. In one study, chondroitin supplements were given one of two ways. In one method, 800 mg of chondroitin sulfate was provided to volunteers in one sitting. In the other method, 400 mg of chondroitin sulfate was given in the early part of the day and another 400 mg was given later in the day. Although both dosing schedules increased blood levels of the compounds associated with this supplement, the once-daily schedule resulted in higher levels.

Don't Give up Too Soon

Don't expect instant relief after starting a regimen of glucosamine and/or chondroitin. Most research has found that these supplements need to be taken daily for at least four weeks in order to derive benefits. You should begin to experience increasing pain relief and increased mobility during this initial month, and many people continue to improve further in subsequent weeks and months.

A "Daily Pain Record" chart is a tool to help you track your pain on a day-to-day basis over a one-month period to determine how much, if at all, the glucosamine and/or chondroitin supplements are helping your osteoarthritis.

DAILY PAIN RECORD

DAY	PAIN LEVEL				
	0	1	2	3	4
1					
2					
3					
4					
5					
6					
7					
8					
9					
10					
11					
12					
13					
14					
15					
16					
17					
18					
19					
20					
21					
22					
23					
24					
25					
26					
27					
28					
29					
30					

What is your level of discomfort today?

0 None	**3** Moderately severe
1 Mild	**4** Severe
2 Moderate	

Consider Cycling On and Off

After taking glucosamine and/or chondroitin for many months or years, you will have reached the peak of your pain relief with these supplements. At this point, it might be appropriate to lower your dosage to a maintenance dose. (For example, to 500–1,000 mg per day of glucosamine and/or 400–800 mg of chondroitin.) You might even be able to stop taking the supplements for a while.

The benefits of these supplements do not stop the day after you stop taking the pills. Several research studies have found that joint relief continues for many weeks, and sometimes up to three months after their use is discontinued. For this reason, some people have found that they can save money and the daily hassle of taking pills by using glucosamine and chondroitin on an intermittent basis.

Avoid Glucosamine Cream

Glucosamine and chondroitin should be used only in oral (pill) form for osteoarthritis. To date, there is no evidence that putting these compounds on the skin over a joint will provide any health benefit whatsoever, so it is probably a waste of money to use glucosamine or chondroitin in topical rub-on cream or gel forms.

The cream form, however, might have some merit for other health conditions. It has been favorably studied for relieving the itchiness of poison ivy and poison oak.

Will Glucosamine Work for You?

While study after study has shown glucosamine and chondroitin to have scientifically measurable benefits in the disease of osteoarthritis, there are no guarantees they will work in a particular individual's case. In general, however, clinical trials comparing glucosamine to a placebo found that glucosamine provided significant pain relief, joint mobility improvement, and other benefits in 52 to 55 percent of those taking it.

Researchers have identified a few criteria that influence who will be a "responder" (versus a non-responder) to supplemental therapy. Those with less severe cases (that is, mild-to-moderate cases of osteoarthritis) are more likely to respond to glucosamine. This makes sense, since the joints still have some amount of normally functioning cartilage that can be "jump-started" with the addition of glucosamine.

There have been reports that obesity hampers a person's response to glucosamine. But, it has yet to be tested whether simply increasing the glucosamine in such cases will overcome the less-than-ideal response.

In addition, there have also been anecdotal reports that people with active peptic ulcers and those taking diuretics are less likely to be among the glucosamine success stories. Again, the use of a "Daily Pain Record" chart can help you determine if you are a responder and if it is worth the trouble and expense to continue taking glucosamine and/ or chondroitin.

Most Important of All, Start Early

It's just common sense: The earlier they are taken in the disease process, the more effective glucosamine and chondroitin are. Mild-to-moderate osteoarthritis has a good chance of being helped by these supplements. In the few studies that included patients with severe arthritis, their response was certainly less stellar than the response of those with more moderate cases of this disease. This is not to say, however, that you can't be helped if you have severe osteoarthritis. Try it; it's worth a test run.

Many people with osteoarthritis fail to seek help until years after symptoms begin. Be advised, though, that the sooner you start taking these supplements, the better your chances of reversing joint damage are.

ADDITIONAL JOINT PROTECTORS

Glucosamine and chondroitin are certainly in the front-lines when it comes to easing pain and healing joints damaged by osteoarthritis, but they are not necessarily the entire army. There are several other vitamins, minerals, and dietary supplements that serve as supporting soldiers to give your joints extra protection.

Low levels of several nutrients are associated with arthritis, although whether this is a cause or a result of arthritis is still a little murky. What is known is that joint pain and stiffness increase when a person is malnourished and symptoms improve when there is an increased intake of nutrients.

In addition, the inflammation common to arthritis can change the lining of the intestines, reducing the absorption of some nutrients, while at the same time increasing nutrient needs. Optimal intake of vitamins and minerals is also important to ensure that the body will have the building blocks necessary to rebuild joints and connective tissues damaged by an arthritis flare-up or by drug therapy.

Added Vitamins and Minerals Give Osteoarthritis a One-Two Punch

In numerous clinical trials, a combination of glucosamine and chondroitin has been shown to manage osteoarthritis, and vitamin C and manganese can support the action of these joint-healing supplements.

Vitamin C is certainly an important nutrient to consider as a supporting player for the health of your joints. The key story with this vitamin is that it is needed for collagen synthesis. In addition, it decreases free radical damage, which is one of the potential causes of osteoarthritis.

The mineral manganese also plays a supporting role in the body's manufacture of chondroitin. Although the role of manganese deficiency in the development of osteoarthritis has not yet been specifically researched, it is known that Western societies are at risk of suboptimal manganese intake.

In fact, approximately one in three Americans has low manganese intake. Why do we fall short with this mineral? For starters, modern farming techniques deplete manganese from the soil of farming lands and, in turn, from the food that is grown there. Furthermore, refined grains (white flour, white rice, and so on) are the predominant food choices in contemporary America and they contain only half the manganese of whole grains. It all adds up to a pretty suspicious situation.

Joint Disease Seen in Animals
In animals, manganese deficiency leads to cartilage problems and a form of joint disease. It has been suggested that the lack of this mineral in the diet, could cause the same problems in people.

Not surprisingly, there have already been several studies that use a combination of glucosamine, chondroitin, vitamin C, and manganese. In one clinical trial using this combination, symptoms of osteoarthritis in the knee were greatly reduced.

In another trial, published in the journal *Osteoarthritis and Cartilage*, ninety-three patients with osteoarthritis of the knee took this combination supplement or a placebo. Those with mild to moderate osteoarthritis who took the supplement showed significant improvement in their symptoms by the end of the six-month study. Those with severe osteoarthritis, however, showed fewer benefits. In an animal model, this same combination made it less likely that animals would even develop arthritis in the first place.

There are formulas on the market that contain the combination of glucosamine, chondroitin, vitamin C, and manganese. However, manganese can be "too much of a good thing." Concerns have been raised that some of these supplements contain excessive amounts of manganese which has prompted several manufacturers to reformulate their products with appropriate, lower amounts of manganese. (See "Mind Your Minerals" in the Safety Profile section for more about manganese toxicity.)

Tips to "B" Healthier

Supplements of certain B vitamins may be just as effective in arthritis as NSAIDs—but without the side effects. In one study of B vitamins in arthritis, twenty-six men and women with osteoarthritis were given a combined supplement of folic acid and vitamin B_{12}, or a placebo, daily, for two months. During the study none of the patients used anti-arthritis drugs or any other supplements.

After taking the B-vitamin supplements for two months, the arthritis patients had better hand grip strength and less joint tenderness than those who were given a placebo. The beneficial effect was equivalent to that expected with

NSAID use. The researcher of this study summed up the benefits of B-vitamin supplements over conventional drugs in the *Journal of the American College of Nutrition*: "Side effects with the vitamin combination were none; side effects of NSAID are many, and the cost of vitamins . . . is lower."

Niacinamide is a form of vitamin B_3. Several decades ago, this form of vitamin B_3 was first reported in the *Journal of the American Geriatric Society* to provide dramatic improvement for those with osteoarthritis, in terms of joint mobility, inflammation, and pain. This original research indicated it might take up to a month to see benefits, but then the improvements would continue for many years while niacinamide was taken. This early research administered 500 mg of niacinamide three to four times per day.

It's taken a long time, but researchers have finally resumed studies with this vitamin. In a recent double-blind study, the benefits originally reported with niacinamide were supported in seventy-two patients with osteoarthritis. Researchers found that niacinamide produced a 29 percent improvement in all symptoms and signs compared to a 10 percent worsening in the placebo group.

Be Careful with Niacinamide
Although niacinamide is generally safe to use, it can cause serious liver-damage problems for a few people. Work with your doctor if you are taking more than 1,500 mg per day.

Niacinamide is generally well tolerated and without side effects. Unlike niacin (another form of vitamin B_3), niacinamide does not produce flushing of the skin. However, with the amounts used for arthritis, it is prudent to have blood tests several times a year to monitor for any possible liver damage.

Not surprisingly then, this supplement should not be used by anyone with pre-existing liver disease. In addition, people with diabetes need to know that niacinamide might alter requirements for insulin. Thus, you should work with your health care provider to monitor blood-sugar levels and adjust your medication, as needed. Since the B vitamins are known to work better as a unit than when taken individually, it is advisable to take a B-complex supplement along with these individual Bs.

Vitamin D Fits the Bill for Prevention

For anyone with osteoarthritis, a low intake of vitamin D is like adding insult to injury. Worsening knee problems are two to four times more likely in vitamin D–deficient osteoarthritics. In another study, people with low blood levels of vitamin D were found more likely to develop osteoarthritis of the hip.

Foods rich in vitamin D, sun exposure, or vitamin D supplements appear to be equally effective in raising the levels of vitamin D enough to hamper the progression of the disease. However, keep in mind that supplementation with vitamin D should be limited to 200–400 mg per day since this vitamin can be toxic in higher amounts.

Fighting Free Radicals

The antioxidant nutrients are particularly important for anyone with arthritis. The inflammatory process causes large numbers of harmful compounds called free radicals to be released. A free radical is missing a vital part of itself—one of its electrons. In an effort to restore the balance of a paired electron, it reacts with any nearby molecule in the body, such as fats, proteins, or even DNA.

Antioxidants: Electron Donors
Antioxidants have the unique ability to donate the much-sought-after electron that free radicals need without becoming free radicals themselves.

The end result is a deadly game of hot potato. As the original free radical passes off its unpaired electron or steals an electron from another molecule, that molecule becomes unbalanced. This newly formed free radical then interacts with yet another molecule in pursuit of stability, and so on. Essentially, antioxidants act as a referee in the body, ending the potentially out-of-hand game of free-radical hot potato that, if left unchecked, can destroy the body.

Vitamin E is an important antioxidant in the body's defenses against free radicals. In one study, patients with osteoarthritis took 600 mg of vitamin E per day, or a placebo, for ten days. Later, they switched to the opposite treatment of either vitamin E or the placebo. A little more than half of those taking vitamin E experienced pain reduction, while only 4 percent of the placebo group could say the same. In other research, vitamin E was compared to the NSAID diclofenac and was shown to be just as effective as that medication for increasing joint mobility and improving walking time.

Dr. Timothy McAlindon at the Arthritis Center, Boston University Medical Center has been studying the protective role of antioxidant nutrients in osteoarthritis. With 640 participants in his Framingham Osteoarthritis Cohort study, it was found that a higher intake of vitamin C, another antioxidant, was related to a threefold lesser risk of disease progression. The benefits of vitamin C were seen in both men and women, at various stages of disease severity, and in both users and non-users of supplements. The benefits of beta-carotene and vitamin E were not as strong in this study.

Dr. McAlindon notes that ". . . the effect of vitamin C appeared stronger and more consistent than that of beta carotene or of vitamin E." This may be explained by the watery environment of certain parts of the joint that would benefit more from a water-soluble, rather than a fat-soluble, antioxidant. (Vitamin C is water-soluble, while vitamin E and beta-carotene are fat-soluable.)

Dr. McAlindon summed up his research by stating that a "high intake of antioxidant micronutrients, especially vitamin C, may reduce the risk of cartilage loss and disease progression in people with [osteoarthritis]."

There are many antioxidant nutrients, but the ones

with documented success in arthritis are vitamin C, vitamin E, and selenium. However, the bioflavonoids, such as quercitin, and the proanthocyanidins in pine bark and grapeseed extract may also be helpful in preventing accumulation of fluids, swelling, and pain in the joints.

The Latest Aids: SAMe and MSM

S-adenosylmethionine (SAMe), which is related to the amino acid methionine, holds a lot of promise for folks with osteoarthritis. While this supplement was being investigated as a treatment for depression, many of the depressed patients who also happened to have osteoarthritis began to report to their doctors that SAMe was giving them relief from their joint troubles.

The Cartilage Builder
SAMe is yet another of the important building blocks needed to make new crops of healthy, strong cartilage.

Since then, several large trials have examined the role of SAMe in osteoarthritis. In the more than 22,000 patients who have now been treated with SAMe in trials, it is clear that SAMe is at least as effective as NSAIDs, according to a review published in the *Alternative Medicine Reviews*. The studies have generally provided 400–1,200 mg per day of SAMe.

SAMe is formed in the body by combining the essential amino acid methionine with adenosine triphosphate (ATP). SAMe is involved in dozens of biochemical reactions in the body, and works with several B vitamins to support certain body functions. More important, this compound is needed for the body to make cartilage components, such as chondroitin sulfate. When the body has a deficiency of SAMe, the joints are less able to maintain their springy, resilient qualities.

SAMe is generally without side effects, although gastrointestinal disturbances and nausea have been occasionally reported. If you have bipolar disorder or Parkinson's disease, you shouldn't take this supplement.

Methylsulfonylmethane (MSM) has recently become popular as a pain reliever for those with arthritis. MSM is related to DMSO—the topically applied substance which saw its heyday in the 1960s and 1970s. Unfortunately, DMSO is associated with many side effects, such as blistering, diarrhea, dizziness, nausea, and rashes, and should be used cautiously.

In contrast, MSM—which is taken orally—has been shown in some research to ease the pain and inflammation of joints without the side effects of DMSO. Animal research suggests that MSM protects against the breakdown of cartilage in joints. MSM (as well as DMSO) is believed to aid in arthritis through its sulfur content, a mineral that is needed for a wide array of body functions.

Joint tissues need sulfur to help stabilize the connective tissue matrix. Research dating back almost a century had indicated that people with arthritis are more likely to be deficient in sulfur. While this is intriguing, there have thus far only been anecdotal claims for MSM as an arthritis treatment; the hard scientific research remains to be done. However, this supplement is safe and you can try one to three grams daily to see if your symptoms would be improved.

Herbal Relief

Cayenne peppers, plants native to Central America, have become one of the hottest arthritis treatments around. Capsaicin—the active ingredient in cayenne peppers—is applied topically as a cream and reduces the pain of arthritis by depleting the nerves of "substance P," a chemical that carries pain sensations to the brain. Topical creams that contain 0.025 percent capsaicin cream are generally used four times per day. They are widely available in health food stores, drug stores, etc.

Pain, Pain Go Away
The hot cayenne pepper, well known for its role in the kitchen, also has a role in your medicine chest. Creams made from cayenne can provide relief from joint pain.

Initially, capsaicin might cause a burning sensation, but this discomfort quickly goes away—as (in many cases) does the arthritis pain. A word of caution: wash your hands after applying capsaicin cream, as it can be painful and irritating if any residual cream on your hands comes into contact with your eyes or other sensitive tissues.

The Devil's claw plant (*Harpagophytum pricumbens*) was given this vivid name in reference to the claw-shaped growths—complete with imposing thorns adorned with several fingerlike growths—which wrap around and protect the plant's seeds. The underground tubers of this plant were used medicinally by indigenous African tribes, primarily for arthritis conditions.

Europeans traveling to Africa heard tales of the health-enhancing properties of Devil's claw and brought samples of it back to Germany and other European countries to test. The clinical research using Devil's claw root for arthritis conditions proved favorable and Devil's claw quickly gained recognition throughout Europe for alleviating arthritis symptoms, particularly for reducing pain and inflammation. More research with this herb is warranted, but you could give it a try if you haven't been able to find adequate pain relief with other methods.

Ginger, a popular food spice, has been used as a folk medicine for numerous maladies. Ginger holds an important place in several traditional systems of medicine. When researchers put ginger to the test in both rheumatoid arthritis and osteoarthritis cases, more than three-quarters of those tested experienced relief from pain and swelling.

Boswellia serrata, an herb from the Ayurvedic tradition, improves blood supply to the joints and prevents tissue deterioration. Boswellia is valuable because, although it acts like a NSAID, it does not produce the side effects of pharmaceutical NSAIDs. One clinical trial of 175 rheumatoid arthritis patients found that Boswellic acid supplements (the active ingredient in *Boswellia serrata*), improved grip strength, morning pain and stiffness, and physical performance in 97 percent of patients after three to four weeks of treatment.

The turmeric plant has long been used in India as a source of spice and clothing dye. Today, *curcumin*—an extract from the turmeric spice—is gaining worldwide recognition for its potent ability to quell inflammation. (As one of the oldest anti-inflammatory drugs used by traditional Indian medicine, turmeric is not actually a new discovery.) Animal studies, as well as some preliminary work with people, show promising results.

Beware of Nightshade Vegetables

Could your arthritis symptoms be traced back to what is served on your dinner plate? It's possible if you are eating foods from the nightshade family. In the 1960s, Dr. Norman Childers, a horticulturist from New Jersey's Rutgers University, noticed a worsening of his own arthritis pain and stiffness after eating vegetables from the nightshade class, and an easing of his symptoms when he avoided these foods.

The Nightshade Family
Nightshade vegetables include bell peppers, eggplant, paprika, potatoes (but not sweet potatoes or yams), and tomatoes. Tobacco is also in this family of plants.

Since Dr. Childers' discovery, the role of nightshade plants in arthritis has been a topic of heated controversy. While many with arthritis give testimony about the strong relationship they have experienced between nightshade plants and joint problems, the scientific community has yet to back up these claims. Various alkaloids found in nightshade plants, such as atropine, nicotine, and scopolamine, have been hypothesized to provoke arthritis symptoms.

Reports vary widely (from five to 66 percent) on the number of people sensitive to nightshade plants. In order to determine if you are among those affected by this class of foods, simply eliminate nightshade plants from your diet. If you are sensitive, it may take up to six weeks to notice a beneficial effect from avoiding these plants.

Hot and Cold Relief

Diathermy or "deep heat" has been reported as a valuable aid for controlling pain and increasing joint mobility in arthritis. It is administered by high frequency sound waves (ultrasound) or electromechanical irradiation (microwave or short wave). The application of heat is thought to increase the pain threshold and relieve pain by reducing nerve-conduction velocity. On the downside, diathermy can be expensive and time consuming.

The Best of Both Worlds
Some people with arthritis find it helpful to alternate heat and cold to maximize the benefits of both.

In recent years, there have been only two randomized clinical trials that assessed the effectiveness of diathermy. Both involved patients with osteoarthritis of the knee, and after the diathermy treatments, there were only slight improvements, which were not great enough to reach statistical significance. For now, therefore, it would seem that this therapy does not provide effective arthritis treatment.

Play It Smart with Heat Therapy
Heat can be very soothing, but don't apply heat to a joint that is already hot and swollen or continue heat treatment for more than about thirty minutes.

Other forms of locally applied heat, such as a heating pad, hot water bottle, or heat lamps, are valued by many with arthritis for the comfort they provide. Heating the skin increases blood circulation and helps the muscles relax.

Some people with arthritis consider the opposite treatment—cold therapy or cryotherapy—effective. Cold therapy is conducted by applying gel-filled, refreezable cold packs or plastic bags filled with ice to the joint, making sure to protect the skin with a layer of cloth, and to limit the treatment to twenty minutes every few hours. This therapy is fairly effective in reducing inflammation.

Hydrotherapy, in baths, spas, springs, tanks, or tubs, is one of the oldest and most enjoyable forms of medical treatment. Although its effects are temporary, they are pleasant and pain relieving. Hydrotherapy basically works by acting as a whole-body heat treatment, warming all the joints at once to ease both pain and stiffness (although it has no effect on inflammation, and heat is not recommended if there is inflammation).

Could Needles Relieve Pain, Instead of Causing It?

Acupuncture is a 2,000-year-old branch of Chinese medicine based on the belief that life force (called *chi*) flows through the body along meridians or channels. Blockage of these meridians leads to ill health, while opening the meridians with the use of needles inserted into the skin restores health. In fact, acupuncture is becoming an increasingly common and effective treatment for osteoarthritis.

Tap Into Your Natural Painkillers
Modern research suggests that acupuncture relieves the pain of arthritis and other conditions by causing the release of endorphins (the body's natural morphine) which act as natural painkillers.

A group of people waiting for a total hip replacement agreed to take part in a study. Half were treated with acupuncture, and the other half were given advice and a set of hip exercises. Over the eight-week study, the acupuncture group showed significant improvement, while the other group experienced no changes.

Other research has documented that real acupuncture, as opposed to sham acupuncture (where needles are inserted in sites not believed to have any health benefit) is more effective for pain relief of knee osteoarthritis than the sham treatment, which is equivalent to a placebo. Thus, this study shows that acupuncture has merit for use in osteoarthritis. Additional research found that acupuncture treatment in thirty-two osteoarthritis patients treated twice weekly for three weeks improved pain by 23 percent and mobility by 28 percent.

USING SUPPLEMENTS AND CONVENTIONAL MEDICINES

The arthritis-drug market is the source of big bucks for the pharmaceutical industry. These drugs bring in $6.6 billion per year, and this astounding number doesn't even include such standards in arthritis relief such as acetaminophen.

With all that money pouring into the pharmaceutical coffers, one would expect osteoarthritis patients to feel great. But the sad fact is that even though they're spending all that money on arthritis drugs, many patients do not get satisfactory relief from their pain and disability. Adding insult to injury, conventional arthritis drugs tend to come with an additional steep price: that of undesirable side effects.

Glucosamine and chondroitin are great, side–effect-free options to explore in place of conventional drugs. But you don't necessarily have to choose one over the other. There's no reason you can't maximize your osteoarthritis relief by taking a combination of both glucosamine/chondroitin and conventional arthritis drugs such as NSAIDs.

Conventional Treatments Fall Short

Although magazines and television are overflowing with ads for over-the-counter and prescription drugs for arthritis, the truth is that conventional medicine continues to fail in their search for a cure to arthritis. Instead they merely offer painkilling medications that only mask the problem (and come with a hefty price in side effects).

Aspirin is the most basic of anti-inflammatory drugs used to combat arthritis. The easing of the inflammation combined with its analgesic quality has made this the drug of choice for many people. Aspirin is a relatively inexpensive drug, but what it offers in reasonable pricing, it makes up for in harmful side effects which can include headaches, nausea, ringing in the ears, and/or stomach pain,.

Nonsteroidal anti-inflammatory drugs (NSAIDs) are used in cases where aspirin is unsuitable. NSAIDs, which include ibuprofen (Motrin), indomethacin (Indocin), fenoprofen (Nalfon), naproxen (Aleve), sulindac (Clinoril), tolmetin (Tolectin), and many others, are less likely than aspirin to cause stomach upset but have other harmful side effects. Newer generations of NSAIDs, such as celecoxib (Celebrex) and rofecoxib (Vioxx), have entered the market, but even these are not without problems.

NSAIDs act as painkillers while also reducing inflammation in the joints and soft tissues; they do not, however, cure or halt the progress of the disease. Their mechanism of action is to block the production of prostaglandins (hormonelike substances in the body that can produce inflammation and pain). The list of adverse effects from NSAIDs is numerous, and in some cases very severe, but the most common side effects are diarrhea, indigestion, nausea, and peptic ulcer.

Corticosteroids act similarly to natural hormones in order to suppress inflammation. However, since inflammation is a necessary process for the body's immune defense system, corticosteroids can impair the body's ability to deal with infections and injuries. These drugs may also suppress activity of the adrenal cortex. Corticosteroids are best used on a short-term basis.

Penicillamine, a synthetic derivative of penicillin, is another conventional treatment for arthritis. As with other conventional treatments, penicillamine can result in serious side effects, including bleeding, gastrointestinal upset, and liver problems.

Artificial Joints: Are They the Answer?

One other option of conventional medicine: radical surgery in which an artificial joint takes the place of the problematic joint. Even this extreme step is not a cure, since the artificial joint has a life span of only about ten years, when the surgery will have to be repeated. (Although there are exceptions, especially with cementless hip replacements where bone and metal fuse.) Despite the generally limited life span of artificial joints, lots of people with arthritis are going under the knife when their symptoms become so severe they feel there is no other option. In fact, joint replacement has become a common procedure. Each year, about 267,000 knee replacements and 168,000 artificial hip surgeries are performed.

A Closer Look at Pain Relievers

As previously stated, NSAIDs work by blocking the production of prostaglandins (hormonelike substances that can trigger inflammation). But blocking these inflammation-promoting prostaglandins is also the source of NSAIDs' side effects. Prostaglandins play other roles in the body; for example, they are needed to control the secretion of gastric juices and the mucus that serves as stomach lining. This

Integrative Medicine
Integrative medicine is based on the philosophy of using what works best for a patient, whether that is conventional or alternative medicine. For the case of osteoarthritis, integrative medicine might mean supplementing with glucosamine/ chondroitin and continuing to take a small amount of NSAIDs.

is why NSAIDs are linked to ulcers and even life-threatening gastric bleeding when used long-term.

NSAIDs cause some disturbing side effects, ranging from indigestion and gastrointestinal hemorrhage to kidney failure. These side effects are serious business, with the NSAID-induced hemorrhages leading to at least 103,000 hospitalizations each year and 16,500 deaths.

The Dark Side of NSAIDs
Nonsteroidal anti-inflammatory drugs (NSAIDs) are commonly used by those with arthritis, but they all too often cause side effects, such as stomach upset and ulcers.

And there is even worse news about standard drugs used for osteoarthritis pain. Aspirin and NSAIDs not only inhibit the repair of cartilage, they actually accelerate cartilage destruction. This means that, over time, aspirin and NSAIDs might actually worsen the disease they are "treating." In other words, although aspirin and NSAIDs might suppress symptoms, they also speed up the progression of the disease—not a worthwhile trade-off.

Cox-2 inhibitors (for example, Celebrex and Vioxx) were thought of as a breakthrough in improved arthritis treatment when they emerged on the market in 1999 because they target the specific prostaglandins that trigger inflammation, and don't affect those that play a role in stomach juices and mucus lining. However, the Cox-2 drugs come with a steep price tag ($3 to $6 per day) and, just recently, reports of a scary risk of side effects.

In the *Journal of the American Medical Association*, a leading cardiologist reported that Celebrex and Vioxx have a connection to heart problems. Specifically, these arthritis drugs could cause a small increase in heart attacks and ischemic strokes, a type of stroke. The cardiologist speculates that this risk is related to the drugs promoting the formation of blood clots.

While this new risk with Cox-2 drugs still requires further study to confirm, it leads one to wonder why anyone would take the unnecessary risk of putting their heart in jeopardy when there are safer, more effective, and cheaper alternatives such as glucosamine and chondroitin. Anyone with a personal or family history of heart disease should be especially careful of the risk that Cox-2 drugs might pose to cardiovascular health.

Glucosamine Works Better Than Conventional Medicine

Numerous head-to-head studies show that glucosamine is as effective as ibuprofen for symptomatic relief of osteoarthritis. For example, a group of 200 people with osteoarthritis of the knee agreed to take part in a one-month study. Half took 1,500 mg of glucosamine daily, and the other half took 1,200 mg of ibuprofen daily. Symptoms, including pain at night, pain after immobility, after standing, and after getting up from a chair, as well as walking dis-

tance and limitation of daily living activities, were recorded as a single score on the Lequesne index.

At the start of the study, the average Lequesne score for each group was sixteen. By the end of the study, both groups had dropped six points. In other words, the glucosamine was just as effective as the drug treatment.

The story is the same with chondroitin. Chondroitin sulfate (1,200 mg per day) was compared to 50 mg daily of the NSAID diclofenac (Voltaren). The Lequesne score dropped 78 percent with chondroitin, and 63 percent with diclofenac. When chondroitin was compared to ibuprofen (both groups took 1,200 mg daily), the chondroitin proved more effective in relieving symptoms.

Lequesne Index
A tool used in medical research to measure the severity of osteoarthritis symptoms. By combining the answers to a series of questions about ability to use a joint, pain, and range of motion, a single score is obtained.

It really makes sense to choose glucosamine and/or chondroitin instead of NSAIDs. You should get the same relief, and you'll skip the side effects.

Slow and Steady Wins the Race

The research is clear and unequivocal that glucosamine and chondroitin are just as effective as NSAIDs for symptomatic relief in osteoarthritis. However, there is a caveat. These supplements have a lag time before benefits are noted, whereas the NSAIDs are pretty much immediately effective.

For instance, in the glucosamine/ibuprofen study discussed earlier, 48 percent of the ibuprofen patients responded in the first week, but only 28 percent of the glucosamine group responded that quickly. By the end of the study, the numbers were neck and neck. Glucosamine and chondroitin take longer to work, but the wait is worth it.

Lessen Your Use of NSAIDs

A handful of studies have provided osteoarthritis patients with either glucosamine or chondroitin, and then let them continue to take their NSAID medication, as needed, for optimal pain relief. Without fail, these studies report that the need for NSAIDs drops with time. For instance, in one such study supplying 800 mg of chondroitin sulfate to those with osteoarthritis of the finger joints, hip, and/or knee, the amount of NSAIDs required to relieve pain was reduced by an impressive 72 percent.

In another study, also based on chondroitin supplements, NSAID use was allowed for severe pain. By the end of the trial, the patients took an average of 2.4 tablets of NSAIDs per month, whereas the placebo group was taking an average of 7.6 tablets.

The effect of glucosamine on inflammation has also been compared to NSAIDs. Remember that the main thing NSAIDs do is reduce inflammation. In an animal model, a combination of glucosamine and NSAIDs is best at reducing inflammation. In fact, this combination allowed the researchers to lower the NSAID dose two to three times and still retain the same amount of inflammation relief.

This means that even if you aren't able to entirely eliminate your use of NSAIDs, at least you will have lessened your risk for NSAID-related side effects by using fewer of these drugs.

Synergy of Treatment

The mechanism by which glucosamine/chondroitin quells inflammation in the body is different than that for NSAIDs. For this reason, some experts have suggested that the combined use of glucosamine/ chondroitin with NSAIDs might have a synergistic effect as anti-inflammatory agents.

The idea here is that glucosamine/chondroitin and NSAIDs, when taken at the same time, each contributes to easing inflammation in its own way. And the net effect is that inflammation vanishes from a swollen joint.

Try Glucosamine and Chondroitin Alone

There have been many examples in this section about how glucosamine and/or chondroitin supplements can work alongside NSAID medications. Even so, from a holistic health standpoint, it makes the most sense to try these supplements alone—that is, without the NSAIDs. NSAIDs always come with a risk of side effects.

If you can possibly cut NSAIDs out of your life, you'll be the better for it. However, that is not a realistic goal for some severe cases of osteoarthritis. In such cases, reducing reliance on NSAIDs would be the next best thing.

OSTEOARTHRITIS AND BEYOND

The lion's share of the research and attention about glucosamine and chondroitin is focused on osteoarthritis. But these supplements have other roles in health. Chances are, you started taking glucosamine or chondroitin for your stiff knee or achy hip, but did you know that your cholesterol levels might be dropping at the same time, and that your spouse may sleep better because you're not snoring? Let's look at the other benefits of glucosamine and chondroitin.

Atherosclerosis

Cardiovascular diseases claim the lives of almost one million Americans each year, more than any other disease. One in five Americans will eventually develop some form of cardiovascular disease. Although the initiation and progression of heart disease is a complex, multifaceted process, most research agrees that elevated cholesterol levels are a major contributor, since cholesterol is closely linked to the development of arteriosclerosis. Arteriosclerosis—com-

monly known as "hardening of the arteries"—occurs when the walls of the arteries lose their elasticity, thus interfering with proper circulation.

Atherosclerosis is the most common type of arteriosclerosis. With atherosclerosis, the hardening is a result of a buildup of fatty deposits. Atherosclerotic arteries are hard, inflexible, clogged with clumps of cholesterol, and more likely to develop high blood pressure. Even worse, when the coronary arteries (which feed the heart) are clogged, then the situation is known as coronary artery disease and the stage is set for a heart attack.

Tracking Your Cholesterol Numbers
The total cholesterol level generally deemed a low risk for heart disease is below 200 milligrams per deciliter of blood. If yours is above 240 mg/dl, there is cause for alarm.

Chondroitin sulfate has a documented role in protecting the health of blood vessels. Although the focus of this part of this book is on the role chondroitin plays in the joints, it is also found in the lining of the blood vessels where it helps prevent the movement of blood across the blood vessel lining, inhibits the clumping of blood platelets, and lowers blood cholesterol levels.

In all these roles, chondroitin contributes to healthier circulation and a lower risk of heart disease. Research has found that chondroitin does, indeed, prevent atherosclerosis in animals and humans, and further lowers the chances of a heart attack in people who already have the disease.

If you're taking chondroitin for an achy joint, it's nice to know that your heart might garner a little protection as well.

Dry Eyes

If your tear ducts don't make enough tears to keep your eyes moist, they can feel continually dry and irritated, with a burning, itchy sensation. Dry eyes are more common in women, especially after menopause. They can even be a symptom of a serious health problem, such as rheumatoid arthritis or lupus, or a side effect of medication.

Artificial tears are a common way to relieve symptoms. And there is research showing that the inclusion of chondroitin sulfate in artificial tear products can improve their ability to lessen the feelings of burning, itching and foreign body sensation. Chondroitin sulfate is not yet commercially available in artificial tear products, but it should be in the not-too-distant future.

Kidney Stones

Kidney stones, which are much more common in Western countries, can be formed when substances in urine, such as calcium, precipitate into stones, calcium oxalate stones being the most common type. Kidney stones result in severe pain, accompanied by chills, fever, and nausea.

Chondroitin can lend a hand since it is naturally present in the urinary system, in such places as the bladder wall lining. One study reports that oral administration of glycosaminoglycans (chondroitin and related compounds) lowers urinary oxalate levels in individuals prone to accumulating oxalates, and lower oxalate levels are presumed to result in fewer kidney stones.

If you are prone to kidney stones, make sure you drink plenty of water, eat a high-fiber diet, minimize your intake of animal proteins, and avoid chocolate, spinach, and rhubarb (all sources of oxalate).

Migraine

Migraines are a regular occurrence for 26 million Americans. These intense headaches are triggered by disturbances of the blood vessels in the head and, on average, last more than seventeen hours. There is an intriguing case report in the medical literature about glucosamine and migraines. It seems that a frequent migraine sufferer was taking glucosamine for osteoarthritis, and in the course of that treatment, the patient's migraines stopped.

To ascertain whether this was a real benefit of glucosamine, or simply a coincidence, ten volunteers who regularly faced migraines were asked to take glucosamine supplements daily. After a four-to-six week period in which no major changes were noted, the volunteers started to report a substantial drop in the frequency and/or intensity of their headaches. Glucosamine's role in blood-vessel-health is hypothesized to be the source of its benefits for migraine.

Snoring

There is an interesting study where chondroitin sulfate was sprayed into the noses of chronic snorers. Because chondroitin sulfate forms a coating on the nasal passages, this is thought to curtail snoring. The study found that it did indeed help—the snorers only snored for two-thirds of their usual snoring time. It is not yet known if oral (pill) forms of chondroitin would provide this same benefit.

TMJ

Temporomandibular joint syndrome (TMJ) is a disorder of the joint in the jaw bone. Chronic neck pain, headaches, "popping" noises when using the jaw, toothaches, and overall pain are the hallmark symptoms of TMJ. The cause of TMJ is often traced to clenching the jaw muscles and tooth grinding, behaviors which, in turn, exert pressure on the jaw joint and can wear down the cartilage there, essentially leading to osteoarthritis in that joint.

There is a report of fifty TMJ patients who were treated with either glucosamine or a mixture of chondroitin and vitamin C. An impressive

Simple TMJ Test
To see if you might have TMJ, put your pinkies in your ears and press forward. Then, open and close your mouth. If you hear a clicking noise and feel your jawbone push against your fingers, you might have TMJ and should consult a health professional.

80 percent of these patients responded to the treatment with a reduction in joint noises, pain, and swelling. These benefits were evident within the first two weeks of the study.

In another study, forty-five TMJ patients were randomly assigned to take either glucosamine or ibuprofen over a three-month period for their TMJ symptoms. Three-quarters of the glucosamine group responded to the treatment, while only 61 percent of the ibuprofen group improved. When the patients who responded to either treatment were examined more closely, it was found that the glucosamine led to a significantly greater pain reduction than the ibuprofen.

Ulcers

Stomach ulcers are a common problem, affecting one out of every ten people in their lifetime. Stomach ulcers (technically known as peptic ulcers) are caused when the mucous membrane of the stomach or upper portion of the intestines become eroded, and are worsened by the constant exposure to acidic stomach juices in the eroded area. NSAID medications irritate the protective mucous membranes, setting the stage for ulcers which cause burning pain and sometimes nausea.

When osteoarthritis patients are able to toss out their NSAID medications in favor of glucosamine, they are at lower risk for ulcers since the ulcer-promoting NSAIDs are no longer in their system. If you are even able to reduce your reliance on NSAIDs by using glucosamine, your stomach stands to benefit. Glucosamine, unlike NSAIDs, does not irritate the GI tract, and it has another benefit: glucosamine stimulates the production of protective gastric mucus which could potentially bolster the stomach's resistance to ulcers.

Wound Healing

The healing of wounds requires, among other things, the raw materials to make replacement skin and other soft tissues. Glucosamine and chondroitin both qualify as such raw materials. Laboratory studies on animals and humans all document that glucosamine and chondroitin promote improved healing of wounds.

SAFETY PROFILE

Glucosamine and chondroitin are made by the body for use in several locations, including the joints. This bodes well for their safety profile because compounds that are not foreign to the body are less likely to cause problems, and this certainly seems to be the case with glucosamine and chondroitin. Even so, there are a handful of safety concerns to consider, particularly if you have shellfish allergies or a sensitive stomach.

Chondroitin might have a mild blood-thinning effect, and for this reason people taking anticoagulant (blood-thinning) drugs should use this supplement with caution, or better yet use a product containing only glucosamine, which does not have this effect.

It's a relief to know that glucosamine and chondroitin supplements have been safely used in osteoarthritis patients with other health problems, such as circulatory disease, depression, diabetes, liver disorders, and lung disorders. In all these cases, the glucosamine and chondroitin supplementation for osteoarthritis did not interfere with the course or treatment of those other conditions.

Slight Stomach Upset Most Common Problem

All the clinical trials of glucosamine and chondroitin include reports on side effects and, in study after study, the research has consistently documented the safety and tolerability of these supplements. For instance, in one study evaluating the tolerability of glucosamine in 1,208 patients, 88 percent of those taking this supplement reported absolutely no side effects. Of the side effects reported by the other 12 percent, all of them were mild. Most common was the approximately 3 to 5 percent of people who reported diarrhea, heartburn, nausea, and/ or stomach upset, a finding that is consistent with the adverse events reported in other studies. Similarly, with chondroitin about 3 percent of users report nausea or stomach upset.

Keep in mind that this slight risk of GI upset is still much lower than the risk of stomach problems seen with the use of NSAIDs. In fact, in one animal model, the researchers found that the toxicity of glucosamine compared to the NSAID indometacin was ten to thirty times more favorable for the glucosamine than for the NSAID.

Diabetics Can Rest Assured

For a while, the safety of glucosamine supplements for people with diabetes came into question. Some rat studies had found that the continuous administration of high doses of intravenous glucosamine led to insulin resistance. However, these very high levels of glucosamine are vastly different from the standard low doses of glucosamine pills taken by people.

Understanding Insulin Resistance
Insulin is a hormone needed to regulate levels of sugar in the blood. When the body is resistant to insulin, blood-sugar levels can increase and interfere with normal body functions.

The definitive word in glucosamine's safety for those with diabetes came from a large, three-year placebo-controlled study of glucosamine. This study carries much more weight than the rat studies since, for starters, it is actually with people instead of animals. In addition, the long duration of this study is another mark in its favor. In this study, people taking standard doses of glucosamine did not show any

increases in blood-sugar levels. In fact, the opposite was true. There was actually a slight decrease in fasting blood sugar levels in the glucosamine users, compared to the placebo group's levels.

And, when analyzed separately, patients who entered the study with baseline blood-sugar levels that were higher than normal showed a tendency for their blood sugar to drop while taking glucosamine.

If you have diabetes and want to be completely safe while taking glucosamine supplements, simply increase your blood-sugar monitoring. If you notice any elevation, stop taking the supplement and see if your blood sugar then drops.

Mind Your Minerals

There have been reports that some glucosamine supplements contain too much manganese, a mineral generally found in combination products as manganese ascorbate. Although there have been no symptoms of manganese toxicity reported by any studies, there is a theoretical risk.

The Tolerable Upper Intake Level for manganese, established by the National Academy of Sciences' Institute of Medicine, is 11 mg per day. In a 2001 study, some glucosamine supplements were found to provide up to 30 mg per dosage. Fortunately, in light of the newly established Tolerable Upper Intake Level for manganese, many manufacturers are reformulating their products to be within recommended levels, and this is unlikely to be a problem in the future.

Signs of Too Much Manganese
Manganese toxicity can cause coughs, hypertension, iron-deficiency anemia neurological problems, tremor, and weakness.

As an interesting aside, many Americans are at risk for too little manganese, rather than too much. It is estimated that 37 percent of Americans have low manganese intake.

Mad Cow Disease: Is It a Concern?

Mad cow disease is the commonly used name for bovine spongiform encephalopathy (BSE), a serious disease affecting cows. BSE is a degenerative neurologic disorder that most recently emerged in Europe in the 1980s. Its appearance in cows has been traced back to the use of diseased sheep parts in cattle feed, since sheep can suffer from a similar disease. But until BSE began appearing in cows, farmers did not know the disease could pass between these two species.

What does a cow's disease mean to you? Well, it seems this disease can also transfer between the species of cow and human. The BSE-related form of this disease that strikes humans is called variant Creutzfeldt-Jakob disease (vCJD), and several cases have been found in Europe.

Chondroitin is manufactured from bovine (cow) trachea. Theoretically, BSE could be transmitted through cow-derived products, such as chondroitin supplements. However, there are numerous safeguards in place to ensure the safety of beef products. For starters, the Food and Drug Administration (FDA) has import restrictions prohibiting the importation of beef or other cow parts for use in foods or dietary supplements from countries with known cases of BSE. Furthermore, protective steps are taken in the manufacturing process, including the use of cows only from certified non-BSE countries and the enzymatic digestion of all proteins (the infective part causing BSE is a protein fragment).

So the bottom line is that you should be no more concerned about the risk of vCJD from dietary supplements than you are from the meat you might eat. Meat and supplements derived from animal sources are held to the same standards to protect the public from vCJD.

Shellfish Allergies: Proceed with Caution

If you have an allergy to shellfish, you should avoid glucosamine supplements. Many glucosamine products are manufactured from crab shells, and there is a slight risk that some of the crabmeat could inadvertently be included along with the shell during the manufacturing process. Even though the risk is small, erring on the side of safety means avoiding these supplements.

Always a Good Idea to Consult Your Doctor

You don't need a doctor's prescription to buy the dietary supplements glucosamine and chondroitin, or the others discussed in this book, such as vitamin C, vitamin D, and SAMe. However, it is a good idea to consult with your physician before treating your osteoarthritis.

For example, it's important to ensure that osteoarthritis is the source of your joint symptoms, rather than a different joint condition such as bursitis, gout, lupus, or rheumatoid arthritis. The following chart shows the main symptoms of these different disorders.

CONDITION	MAIN SYMPTOMS
Bursitis	Pain and swelling in a joint caused by inflammation of a bursa, a saclike membrane between bone and tissues near a joint. Often traced to a sports injury.
Gout	Metabolic disorder most frequently affecting the big toe. Sudden, sharp, painful attack of tenderness in the joint. Most common in men over age forty who have a family history of this condition.

CONDITION	MAIN SYMPTOMS
Lupus	Joint pain, redness, and swelling, that varies from day to day, most often affecting the fingers and wrists. Chest pain, coughing, fatigue, rashes, and sunlight sensitivity often present. Women in their twenties and thirties are most often affected.
Osteoarthritis	Joint pain, limited range of motion, stifness. Usually starts in just one joint, often after an injury or overuse. More common with increasing age.
Rheumatoid arthritis	Autoimmune disorder, with joint inflammation as key manifestation. Loss of motion, pain, redness comes and goes.

CONCLUSION

If dietary supplements have a good chance of helping you and cause no harm—why wouldn't you give them a try? Such is the case with glucosamine and chondroitin for osteoarthritis. The argument for trying these supplements is bolstered by the fact that they can replace, or at least reduce, your use of NSAID medications that have a clearly documented potential for harm.

Sir William Osler, a nineteenth century British physician, stated his disappointment over not having a viable treatment for arthritis: "When a patient with arthritis walks in the front door, I feel like leaving out the back door." In the many years since he made that statement, not much has changed in terms of any success for conventional medicine in treating arthritis. This lack of success is not for lack of trying. Most of those with arthritis are overwhelmed by one side–effect-provoking medication after another. But until one of these drugs is able to treat arthritis without excessive side effects, arthritis will remain conventional medicine's failure.

This is where glucosamine, chondroitin, and other dietary supplements come in. While these supplements can't promise to be a magic bullet, they do have a lot to offer—from decreasing reliance on NSAIDs to doing what doctors can't: relieving the inflammation, mobility impairments, and pain of arthritis while actually promoting the growth of new, healthy cartilage.

If you are among the more than one in ten Americans currently suffering from osteoarthritis, relief cannot come too soon. Give glucosamine and/or chondroitin a try.

PART EIGHT

ST. JOHN'S WORT

LAUREL VUKOVIC, MSW

Everyone suffers from passing moods. True, it doesn't feel good to be sad, blue, or down-in-the-dumps, but changing emotions are a part of what makes us human. It's not realistic to expect to always be happy, or to always feel good. Feelings of sadness and loss are a normal part of life.

However, severe or persistent feelings of sadness or hopelessness erode well-being and significantly interfere with the enjoyment of daily life and the ability to function normally. According to the World Health Organization, major depression is the leading cause of disability in the United States and throughout the rest of the world. The National Institute of Mental Health reports the sobering fact that approximately 17 million American adults suffer from depression each year—more than are stricken with cancer or heart disease.

Fortunately, depressive disorders are highly treatable illnesses. Great strides have been made in recent decades in the physiological and psychological treatment of depression, including natural approaches to treating depressive disorders. By reading this book, you'll gain an understanding of depression and the many things that you can do to alleviate these debilitating conditions.

In this part of *User's Guide to Nutritional Supplements*, you'll learn about depression and who it affects. You'll find clear descriptions of the symptoms of depressive disorders, along with a simple self-test for depression. Most important, you will learn a great deal of information about effective treatments for depressive disorders. You'll discover the pros and cons of the prescription drugs that are so commonly prescribed for treating depression, and you'll gain a solid knowledge of the natural alternatives available. You'll understand why one of the most highly regarded, well-researched, effective, and safe alternatives to prescription antidepressants is the herb St. John's wort.

In this part of the book, you'll find in-depth and simple-to-understand answers to your questions about St. John's wort. You'll find out how to safely use St. John's wort, and you'll be informed about the most effective forms and dosages of this herb. There are many scientific studies that support the use of this valuable herb for the treatment of

depression, and you'll learn about some of these important studies in these pages.

First things first. Read on to discover more about exactly what St. John's wort is, and how it has come to be a renowned herbal treatment for depression.

SO YOU'RE CURIOUS ABOUT ST. JOHN'S WORT

If you're reading this part of the book, you've most likely heard something about St. John's wort. You've probably heard that it can help alleviate feelings of depression. And you might be wondering if St. John's wort could be helpful for you or someone you know.

Perhaps you've been feeling blue lately or have struggled with depression for a long time. Or you might be feeling anxious and are having difficulty sleeping. You might even have tried antidepressant medications, but are unhappy with the side effects or would like to try a more natural approach.

If you are suffering from depression, St. John's wort, an herb with a long history of use in the treatment of emotional distress, may be helpful for you. In a nutshell, it has been found to be most beneficial for people suffering from mild to moderate depression. It's also been found to be helpful for alleviating anxiety and insomnia related to depression, and for depression related to premenstrual syndrome (PMS), menopause, and seasonal affective disorder (SAD).

What Is St. John's Wort?

A perennial plant native to Europe, St. John's wort (*Hypericum perforatum*) has naturalized and grows abundantly along roadsides and other sunny open spaces throughout North and South America, Asia, Africa, and Australia. It was most likely introduced to North America by early European colonists, and is now grown commercially because of its valuable medicinal properties.

St. John's wort is a nondescript, weedy looking plant that

is easy to overlook until mid-summer, when it bursts into a flush of tiny, bright yellow star-shaped flowers. The small, oval leaves are dotted with tiny perforations, hence the species name, *perforatum*.

If you crush a fresh flower bud, it will release a deep reddish purple oil. This substance is called hypericin, and is considered to be one of the primary active ingredients that gives St. John's wort its healing properties.

Hypericin
A natural chemical compound found in St. John's wort that is considered to be one of the herb's primary active ingredients.

One theory as to the origin of the common name of the herb is that early Christians named St. John's wort in honor of John the Baptist. The plant blooms around the time of St. John's Day (June 24) and the herb was traditionally collected on this day, steeped in olive oil to release its blood-red color, and used as an anointing oil to symbolize the blood of the saint. The Latin botanical name *Hypericum* is derived from the Greek word *yper*, which means "upper," and the word *eikon*, which means "image." Early Greeks and Romans placed St. John's wort in their homes above statues of their gods as a protection against evil spirits.

Historical Uses of St. John's Wort

In ancient Europe, St. John's wort was believed to have protective powers against the unseen forces of evil. In Greece and Rome, the herb was used for protection against sorcerer's spells, and early Christians believed that St. John's wort drove away evil spirits. It may be that the people who were considered to be possessed by evil spirits were actually suffering from mental illness and were helped by using St. John's wort. By the time the colonists brought St. John's wort to America, the herb had a reputation for being effective as an antidepressant and for topical wound healing.

Throughout more than 2,000 years of use as a healing herb, St. John's wort has been valued for treating nerve injuries, inflammation, sciatica, ulcers, and burns. But the most compelling use that has brought St. John's wort to the forefront of herbal medicine and the attention of millions of people was the confirmation of the herb's remarkable effects as a natural antidepressant.

Since 1979, St. John's wort has been the subject of more than two dozen rigorous, double-blind, controlled clinical studies. Most of these studies were conducted in Europe, which has a long history of using herbs as alternatives to drugs in the treatment of mental and physical diseases. These well-designed studies have shown that St. John's wort is just as effective as pharmaceutical drugs for treating mild to moderate depression. As a result, St. John's wort is one of the most prescribed treatments for mild to moderate cases of depression in Germany, and has become one of the top ten best-selling dietary supplements in the

United States. In 1998, United States consumers purchased $170 million dollars worth of St. John's wort.

St. John's Wort—A Hidden Healer

Although St. John's wort was known as a valuable healing herb for thousands of years, it's only been within the past few years that the herb's value has been fully recognized in the United States. That's because herbal medicine, along with other forms of healing, like homeopathy, that are now considered "alternative medicine," were edged out of popular use by the rise of the conventional medical establishment many decades ago.

From the mid-1800s through the 1930s, there were two primary schools of medicine practiced in the United States. The orthodox physicians (known as "regulars") practiced conventional medicine, while the Eclectic physicians relied heavily on the use of herbs for healing, much as naturopathic physicians do today. With the discovery of pharmaceutical antibiotics, which appeared to work miracles, orthodox medicine gained a position of power in the United States and drove out the Eclectics.

Naturopathy
A method of treating illness that relies on herbs, diet, and other natural approaches to restore the body to health.

But as we've seen in recent decades, so-called miracle drugs can be a double-edged sword. The antibiotics that were hailed as cures for contagious and often deadly diseases did, in fact, cure individuals. But the overuse and overprescribing of those drugs have created strains of even deadlier antibiotic-resistant bacteria. Epidemiologists and scientists warn that these bacteria could cause mass epidemics, which essentially puts us back at square one in the fight against contagious disease.

The same thing is happening with the medical establishment's reliance on antidepressant drugs. These drugs, especially the most recent varieties, have been prescribed as mood-enhancers for millions of Americans. Touted as safe and effective, three antidepressant medications (Prozac, Zoloft, and Paxil) are among the top-ten selling prescription medications in the United States. But the backlash of overprescribing antidepressants is now being recognized, as more and more stories about unpleasant and lethal side effects—including suicide—and the difficulties of withdrawing from these drugs are coming to light.

How St. John's Wort Gained Recognition

Fortunately, herbal medicine never took a beating in Europe the way it did in the United States. European doctors have always regarded herbs as legitimate medical treatments, and herbal products are commonly sold in European pharmacies. The consumer-driven trend toward natural medicine, including herbal medicine, has fueled the popularity of herbs, including St. John's wort. The long history of St. John's wort as a safe and effective treatment for depression and the dozens of well-researched studies that provide scientific support for St. John's wort make it a logical choice as a natural remedy for alleviating mild to moderate depression.

St. John's wort is the most thoroughly researched of all natural antidepressant remedies. It has been shown to relieve the sadness, irritability, anxiety, hopelessness, sleep disturbances, exhaustion, and other symptoms of depression as well as prescription antidepressants. There are several advantages to using St. John's wort instead of pharmaceutical drugs: St. John's wort has far fewer side effects than drugs (and when side effects do occur, they tend to be minor), St. John's wort extracts cost significantly less than pharmaceutical antidepressants, and patients tend to report greater satisfaction with St. John's wort than with drugs.

Today, St. John's wort is approved by the German Commission E, a regulatory agency similar to the U.S. Food and Drug Administration (FDA), for internal use for the treatment of depression and anxiety, and externally for the treatment of wounds, burns, bruises, and muscle pain.

UNDERSTANDING AND DIAGNOSING DEPRESSION

Occasional feelings of sadness in response to life situations and disappointments are a normal part of being human. Losing a job, moving and leaving behind friends, relationship difficulties, children leaving home, a serious or chronic illness, or the death of a loved one all can bring on feelings of sadness and loss. However, these passing states, although commonly labeled as depression, are very different from the serious illness known as a depressive disorder.

SYMPTOMS OF DEPRESSION

- Prolonged sadness or unexplained crying spells.
- Significant changes in appetite or sleep patterns.
- Irritability, anger, worry, agitation, anxiety.
- Pessimism, indifference.
- Loss of energy, persistent tiredness.
- Feelings of guilt, worthlessness.
- Inability to concentrate, indecisiveness.
- Inability to take pleasure in former interests.
- Unexplained aches or pains.
- Recurring thoughts of death or suicide.

Sadness versus Depression

Distinguishing between normal feelings of sadness and clinical depression is an important first step in recognizing and treating a depressive disorder. It can be a challenging task, because the fluctuating moods that are typical of everyday life can make differentiating between normal and abnormal challenging. Psychiatrists and psychotherapists diagnose someone as being clinically depressed if the person has had at least five specific symptoms of depression for at least two weeks, or if the symptoms have significantly impaired the person's ability to function at work, at school, or in relationships. (In the next section, you'll find out more about these specific symptoms.)

Although we tend to think of depression as involving the mind, it also has a significant effect on the body. Depression impairs well-being on many levels, and interferes with normal patterns of sleeping, eating, exercise, work, relationships, and leisure. Depression significantly affects thoughts, moods, and behaviors. It's not uncommon for a person who is depressed to lose interest in life, even to the point of thinking about suicide.

It's important to realize that anyone can suffer from depression. Certainly, depression is not a sign of weakness, nor is it something of which to be ashamed. In fact, some very prominent people in history—including Abraham Lincoln, Ludwig von Beethoven, Mark Twain, Georgia O'Keefe, and Vincent Van Gogh—have suffered from depression. No one is guaranteed immunity—people of every age, religion, race, and economic and social group are stricken with depression.

Fortunately, through medical research and modern psychotherapy, we have learned a great deal about depression and how to effectively treat it. According to the American Psychiatric Association, up to 90 percent of all cases of depression can be treated. But it's essential to recognize the need for help. The National Institute of Mental Health reports that two of every three people who suffer from depression don't get the help they need.

Some people simply aren't aware that they are suffering from a depressive disorder. They know that they aren't feeling well, but may think that their symptoms are caused by fatigue or stress. Others are too ashamed to seek help, or may be so worn down by their depression that making the effort to get help is too overwhelming to consider. And according to the National Alliance for the Mentally Ill, professionals may even have a difficult time making a clear diagnosis of a depressive disorder. They report that, on average, it takes almost eight years from the onset of depression for an individual to obtain a proper diagnosis.

The Different Faces of Depression

The most common types of depression are major depression, dysthymia, and bipolar disorder. Major depression (also known as unipolar depression) tends to occur in episodes, and can be so debilitating that it becomes difficult for the sufferer to perform the basic tasks of daily life, or even to get out of bed. This severe form of depression tends to be a chronic, recurring illness.

Although a traumatic life event can provoke a major depressive episode, not all stressful events cause depression, and not all depressive episodes are triggered by a stressful event. According to the U.S. Department of Health and Human Services, major depression affects approximately 15 percent of Americans at some time in life. In economic terms, depression costs the United States approximately $43 billion a year in lost productivity, absenteeism, and medical costs, estimates the National Depressive and Manic Depressive Association. The costs to a human life are immeasurable. Tragically, approximately 15 percent of those who suffer from chronic depression will eventually commit suicide.

Major Depression
A form of depression that tends to occur in episodes; so debilitating that it becomes difficult for the sufferer to perform the basic tasks of daily life.

Symptoms of depression include persistent feelings of sadness, crying spells, feelings of hopelessness, a loss of pleasure in activities that previously were enjoyed, significant changes in appetite or body weight, difficulty sleeping or sleeping excessively, decreased energy, loss of sexual desire, difficulty concentrating or making decisions, restlessness and irritability, feelings of worthlessness or guilt, and thoughts of death or suicide. Recurring physical symptoms such as headaches, chronic pain, and chronic digestive disorders can also be part of the profile of depression. A person is diagnosed with major depression (also called major depressive disorder or unipolar major depression) if they have five or more of these symptoms persisting for two weeks or longer.

Dysthymia is a less severe form of depression that takes the form of chronic symptoms that can persist for years. People with dysthymia often suffer from low energy, fatigue, sleep disturbances (either oversleeping or insomnia), and appetite disturbances (either poor appetite or overeating).

Dysthymia
A milder form of depression with chronic symptoms that can persist for years.

An individual suffering from dysthymia can generally go about the business of attending to the necessities of daily life, but she feels a persistent lack of pleasure or joy, does not function at her best, and may frequently be irritable and complain of stress. Because they are able to function in daily life, many people with dysthymia are unaware that they are suffering from a depressive disorder. As a result, they don't seek help, but endure the symptoms of depression and the subsequent loss of pleasure and productivity that characterize a healthy life.

Approximately 10 million Americans suffer from dysthymia

each year. A diagnosis of dysthymia is made when a depressed mood in an adult persists for at least two years (one year in children or adolescents) and the mood is accompanied by at least two other symptoms of depression.

Bipolar disorder, more commonly known as manic-depressive illness, is less common than the other types of depression, and affects only about one percent of Americans. There is often a family history of manic depression in people who develop this illness. Bipolar disorder usually strikes in late adolescence, often first appearing as depression. But it can also develop in early childhood, or the initial episode may occur in mid-life.

Bipolar disorder is characterized by episodes of major depression that alternate with excessively elevated moods known as mania. Symptoms of mania include irritability, excessive talking, a decreased need for sleep, racing thoughts, agitation, overly inflated self-esteem, inappropriate social behavior, and impulsive behaviors that may involve dangerous activities.

The depressive symptoms of bipolar disorder parallel those of major (unipolar) depression. Because of this, and the fact that manic episodes don't often make an appearance until a person reaches their mid-twenties, people with bipolar disorder may be diagnosed simply with depression. This can be problematic, because the use of antidepressants can bring on a manic episode in someone who actually has bipolar disorder. Working closely with a mental health professional who is skilled in the treatment of bipolar disorder is essential.

Bipolar Disorder
A depressive disorder characterized by episodes of major depression that alternate with excessively elevated moods known as mania.

Although the mood shifts between depression and mania can be sudden, they most often take place gradually over a period of weeks or months. Many people who have bipolar disorder notice that they tend to feel depressed more often in the winter and have symptoms of mania more frequently in the spring.

It's important to note that depression varies from person to person, and that not everyone who is depressed experiences every symptom. Other variables in depression include the severity of symptoms and the response of the individual to treatment. In the vast majority of cases, however, depression is treatable.

What Causes Depression?

Depression has many different causes, and researchers and mental health professionals are still attempting to understand this complex disorder. Many studies indicate a biochemical and genetic basis for some types of depression. That's why depression sometimes appears to run in families, with depression recurring through the generations. Studies of identical twins support the theory that depression has a genetic basis. Researchers have found that if one twin suffers from depression, the other has a 70 percent chance of also being depressed (this holds true even if the twins are separated at birth and raised apart from each other).

But not everyone who has a family history of depression will necessarily fall prey to the illness. And many people with no family history of depression become depressed. A variety of other factors, such as a significant loss, or relationship, family, work, school, financial, and social stresses can trigger the onset of depression.

Genetic
A hereditary tendency passed down from one generation to another through the genes.

Coping Styles and Depression

Personality characteristics and coping styles also play a critical role in depression. People with low self-esteem or those who tend to have a pessimistic outlook are more likely to suffer from depression, as are those who have a low tolerance for the stresses of everyday life. A psychological theory of depression developed by Martin Seligman, Ph.D., in the 1960s (known as the "learned helplessness model") demonstrated that animals who were subjected to situations where they were helpless became depressed, and exhibited changes in brain chemistry that were indicative of depression.

When the dogs in his study were given antidepressant drugs, their brain chemistry changed for the better and their depression lifted. However, when the dogs were taught how to gain control over their environment, their brain chemistry also became normal. This study is significant in that it supports the theory that people who feel helpless and hopeless undergo brain chemistry changes that are associated with depression, and that learning to be self-empowered can alleviate depression.

Depression Is Not a Character Flaw

It's important to remember that depression is not a sign of personal weakness, nor is it a character flaw. Genetics may play a role in personality structure, but for the most part, these behavioral styles are learned at an early age in the individual's family of origin. An emphasis on learning new behavior and thinking patterns is one of the primary psychological approaches to alleviating depression.

Many physicians immediately prescribe drugs to treat depression, but psychotherapy may work just as well, at least in cases of mild to moderate depression. Teaching people to be more optimistic is one of the most powerful techniques for shifting brain chemistry into a healthy balance. In his studies, Seligman observed that optimistic people rarely, if ever, became helpless and depressed. On the other hand, people who had a pessimistic view of life were highly likely to sink into depression when they encountered challenging life stressors.

Behavioral and attitude changes also generally take time and practice, and the appropriate use of antidepressant medications can help to ease the immediate symptoms to make psychological work more beneficial. St. John's wort is an excellent alternative to psychiatric medications because the lack of side effects makes it easier for many patients to tolerate.

Physical Causes of Depression

In addition to genetic causes and learned behavioral styles, physical illness can also be at the root of depression. Serious illnesses such as a heart attack, stroke, cancer, and rheumatoid arthritis are commonly accompanied by feelings of depression. For example, according to the U.S. Department of Health and Human Services, a person who has suffered a heart attack has a 40 percent chance of becoming depressed. Changes in body chemistry, such as the hormonal shifts that occur during menopause and pregnancy, also can trigger depression.

It's essential to check for the possibility of an underlying physiological cause for depression. If the physical causes aren't addressed, then any attempt at treating the depression will be less successful. Some of the common underlying physical disorders that can cause or contribute to depression include nutrient deficiencies, hypoglycemia, hormonal imbalances (particularly insufficient thyroid or adrenal hormones), allergies, and drug use (including alcohol, caffeine, and prescription drugs).

Hormonal Aspects of Depression

A number of hormones have a significant influence on mood. Many times, physicians neglect to consider hormone levels as an important factor in the treatment of depression. For example, low thyroid function (also known as hypothyroidism) is frequently overlooked by physicians as a cause of depression. Even minute decreases in thyroid hormones can negatively affect the body and mind. Other symptoms of hypothyroidism include fatigue, skin dryness, constipation, feeling cold, difficulties concentrating, and weight gain. If you suspect that your thyroid might not be functioning up to par, ask your doctor to perform a complete endocrine workup, including testing for thyroid hormones.

Hypothyroidism
A common condition of low thyroid function that can cause depression.

Adrenal hormones also play a critical role in depression. Long-term stress, which is frequently a precipitating factor in depression, affects the hormonal output of the adrenal glands. An increased level of cortisol (a hormone released during times of stress) causes mood changes such as nervousness, insomnia, anxiety, and depression. Living under highly stressful condi-

Cortisol
A hormone secreted by the adrenal glands in response to stress; causes mood changes such as anxiety and depression.

tions, or not having adequate coping skills, can cause the adrenal glands to continue secreting cortisol even when the stressful events have subsided.

The use of alcohol, recreational drugs, and even prescription drugs can bring on a depressive disorder in susceptible people. And depressive disorders are a common factor in other emotionally based illnesses such as eating disorders, substance abuse, and anxiety disorders.

Even the change of seasons, from summer to winter, can bring on a type of depression known as seasonal affective disorder, or SAD. The symptoms generally begin in the fall, as the days grow shorter and daylight decreases, and last until spring. Seasonal affective disorder is characterized by fatigue, oversleeping, overeating, and anxiety. Researchers believe that this depressive disorder is triggered by a decline in natural mood-enhancing brain chemicals and is associated with the decrease in sunlight during the winter.

Seasonal Affective Disorder
A depressive disorder associated with the decrease in sunlight during the winter.

In many cases, the first episode of a depressive disorder is triggered by a combination of situational and psychological stressors as well as a possible genetic predisposition toward depression. Subsequent episodes of depression may occur in response to mild stressors or without any apparent cause.

WHO SUFFERS FROM DEPRESSION?

Anyone can suffer from depression. According to the National Institute of Mental Health, depressive disorders most often first occur between the ages of twenty and fifty, with the average age of onset about forty. But people of any age can suffer from depression. There are certain characteristics that seem to apply to specific groups of people.

Depression in Women

Women are far more likely than men to be depressed. In fact, women are twice as likely as men to suffer from depression, and approximately one of every four women will experience clinical depression at some time during her life. This statistic holds true regardless of racial or ethnic background or economic status. In women, depression often appears as a pervasive feeling of helplessness and hopelessness.

Fluctuating hormones during the menstrual cycle, pregnancy, and menopause play a role in a woman's susceptibility to depression. As many as one in ten mothers experience depression after childbirth. These feelings range from a relatively mild case of the blues to major clinical depression; in many cases, women who suffer major depression postpartum have often had prior episodes of depression, although they may not have been diagnosed or treated.

Postpartum Depression
Depression in women that occurs after childbirth.

Because they feel badly about feeling depressed at a time when they think they should be especially happy, women may have difficulties seeking help. Not surprisingly, many women also find the increased stresses of juggling work, family, and household responsibilities cause anxiety and depression.

Depression in Men

Although men are not diagnosed with depression as often as are women, the incidence of depression in men may be higher than it appears. Men are less likely to acknowledge feeling depressed, and tend to cover up their feelings with excessive alcohol or drug use. Many men also bury their depressed feelings in working long hours.

Because depression in men often takes the form of anger, irritability, and emotional withdrawal, others may not realize that a man is depressed. Even physicians are less likely to suspect depression in a man than in a woman. To complicate matters, although a man may be aware of feeling depressed, he is much less inclined than a woman to seek help. This may be the reason why the rate of suicide in men is four times that of women, despite the fact that more women make suicide attempts.

Depression in Children

It's only recently that depression in children has been recognized as a serious problem. Mental health professionals estimate that as many as one of every thirty-three children and one in eight adolescents suffers from depression. Children manifest depression in various ways that may not look on the surface like a depressive disorder. Young children may feign illness, resist going to school, or be excessively fearful. Older children may get into trouble at school, do poorly in classes, exhibit an overall negative attitude, and have difficulty getting along with others.

Depression in children can be difficult to recognize because children naturally go through various stages that can be trying for the child and the parent. A warning sign that something is awry is if symptoms of fear, school problems, or a negative attitude persist. Other behaviors to be aware of include frequent absences from school, isolation from peers, or reckless behavior.

Depression in the Elderly

As a group, the elderly have perhaps been the most neglected in both the recognition and treatment of depression. Because so many older people suffer from depression, some people mistakenly believe that depression is a normal part of aging. This is not true, although approximately one-sixth of Americans over the age of sixty-five suffer from a depressive disorder. Because the symptoms may primarily manifest under the guise of fatigue or other physical complaints, depression is often overlooked in the elderly.

For many older people, depression takes the form of a loss of interest in activities that were formerly pleasurable, a sense of hopelessness about the future, and persistent feelings of sadness. Depression is often triggered by the loss of a spouse or chronic health problems. In the elderly, a depressive disorder has the potential for the most serious health consequences. Those who do not receive treatment for depression are more likely to have poor outcomes associated with the treatment of other illnesses such as heart disease and diabetes. In addition, untreated depression is the primary cause of suicide in the elderly.

Depression Is Treatable

A depressive disorder is a serious illness, and it's not likely to go away without some type of treatment. Depression affects the body, mind, and spirit, and permeates all aspects of an individual's life. Without treatment, depression can linger for years, and cause severe suffering for the individual and those who care about him.

Unfortunately, many people who are depressed do not seek help. Many people are not aware that depression is treatable, or they may feel uncomfortable admitting to feelings of depression. It's important to realize that depression is not a sign of weakness, nor is it a passing mood. A person who is depressed cannot simply pull himself together and shake off depression. With appropriate treatment, however, most people who suffer from depression can be helped. The next section will help you determine if you, or someone you know, is suffering from depression.

Helping Someone Who Is Depressed

Many times, people who are depressed do not realize that they are suffering from a depressive disorder. If you suspect that someone you care about is depressed, the most important thing you can do is to help her receive appropriate treatment. Encourage her to seek help, and be willing to take the initiative to make and even to take her to appointments.

Offering emotional support is essential. Try to engage the person in conversation, and pay attention to what she is saying. However, don't try to act as a therapist, and resist the urge to try to solve her problems. Instead, just listen and give the person an opportunity to share her feelings. As trying as it can be to relate to a depressed person, be as patient as possible and remember that someone suffering from a depressive disorder cannot just "snap out" of her depression.

A depressed person needs to know that he has the loving support of his family and friends. Offer encouragement and try to engage the depressed person in simple activities such as a walk or going to a movie. Even if he resists, be persistent in a supportive, gentle, and encouraging manner. Don't be too pushy, because if the person feels like he cannot live up to your expectations or demands, he will feel like a failure and may become more depressed. Remember—and remind the depressed person—that with time and appropriate treatment, he will begin to feel better.

If at any time a depressed person talks about suicide, report this to his therapist. If you suspect that the person may be planning a suicide attempt, call 911 and his therapist right away.

ARE YOU DEPRESSED? A SIMPLE SELF-TEST

If you suspect depression in yourself or in someone you know, this simple self-test can serve as a gauge to help you decide whether or not to seek professional help. There are no right or wrong answers to this test. The more truthful you can be, the more accurately you can determine your emotional state.

Please note that this test is not a substitute for a therapeutic evaluation. Only a properly trained health professional can accurately diagnose whether or not you are suffering from a depressive disorder. But answering these questions can help you sort through your feelings and communicate your symptoms to your doctor or therapist.

Answer the following questions about how you have been feeling during the past two weeks.

Self-Test for Depression

1. I've been feeling sad or unhappy.

_____ Never or rarely   _____ Sometimes

_____ Often   _____ Most of the time

2. I feel tired and don't have much energy.

_____ Never or rarely   _____ Sometimes

_____ Often   _____ Most of the time

3. I'm sleeping more than usual (or less than usual).

_____ Never or rarely   _____ Sometimes

_____ Often   _____ Most of the time

4. My sleep is restless and disturbed.

_____ Never or rarely   _____ Sometimes

_____ Often   _____ Most of the time

**5. I'm eating more than usual
(or less than usual).**

_____ Never or rarely   _____ Sometimes

_____ Often   _____ Most of the time

6. I feel restless and irritable.

_____ Never or rarely   _____ Sometimes

_____ Often   _____ Most of the time

**7. I find it difficult to concentrate or
to think clearly.**

_____ Never or rarely   _____ Sometimes

_____ Often   _____ Most of the time

**8. I don't enjoy activities that I used to
find pleasurable.**

_____ Never or rarely   _____ Sometimes

_____ Often   _____ Most of the time

**9. I'm not interested in sex, or I'm having
sexual difficulties.**

_____ Never or rarely   _____ Sometimes

_____ Often   _____ Most of the time

**10. I have headaches or other pains
and my doctor can't find a cause.**

_____ Never or rarely   _____ Sometimes

_____ Often   _____ Most of the time

**11. I feel as though no one really
likes me.**

_____ Never or rarely   _____ Sometimes

_____ Often   _____ Most of the time

12. I feel unattractive.

_____ Never or rarely   _____ Sometimes

_____ Often   _____ Most of the time

13. I feel guilty without any real reason.

_____ Never or rarely   _____ Sometimes

_____ Often   _____ Most of the time

14. I feel fearful and anxious.

_____ Never or rarely   _____ Sometimes

_____ Often   _____ Most of the time

**15. I have negative, critical thoughts
about myself.**

_____ Never or rarely   _____ Sometimes

_____ Often   _____ Most of the time

16. I feel hopeless.

_____ Never or rarely   _____ Sometimes

_____ Often   _____ Most of the time

17. I feel like a failure in life.

_____ Never or rarely   _____ Sometimes

_____ Often   _____ Most of the time

**18. My life feels empty and nothing seems
worth doing.**

_____ Never or rarely   _____ Sometimes

_____ Often   _____ Most of the time

19. I don't feel like I will ever feel better.

_____ Never or rarely   _____ Sometimes

_____ Often   _____ Most of the time

20. I have thoughts of death or suicide.

_____ Never or rarely   _____ Sometimes

_____ Often   _____ Most of the time

When you finish taking the test, tally up your responses in each category. Assign each "Never or rarely" answer 1 point; each "Sometimes" answer 2 points; each "Often" answer 3 points; and each "Most of the time" answer 4 points.

If you scored below 30 points, you are probably not depressed. If you scored between 30 and 50, you are likely mildly or moderately depressed, and should consult a therapist or your doctor for guidance. If you scored over 50 points, you may be suffering from serious depression, and should consult your doctor for help without delay. Preferably, consult a doctor who is open to treating depression in a holistic way.

CONVENTIONAL TREATMENTS FOR DEPRESSION

If you think that you or someone you care about is suffering from depression, the first step is to see a doctor for a thorough examination. It's important to rule out physical conditions that can mimic depression. For example, a lingering viral infection can cause fatigue, lethargy, and other symptoms associated with depression. If your doctor finds no physical reason for your symptoms, the next step is to consult a psychologist, psychiatrist, or psychotherapist who can evaluate your symptoms and make a diagnosis.

Diagnosing Depression

During a psychological evaluation, you can expect to be asked about the history of your depression, including the symptoms you are experiencing, when they began, and if you have ever suffered from depression in the past. A thorough evaluation will also include questions about drug and alcohol use, any family history of depressive disorders, and previous treatments you may have received for depression. It's important to distinguish between situational depression, which is related to external events such as the loss of a spouse or other stressful life situations, and endogenous depression, which arises internally and is independent of life stressors.

Endogenous Depression
Depression that originates from within without apparent relation to external life events.

A variety of different medications and treatments are available for treating depressive disorders. Milder forms of depression often respond well to psychotherapy and the use of antidepressants when necessary. People suffering from moderate to severe depression generally do best with a combination of antidepressant medication and psychotherapy. Antidepressants help to shift brain chemistry to alleviate feelings of depression, and psychotherapy provides the opportunity to learn more effective ways of managing life stressors.

Conventional Medical Treatments

The most common conventional medical treatment for depressive disorders is medication; so commonly are these medications prescribed that more than 28 million Americans take antidepressant drugs or anxiety medications. Scientists generally regard depression as caused by disordered brain chemistry, and a number of studies support the view that depressed people have imbalances in neurotransmitters, the chemicals in the brain that facilitate communication between nerve cells.

Two neurotransmitters that are thought to be especially important are serotonin and norepinephrine. Both of these brain chemicals are generally found in short supply in people who are depressed. Serotonin is often referred to as the brain's natural mood-elevating drug. It also has relaxing and sedative properties. People who have high levels of serotonin tend to be optimistic, calm, patient, and good natured. They also tend to be focused, creative, and have a good ability to concentrate. Physiologically, they usually sleep well, and do not have an undue craving for carbohydrates.

Neurotransmitters
Molecules used as chemical messengers in the body.

On the other hand, people with low serotonin levels tend to be depressed, anxious, irritable, and impatient. They typically crave sweets and high-carbohydrate foods, and often suffer from insomnia. The lowest levels of serotonin are found in people who have attempted suicide.

Scientists believe that some people are genetically programmed to produce less serotonin, which can predispose them to depression. But not everyone with this genetic tendency will become depressed, and there are plenty of people who produce sufficient levels of serotonin who are depressed. Clearly, although serotonin plays an important role in depression, there are many other factors involved in the disorder.

Medications for Depression

The U.S. Food and Drug Administration has approved dozens of medications for treating depressive disorders. The medications are classified according to their effects on the various chemicals in the brain. The older antidepressants, first prescribed in the 1950s, include tricyclic antidepressants such as Tofranil (imipramine) and monoamine oxidase inhibitors (MAOIs) such as Nardil (phenelzine). Newer antidepressants, known as selective serotonin reuptake inhibitors (SSRIs), include Prozac (fluoxetine), Zoloft (sertraline), Paxil (paroxetine), Wellbutrin (bupropion), Effexor (venlafaxine), Remeron (mirtazapine), and Serzone (nefazodone). These newer drugs work by increasing serotonin levels.

Understanding how serotonin works in the body helps in understanding something about how these drugs work.

Serotonin is manufactured naturally in the brain, and then is stored in nerve cells until it is needed. The job of serotonin is to carry messages to nerve cells. When serotonin is released, it transmits a chemical message to a nerve cell by attaching to a receptor site on the nerve cell. At the same time that serotonin is being released, enzymes in the body go to work either to break down the serotonin or to help it be taken back into the brain cells. Both of these processes reduce the effect of serotonin in the body. The drugs developed to alleviate depression work by either preventing the breakdown of serotonin or inhibiting the reuptake of serotonin into the brain. This means that there is more serotonin available in the body to produce a natural mood-enhancing effect.

While these drugs have demonstrated effectiveness for treating depression, they may not be necessary for mild or moderate cases of depression. There are a number of effective alternatives to antidepressant drugs, including diet and lifestyle changes that help to naturally increase serotonin levels. These factors include balancing blood sugar levels, eating a diet rich in foods that support nervous system health, and regular exercise. You can read more about this later.

In addition, addressing the underlying psychological causes for depression and learning new and more positive ways of coping with life stressors also helps to increase serotonin levels naturally. Later, I'll go into detail about the many ways that you can help yourself overcome depressive disorders.

Lifestyle changes and psychotherapy approaches are not magic wands, however. They take time and consistent effort, and results generally do not occur overnight. In the meantime, St. John's wort offers a natural, safe, and effective alternative to antidepressant drugs for providing a boost of serotonin, which helps to ease the symptoms of depression and supports the effort necessary for making life changes.

How Antidepressants Work

Researchers aren't exactly sure how antidepressants work, but they do know that these drugs help to restore chemical balance in the brain, which in turn, helps to alleviate depressive symptoms. For most patients, it takes between four to eight weeks for the drug to fully take effect. To avoid a relapse, many patients remain on antidepressants for six months to one year following a major depressive episode.

No one treatment works best for everyone, and discovering the most effective treatment involves working closely with a doctor who can adjust medications or combinations of medications as needed. Physicians often try a variety of antidepressant medications to find the most effective medication or combination of medications. In general, it takes anywhere from one to two months to obtain the full therapeutic benefit of the drug.

Antidepressants are usually prescribed for at least four months, and in the case of a chronic major depressive disorder or bipolar disorder, medication may need to be taken indefinitely to prevent a recurrence of symptoms. Antidepressants should never be discontinued abruptly; to do so can cause unpleasant withdrawal symptoms.

Although prescription antidepressants can be remarkably effective for treating depression, they are not a cure-all nor are they benign substances. For one thing, the drugs don't alleviate depression for everyone. For some people the relief provided by drugs merely softens the edge of depression. It's not unusual for antidepressants to cause side effects. The primary side effects of tricyclic antidepressants are dry mouth, constipation, blurred vision, dizziness, drowsiness, sexual problems, and difficulty urinating. Monoamine oxidase inhibitors (MAOIs) can cause a fatal rise in blood pressure if combined with certain foods or medications. The most common side effects of SSRIs include headache, nausea, agitation, insomnia, and sexual difficulties.

Withdrawal from Antidepressants

One of the most disturbing and least talked about problems with antidepressants is the issue of withdrawal. The brain becomes accustomed to certain levels of serotonin, and some people suffer distress when they either stop taking or take lower doses of serotonin-boosting antidepressants.

In fact, studies indicate that up to 85 percent of patients who take prescription SSRIs have some type of withdrawal symptoms when they stop taking the drug. The symptoms include balance problems, nerve tingling, nausea, flulike symptoms, difficulties sleeping, anxiety, and depression. Many patients continue taking antidepressant drugs unnecessarily because they assume their withdrawal symptoms signify a relapse of depression. Disturbingly, many doctors are not aware that stopping antidepressants can cause such symptoms.

Often, doctors routinely prescribe antidepressants for patients who show any sign whatsoever of depression. In fact, Prozac, which has been on the market since 1988, is the third top-selling drug in the United States. Zoloft, introduced in 1992, is seventh on the list, and Paxil, brought to the market in 1993, is in ninth place. Hailed as the miracle drugs of modern psychiatric medicine, these antidepressants have been prescribed for at least 28 million Americans. But the drawbacks of Prozac and similar antidepressants are now being recognized, just as the problems with Valium and amphetamines (both also used as mood enhancers in the past) came to light a couple of decades ago.

Experts Criticize Antidepressant Drugs

Critics of antidepressant drugs maintain that far too many prescriptions for these drugs are being written. Joseph Glenmullen, M.D., a Harvard psychiatrist and author of *Prozac Backlash*, maintains that the long-term effects of antidepressants have not been considered. He also criticizes the managed health care system in this country for putting people on antidepressants because it's cheaper than paying for psychotherapy. Although he acknowledges that antidepressants can be helpful for people with serious depression, he recommends that people with mild depression should avoid prescription antidepressants, and suggests St. John's wort and psychotherapy as alternative approaches.

Problems arise when people who suffer from mild depression or even those who are simply experiencing an intense period of life stress are started on prescription antidepressants by their doctors, and then suffer withdrawal symptoms when they try to get off of the medication. When they decrease their dosage of the drugs, it can be difficult for the doctor to determine whether the patient's symptoms are caused by withdrawal from the drug, or if the symptoms of the depression are recurring.

The cycle of trying to wean a patient from antidepressants can potentially go on for years, with patients being switched from one drug to another in an attempt to alleviate symptoms. The truth is that very little is known about the long-term effects of modern prescription antidepressants. These drugs were initially approved by the Food and Drug Administration, the government agency responsible for protecting the health of consumers. But once a drug is on the market, the FDA does little in the way of tracking the side effects of long-term use. The FDA itself estimates that only 1 percent to 10 percent of all drug side effects are reported to the agency.

Doctors have the responsibility of informing their patients about the potential adverse effects of antidepressants, as well as how to safely stop taking the drugs. But a report in the *Journal of Clinical Psychiatry* showed that as many as 70 percent of general practitioners and 30 percent of psychiatrists aren't educated about the withdrawal effects of stopping serotonin-boosting antidepressants such as Prozac, Zoloft, and Paxil. Of the doctors who are aware, only 17 percent of general practitioners and 20 percent of psychiatrists inform their patients of the correct way to wean themselves from the drugs.

Clearly, as effective as modern antidepressant drugs can be for treating depressive disorders, they are not a panacea, nor do they come without risks. There are, however, a number of alternative approaches to depression that have been shown to be as effective as pharmaceutical drugs, but with few or no side effects. One of the most promising of these alternatives is the herb St. John's wort.

How St. John's Wort Can Help You

Not only is St. John's wort a popular treatment for mild to moderate depression, but it can also be helpful for anxiety, sleep disorders, the mood swings associated with premenstrual syndrome (PMS) and menopause, and seasonal affective disorder (SAD).

A quick recap of depression: People suffering from depressive disorders have an imbalance of specific brain chemicals known as neurotransmitters. This imbalance causes a variety of physical, emotional, and mental symptoms. Physically, these symptoms manifest as changes in sleep, appetite, and energy. Emotionally, the person may feel a sense of hopelessness, irritability, or a lack of interest in work, socializing, or hobbies. And mentally, the person may have difficulties concentrating or making decisions. St. John's wort has proven helpful for alleviating all of these symptoms. As a result, this herb is highly regarded as an alternative to conventional medications for depressive disorders.

St. John's wort plays a prominent role in European herbal medicine, particularly in Germany, where doctors prescribed almost 66 million daily doses of the herb in 1994 for psychological disorders. St. John's wort is clearly the treatment of choice for depressive disorders in Germany—physicians there prescribe extracts of the herb twenty times more often than they do Prozac.

Prescribing St. John's wort as an alternative to pharmaceutical antidepressants makes sense. Pharmaceutical drugs have numerous side effects, including dry mouth, nausea, fatigue, headache, gastrointestinal distress, sleep disturbances, and impaired sexual functioning. In contrast, St. John's wort carries little risk of side effects, and those that are reported, such as gastrointestinal upset, tend to be minor. St. John's wort also costs far less than prescription antidepressants. And St. John's wort does not require a prescription.

If you are currently taking prescription medication for the treatment of a depressive disorder, do not begin taking St. John's wort without consulting with your doctor. The combination of St. John's wort and standard antidepressants can cause side effects. And never discontinue antidepressants without talking with your doctor. While many people have switched from antidepressant drugs to St. John's wort, you should only do so under the supervision of your doctor.

How St. John's Wort Works

The primary compounds in St. John's wort include flavonoids (hyperoside, quercetin, isoquercitrin, and rutin), hyperforin, hypericin, pseudohypericin, polycyclic phenols, kaempferol, luteolin, and biapigenin. Researchers have not determined which of these compounds are the active ingredients, but there is some consensus that hyperforin has effects on mood. Many St. John's wort products are standardized to contain specific amounts of hypericin and hyperforin, which guarantees that the supplement contains what has been judged by researchers to be a sufficient amount of the herb to have a beneficial effect.

Hyperforin
A naturally occurring chemical compound in St. John's wort that has been identified as having antidepressant effects.

Researchers are still studying St. John's wort to determine exactly how it manages to alleviate depression. Although many clinical studies have proven the effectiveness of St. John's wort in relieving depression, scientists like to have a clear picture of exactly how the herb affects the body and brain. The theories are fairly complex, and it appears that St. John's wort may operate in somewhat roundabout ways to ease depressive symptoms. Some research indicates that St. John's wort acts in a similar way to antidepressive drugs in that it inhibits the rate at which brain cells reabsorb serotonin (the neurotransmitter that aids communication between nerve cells and acts as the body's natural feel-good chemical). People who are depressed often have low levels of serotonin.

Another theory about the beneficial effect of St. John's wort is that it seems to reduce levels of interleukin-6, a protein that plays a role in the communication between cells in the body's immune system. Increased levels of interleukin-6 may stimulate the increase of adrenal regulatory hormones, which are a biological marker for depression. It may be that by reducing interleukin-6, St. John's wort helps to treat depression. More studies are needed (some are currently in progress) to determine precisely what are the active ingredients in St. John's wort, and to figure out exactly how these compounds work. Meanwhile, the following are some of the depressive disorders for which St. John's wort has been found helpful.

St. John's Wort and Anxiety

Anxiety often plays a prominent role in depressive disorders, manifesting as feelings of restlessness, irritability, and insomnia. Other common symptoms of anxiety include muscle tension, digestive upsets, and heart palpitations. A certain level of anxiety is a normal reaction to specific situations—for example, most people feel anxious when faced with a dangerous situation. But constant, chronic anxiety impairs the quality of life and can become debilitating.

Physicians often prescribe benzodiazepine medications such as Valium and Xanax for treating anxiety. These drugs have numerous side effects (including lethargy, drowsiness, and mental impairment) and a high potential for addiction. They can also trigger depression. A much safer alternative is to follow the lifestyle suggestions in this book, making sure to avoid all stimulants such as caffeine. St. John's wort has been found to be as helpful as prescription medications in easing anxiety, but without the harmful side effects.

SAD Relief with St. John's Wort

St. John's wort is not only helpful for chronic depression, but it can also be valuable for treating seasonal affective disorder, also known as SAD. People with this condition are strongly affected by the onset of winter, and suffer from feelings of fatigue, irritability, and depression. The condition is related to the diminishing sunlight that typically occurs during the winter months. Although it's not uncommon to feel the urge to "cocoon" during the winter, people with SAD may become so withdrawn that they find it difficult to perform the normal tasks of daily life. They may also tend to overeat, especially carbohydrates, and spend a greater amount of time sleeping than usual. The symptoms of SAD usually disappear with the return of spring and increasing daylight, but the winter months can become unbearable for those who suffer from the disorder.

One of the most effective treatments for SAD is to spend time every day in full spectrum light, which duplicates the beneficial mood-enhancing properties of sunlight. Light boxes made especially for this purpose are widely available, and symptoms are generally relieved within a week or two of daily exposure. It usually takes at least thirty minutes of daily early morning light therapy for best results. In addition, engaging in regular exercise at midday is helpful for obtaining as much natural light as possible during the winter months.

Photosensitivity
An allergic skin reaction that occurs with exposure to ultraviolet rays.

Prescription antidepressants are often recommended for people suffering from SAD. St. John's wort can be an effective, natural alternative. You may have heard cautions concerning the combination of St. John's wort and sunlight. It's true that St. John's wort can cause photosensitivity (an allergic reaction that occurs with exposure to the ultraviolet rays of sunlight) but it's unlikely to occur in humans. There's absolutely no need to be concerned about the combination of light box therapy and St. John's wort, because light boxes do not produce ultraviolet light.

St. John's Wort and PMS

Premenstrual syndrome (PMS) is one of the most widespread problems afflicting women. By some estimates, as many as 90 percent of women in their reproductive years are affected to some degree by PMS. Mood swings, irritability, insomnia, and depression commonly occur during the week to ten days prior to the onset of menstruation. For some women, PMS symptoms can occur during most of the month.

A study of nineteen women at the University of Exeter in the United Kingdom showed that two-thirds of the women found significant relief when taking St. John's wort. They were given 900 mg of the herb daily for two complete menstrual cycles, and found that their PMS-related symptoms of depression, anxiety, nervous tension, confusion, and crying were diminished by more than half.

St. John's Wort and Menopause

Menopause is a time of great change on many levels. It's not uncommon for a woman to experience situational depression associated with midlife and the many adjustments that accompany this life transition, such as children leaving home, relationship changes, the loss of youth, and of course, the actual physiological changes of declining hormone levels. Many women find that the perimenopausal and menopausal years bring profound emotions to the surface.

Christiane Northrup, M.D., author of *Women's Bodies, Women's Wisdom,* points out that menopause is often a time when women find themselves facing the "unfinished business" of the first half of their lives. Many women may find that they have spent years denying their real wants and needs, and depression may be a cry from the inner self for acknowledgment. A woman may find that she grieves paths not taken, opportunities missed, and the loss of youth. It's important during this time to not suppress feelings, but to pay attention to them. There is often wisdom and greater self-understanding lying beneath the surface of depression.

Giving yourself the time to fully explore your feelings will help you to free yourself from regrets and to make decisions as to how you want to live the second half of your life. "If a woman is willing to deal with her own unfinished business, she will have fewer menopausal symptoms," says Northrup. "She will find that her symptoms are messages from her inner guidance system that parts of her life need attention." In addition to self-exploration, dietary improvement, and exercise, Northrup also suggests St. John's wort for supporting a woman who needs extra help alleviating menopausal depression.

Unfortunately, many doctors are too quick to prescribe prescription antidepressants for treating menopausal depression. Lifestyle changes, psychotherapy, and natural remedies present a far safer and healthier alternative. It is much better to avoid drugs, especially in cases of mild to moderate depression, and to use natural therapies combined with appropriate emotional work for healing the underlying psychological distress.

SCIENTIFIC SUPPORT FOR ST. JOHN'S WORT

The benefits of St. John's wort compared to pharmaceutical prescription drugs have been clearly demonstrated in a number of well-designed clinical studies. A handful of these studies are outlined here to give you an idea of the scientific support for St. John's wort.

Not only has the herb been found to be as effective as prescription drugs such as Prozac and Zoloft, but it also has far less incidence of side effects, and the side effects that do occur, such as dry mouth, tend to be minor. Other studies that you will find mentioned in this section include the usefulness of St. John's wort for treating depression in children, and the beneficial effects of St. John's wort on premenstrual depression and menopause in women.

Why Doctors Prescribe Drugs

Unfortunately, even with the numerous studies that have demonstrated the effectiveness and safety of St. John's wort for treating mild to moderate depression, many physicians continue instead to prescribe drugs. There are several possible reasons for this. Pharmaceutical companies spend billions of dollars advertising their antidepressant drugs, including ads in the popular media, which influence not only what physicians prescribe, but also what patients request from their doctors. In addition, pharmaceutical companies are generally not interested in researching botanical medicines because they would have difficulties obtaining a patented formula. And the fact that herbal remedies are widely available over the counter in natural food stores and pharmacies significantly limits marketing potential, sales, and income for pharmaceutical manufacturers.

Some physicians also hesitate to prescribe St. John's wort because they aren't accustomed to using herbal remedies. And other doctors may be uncomfortable because all of the precise active ingredients in St. John's wort have not been identified. This is not unusual with botanical medicines. Typically, they contain a wide array of compounds that act in harmony with one another. Trying to isolate one compound and dismissing the rest as unimportant is a short-sighted view that has plagued modern medicine.

As many herbalists and botanical researchers point out, herbs contain a variety of compounds that act synergistically to create a physiological effect in the body, and the complete herb has greater potential for healing than just one isolated chemical constituent. For example, while hyperforin may indeed be the primary active ingredient in St. John's wort that helps to relieve depression, there are other compounds that support the action of hyperforin, and still others that buffer the active ingredients to prevent side effects.

The important point that you will see from the studies described below is that St. John's wort is clearly effective for the treatment of mild to moderate depression. It alleviates symptoms, and it does so without harm to the patient, which undoubtedly meets anyone's criteria for good medicine.

St. John's Wort versus Placebo

In a study of seventy-two patients comparing St. John's wort to a placebo, German physicians gave patients either 900 mg of St. John's wort extract or a placebo daily for forty-two days. They found that the patients' scores on the Hamilton Depression Scale (a standard test used to measure depression) declined by 55 percent among those taking St. John's wort, and dropped only by 28 percent among those taking the placebo. Those who were given St. John's wort also showed improvement in symptoms after only one week of taking the herb, and showed significant positive response after twenty-eight and forty-two days. The patients reported no side effects.

In addition, an overview of twenty-three clinical trials published in the *British Medical Journal* found that St. John's wort extracts were significantly superior to a placebo in relieving depression, and as effective as standard antidepressants. The studies involved a total of 1,757 outpatients with mild to moderately severe depressive disorders.

St. John's Wort versus Prozac

In a six-week German study, 240 patients suffering from mild to moderate depression were given either 500 mg of St. John's wort daily or Prozac. The patients were assessed using the Hamilton Depression Scale. Both groups showed approximately a 12 percent decline in depressive symptoms at the end of the six weeks.

Patients were also tested using the Clinical Global Impression Scale, which showed that St. John's wort was significantly more effective in relieving depression than Prozac. Only six of the patients taking St. John's wort complained of side effects, and these were gastrointestinal symptoms. But thirty-four of the patients taking Prozac reported side effects, including gastrointestinal problems, vomiting, agitation, dizziness, and erectile dysfunction.

St. John's Wort versus Zoloft

In a seven-week study of thirty depressed patients conducted by Ronald Brenner, M.D., and associates of the St. John's Episcopal Hospital in Far Rockaway, New York, St. John's wort was found to be comparable to Zoloft in relieving depressive symptoms. The patients were given either the prescription antidepressant Zoloft or 600–900 mg of a standardized extract of St. John's wort daily. Depression was measured using the Hamilton Depression Scale and the Clinical Global Impression Scale.

Brenner reported significant improvements in the patients taking St. John's wort within two weeks. Measurements after six weeks showed that depressive symptoms were reduced by an average of 40 percent in patients taking Zoloft, and 47 percent in those taking St. John's wort. Two of the patients taking Zoloft reported symptoms of

nausea or headache, and two patients taking St. John's wort reported dizziness.

St. John's Wort versus Tofranil

In two clinical studies, St. John's wort has been shown to be as effective as Tofranil (imipramine), one of the most frequently prescribed tricyclic antidepressants. In a study at the Imerem Institute for Medical Research Management and Biometrics in Nuremberg, Germany, psychiatry professor Michael Philipp, M.D., and his colleagues gave 1,050 mg of St. John's wort extract, Tofranil, or a placebo daily for eight weeks to 263 patients (66 men, 197 women) suffering from moderate depression.

The results, published in the *British Medical Journal*, showed that St. John's wort was superior to the placebo and comparable to Tofranil in relieving the patients' depressive symptoms. Results were measured by the researchers using the Hamilton Anxiety Scale, the Clinical Global Impression Scale, and the Zung Self-Rating Depression Scale. The patients who were given St. John's wort had one-third the incidence of side effects as those taking Tofranil. The chief side effect reported was dry mouth. The researchers noted that St. John's wort is a safe treatment for depression and that it improves quality of life for patients.

St. John's wort also compared well to Tofranil in another German study of 324 patients with mild to moderate depression. Helmut Woelk, M.D., of the University of Giessen, Germany, and his colleagues gave St. John's wort or Tofranil daily to the patients for six weeks. They found that both St. John's wort and Tofranil decreased the symptoms of depression by half. St. John's wort exceeded Tofranil in reducing anxiety, however. The researchers also noted that almost half of the study participants experienced side effects while taking Tofranil, primarily complaining of dry mouth and nausea. In contrast, only 20 percent of the patients taking St. John's wort suffered side effects, most commonly dry mouth.

St. John's Wort and PMS

Many women suffer from depressive symptoms in the week or two prior to menstruation. The Food and Drug Administration has recently approved a form of Prozac, called Serafem, as a treatment for depression associated with premenstrual syndrome. Serafem and St. John's wort have not been directly compared in a clinical study, but St. John's wort has been shown to be an effective treatment for alleviating premenstrual depression.

A study of nineteen women at the University of Exeter in the United Kingdom conducted by Edzard Ernst, M.D., showed that two-thirds of the women found significant relief when taking St. John's wort. They were given 900 mg daily for two complete menstrual cycles, and found that their PMS-related symptoms of depression, anxiety, nervous tension, confusion, and crying were diminished by more than half. No significant side effects were reported by the study participants.

St. John's Wort and Menopause

Depressive symptoms occur frequently in the pre- and postmenopausal years, and cause significant distress for many women. A German study of 111 women found that St. John's wort provides substantial improvement in the psychological and psychosomatic symptoms of menopause.

The women studied were between forty-three and sixty-five years old with symptoms characteristic of the pre- and postmenopausal years. They were given 900 mg of St. John's wort extract (300 mg three times a day) for twelve weeks, and their symptoms were evaluated using the Clinical Global Impression Scale and the Menopause Rating Scale. Symptoms were evaluated after five, eight, and twelve weeks of treatment.

The researchers found that there was significant improvement in menopausal problems, with menopausal complaints diminishing or disappearing completely in the majority of women. The women self-rated their improvement at 76 percent, and their physicians rated the women's improvement at 79 percent. The researchers also noted that the women's sexual well-being was enhanced as a result of treatment with St. John's wort.

St. John's Wort for Childhood Depression

At least one in thirty-three children under the age of twelve suffers from depression, and researchers have found that St. John's wort is as effective and safe for treating childhood depression as it is for adults.

A recent German study by Wolf-Dietrich Huebner, M.D., and Tilman Kirste, M.D., at thirty-five pediatric clinics in Germany evaluated seventy-four children suffering from depressive symptoms, including anxiety, irritability, restlessness, poor concentration, sleep disturbances, feelings of dejection, and lack of motivation. The children, ranging in age from one to twelve, were given 300–1,800 mg of St. John's wort extract daily for four to six weeks.

The study found that 72 percent of the children were "good" or "excellent" responders after only two weeks of taking the herb. After four weeks, the number of positive responses rose to 97 percent, with a full 100 percent evaluated as "good" or "excellent" responders at the end of six weeks. The parents also evaluated their children, and their ratings were almost identical to those of the researchers. While St. John's wort improved most of the children's depressive symptoms, it did not appear to have an affect on their ability to concentrate. There were no side effects noted. However, one child showed an increase in depressive symptoms after starting St. John's wort, but subsequently improved over the following two weeks of taking the herb.

Challenge to St. John's Wort

Last year, a study came out that seemed to dispute the credibility of St. John's wort. The study was published in the *Journal of the American Medical Association,* and the ensuing newspaper headlines reported that St. John's wort had been found useless for the treatment of depression. Unfortunately, this study was very misleading. It was conducted on people suffering from severe depression, for which St. John's wort has never been purported to be the most effective treatment. St. John's wort has been recommended for treating mild to moderate cases of depression, for which it has been found very successful.

It is important to note that this study was funded and organized by Pfizer, the same pharmaceutical company that makes Zoloft, which is one of the most often prescribed conventional antidepressant drugs.

Numerous previous clinical studies have supported the use of St. John's wort for the treatment of depression. These studies have demonstrated that St. John's wort is not only as effective as prescription antidepressants, but it has far fewer and much less severe side effects. And even this controversial study did acknowledge that a few patients, although they suffered from severe depression, did actually benefit from taking St. John's wort.

ALLEVIATE DEPRESSION WITH DIET AND EXERCISE

It's not news that nutrition has a direct effect on your physical well-being, as many studies over the past few decades have proven. Heart disease, high blood pressure, cancer, and diabetes are a few of the many diseases that have been shown to be directly affected by diet. But many people are unaware that food choices also play a significant role in emotional and mental well-being.

Eat Right to Combat Depression

Nutrition affects not only your daily moods, but is also a factor in the onset and progression of depression. Your brain requires an adequate and steady supply of nutrients and quickly shows signs of stress when your diet is inadequate. While people vary somewhat in their dietary needs, the following guidelines are usually helpful for most people who suffer from mood swings and depression.

Keeping blood sugar levels balanced is essential for those who are prone to depression. The brain and nervous system are highly sensitive to blood sugar fluctuations. In addition, keeping blood sugar stable ensures a constant supply of energy for the body, which helps to prevent fatigue. To keep blood sugar levels on an even keel, avoid sugary foods and refined carbohydrates, which are quickly converted to sugar in the body. Obviously, desserts and sweets are usually loaded with sugar, but other foods such as salad dressings and dry cereals often contain large amounts of sweeteners.

Some of the many guises of sugar include sucrose, glucose, maltose, dextrose, and corn syrup. Even sweeteners that are thought to be healthful alternatives, such as honey, maple syrup, barley malt, and molasses have a detrimental effect on blood sugar. Ideally, eat sugar primarily as it occurs in whole foods, such as fresh fruits and sweet vegetables such as carrots, winter squashes, and sweet potatoes, and reserve concentrated sweets for occasional treats. Other foods that interfere with healthy blood sugar levels include refined carbohydrates made from white flour, which are rapidly broken down into simple sugars during digestion.

Also avoid caffeine and alcohol, which cause blood sugar fluctuations and have other negative effects on the body. Caffeine is a powerful stimulant drug that stresses the nervous system and contributes to anxiety, irritability, and insomnia. It overstimulates the adrenal glands, creating a state of chronic stress, and results in fatigue after the initial stimulant effect wears off.

To ensure a constant supply of nutrients that keep blood sugar levels balanced, eat small meals several times a day. Choose from high-complex carbohydrates, lean proteins, and healthful fats. High complex carbohydrates, such as legumes, whole grains, nuts, seeds, vegetables, and fruits provide a steady source of energy for the body and brain. Avoid skipping meals or going for more than three hours without eating. For optimal blood sugar control, eat three moderate meals daily plus a mid-morning, mid-afternoon, and a before-bed snack.

Natural Antidepressant Foods

Keeping blood sugar levels in balance is important for stabilizing mood and increasing energy and well-being. But don't stop there. The foods you choose to eat on a daily basis can actually have a significant antidepressant effect.

Nerve cells in the brain communicate through chemicals called neurotransmitters, which are dependent upon specific nutrients in the blood. Prescription antidepressants work by increasing levels of neurotransmitters, but you can also increase these mood-elevating substances with foods and nutritional supplements. Protein-rich foods such as chicken, turkey, fish, eggs, lentils, almonds, tofu, and yogurt are made up of amino acids, which are the building blocks for neurotransmitters. To ensure an adequate supply of protein in your diet, eat a small serving of protein at each meal and include a bit of protein (such as a few nuts or a small piece of cheese) with each snack, for a total of approximately 8 to 10 ounces of protein daily.

Essential fatty acids are another important nutrient for alleviating depression. They play a critical role in maintaining healthy cell membranes, which are involved in the synthesis and transmission of neurotransmitters. Depression is associated with low levels of essential fatty acids, particularly omega-3 fatty acids and gamma-linolenic acid (GLA). Omega-3 fatty acids are thought to enhance the responsiveness of nerve cells to serotonin, the brain's natural mood-uplifting chemical.

Omega-3 fatty acids are found in cold-water fish such as salmon, mackerel, sardines, trout, and albacore tuna; walnuts; and flaxseeds. To obtain sufficient amounts of omega-3 fatty acids, eat cold-water fish at least three times a week (daily is better if you are suffering from depression), and eat a small handful of raw walnuts or one tablespoon of flaxseed oil daily. If you use flaxseed oil, buy it fresh in a dark bottle, keep it refrigerated, use the oil within six weeks after opening, and don't heat it. Flaxseed oil is highly susceptible to deterioration when exposed to heat, light, or oxygen.

Gamma-linolenic acid is an essential fatty acid that is not readily found in foods. Under ideal circumstances, the body makes GLA from fats and oils in the diet, but in reality, many factors interfere with the production of this important nutrient. The best and most reliable source of GLA is to take capsules of evening primrose, black currant, or borage seed oil. Take enough capsules so that you are obtaining between 120 and 240 mg of GLA daily.

Supplements for Overcoming Depression

Because low levels of many nutrients are associated with depression, it's helpful to take a high-potency vitamin and mineral supplement daily. The B-complex vitamins are particularly important in the treatment of mood disorders because they are critical for the production of neurotransmitters and a healthy nervous system.

Vitamin B_6 helps to regulate mood, and is involved in the production of serotonin, a brain chemical that promotes feelings of well-being. People who are prone to depression tend to have low levels of both B_6 and serotonin. Foods rich in B_6 include whole grains, dark leafy greens, bananas, chicken, and avocados.

Vitamin B_{12} is also essential in the prevention and treatment of depression. This vitamin is found in animal proteins, but many people have deficiencies of vitamin B_{12} because it is not easily absorbed through the digestive tract. With age, the ability to absorb B_{12} becomes even weaker. If you suffer from depression, you may want to consider taking sublingual tablets of B_{12} in addition to a B-complex supplement. Sublingual tablets are dissolved under the tongue and absorbed directly into the bloodstream. Take one milligram of vitamin B_{12} every other day.

A lack of folic acid, another B vitamin, also causes depression and changes in personality. Folic acid occurs abundantly in leafy green vegetables, but because not many people eat sufficient amounts of leafy greens and the vitamin is destroyed by cooking, few people get sufficient amounts of this important vitamin. To ensure that you are getting adequate amounts these essential nutrients, buy a B-complex supplement that supplies 50–100 mg per day of B_1, B_2, B_3, B_5, and B_6, plus 400 mcg (micrograms) of folic acid.

Specific minerals also play a significant role in alleviating depression. Calcium and magnesium are two of the most important, and both help to calm the nervous system. Foods rich in calcium include dairy products, broccoli, kale, oranges, sesame seeds, sardines, and almonds. To ensure sufficient amounts of calcium, take 800–1,200 mg of supplemental calcium daily in the form of calcium citrate, which is the most easily absorbed form. For best assimilation, divide into two or three doses and take with meals.

Good dietary sources of magnesium include legumes, nuts, seeds, and whole grains. Again, to ensure sufficient levels of this necessary mineral, take 400–600 mg of supplemental magnesium daily in the form of citrate, malate, aspartate, gluconate, or lactate. Don't take more than 600 mg daily because excessive magnesium can cause diarrhea.

Diet and Lifestyle Stressors

Alcohol, tobacco, and caffeine all are contributing factors to depression and are best avoided in the quest for improved mental and physical well-being. Alcohol is a significant depressant (that's why many people have a drink to relax). Although a drink or two several times a week may have some health benefits such as reducing cholesterol levels, if you are prone to depression, you are probably better off not drinking. Alcohol stimulates the production of adrenal hormones, which can increase feelings of anxiety. It also interferes with normal sleep cycles, and can contribute to insomnia. Drinking alcohol also causes blood sugar levels to drop, which contributes to hypoglycemia and mood swings.

Although caffeine is a socially acceptable beverage, it is a powerful and highly addictive drug. The stimulant effects of caffeine may be especially appealing to someone suffering from depression. Caffeine provides a momentary boost of energy and can help to clear thinking. However, people who are subject to anxiety or depression tend to be particularly susceptible to the effects of caffeine, and often experience nervousness, irritability, heart palpitations, and anxiety as a result. Several studies have found a direct correlation between coffee intake and depression. For some people, even the minute amount of caffeine found in decaffeinated coffee is enough to trigger anxiety and depressive symptoms.

Cigarette smoking is not generally considered as a factor in depressive disorders. However, nicotine stimulates the secretion of adrenal hormones, including cortisol, the stress hormone. One of the effects of increased cortisol is to interfere with the amount of tryptophan that is delivered to the brain. Because serotonin levels are dependent upon tryptophan, serotonin is reduced.

Tryptophan
An essential amino acid that plays a role in the synthesis of serotonin.

At the same time, cortisol hinders serotonin receptors in the brain and makes them less responsive to the available serotonin.

Overcome Depression with Exercise

Exercise is one of the most powerful tools you have available for overcoming depression and keeping it at bay. In fact, regular daily exercise has been proven to be as effective as antidepressant drugs for relieving mild to moderate depression. In contrast to pharmaceutical drugs, the only side effects of exercise are beneficial and life-enhancing—exercise almost immediately changes your brain chemistry, and it provides a boost for your self-esteem.

Although all forms of exercise are helpful, aerobic exercise such as brisk walking, dancing, cross-country skiing, swimming, and bicycling appears to be the most beneficial for alleviating depression. Vigorous exercise stimulates the release of endorphins, the body's natural mood-elevating compounds.

Endorphins
Natural mood-elevating compounds produced naturally by the body in response to stimulus such as exercise.

In addition, aerobic exercise offers a healthy outlet for relieving feelings of irritability, frustration, and anger and encourages the shift to a more positive frame of mind. Studies have shown that people who exercise regularly not only have decreased symptoms of fatigue, anxiety, and depression, but they also have higher self-esteem than people who do not exercise. For the greatest benefit, exercise in the daylight. A moderate amount of sunlight improves mood by stimulating the production of mood-enhancing hormones and brain chemicals.

If you are depressed, you may feel lethargic and fatigued and not at all interested in exercising. But it's important to exercise even if you don't feel like it. Simply go out for a half-hour walk every day. If you are mildly depressed, you will probably feel your mood shift immediately. If you are suffering from more serious or chronic depression, it may take a few weeks of consistent exercise to notice a definite difference in your mood. Not only does exercise help to change your body chemistry to relieve depression, but establishing and following through with a regular program of exercise improves your self-confidence and enhances your ability to cope with the challenges that life presents.

The minimum amount of exercise that appears to be effective for preventing and relieving depression is approximately thirty minutes of activity five days a week. Early morning exercise seems to be most helpful for establishing a balanced and positive mood for the day, but exercise is beneficial at any time.

A HOLISTIC APPROACH TO DEPRESSION

Approaching depression from a holistic standpoint involves considering the complex interaction of the body, mind, and spirit. Depressive disorders create ripples of pain that affect a human being on all levels—physical, mental, emotional, and spiritual. While medication can alleviate symptoms, no pill is a magic cure. From a holistic point of view, depression is an opportunity for self-empowerment and transformation.

The Deeper Meaning of Depression

The idea that depression may be a message from the soul has intrigued philosophers, poets, spiritual teachers, and psychotherapists for centuries. In our society, we idealize happiness, and busy ourselves with productivity to keep feelings at bay. There is little room for the sadness, emptiness, and loss that are also a part of normal life. But embracing these feelings and integrating them into our beings allows us to experience the full depth of our human nature, and contributes to our maturity.

Depression almost always carries a deeper message, and covering up or denying the feelings does not allow this deeper wisdom to rise to the surface of conscious awareness. Learning to tolerate feelings of sadness, grief, loneliness, anger, and the myriad of other emotions that we don't classify as "happy" can teach us much about ourselves.

This is not to say that you should live with debilitating depression. If you suffer from longstanding or severe depression, you should seek professional help. At the same time, begin to regard your depression as a messenger. Experiment with viewing melancholy as an opportunity for reflection. Take time to be quiet, to nurture yourself, and to ask your depression what it is trying to tell you.

Journaling for Self-Understanding

Depression is a signal that something is out of balance in your life. What is disturbing you? What feels overwhelming? What is dissatisfying about your life at this time? Writing down your feelings can be immensely helpful in this process of self-exploration. In fact, journaling on a regular basis has been shown in clinical studies to provide relief from depression and anxiety.

If you want to try journaling as a practice to ease depression, set aside approximately twenty minutes at a time when you can be alone. Write about your deepest thoughts and feelings, without consideration for grammar or spelling. Bypassing the intellect is essential for being able to access emotions. While you don't have to adhere to a schedule to benefit from journal writing, it does help to write frequently. Some people enjoy writing in the early morning, while others like to journal just before sleeping in order to process the day's events.

As scientists have pointed out, there does seem to be a definite link between disordered brain chemistry and depressive illness, but which comes first? The answer is most likely that sometimes, the depressed state comes first, which inhibits the production of feel-good brain chemicals. Other times, there is a genetic predisposition to low levels of mood-enhancing neurotransmitters, which can trigger depression. Either way, taking the time for self-reflection and giving your body, mind, and spirit the opportunity to come into a state of balance can only be beneficial and healing.

Meditation as a Path to Healing

Meditation is another helpful path to calming the mind and body. The regular practice of meditation helps you learn to observe the thoughts that pass through your mind, and to learn a healthy detachment from them that allows you to see the bigger picture. Meditation can help you recognize that your thoughts are simply thoughts—they are not you, they are not reality, they are simply the activity of your mind. In learning to meditate, you cultivate the ability to access a place of well-being in the midst of whatever may be going on in your life.

In addition, meditation helps in achieving an internal sense of balance and moderation, something that is sorely lacking in our society. Andrew Weil, M.D., is an advocate of meditation for alleviating depression. According to Weil, depression could just as easily be the result of disordered thinking causing biochemical brain changes—instead of current psychiatric theories, which maintain that disordered brain chemistry causes depression. He maintains that the result of constantly seeking the "highs" of life leads to depression because people then don't know how to live with the "lows" that necessarily follow. He suggests daily meditation as an alternative to constantly seeking stimulating experiences.

Focusing on your breath is an uncomplicated meditation practice. Your breath connects your mind and body, and when you consciously focus your attention on your breathing, you immediately and positively influence your physical and emotional well-being. By paying attention to your breathing and learning to consciously influence the rate and depth of your breath, you can significantly alter your emotional state.

To begin breathwork practice, find a quiet place where you will not be disturbed, and sit in a comfortable position. Bring your attention to your breathing. Relax, and inhale through your nose to a count of five, counting at a pace that is comfortable for you. Hold your breath for a count of five. Open your mouth slightly, and exhale to a count of ten, keeping your exhalation smooth and controlled. Repeat the exercise for a total of five complete cycles.

For a basic meditation practice, try focusing on a word or a phrase that you find calming and relaxing. You might try, "I am calm," or any other word or phrase that appeals to you. Sit or lie in a comfortable position, close your eyes, and take three slow, deep breaths, exhaling completely. Begin saying to yourself, "I am calm," with each exhalation. When your mind wanders, gently bring your attention back to your breathing and your calming phrase. Continue for twenty minutes, imagining waves of relaxation and well-being flowing throughout your body. The more you practice, the easier meditation becomes.

Focusing your complete awareness on a task such as bathing, cooking, or washing dishes is a way of bringing the principles of meditation into everyday life. To try this meditation practice, choose a routine task and focus your attention completely on what you are doing. Slow your movements down to about half of your normal pace. Pay close attention to your body, to each movement, and notice any feelings of tension or discomfort. Breathe into any tightness that you discover and consciously release the tension.

We often habitually perform daily tasks with much more effort than is needed. By paying close attention to your movements, you can learn to do whatever you need to do with the optimal expenditure of effort. This leaves your body relaxed and prevents the unnecessary buildup of stress and tension. This meditation practice is also a way of focusing your attention in the moment, and not allowing your mind to play the negative tapes that it is accustomed to running.

Psychotherapy and Depression

Psychotherapy, also known as "talk therapy," plays a central role in the successful treatment of a depressive disorder. In fact, in some cases of mild or even moderate depression, psychotherapy can be sufficient for alleviating depression. Many doctors still prescribe medication because of the quick symptom relief that can occur. But in most cases of depression, psychotherapy is necessary to address aspects of the illness that drugs do nothing to heal.

Drugs, including the natural alternative St. John's wort, can help to ease the physiological aspects of depressive disorders—the imbalance in brain chemistry that can make everyday functioning so difficult. But for long-term healing, people often need to learn more healthful ways of interacting with their environment. Healing the deep inner wounds that are often at the core of a depressive disorder generally requires intense inner work. A good therapist can help you understand and work through your feelings, and can also help you learn new ways of coping with life stressors that contribute to depression.

There are many different styles of psychotherapy. It's important to find a style of psychotherapy that works for you, and to find a therapist with whom you feel comfortable. Psychotherapy involves sharing your deepest thoughts and feelings, and you need to work with someone that you trust. Although psychotherapists (including psychologists and clinical social workers) are highly trained professionals, they cannot prescribe medication. If you or your therapist believe that medication would be beneficial in the treatment of your depressive disorder, you must see your medical doctor or a psychiatrist for a prescription. If you are interested in trying St. John's wort, no prescription is necessary.

Cognitive therapy is one of the most successful of the psychotherapy approaches for alleviating depression. In cognitive therapy, the focus is on identifying and changing the thinking and behavior patterns that lead to depression. Depression is often related to low self-esteem and negative, self-defeating thoughts. In cognitive therapy, you learn to recognize and dispute the unconscious negative beliefs that permeate your thinking and to replace them with more realistic and self-affirming thoughts. It is often helpful to write down the thoughts as they occur, which helps in identifying and challenging the negative thoughts that run like cassette tapes through the subconscious mind. In cognitive therapy, you learn to change the way that you think about yourself.

One Step at a Time

Depression can be debilitating, both physically and emotionally. It's important to take steps to overcome depression, but at the same time, remember to be gentle with yourself and to set reasonable goals. Here are some things that can help.

Make a list each day of what you want to accomplish. Keep it simple and specific so that you don't end up feeling overwhelmed. Recall the activities that you enjoyed in the past, and make plans to engage in at least one activity each week, even if you don't feel like it. Schedule in at least thirty minutes of aerobic exercise every day—even a brisk walk is sufficient. Spend time with people that you like, and share your feelings with someone that you trust.

Don't expect your mood to change immediately, but cultivate awareness of small improvements in how you feel and the ways that you engage in life. You may find it encouraging to make a list at the end of each day, noting the positive steps you took during the day to help yourself feel better.

Take Time to Nurture Yourself

Time for self-nurturing is often last on the list of things to do in our overly busy, productivity-obsessed society. But without some regular time out from the activities of daily life, it's easy to become exhausted physically, mentally, and spiritually. With the challenges of juggling family, career, home, and social responsibilities, it's even more essential to set aside time for yourself to indulge in the activities that you find restorative for your body, mind, and soul. Neglecting this important aspect of self-care sets the stage for the emptiness and fatigue that we label as depression.

Make self-nurturing a priority, and you will most likely find that you have more energy and enthusiasm for engaging in daily life. Begin by making a list of your favorite ways of caring for yourself, the things that bring you pleasure and make you feel glad to be alive. Include things for your body (receiving a massage, soaking in an aromatherapy bath, talking a walk in nature); for your mind (reading a new book, going to a lecture that interests you, watching a favorite movie); and for your soul (listening to sacred music, talking intimately with a friend, visiting an art gallery).

Each week, set aside time for engaging in at least one activity for each aspect of your being—one thing to nurture your body, one for your mind, and one for your soul. Schedule your appointments for self-nurturing on your calendar, just as you would any other important engagement.

Establish Community

People who are depressed often report a sense of isolation and loneliness. The sense of separation from others that characterizes our modern society is a recent phenomenon. Human beings naturally gravitate toward living in community, and when deprived of close contact, begin to feel disconnected and alone. Even if your family of origin is not made up of people that you would choose as close friends, you can still create a sense of family and intimacy in your life.

Building a network of loving support and friendship takes time and effort, and you might find it difficult to reach out if you're feeling depressed. Start slowly, but make it a goal to do one thing each day to connect with someone that you think you might like to know better. Invite a neighbor over for tea; attend a lecture or meeting on something that interests you and stay around afterward to socialize; join a group or service organization; attend a church, synagogue, or other religious service; join a health club, exercise class, or yoga class; volunteer for a cause you believe in. Make it a goal to have at least a half-dozen people in your life with whom you can share your deepest thoughts and feelings, and with whom you enjoy spending time.

SAFETY AND PRECAUTIONS

Because St. John's wort is marketed as a nutritional supplement and not as a drug, it does not fall under the regulation of the Food and Drug Administration (this is true for all herbal supplements). To further complicate the issue, most conventionally trained doctors do not receive training in botanical medicine. This means that your doctor may not be fully aware of the beneficial properties of St. John's wort and may not know exactly how to prescribe it, or what cautions should be observed.

Herbs Are Powerful Medicines

Many people have the erroneous belief that because a substance is derived from a plant, it cannot be harmful. Herbs have healing benefits because they contain compounds that have measurable biological effects on the body. Some of these compounds are potentially harmful if the plant is used improperly.

The renaissance of interest in herbal medicine in this country indicates that the general public is tired of the side effects and costs of prescription medications, and that people are interested in a more natural, less invasive approach to healing. Herbal remedies also offer the opportunity for a more empowered role of health care, one that enables individuals to assume a more active role in their healing. This freedom also means that it is essential to be educated about the substances that you take into your body, whether these substances are prescription drugs or herbs.

Possible Side Effects of St. John's Wort

The long history of safety of St. John's wort makes it a valuable alternative to prescription antidepressants for many people. Most people can use St. John's wort safely, but as with any medicinal herb or drug, certain precautions should be observed. If you are taking St. John's wort, be sure to tell your doctor, because the herb may affect other medications that you are taking. Do not take St. John's wort if you are pregnant without consulting your doctor.

Side effects occasionally occur with St. John's wort, but they tend to be minor and uncommon. Some people report mild stomach upset while taking the herb. Taking St. John's wort with food can help to prevent digestive upset. More rarely, some people experience allergic reactions, fatigue, or restlessness while using St. John's wort. If you notice any of these symptoms, consult your health care practitioner for advice before continuing to use the herb.

At one time, St. John's wort was thought to act in a similar way to monoamine oxidase inhibitors (MAOIs), an older class of antidepressant drugs. For this reason, people taking St. John's wort were cautioned to avoid foods high in the amino acid tyramine (such as red wine, aged cheese, and chocolate) because the interaction of these foods with MAO inhibitors can cause blood pressure levels to become dangerously elevated. Symptoms of this reaction include headaches, palpitations, and nausea. But more recent research has not confirmed that St. John's wort is an MAO inhibitor. Instead, St. John's wort is thought to act more like the more recent class of antidepressant drugs that increase levels of serotonin in the brain.

St. John's Wort and Photosensitivity

St. John's wort is classified as toxic to livestock because it can cause severe photosensivity (adverse reaction to sunlight). Although this reaction is uncommon in humans, there have been a few reports of photosensivity in people taking therapeutic amounts of St. John's wort.

Symptoms of photosensitivity include skin rash, unusual susceptibility to sunburn, or pain or burning of the skin when exposed to ultraviolet light. Fair-skinned people are most vulnerable, as are people who have experienced reactions to ultraviolet light when taking other types of medications. If you are at risk for photosensitivity, take care to avoid excessive sun exposure, tanning lamps, or other sources of ultraviolet light while taking St. John's wort.

The Effect of St. John's Wort on Prescription Drugs

Research reported by the National Institutes of Health in early 2000 revealed that St. John's wort may reduce the effectiveness of some prescription drugs. As a result, the Food and Drug Administration asked health care professionals to caution patients about the potential risks of combining St. John's wort with other medications. However, this does not mean that St. John's wort can never be used in combination with prescription drugs. It simply means that to be safe, you should always let your doctor know about any herbal supplements that you may be using to avoid the possibility of harmful drug interactions.

St. John's wort appears to speed up metabolic activity in a key pathway that is responsible for the breakdown of some prescription drugs. Basically, this means that the body processes the drugs more quickly, which lowers blood levels of the medications and decreases the effectiveness of the drugs.

Specifically, St. John's wort has been found to affect indinavir and other protease inhibitors, which are antiviral drugs used to treat HIV infection. St. John's wort also apparently affects cyclosporin, which is used to help prevent organ rejection in patients who have undergone transplants. In addition, St. John's wort may affect other immunosuppressant drugs and other medications that work through the same pathway. This includes birth control pills, cholesterol-lowering medications such as Mevacor (lovastatin), other drugs used in heart disease such as digoxin, some cancer medications, seizure drugs, and blood thinners such as Coumadin (warfarin). If you are taking these drugs, taking St. John's wort may interfere with their effectiveness and could potentially cause dangerous changes in drug effects. To be safe, always inform your doctor about any herbs and supplements that you are taking.

St. John's Wort and Antidepressants

If you are currently taking antidepressant medications, it is essential that you work with your doctor if you are interested in taking St. John's wort. Do not attempt to abruptly discontinue antidepressants, but instead, work with your doctor to gradually wean yourself from prescription medications. Also, be aware that in some cases (especially for people with major chronic depression and those with bipolar disorder) prescription medications are probably necessary. Hyla Cass, M.D., offers a protocol helpful for physicians and patients for substituting St. John's wort for antidepressants in her book *St. John's Wort: Nature's Blues Buster.*

HOW TO BUY AND USE ST. JOHN'S WORT

St. John's wort is a top-selling herb and is widely available in natural food stores and pharmacies. Choosing among the dozens of St. John's wort products can be confusing. In this section, you will learn how to identify good-quality products and understand the differences among the various herbal formulations. With this information, you will be able to make an informed decision that will help you choose a product that best meets your needs. You will also learn how to take St. John's wort and the dosages that are most effective.

Please note that if you are suffering from anything other than very mild depression, you should be working with a health professional who can provide you with appropriate support and guidance.

Finding an Effective Supplement

There can be a vast difference in the way that St. John's wort is grown, harvested, and processed. As a result, there can be significant differences in the quality of commercial St. John's wort products. While some products are good sources of the beneficial compounds that make St. John's wort so effective, others may contain little or none of the active ingredients. While all parts of the plant contain some degree of plant chemicals, the flower buds of St. John's wort contain the highest concentrations of the active ingredients.

In 1998, the *Los Angeles Times* commissioned laboratory tests on ten different St. John's wort products. The researchers found that the potencies of the products were very different from what was claimed on the label. Because manufacturers want consumers to have confidence in the herbal products they are buying, the herbal industry is moving toward third-party certification, such as is provided by the U.S. Pharmocopeia, a nonprofit group that establishes drug standards, and NSF International, a nonprofit group that sets health standards. This means that herbal products are tested by an independent group to ensure that the products meet certain standards. In the process, the consumer is assured of a quality product.

Different Forms of St. John's Wort

St. John's wort is available in many different forms, including as teas, capsules, tablets, and liquid extracts. You'll even find St. John's wort included in some foods, such as breakfast cereals and snacks. The addition of St. John's wort to food products is a marketing strategy that capitalizes on the popularity of St. John's wort, and is not meant for the treatment of depressive disorders.

St. John's wort has traditionally been used as a tea and as a tincture (a liquid extract made by crushing and steeping the herb in food-grade alcohol). Teas made from St. John's wort are not recommended for treating depression, because the active ingredients are not adequately extracted in hot water. Tinctures (now labeled as liquid extracts by manufacturers) do extract the active chemicals. Of course, this depends on the initial quality of the plant material and the care of the manufacturer during the processing of the plant.

The amount of active ingredients can vary greatly in liquid extracts. If you want to try taking a liquid extract, the Herb Research Foundation suggests taking 20 to 30 drops three times a day. Dilute the extract with a small amount of warm water or add to juice, and take it with meals.

Standardized Extracts

All of the research on St. John's wort has been conducted using standardized extracts, which makes it easier for researchers to maintain consistency in their studies. While St. John's wort products do not have to be standardized to be effective, if you want to be sure that you are obtaining adequate levels of the active compounds, your best bet is to buy products that are labeled as standardized extracts.

Standardization
Standardized extracts are herbal products guaranteed to contain a specified amount of the herb's primary active ingredients.

Standardized extracts are herbal products that are guaranteed to contain a specified amount of what is currently believed to be the herb's primary active ingredient. Various processes are used to obtain the specified concentration, including removing what are considered to be unimportant constituents and adding high concentrations of the isolated active ingredients.

St. John's wort extracts are typically standardized to contain 0.3 percent hypericin and 5 percent hyperforin. If you are using a standardized extract, buy products that state on the label that they contain these percentages of active ingredients.

Although most of the research on St. John's wort has used 900 mg daily of St. John's wort (usually taken as 300 mg three times a day), people vary in their response to the herb and you can adjust the dosage as needed. Some people respond well to lesser amounts of the herb, while others need more.

It's safe to take as much as 1,800 mg of St. John's wort daily, but you should give the herb at least two months at the standard amount of 900 mg before increasing your dosage. To increase the amount you are taking, add an additional 300 mg daily for one month, and then continue adding an additional 300 mg daily dosage each month until you reach 1,800 mg. Working with a health practitioner who is familiar with St. John's wort can be helpful in determining the dosage that is most appropriate for you.

It's best to take the full amount of the herb in three equal doses, one with each meal. Taking the herb with a meal helps to prevent the possibility of any digestive upset. Taking St. John's wort at regular intervals throughout the day keeps a steady supply of the active ingredients available to your body. Many people notice a significant difference within a couple of weeks of taking St. John's wort, and report improvements in sleep quality, energy levels, and appetite. But don't be discouraged if you don't notice changes right away. It can take several weeks for the full effects of St. John's wort to kick in.

Seeing Results from St. John's Wort

The most common mistake that people make when taking herbal supplements is in not giving the herb sufficient time to have a physiological effect on the body. You should expect definite results, but be patient and give the herb at least six weeks before making a decision about whether or not to continue taking it.

It's important to take the herb regularly, not just when you're feeling depressed. St. John's wort has a cumulative positive effect on depression, and interrupting your regular schedule of taking the herb can diminish the benefits. However, don't fret if you happen to miss a dosage. Just try to keep as much as possible to a regular schedule of taking the herb. If necessary, you can always double up on a dosage if you happen to miss one.

If you're not getting positive results from St. John's wort within six to eight weeks, it's possible that the supplement you are taking may not contain adequate amounts of the active compounds to be effective. For this reason, it is essential to buy quality herbal products from a reputable company. Ask your doctor, pharmacist, or a qualified herbalist for recommendations.

How Long to Take St. John's Wort

As your depression lifts and your mood stabilizes, you may want to consider beginning to taper off of St. John's wort. For most people, staying on the herb for at least one month after depressive symptoms have abated is helpful. Although there are generally no negative side effects associated with discontinuing St. John's wort, you may want to taper off of it gradually, lessening your dosage by 300 mg at a time over a period of weeks. While many people do take St. John's wort for brief periods, others find that they do best when they take the herb for months, or even years. St. John's wort can be taken for as long as is necessary and can be used safely for an indefinite period of time.

Because it can be difficult to self-evaluate progress in depressive disorders, you may find it useful to retake the depression test in this book once a month while you are using St. John's wort, and also during the time when you are decreasing your dosage of the herb. It's also best to work with a mental health professional who can guide you in your treatment plan.

Depressive disorders are complex, and the successful path to a satisfying way of life requires a commitment to healing on all levels. Combined with attention to your physical, emotional, and spiritual well-being, St. John's wort can be a valuable ally in your journey.

GINKGO BILOBA

HYLA CASS, M.D., & JIM ENGLISH

Ginkgo biloba is the best-selling prescription herb in Europe, the fifth most widely used herb in the United States, and one of the most highly sought-after herbs in the world, all for good reason. It became one of the most highly prized natural supplements because of its proven effectiveness for enhancing memory and mental function, improving blood circulation to the brain, reducing inflammation, relieving allergies and asthma, and protecting the body from the effects of aging. Ginkgo's well-earned reputation is supported by more than thirty years of scientific and clinical research. In Part Nine of this book, we are going to outline a number of these studies and let you see for yourself the important benefits this magnificent herb has to offer.

A major health threat facing humans, especially aging baby boomers now entering middle age, is the decline in their mental abilities. The decline was traditionally accepted as a normal part of the human aging process, but that idea is now being discarded as an outmoded concept, and treatment for this formerly accepted process is now regularly sought out. The result is that healthcare providers and medical professionals are struggling to cope with the growing flood of older people and their caregivers all looking for ways to treat dementia, memory impairment, and other age-related cognitive dysfunctions. To solve this crisis, medical researchers from around the world have engaged in a desperate search for new treatments to help prevent or treat Alzheimer's disease and other degenerative brain conditions.

For years, American doctors dismissed the value of herbs, preferring instead to prescribe expensive drugs. European doctors, on the other hand, have always prescribed "phytomedicines," or herbal medicines, alongside the pharmaceuticals. And there has been enough research done on these herbs in Europe that physicians in the United States are beginning to take notice.

One of the most impressive bodies of research growing out of this medical challenge to find new treatments consists of several thousand published studies on ginkgo biloba. In China, extracts of the fruit and leaves of the ginkgo tree have been used for more than 5,000 years to treat asthma, cardiovascular diseases, and poor memory. And over the last fifty years, clinical studies have documented the many attributes of this ancient tree herb.

It has been found to alleviate angina pectoris (chest pain) due to coronary artery disease; asthma; depression; intermittent claudication (leg pain due to poor blood flow when walking); macular degeneration; PMS symptoms, including edema (swelling); and tinnitus (ringing in the ears).

It can also:

- Improve memory in both normal adults and those with Alzheimer's disease; pulmonary function; sexual function and desire in both men and women; and visual acuity.

- Inhibit platelet aggregation and the tendency for blood to clot abnormally.

- Reduce or eliminate vertigo (dizziness and instability).

- Reduce elevated blood pressure.

Ginkgo has been able to perform this myriad of beneficial effects because of its antioxidant properties, its ability to enhance blood flow in your arteries and capillaries, and its amazing ability to inhibit the platelet-activating factor (PAF), and thereby prevent abnormal blood clots from forming.

In the following sections, we will outline the history of this ancient healing herb for you, and examine the growing list of its remarkable health benefits, which includes the ability to boost mental functions, strengthen the cardiovascular system, and fend off the ravages of aging.

DISCOVERY OF A LIVING FOSSIL

If you were to search for a natural compound that could offer protective benefits against the effects of aging, ginkgo would crop up as a most likely candidate. Not only is ginkgo one of the most ancient surviving species in the world—its fossils from the Triassic period date back almost 200 million years—but it is also one of the most long-lived of all plants. There are ginkgo trees that have lived for more than 1,000 years—and they are *still* living.

When the unusually shaped impressions left in ancient shale deposits were first discovered, botanists identified the plant as a gymnosperm, a plant family that includes pines, cedars, and firs. Eventually, fifteen different types of the Ginkgoaceae tree family were identified, but only from fossil records, so it was believed that all these plants were extinct, the victims of massive climatic changes during the last major ice age.

In the early 1700s, all this changed when Western researchers were stunned to learn that a species of ginkgo had been found *thriving* in China and Asia. The discovery created quite a sensation at the time, particularly as reports about the medicinal uses of this "sacred plant" had begun to surface in the West.

The "Way of Long Life"

The name ginkgo was first given to the newly discovered plant in the early 1700s by a German surgeon working in Asia for the Dutch East India Company. He coined the name ginkgo from the phonetic transcription of a Japanese variation on the Chinese word *yinhsing,* which means "silver apricot." In 1771, the famed Swedish botanist Carolus Linnaeus, recognized as the Father of Taxonomy for his system of classifying plants, renamed the plant ginkgo biloba, ("ginkgo with two lobes") based on the unique division of the leaves into two lobes. The ginkgo tree is also sometimes referred to as the kew or maidenhair tree, because the leaves also bear a likeness to the fronds of maidenhair ferns.

The West soon learned that, in addition to being revered as a sacred plant that was commonly planted around Buddhist temples, the leaves and fruit of the ginkgo tree had been used in traditional Chinese medicine for more than 5,000 years. The discovery of the health-enhancing effects of ginkgo is attributed to the legendary emperor Shen Nong Shi (2,852–2,737 B.C.) who taught primitive farmers to make farming tools and grow crops. Following the "Way of Long Life," Shen Nong devoted himself to the study of various plants and became an expert in the properties of herbal medicines. Since there were no written records at the time, his discoveries were passed down by word of mouth until, almost 2,000 years later during the Han dynasty (206 B.C.–A.D. 220), his teachings were committed to text in the *Pen T'sao Ching* (The Classic of Herbs). Also referred to as the *Materia Medica of Shen Nong,* this earliest recorded text of herbal treatments recommended ginkgo leaves as especially helpful for treating failing memory and relieving the symptoms of asthma and cough.

Shen Nong is also credited with establishing the concept of opposing principals of nature that are recognized today as the "yin" and "yang" forces of nature. In keeping with this philosophy, ginkgo is considered a dry agent that is best used to counter and balance wet diseases. Then, as now, Chinese healers used the leaves, bark, seeds (or nuts), and the fruits of the ginkgo tree. The leaves were prepared either as a tea or, mixed with rice wine, as a concoction useful for treating angina pectoris, bronchitis, elevated blood fats, fading mental powers, hangovers, or parasites, and for improving blood circulation. The bark was used to treat discharges from the sexual organs, or was applied to the skin as a poultice to prevent infections.

Using the fruit of the ginkgo tree is problematic, as the seeds contain a group of terpene compounds that can irritate the skin and cause a rash. If eaten, the fruit and seeds can irritate the gastrointestinal tract and cause painful spasms and nausea, or can even lead to kidney and liver damage. In order to remove these harmful terpenes, Chinese herbalists learned to prepare ginkgo fruit by boiling it first, then using the seeds to treat conditions such as asthma and diarrhea.

The Ornamental Origins of Ginkgo

The ginkgo was first imported to the United States in 1784 as an attractive ornamental plant that was highly regarded for its extraordinary resistance to insects and disease. Its legendary medical properties were largely unrecognized by the West at the time. The ginkgo is so resistant to damage, in fact, that one ginkgo tree actually survived the atomic bomb dropped on Hiroshima, and is reportedly still alive and growing near the epicenter of the explosion.

One minor problem with the introduction of the ginkgo is that the species is dioecious, meaning that the trees are composed of two distinct sexes that reproduce when wind-born pollen from the male tree fertilizes the female tree. Both trees are equally attractive, but the female bears a small fruit with a highly objectionable, foul smell that has been compared to rancid butter or dog droppings. To get around this problem, horticulturists and gardeners simply choose to plant the male ginkgo tree.

Dioecious Trees
"Di" meaning two, is combined with "oecious," from the Greek word oikos for house, to refer to the two houses representing a separate house, or tree, for each of the sexes.

Ginkgo's Unique Chemistry

As ginkgo trees grew in popularity, they spread across urban settings in Europe and America, flourishing in places where other species, less resistant to pollution, diseases, and insects, failed to thrive. Modern research on ginkgo arose from a scientific interest in its adaptive properties, and in the 1950s, German researchers began to study ginkgo in earnest, searching for unknown compounds that might reveal the secret to its unique longevity.

One of the pioneers in ginkgo research was Willmar

Schwabe, Ph.D., a West German researcher who set out to isolate the active constituents of the ginkgo leaf and determine if they possessed any medicinal benefits. What Schwabe and his colleagues discovered were a *number of potent compounds that are completely unique to the ginkgo plant and are not found anywhere else in nature.*

Ginkgo's Active Compounds

Flavone Glycosides. Researchers have identified a number of complex molecules in the ginkgo, including a group of special antioxidant compounds known as flavone glycosides, a type of flavonoid (also called bioflavonoids) found in many plants. These compounds act as powerful antioxidants to quench the activity of free radicals—these destructive oxidizing molecules produced normally in the body, and by air pollution, cigarettes, and radiation. Left uncontrolled, free radicals wreak havoc with cells and can damage DNA, setting the stage for degenerative diseases, initiating cancer, and accelerating the aging process. The flavone glycosides isolated from the ginkgo consist of three bioflavonoid compounds known as quercetin, kaempferol, and isorhamnetin. In addition to acting as antioxidants, these flavone glycosides also work together with vitamin C, sparing it from free radical damage and increasing its effectiveness in the body.

Antioxidants
Molecules that donate electrons to stabilize damaging free radicals and render them harmless.

One of the most important benefits of the flavonoids is their ability to protect blood vessels. Old age, infection, use of steroid drugs, and nutritional deficiencies common to the elderly all set the stage for weakened blood vessels. These fragile blood vessels are, in turn, more prone to damage, resulting in bruising, even from minor bumps. Flavonoids like those found in ginkgo have been shown to enhance capillary walls, thereby protecting vessels from rupture, preventing seepage of blood into surrounding tissues, and reducing inflammation.

Terpene Lactones. A second group of active ingredients isolated from the roots and leaves of ginkgo biloba are several terpene compounds, including terpene lactones. Several studies have found that the terpenes found in the ginkgo protect brain tissues by acting as free radical scavengers outright, while also reducing the formation of free radicals by protecting your brain and nerve cells from the damaging effects of hypoxia (impaired flow of oxygen to the brain). This activity most likely accounts for ginkgo's ability to help in recovering from a stroke.

Stroke
The third leading cause of death in the U.S. It occurs when a region of the brain loses blood flow, usually from an obstructed blood vessel. Each year about 400,000 cases of stroke and approximately 150,000 deaths from it are reported in the U.S.

Terpene lactones also enhance energy by increasing the body's absorption of glucose (blood sugar) and by boosting the body's production of adenosine triphosphate (ATP), the universal energy molecule. This combination of increased glucose intake and ATP production results in increased brain metabolism and physical energy.

Cerebral Hypoxia
A condition in which oxygen flow to the brain is impaired. The reduced flow of oxygen does not always involve a diminished flow of blood. This fact emphasizes blood's important role in supporting the brain cells outside of oxygen delivery.

Platelet–Activating Factor (PAF) and Ginkgo

Ginkgolide B, one of the terpenes in ginkgo, is particularly important in reducing blood clotting because of its regulatory effects on platelet-activating factor (PAF). Normally, when a wound or injury occurs, the platelets in the blood are stimulated by PAF to become sticky, gather together, and form clots that block the flow of blood. This is a good thing because it protects us from bleeding to death.

But, while a little PAF is necessary for normal clotting, too much PAF can promote sticky blood, and this can lead to a number of health problems, for example, restricting the flow of blood to the brain, thereby reducing the amount of oxygen it receives. Excess PAF also increases free radical production, damages nerve tissues, initiates rejection of transplanted organs, and promotes inflammation and bronchial constriction. Additionally, the excess platelet aggregation that is triggered by PAF leads to an increased formation of blood clots (thromboses). These can, in turn, lead to heart disease, strokes, and peripheral vascular disease— including intermittent claudication, a painful condition due to impaired circulation in the legs that restricts walking.

Platelet–Activating Factor
Stimulates platelets in the blood to gather together and form clots to block the flow of blood.

Excess production of PAF is believed to be caused by elements of our contemporary lifestyle—a diet high in processed (hydrogenated) fats, chronic exposure to allergens, and stress, for example.

Ginkgolide B has been shown to inhibit PAF and prevent platelet clumping by preventing PAF from binding to the platelets.

The Synergy of Ginkgo

In ancient traditional Chinese medicine, healers used the seeds and leaves of ginkgo to treat their patients. And although the various active compounds isolated from the ginkgo were shown to be effective, researchers determined that these ingredients worked more effectively when taken together, a phenomenon referred to as *synergy.*

Recognizing that the health effects of ginkgo require the right synergistic balance of its active components, German researchers concentrated their efforts on arriving at a standardized extract. Only by guaranteeing that the final extract contained the correct ratio and potency of the purified active ingredients could a reliable extract be produced for consistent health benefits.

One of the major problems in arriving at a standardized extract is the wide variation and inconsistency in the percentages of active ingredients that may be present in any given crop of harvested ginkgo. Whereas it was traditionally harvested from fallen leaves in ancient China, today's ginkgo is harvested from trees grown on plantations in China, France, and the United States. The leaves are harvested once a year, and only in the fall.

A number of factors can influence the quality and the quantity of the flavonoids and terpene lactones, including the age of the plants, the abundance, or lack, of rainfall, the soil acidity, the growing temperature, and a number of other natural factors. Even under the most strictly controlled growing conditions, the final content of active ingredients can vary enormously.

After years of experimentation, Dr. Willmar Schwabe of Schwabe GmbH, the largest phytomedicine company in Germany, was able to establish a process for producing a guaranteed, standardized extract known as EGb 761. This process allowed for consistent and reproducible manufacture of a standard potency product that could then be used use in clinical trials. The process starts with the harvesting of green leaves from the male plant in the late summer or early fall, when the flavonoid content is at its highest levels. After harvest, the leaves undergo a complex process involving twenty-seven distinct steps. Over a period of two weeks, fifty pounds of raw leaves are dried and pressed, and the active ingredients are then isolated and balanced.

All this precise work results in a final, purified, and standardized extract that weighs a mere one pound. Called ginkgo extract, or GBE, it is standardized to contain between 22 and 27 percent ginkgo flavone glycosides, or flavonoids, and 5 and 7 percent terpene lactones. This process has been further standardized. As a result most ginkgo extracts available on the market currently contain ratios of 24 percent ginkgo flavonoids, 6 percent terpene lactones, and 1 percent bilobalide.

GINKGO BILOBA AND THE BRAIN

The human brain is one of the most complex wonders in all of nature. For sheer complexity and processing power, no other organized structure can begin to match this mysterious organ. Composed of some 10 billion neurons and their supportive network, the human brain controls virtually all of our life systems, while generating the flood of thoughts, dreams, and feelings that define our identity and color our very perception of reality. Virtually every thought, concept, opinion, belief, and emotion you have is derived from the millions of chemical and electrical reactions that occur in your brain every minute. And to power all this activity, your brain places a huge demand on your body's energy reserves. Though it accounts for a mere 2 percent of the body's weight, your brain greedily consumes more than 20 percent of your body's available energy in the form of oxygen and glucose. And when your brain activity increases, so too does the demand for energy.

A Matter of Balance

Yet for all of its impressive complexity, your brain is also an extremely delicate organ that depends entirely on the other organs of your body for its existence. The lungs must work continuously to deliver vital oxygen to brain cells, while the liver converts carbohydrates into glucose for energy production. And your heart and cardiovascular system must work tirelessly to keep blood flowing into your brain to deliver these vital nutrients and remove the resulting waste products. Any condition that interrupts or impairs the flow of blood and oxygen to the brain can cause irreparable damage—and even death—in minutes.

The Aging Brain

Time takes a major toll on the human brain. On average, by age seventy, we lose about 10 percent of our original brain cells from the effects of normal aging. And while our other body tissues, such as the skin and liver have the capacity to regenerate, this trait is not shared by our brain cells—once a brain cell is lost, it is gone forever. With the passage of time, this continual loss of brain cells is further aggravated by damage from by other age-related conditions, such as arteriosclerosis (hardening of the arteries), diabetes, hypertension, and cerebrovascular diseases (CVD), such as cerebrovascular insufficiency, strokes, and multi-infarct dementia (MID).

Brain-Protective Effects of Ginkgo Biloba

Intrigued by historical reports of ginkgo protecting mental functions, European researchers began to study this compound in the 1950s. Initial studies revealed that the unique compounds found only in ginkgo could enhance normal brain functions and aid in the prevention and treatment of a number of brain disorders, including Alzheimer's disease, cerebrovascular insufficiency, and depression, as well as a number of degenerative aging diseases. Their research to date, published in hundreds of studies, has shown that ginkgo biloba is one the safest and most effective agents available for treating age-related mental disorders.

Cerebrovascular Insufficiency

In 1992, a team of German researchers coined a new term—cerebrovascular insufficiency—to describe twelve symptoms common to older people that result from chronically impaired blood flow to the brain. These symptoms include:

- Absent-mindedness
- Anxiety
- Confusion
- Decreased physical performance
- Depression
- Dizziness (vertigo)
- Fatigue
- Lack of energy
- Poor concentration
- Poor memory
- Tinnitus

In addition to causing distress and impairing normal activities, these symptoms are also thought to predict the later onset of dementia or other degenerative diseases.

How Ginkgo Helps Treat Cerebrovascular Insufficiency

Cerebrovascular insufficiency is caused by a reduction in the flow of blood to the brain. This impairment, in turn, reduces the amount of oxygen reaching the cells, which causes an increase in the production of harmful free radicals. This leads to further tissue damage, particularly to the outer membrane of brain neurons.

In Germany, ginkgo has been approved and licensed for the treatment of cerebral insufficiency based on the positive results of a series of clinical studies. Researchers believe that the positive brain-protecting effects of ginkgo are due to the ability of ginkgo leaf extract to improve blood circulation and oxygen delivery, particularly in the micro-capillaries, and to protect the brain cells against further damage from free radicals. In one study, researchers measured a 57 percent increase in blood flow through capillaries within sixty minutes of giving ginkgo extract to volunteers.

In 1988, in one of the first clinical trials, 166 people over age sixty were given ginkgo as part of a study on the herb's effectiveness in treating cerebral insufficiency. After just three months of treatment, the authors of the study concluded that these test subjects had improved and that the results "confirmed the efficacy of ginkgo extract in cerebral disorders due to aging."

In another early study, reported in 1990, German scientists gave 160 mg of ginkgo extract to a group of sixty hospitalized patients with cerebral insufficiency and depression. Remarkably, the patients given the ginkgo began to show marked improvement after only two weeks, with a significant reduction in many of their symptoms. Over the course of the following four weeks, the researchers noted that eleven of the twelve symptoms listed above had improved significantly in the patients treated with ginkgo extracts, leading to the conclusion that "ginkgo extract can be given to patients with mild to moderate symptoms of cerebral insufficiency."

Again, in 1994, researchers continued to find significant improvements in mental performance after conducting a placebo-controlled, double-blind trial of ninety people with cerebral insufficiency. As in the earlier studies, after only six weeks of treatment with a standardized ginkgo extract, those tested showed marked improvements in their conditions, including significant increases in both short-term memory and concentration.

Placebo
An inactive substance that is used as a control in clinical studies instead of a drug or nutrient.

Dementia, Alzheimer's Disease, and Age-Associated Memory Impairment (AAMI)

Dementia is defined as the loss of intellectual functions. Unlike occasional forgetfulness, dementia is marked by a profound impairment of memory, as well as the loss of additional, complex abilities required for problem-solving, decision-making, spatial orientation, and even the ability to put simple words together to communicate. Dementia is a permanent, progressive disease that mostly affects older people, who may eventually lose the ability to function normally and require round-the-clock care. It is estimated that up to 8 percent of all people over age sixty-five have some form of dementia. That number doubles every five years, leading to an estimate of anywhere from 20 to 50 percent of people in their eighties with dementia. There are close to fifty different causes of dementia, including neurological disorders (Alzheimer's disease), vascular disorders (multi-infarct disease), inherited disorders (Huntington's disease), and infections (viruses such as HIV).

A common factor in all these disorders is a reduced flow of blood and oxygen to the brain. Aside from starving the brain cells of needed fuel, reduced blood flow also increases the production of free radicals, which further damage cell membranes and accelerate brain-cell death. As the number of lost brain cells grows, either from the ravages of age or the debilitating effects of degenerative diseases, mental deterioration continues. Memories begin to fade and the ability to form new thoughts and solve problems is further reduced. Depression, disorientation, incontinence, muscle weakness, speech disturbances, tinnitus (ringing in the ears), tremor, and loss of both visual acuity and coordination also increase as the conditions progress.

Alzheimer's Disease

Alzheimer's disease (also called "senile dementia of the Alzheimer type") is a chronic and progressive, degenerative neurological condition. More than 4 million people in the United States are currently diagnosed with the disease, and it accounts for up to 60 percent of all cases of dementia. Alzheimer's usually appears after age fifty, and from age sixty-five on, the risk of developing the disease doubles every five years. As if these numbers weren't bad enough, they are expected to almost double in the coming decades, placing a further drain on healthcare resources, and leaving almost no family untouched.

While there is currently no cure for Alzheimer's disease, exciting new research shows that ginkgo extract can help in halting the destructive progression of dementia and can offer improvement in the cognitive functions of those with Alzheimer's disease or other forms of dementia.

Alzheimer's disease is associated with a naturally occurring key protein called amyloid. In Alzheimer's, this protein accumulates to form unusual plaques and tangles throughout the brain, leading to dementia, behavioral symptoms, and loss of brain tissues. There is new evidence that the increased production of free radicals seen with aging may be partly responsible for both plaque build-up and the death of brain cells seen in Alzheimer's disease.

Ginkgo Benefits Alzheimer's Patients

Researchers have found that ginkgo can be especially helpful when given to patients at the first sign of symptoms. In one published study, German scientists gave a daily dose of 120 mg of ginkgo to twenty older men and women exhibiting various early symptoms of dementia. The results were dramatic—those receiving ginkgo showed impressive improvements in a variety of clinical tests, as compared to others receiving only a placebo, or dummy pill.

In one large 1996 study, German researchers tested ginkgo extract on a group of 222 people, fifty-five or older, who were diagnosed with a mild to moderate dementia caused either by Alzheimer disease or multi-infarct dementia. They were given either 240 mg of ginkgo biloba extract, twice a day before meals, or a placebo, for the duration of the six-month trial. At the conclusion of the study, the researchers reported those receiving the ginkgo showed a remarkable overall improvement in their condition, including a 300 percent increase in memory and attention, as compared to the others receiving the placebo pills. The researchers concluded their report by stating that, in cases of dementia, ginkgo extract could improve the quality of life while preserving independence and postponing the need for, and expense of, full-time care.

A second German study confirmed the effectiveness of ginkgo in treating people with Alzheimer's disease. Researchers again divided 216 people, all of them suffering from mild to moderate symptoms of Alzheimer's, into two groups. The first group received 240 mg of ginkgo each day, and the other group received a placebo pill. While this trial lasted for only a month, at its conclusion those receiving the ginkgo again exhibited impressive improvements on tests designed to measure mental functions, showing improvements in alertness and overall mood.

Multi-Infarct Dementia

The second most common cause of dementia in older people is multi-infarct dementia (MID), a condition that accounts for about 15 percent of all cases of dementia. Multi-infarct dementia usually affects people between the ages of sixty and seventy-five, and men are more likely to have multi-infarct dementia than are women. MID is typically caused by a series of mini-strokes, also referred to as transient ischemic attacks (TIAs), that can occur when an artery in the brain either becomes blocked or ruptures. Strokes are generally caused by high blood pressure, high blood cholesterol, diabetes, or heart disease. Of these causes, the most important risk factor for multi-infarct dementia is untreated high blood pressure. In fact, it is extremely rare for a person to develop multi-infarct dementia without also having high blood pressure.

While these mini-strokes may or may not be noticed at the time, the effect on the brain is the same—brain cells become damaged by a lack of oxygen and die. Over time, mini-strokes can begin to destroy the substantial portions of the brain that control speech and visual processing.

As with Alzheimer's disease, ginkgo has been shown to help people with MID by enhancing memory, alertness, and overall quality of life. Additionally, given the underlying disorders that cause blood vessels to rupture, ginkgo can also benefit people with MID by restoring elasticity and strength to their stiff, weakened blood vessels.

GINKGO AND THE HEART

The human heart is an organ of remarkable precision and reliability. Every minute, this small pear-shaped organ beats seventy-two times to completely recycle approximately five quarts of blood throughout the body. In an average lifetime, the heart will steadily pound out more than 2.5 billion beats, a number most of us remain blissfully ignorant of, until something interrupts this tireless muscle and its life-giving rhythm.

Just as ginkgo supports cerebral blood circulation and increases the flow of oxygen to the brain, it also protects the circulatory system and enhances the delivery of oxygen to the heart and skeletal tissues. Not only does ginkgo improve the overall performance of the circulatory system, but it has also been effective in strengthening weakened blood vessels while restoring some of the elasticity that veins commonly lose with age. In fact, German researchers have shown that taking ginkgo over the long term can protect your heart tissues and reduce your risk of developing heart disease and high blood pressure.

The Circulatory System

The circulatory system carries blood throughout your body. Driven by the pumping actions of the heart, the arteries are the large blood vessels responsible for distributing oxygen and nutrients throughout your body. As the arteries branch off into smaller vessels that continue through the body, the vessels grow smaller and smaller until they reaching the micro-capillaries, which are so small that blood cells must pass through passageways finer than a human hair. As the blood cells deposit their cargo of vital nutrients and oxygen, they exchange them for the cellular waste products they pick up for disposal. Then, as the blood makes its way back up the system, it moves through increasingly larger veins until it reaches the lungs where the waste carbon dioxide is exchanged for fresh oxygen, and the cycle starts all over.

In 1965, the German physician Dr. Willmar Schwabe III identified the beneficial effects of ginkgo on the circulatory system as part of his interest in developing a concentrated extract to be used in clinical study. Schwabe and other researchers found that ginkgo had a number of effects on the human circulatory system. Shortly after ingesting ginkgo, it can be detected in the plasma that accounts for most of the blood's volume. As ginkgo levels rise in the plasma, ginkgo begins to do its work of supporting the myriad cells and tissues that make up the circulatory system.

Ginkgo has improved the circulatory system by helping to strengthen the blood vessels and restore the elasticity that is lost with advancing age. It also acts as a powerful antioxidant that protects the heart and blood vessels from a number of highly reactive and damaging free radicals.

As discussed elsewhere, ginkgo also inhibits the actions of platelet-activating factor (PAF), improving circulation and keeping the blood flowing freely. This enhances the delivery of oxygen to the brain and central nervous system while reducing the risks of both clot (thrombosis) formation and coronary artery spasms that can lead to heart attacks.

Ginkgo and High Blood Pressure

High blood pressure (hypertension) is one of the most common forms of cardiovascular disease, affecting an estimated 25 percent of Americans. Hypertension is associated with atherosclerosis, congestive heart failure, hypertensive renal failure, "myocardial infarction," or heart attack, and stroke. Although hypertension has been extensively studied, more than 90 percent of all cases are referred to as essential hypertension, meaning the cause of the elevated blood pressure is unknown.

A group of Japanese researchers tested the effects of using ginkgo extract to treat hypertension in rats. After feeding ginkgo to the animals for twenty days, the team reported that the rats' high blood pressure was significantly reduced. Additionally, they noted that the rats didn't show any increase in the size of their hearts, a known sign of sustained high blood pressure. Ginkgo's effect appeared to normalize only high blood pressure; there were no changes in the rats with normal blood-pressure levels.

Ginkgo and Arrhythmia

Any change in the regular beating rhythm of the heart is defined as arrhythmia, called tachycardia when the heart beats very fast, and bradycardia when it beats very slowly. Arrhythmias are the result of interference with the electrical pathways that produce the heart's rhythmic muscular contractions. They are responsible for more than 400,000 deaths each year, and are the cause of death for more than two-thirds of heart-disease victims, killing more men in the Western world than any other disease.

While heart disease is a primary cause of arrhythmias, they can also occur in people with no underlying heart disease, caused by such external factors as alcohol, caffeine, cold medications, diet pills, stress, and tobacco.

A large body of research shows that ginkgo leaf extract can protect heart tissues from arrhythmias and the free radical damage caused by the interruption of oxygen and blood flow during a heart attack. In 1994, experimental heart attacks were induced in rat hearts and ginkgo extract not only protected the heart tissues from damage caused by the prolonged lack of oxygen over the forty-minute test period, but it also prevented the occurrence of any arrhythmias normally present following a heart attack.

Heart Attack

Sudden cardiac death is the leading cause of death in the United States, claiming the lives of about 280,000 people each year. It occurs most often in people who have had past heart attacks (myocardial infarctions), but it can also occur in young, healthy individuals. When the heart muscle doesn't get enough oxygen and blood to contract properly and keep pumping blood to the rest of the body, ischemia (lack of oxygen to the heart) results. Ischemia causes problems such as angina pectoris (chest pain), and can lead to cardiac arrest, a fatal heart attack.

Sudden cardiac death also occurs in individuals with no evidence of heart disease. In these people, a silent ischemia caused by coronary artery spasms may be the cause of cardiac arrest. According to investigators, even in the absence of early chest pain and coronary artery disease, transient ischemia can be severe enough to cause life-threatening arrhythmias.

Ginkgo Protects Heart Tissues

Chinese researchers conducted a study to determine if ginkgo could protect heart tissues from the damaging effects of free radicals caused by the lack of oxygen that occurs during heart attacks. In their 1995 study, ginkgo extract was injected directly into the stressed coronary arteries of rabbits suffering from induced oxygen deprivation. Not only did ginkgo protect the heart, but it also significantly reduced the amount of damage to the tissues. According to the study, published in *Biochemistry and Biology International,* these results indicate that the antioxidant properties of ginkgo protected heart tissues from free radicals while helping the damaged tissues to heal from the effects of oxygen deprivation.

A similar study conducted by researchers at the University of California–Berkeley found similar results, indicating that ginkgo is effective in protecting tissues in the heart wall following an interruption in the delivery of oxygen.

Ginkgo Inhibits PAF

One of the greatest health benefits of ginkgo is its ability to increase blood flow—and oxygen delivery—throughout the entire body. One of the primary ingredients in ginkgo is the terpene ginkgolide B and it is able to block the effects of platelet-activating factor (PAF). Under normal circumstances, PAF assists the body in times of trouble by causing platelets to become sticky and come together to form clots that can stem the loss of blood in times of trauma. Unfortunately, when levels of PAF are elevated, due to stress, the consumption of hydrogenated fats, or an exposure to allergens, this life-saving compound can turn into a serious, life-threatening problem. Excess PAF causes blood to thicken too much, increasing the workload for the heart, and restricting the flow of blood throughout the entire body. As if this weren't bad enough, PAF also increases the production of free radicals, causing more damage to the heart and blood vessels. Adding insult to injury, PAF also promotes inflammation which can stress the cardiovascular system and further restrict the delivery of blood and oxygen.

As discussed previously, the excess platelet aggregation triggered by PAF also leads to an increase in the formation of blood clots (thromboses) that are involved in heart disease, strokes, and peripheral vascular diseases, such as intermittent claudication (see page 207).

Ginkgo Enhances the Delivery of Blood and Oxygen

The good news is that ginkgo has been effective in inhibiting PAF from binding to platelets and turning blood into a viscous, thick, sludge-like fluid that flows with extreme difficulty. By preventing PAF from binding to platelets, ginkgo also reduces the risks of thrombosis formation and prevents coronary artery spasms, heart attacks, and stroke.

Researchers measured the positive effects of ginkgo on blood viscosity by measuring changes in the speed of blood flowing through the capillaries of ten healthy volunteers. Microcirculation and blood flow were carefully measured before and during a four-hour period following treatment with ginkgo extract. The blood velocity was determined by monitoring circulation in the tiny capillaries located in the nail-fold on the fingernails. One hour after receiving a single dose of 112 mg of ginkgo extract, the researchers found that blood flow had increased by an amazing 57 percent in the test subjects. The researchers found no changes in the quantity of plasma or blood cells. Nor did they find any alterations in blood pressure, capillary diameter, or heart rate. No side effects were reported by any of the patients, and the enhanced blood-circulating effects disappeared after three hours. These findings support many other studies, which show that, by reducing the stickiness of blood cells, which allows an increase in blood flow and the delivery of oxygen to the tissues, ginkgo benefits a variety of conditions.

Another way that ginkgo can help to increase circulation is by its ability to relax (dilate) constricted arteries. A number of animal and human studies have shown that ginkgo is more effective than many standard drugs in relaxing arteries and improving blood circulation. In one human trial, researchers compared ginkgo with standard drugs used to treat vasoconstriction. Twenty-five people were treated with ginkgo and were compared with 300 other people receiving standard medications. By measuring the increase in arteriolar dilation in the big toe of volunteers, the researchers determined that the standard drugs resulted in a 39 percent increase in artery dilation, compared with a 44 percent increase in the group receiving ginkgo.

Ginkgo for Peripheral Arterial Occlusive Disease (PAOD)

Peripheral arterial occlusive disease (PAOD), also known as atherosclerosis obliterans, is a disease caused by thick deposits of plaque forming on the interior lining of the peripheral arteries (atherosclerosis) and the abdominal aorta. In PAOD, the interior diameter of the arteries is so narrowed (generally by 60 percent or more) and constricted that it causes a bottleneck as blood tries to flow out to the arms and legs.

The first symptoms of PAOD often appear as painful aches, tired muscles, and a cramping of the muscles in the arms and legs triggered by exercise. This cramping and pain is referred to as intermittent claudication. As PAOD progresses, walking becomes more difficult due to pain. In time, the pain can grow worse when the limb is elevated, becoming severe enough to prevent sleep. The best treatment for PAOD is usually exercise, but with the extreme pain cause by the condition, this option is not always possible.

Ginkgo for Intermittent Claudication

Given ginkgo's ability to increase blood flow, it's not surprising to learn that painful leg cramping caused by intermittent claudication can be relieved by ginkgo extract. In fact, based on the large number of studies showing ginkgo to be highly effective in treating PAOD and intermittent claudication, both Germany and the World Health Organization have approved ginkgo use as a recognized treatment for these and other related conditions.

Clinical studies have found ginkgo to be highly effective for relieving pain in approximately 75 percent of cases of intermittent claudication. Researchers gauged the effectiveness of ginkgo to increase the flow of blood and oxygen to leg muscles by measuring the maximum distance patients could walk on a standardized treadmill before being forced to stop due to pain. Most studies found that doses between 120 and 240 mg of ginkgo extract led to beneficial effects within about eight weeks, though a more recent study suggests that the higher daily dose of 240 mg of ginkgo is significantly more effective than the lower dose.

Based on these and numerous other studies on leg cramps caused by intermittent claudication, researchers believe that, in addition to improving circulation to the peripheral arteries and restoring oxygen, ginkgo also scavenges the free radicals produced by the previously oxygen-deprived muscles.

Intermittent Claudication

Claudication refers to Emperor Tiberius Claudius Drusus Nero Germanicus who, despite suffering serious birth defects that left him with a lifelong limp, ruled Rome from A.D. 41 to 54.

GINKGO AND SEXUAL ENJOYMENT

In previous sections, we've seen that ginkgo effectively improves blood flow and oxygenation of tissues, protects blood vessels from the ravages of free radicals, and restores elasticity and tone to the entire circulatory system. These same properties are of great importance to the sexual functioning and health of both men and women. In this section we'll discuss the reproductive organs and the role ginkgo plays in enhancing sexual function and enjoyment.

The Poor State of Sexual Satisfaction

The October 1995 *Journal of the American Geriatrics Society* reported that sexual satisfaction and performance in men declines with age. The study by researchers at the Mayo Clinic was based on information obtained from 2,115 men, ranging in age from forty to seventy-nine years. The study evaluated five main factors of sexual health:

- Ability to have erections.
- Changes in sex drive.
- Changes in sexual performance during the previous year.
- Satisfaction with sexual activity.
- Worries or concerns about sexual performance.

The Mayo researchers found that 25 percent of men in their forties were already concerned with their sexual performance. This number rose with age, with 47 percent of men in their seventies reporting they were concerned about their declining sexual function. Key findings of the Mayo study include:

Responses to Questionnaire	Men aged 40–49	Men aged 70–79
Concerned about sexual function	25%	47%
Performance worse than the previous year	10%	30%
Dissatisfied with sexual performance	2%	11%
No sex drive	1%	26%
Difficulty or inability to maintain erections	<1%	27%

The Mayo researchers concluded that decreased satisfaction with sex could be accounted for by age-related increases in erectile dysfunction, decreased libido, and the interaction between erectile dysfunction and decreased libido.

Healthy Sexual Functioning

A normal sexual response in men and women begins in the presence of sexually oriented stimulation. When the mood is right, the body responds by releasing a cascade of chemicals that direct the flow of blood into the sexual organs. In women, this leads to engorgement and lubrication of the organs as the body prepares for intercourse. In men, this rush of blood is directed into a pair of pockets, known as the corpus cavernosum, that run inside the shaft of the penis. This inflow of blood is critical to the enlargement and stiffening of the penis.

This engorgement is triggered by a unique neurotransmitter called nitric oxide (NO). Nitric oxide, in turn, stimulates the production of another signaling enzyme

Neurotransmitters
Molecules used as chemical messengers in the body. Serotonin and dopamine are well-known neurotransmitters.

called cyclic guanosine monophosphate, or cGMP for short. Under normal circumstances, cGMP signals the smooth muscles surrounding the arteries of the penis to relax and allow blood to flow into the penis. Any condition that interferes with the signaling of these messenger enzymes can quickly lead to the breakdown of the entire process and cause impotence.

Impotence/Erectile Dysfunction (ED)

According the National Institutes of Health, impotence, or erectile dysfunction, is defined as the inability to attain or sustain an erection adequate for satisfactory sexual intercourse. Experts believe impotence affects between 10 and 15 million American men. In 1985, the National Ambulatory Medical Care Survey counted 525,000 doctor-office visits for erectile dysfunction, and that number has greatly increased since then.

Impotence usually has a physical cause, such as disease, injury, or drug side effects. Any disorder that impairs blood flow in the penis has the potential to cause impotence. It occurs as men age: about 5 percent of men at age forty, and between 15 and 25 percent of men at age sixty-five experience impotence. Yet, it is not an inevitable part of aging.

Viagra

In 1998, the FDA approved the prescription drug Viagra (sildenafil citrate) as a treatment for men suffering from nonorganic impotence due to conditions such as diabetes, radical prostatectomy, spinal cord injury, and vascular disease.

Viagra was originally investigated as a potential antiangina medication based on its ability to release nitric oxide and increase blood flow to the heart. Although Viagra failed as a heart medication, researchers in London noted that many of the men in the clinical trials reported the frequent occurrence of unaccustomed erections and improved sexual performance. Following this serendipitous finding (and five years of clinical trials), Viagra was finally granted approval as a treatment for men who had difficulty achieving erections because of conditions such as diabetes, radical prostatectomy, spinal cord injury, and vascular disease.

Enzymes
Specialized proteins that act as catalysts to promote the billions of biochemical reactions necessary for virtually all life processes.

Viagra was found to help men achieve and maintain erections by (1) enhancing the effects of the neurotransmitter nitric oxide (NO), and (2) maintaining higher levels of the enzyme cGMP, the two key players in penile erection. Viagra does this by selectively inhibiting the enzymes that destroy cGMP, leading to elevated cGMP levels. This, in turn, increases blood flow to the genitals and leads to stronger erections and intensified sensation.

Viagra was found to help 80 percent of men suffering from nonorganic impotence. Additionally, Viagra also seems to enhance sexual performance and enjoyment, and reduce the latent period between erections, even in men who have no dysfunction.

Women and Viagra

Viagra has also gained a reputation with women, which makes sense when one considers that the clitoris, which is structurally similar to the penis, becomes engorged with blood during sexual arousal. Viagra may provide similar benefits to women, by stimulating the release of NO to encourage the flow of blood and enhance their sexual sensation and orgasmic enjoyment.

Serious Side Effects of Viagra

While Viagra is effective for millions of men, the side effects for many—facial flushing, headaches, and indigestion—are too troublesome for continued enjoyment. And, more seriously, soon after its introduction, vision problems began to surface in men taking viagra, leading to warnings for people with retinal eye conditions, such as macular degeneration or retinitis pigmentosa, to use the drug with caution.

In addition to eye problems, both the FDA and the manufacturer began to issue warnings against taking Viagra with any nitrate-based cardiac medications (that is, sublingual nitroglycerin tablets, nitroglycerin patches, and the like). Doctors were warned that heart patients should not be treated with nitroglycerin if the patient had used Viagra in the previous twenty-four hours. Additionally, the manufacturer reported several cases where patients who received both drugs died after developing irreversible hypotension (a severe drop in blood pressure).

As safety issues with Viagra began to arise, researchers once again began to seek out safer alternatives for treating impotence.

Ginkgo Offers a Safer Alternative

Many current pharmaceuticals have evolved from the historical search for herbal compounds to cure or reverse sexual dysfunction. Often, traditional nostrums rely on purely magical (placebo) effects, such as the phallic-influenced belief in the effect of rhinoceros horn—which, in fact, offers no benefit to humans and is fatal for the unfortunate rhino. Conversely, many plant-based traditional treatments, using herbs such as damiana, maca, muira puama, tribulus, and yohimbe, have been explored for their effectiveness in treating sexual dysfunction.

Armed with the fresh body of knowledge revealed by the success of Viagra, researchers once again turned their attentions to the ginkgo extract.

Ginkgo Enhances Sexual Function

Recognizing that circulatory problems are a major cause of impotence, it comes as no surprise that ginkgo has been effective in treating erectile dysfunction caused by impaired blood flow. In one study, ginkgo was found effective in improving erectile dysfunction in a group of impotent males taking 60 mg of ginkgo extract for six months. Researchers suggested that ginkgo worked by stimulating the release of nitric oxide (NO), which, as described above, signals the blood vessels to dilate and sends blood to the corpus cavernosum to achieve and maintain an erection.

Ginkgo's positive effects on impotence were further established by a second study, reported in the *Journal of Urology*, in which researchers found that ginkgo was highly effective in helping men achieve and maintain erections. What was remarkable about this study is that it was involved sixty men who had previously failed to respond to papaverine, an injectable prescription medication commonly used to treat male sexual dysfunction. The men were given ginkgo extract, 60 mg per day, for up to eighteen months. The first signs of improvement were noticed after only six weeks. After six months of therapy, 50 percent of the men were able to achieve erections and engage in sex. By the end of the study, fully 95 percent of the men receiving ginkgo extract showed significant improvements in penile blood flow. According to the study authors, the improvements were due to the direct effect of ginkgo extract to enhance blood flow in arteries and veins.

Ginkgo and Antidepressant–Induced Sexual Problems

Millions of people have been helped by a variety of medications commonly used to treat clinical depression. Unfortunately many antidepressants, especially the class of drugs known as selective serotonin reuptake inhibitors (SSRIs), have a negative effects on a person's sexual libido and satisfaction. Antidepressant-related sexual problems include decreased sexual drive, delayed ejaculation, and difficulty achieving orgasm. It's been estimated that sexual problems related to antidepressants occur in more than 70 percent of patients, though embarrassment leads to underreporting by both doctors and patients.

Ginkgo has been an effective treatment for sexual problems related to the use of the commonly prescribed antidepressant drugs. Researchers tested the effects of ginkgo extract on a group of thirty men and thirty-three women who were suffering from sexual side effects attributed to the use of antidepressant drugs, such as the selective serotonin reuptake inhibitors (SSRIs). Sexual side effects ranged from decreased libido and erectile difficulties to delayed or inhibited orgasm.

Each person received ginkgo extract in doses ranging from 80–120 mg daily. After only four weeks, 84 percent of those tested reported positive results in all phases of the sexual response cycle. A major point of interest with this study is that women responded better than men, with 91 percent of the women reporting improvements in the sexual response, as compared to 76 percent of the men indicating success. No adverse effects were reported and the use of ginkgo biloba appeared to be compatible with antidepressant therapy. As in most other studies, the researchers reported that many subjects also experienced improved cognitive functioning, mental clarity, and memory, and increased energy. And, as with other studies on ginkgo and sexual dysfunction, the researchers of the study attributed the success to ginkgo's ability to aid circulatory function.

Ginkgo as an Aphrodisiac?

Given ginkgo's proven ability to dilate blood vessels and improve blood flow to the penis, it is not surprising to note that many aphrodisiac formulas contain ginkgo extract. According to Dr. Stephen Karch, a specialist in cardiac pathology and author of *The Consumer's Guide to Herbal Medicine*, ancient Chinese herbalists referred to ginkgo as an aphrodisiac. Karch reports that ginkgo enhances nitric oxide (NO) production. Nitric oxide is the primary messenger molecule that is affected by Viagra, and is the key factor in helping achieve erections by informing certain blood vessels to relax.

GINKGO AND VISION

Ginkgo has been studied extensively for its ability to treat a wide variety of vision-related conditions. Age-related cataracts, glaucoma, macular degeneration, and diabetic retinopathy are among the leading causes for loss of vision. Unfortunately, standard medical approaches to preserving sight haven't offered much hope for treatment of these blinding eye diseases. Ginkgo is believed to benefit these and other vision problems by preventing the damage caused by free radical activity and by enhancing the delivery of blood and oxygen to the retina to help repair tissues.

The Eye as a Camera

The inside of the eye has been compared to a camera. Light enters through the lens and is focused onto the retina, a layer of tightly packed and highly sensitive photoreceptors that line the interior back surface of the eyeball. The retina contains millions of light-sensitive cells, called rods and cones, that enable us to pick out colors and fine details. When light hits any of these cells, there is a biochemical reaction to the varying intensities of light and color. The cells then transmit electrical signals along nerve cells to the brain where all the information is assembled and processed to form a picture that we experience as vision.

The cells lining the retina expend a great deal of energy, and require a constant supply of oxygen, glucose, and other nutrients. Consequently, the retina is supplied by a dense tangle of blood vessels that provide one of the highest rates of blood flow found anywhere in the body.

The retina is a delicate structure that is highly vulnerable to oxidative damage from free radicals. The tissues of the retina are also rich in polyunsaturated fatty acids, which are particularly attractive to free radicals.

Ginkgo for Healthy Vision

Because ginkgo extract is such a potent free radical scavenger, scientists believed it would support healthy vision by preventing the age-related accumulation of free radical damage that is commonly blamed for eye diseases, such as macular degeneration and diabetic retinopathy.

To test their theory, German scientists studied ginkgo's protective effects on the retinas of twenty-five older people. They found that just 160 mg per day of the extract resulted in dramatically improved vision for all of these subjects after only four weeks of treatment. According to the researchers, the ginkgo caused a "significant increase in retinal sensitivity."

Ongoing studies show that the greater the damage to retinal tissues, the more profound an effect the ginkgo has on improving vision. A significant finding was that ginkgo had virtually no side effects and that normal retinal functions were unaffected, proving the safety of the herb. These studies showed that ginkgo was not only effective in improving vision, but, in cases where the vision was damaged by poor circulation, the damage could be significantly reversed.

Another form of age-related eye deficiency is the gradual loss of an ability to tell the difference between certain colors. This skill peaks in middle age and, like so many other human abilities, declines with age, reducing once-vibrant colors to more muted shades of pastel or gray.

Again, research has found that ginkgo can help here. After French scientists gave twenty-nine older volunteers ginkgo extract for six months, tests revealed that their ability to distinguish differences in shades of color had improved.

Diabetic Retinopathy

Diabetic retinopathy is a serious complication of diabetes that damages the small blood vessels of the retina. People with diabetes are at increased risk of developing eye problems, such as cataracts and glaucoma, but diabetic retinopathy is the number one vision threat for diabetic patients, affecting half of all diabetics in America. If left untreated, about half of those with the advanced form, proliferative retinopathy, will become blind within five years, compared to just 5 percent of those who receive treatment.

In the early stages of the disease—called non-proliferative, or background retinopathy—the small blood vessels of the retina weaken and develop bulges (micro-aneurysms) that can leak blood (hemorrhage) or fluid (exudates) into the surrounding tissues. The person's vision is rarely affected during this stage of retinopathy.

In the advanced, proliferative stage of retinopathy, circulation problems resulting from damaged and narrowed blood vessels cause the retina to become oxygen-deprived. To cope with this, the circulatory system attempts to maintain adequate oxygen levels within the retina by forming fragile new blood vessels that can grow on the retina and extend into the vitreous (the jellylike substance inside the back of the eye).

Retinal Detachment
A retinal detachment occurs when the retina is pulled away from the back of the eye, leading to blurred vision and blindness if not treated.

These fragile vessels can rupture and release blood into the interior of the eye, leading to blurred vision or temporary blindness. The resulting formation of scar tissue here can eventually pull the retina away from the back of the eye (retinal detachment), and lead to permanent vision loss. In addition, at any stage of retinopathy, a condition called macular edema can occur. This is a severe blurring of the vision when fluid accumulates around the macula, which is the most sensitive part of the retina, and the one that is crucial for seeing fine detail.

All people with diabetes—including type I (juvenile onset) and type II (adult onset)—are at risk for developing diabetic retinopathy. Controlling diabetes is no guarantee that you will not develop retinopathy, either, so you must always be on guard. Pregnant women with diabetes are more prone to developing diabetic retinopathy, so dilated eye examinations each trimester are recommended for these women, to protect their vision.

In standard conventional medicine, both macular edema and peripheral retinopathy are treated with focal laser photocoagulation, a procedure that uses a laser in the vicinity of the macula to seal the leaking blood vessels. Pan-retinal photocoagulation is another, related procedure used by conventional medicine to minimize proliferative retinopathy. It works by targeting hundreds of spots across the retina in order to stop the bleeding from abnormal new vessels and prevent their further growth.

Ginkgo and Retinopathy

A number of experimental studies suggest that ginkgo extracts are potentially useful for treating retinal damage induced by a variety of disorders. Many of the results point to antioxidants as the reason for the protective effects of the extract. In addition, it is suspected that ginkgo's ability to inhibit the platelet-activating factor (PAF), is involved in protecting eye tissues from retinopathy, since ginkgolide B, a known PAF antagonist, has been shown to reduce experimentally induced retinal lesions in animals.

In 1992, a group of researchers tested ginkgo to see if it could protect retinal tissues from the destructive effects of free radicals involved in diabetic retinopathy. After conducting several experimental studies to establish that free radicals were indeed an important cause of the damage seen in diabetic retinopathy, they tested a group of diabetic rats that were fed ginkgo (100 mg/kg) daily for two months. At the end of the study, they concluded that ginkgo was a highly effective free radical scavenger that prevented the retinopathy associated with diabetes.

Human studies also support the use of ginkgo extract in treating retinopathy. In one double-blind trial, researchers gave daily doses of 160 mg of a standardized ginkgo extract to a small group of people with mild diabetic retinopathy. After six months, these volunteers had a noticeable improvement of their pre-existing impaired vision.

Double-Blind Study

In double-blind studies, neither the researchers nor the study participants are aware of who is taking which product until the end when the code is broken and the results are tallied.

A second double-blind, placebo-controlled trial, using twenty-nine people with early diabetic retinopathy, found similar protective effects. Half of the participants (fourteen) were given 80 mg per day of ginkgo extract for six months, while the other half (fifteen) received a placebo. At the end of the trial, those who had received the ginkgo extract showed a small but significant increase in their color vision, indicating a reversal of retinal damage, while the vision of the group receiving the placebo was worse than at the beginning of the study.

Macular Degeneration

Macular degeneration is a term for a group of disorders that all involve the slow destruction of the macula, the central region of the retina. Most cases of macular degeneration occur in people over age sixty and are therefore referred to as age-related macular degeneration (ARMD). ARMD is a major cause of blindness affecting up to 15 million people over age sixty.

As we said, the macula is a crucial part of the center of the retina. It contains an extraordinary array of photosensitive cells that enable us to perceive color and fine details. In ARMD, the macula slowly deteriorates, eventually leading to almost complete blindness in our central visual field and leaving us with only the very edges of peripheral vision. Mainstream medicine can only offer laser surgery or radiation as last-ditch solutions to halting any further loss of vision after the disease has progressed to the point of imminent blindness.

Macular degeneration causes different symptoms in different people, and in its early stages there may be few noticeable changes in vision. Often there is only loss of vision in one eye while the other eye continues to see well for many years. But when both eyes are affected, reading and close-up work can become difficult.

Ginkgo and Age-Related Macular Degeneration

ARMD, like atherosclerosis, is a disease caused by poor circulation. If blood flow is affected by atherosclerosis, diabetes, or any other age-related health problem, the macula slowly atrophies and dies. This process is further hastened by the accelerated production of free radicals that accumulate in the retina when there is reduced blood flow.

Atherosclerosis

A disorder characterized by the buildup of blood fats on the damaged lining of artery walls, leading to plaques that block blood flow.

Smoking contributes to the progression of ARMD by reducing the supply of blood, narrowing the blood vessels, and thickening the blood. A high-fat, high cholesterol diet leading to fatty plaque deposits in the macular vessels also hampers blood flow. Additionally, a shortage of antioxidants may also increase the tendency for ARMD.

Armed with these insights, scientists speculated that ginkgo extract might slow the progression of ARMD by increasing blood flow to the retina and by halting the free radical damage to the photosensitive cells. To test this theory, researchers conducted a double-blind trial in 1988 to see if the antioxidant and circulatory effects of ginkgo extract could reverse or halt the progression of macular degeneration. Twenty volunteers were given either 160 mg of ginkgo extract, or a placebo pill, every day for six months. At the end of the study, the group receiving ginkgo showed significant improvements in their long-distance visual focus. There was no improvement in the group receiving the dummy pill.

Glaucoma: The "Sneak Thief of Sight"

According to the American Academy of Ophthalmology (AAO), more than 1 million people in the United States are at risk for going blind because they don't know they have glaucoma. Once thought of as a single disease, glaucoma is actually the term for damage to the optic nerves (the bundle of nerve fibers that carries information from the eye to the brain) caused by elevated pressure inside the eye. It is estimated that about 50 million people worldwide have impaired vision, if not complete blindness, from glaucoma. In the United States, about 300,000 new cases are diagnosed each year, adding to the more than 3 million cases already on record.

Glaucoma is called the "sneak thief of sight" because it strikes without obvious symptoms. People with glaucoma are usually unaware of it until they have a serious loss of vision. In fact, about half of those who have glaucoma do not know it. Currently, that damage cannot be reversed.

While there are usually no warning signs, some symptoms may occur in the later stages of the disease, such as a loss of peripheral vision, difficulty focusing on close work, seeing halos around lights, and frequent changes of prescription glasses. Unfortunately, though, once the vision is lost, it is gone forever.

African Americans are at a higher risk of developing glaucoma than other racial groups. Others at risk include:

- Anyone with a close relative who has glaucoma.

- Seniors.

- Those with diabetes.

- Those who have been taking steroid medication for a long time.

Ginkgo to the Rescue for Glaucoma

Ginkgo extract can increase the circulation of blood to the eyes, and in some cases, it can help lower the intraocular pressure in the eyes. In one double-blind, placebo-controlled study of older people with macular degeneration, there was a significant improvement in their vision following treatment with ginkgo extract.

In 1999, there was a second study to test the therapeutic effects of ginkgo extract on people with glaucoma. Eleven healthy volunteers were treated with either 40 mg of ginkgo extract, or a placebo, three times daily for two days. Using Doppler imaging, a technique that uses a low-power laser beam, to measure the flow of blood in the eyes before and after treatment, the researchers found a significant increase in blood flow in the main eye artery in those receiving ginkgo. No change was noted in the placebo group. The results indicate that ginkgo effectively increased the blood flow in the eyes which helped lower the intraocular pressure, thereby slowing the progression of the disease.

Ginkgo Protects against UV–Induced Eye Damage

You have only one pair of eyes, and protecting them from excess sunlight is every bit as important as protecting your skin. Overexposure to intense ultraviolet (UV) radiation produced by the sun can cause damage to the cornea, leading to a painful condition known as photokeratitis. Ultraviolet radiation also contributes to the development of other serious eye disorders, including cataracts, degenerative corneal changes, and skin cancer around the eye. It may also contribute to age-related macular degeneration.

Results from a dozen studies over the last ten years suggest that spending time in direct sunlight without wearing proper eye protection can significantly increase your chances of developing any of these serious eye diseases.

UV actually refers to three types of ultraviolet light—UV-A, UV-B, and UV-C. The milder form of radiation, UV-C

rays, are normally screened out by the ozone layer and don't present much of an immediate health threat. The more powerful UV-A rays are composed of longer wavelength radiation that causes skin tanning and premature skin aging. UV-A rays can reach the retina, and long-term exposure to them may greatly increase your incidence of macular degeneration. UV-B light, the active, shorter wavelengths of radiation, are responsible for blistering sunburns and skin cancer, and they cause the greatest damage to your eyes.

Ginkgo can protect your retina from damaging exposure to sunlight. Researchers found that when experimental rats were fed ginkgo two to four weeks prior to exposure to intense light, the antioxidant activity of the ginkgo protected the retinal cells from oxidative damage. The untreated animals fared poorly. There was extensive damage to their retinal tissues, leading to a loss of photoreceptors, fragmentation of their cells, and extensive cell death in their maculas. Ginkgo also prevented a reduction in the thickness of the retinal layer, suggesting that ginkgo was effective in protecting the cells from free radical damage, both from sunlight and as a response by the body's immune system.

Immune System
A complex system of responses that fight invaders, such as bacteria and viruses.

Ginkgo and Cataracts

Cataracts, a cloudiness of the lens inside the eyes that occurs over a period of many years, are a major cause of visual impairment and blindness worldwide. Studies have implicated UV radiation in the development of cataracts, and have also shown that certain types of cataracts are linked to a history of higher exposure to UV rays, especially UV-B radiation.

Since UV-B radiation is reflected off bright surfaces, such as sand, snow, and water, the risk is particularly high on the beach, in mountain areas, or while boating. The risk is greatest during the midday hours, during the summer months, and at high altitudes any time of year. Ultraviolet radiation levels also increase as you get nearer the equator, so residents in the equatorial countries and parts of Northern Australia are at greater risk than those living in temperate zones.

Since the human lens absorbs UV radiation, individuals who have cataract surgery are at increased risk of retinal damage from sunlight. And people with retinal dystrophies or other chronic retinal conditions may be at an even greater risk since their retinas may be less resilient to normal exposure levels to begin with.

Ginkgo is believed to be protective because it helps prevent the free radical damage caused by lifelong exposure to sunlight. To date, there has been only one small study conducted with ginkgo and cataracts, but it showed promising benefits. More research is being done in this area.

GINKGO AND HEARING DISORDERS

More than 28 million Americans are deaf or have hearing problems, and 30 million more are at risk of losing their hearing from exposure to dangerous levels of noise. Our ears can detect frequencies ranging from 20 Hz to 20,000 Hz, but it is most sensitive to the sounds commonly used for speech, which range from 1,500 Hz to 3,000 Hz. Hearing deficits can occur for the following reasons:

- Sound waves are not properly conducted to the cochlea in the ear.

- Scar tissue hampers the cochlear nerves.

- Sound processing in the brain is damaged.

Hearing losses can range from a minor nuisance, such as a difficulty understanding light conversation, or enjoying a full range of musical notes, to total deafness. Older people are the largest group of Americans with hearing loss. It affects 30 to 35 percent of the United States population over age sixty-five, and up to 50 percent of the population over eighty-five. But hearing problems are not exclusive to these groups—in the United States about 1 million school-age children have some degree of hearing loss or total deafness. The most common cause of hearing loss in children is otitis media (middle ear infection) and that primarily affects infants and young children.

Cochlea
So named for its snaillike spiral shape, it transmits auditory information to the part of the brain that processes sound.

Hearing affects how we communicate and interact with the world around us. With the seemingly inevitable age-related loss of hearing, older people can become withdrawn in an attempt to avoid the embarrassment and frustration of appearing confused, unresponsive, or uncooperative. This isolation often leads to depression as well.

During the last decade, important progress has been made in understanding the human ear and the hearing processes. In this section, we will discuss some positive studies that have been conducted on ginkgo and hearing disorders, such as deafness, tinnitus, and vertigo, that are associated with cerebral insufficiency or a reduction in the flow of blood to the inner ear.

Ginkgo Improves Hearing in Sudden Deafness

A number of studies have shown that ginkgo is highly effective in improving hearing, particularly when hearing losses are caused by very loud sounds. Researchers believe that, by restoring circulation to the tiny blood vessels damaged by a lack of oxygen, ginkgo protects and restores function to the cells and blood vessels in the ear.

A French study in 1986 found that ginkgo effectively improved the hearing in the test subjects who all had acute cochlear deafness. This type of deafness, which keeps sound vibrations from getting to the brain, is the result of an insufficient flow of blood to the cochlea. Eighteen people in this double-blind trial received either 320 mg of ginkgo extract daily for thirty days, or nicergoline (Semion), a migraine medication that acts as a vasodilator. While both groups showed improvements, 52 percent of those receiving the ginkgo showed significant improvements in their hearing, compared to only 35 percent in the nicergoline group.

Vasodilator
A vasodilator relaxes the blood-vessel walls, causing them to dilate, and allowing blood, oxygen, and nutrients to pass through them more easily.

In a second clinical study in 1986, German researchers evaluated a group of fifty-nine people with sudden deafness who were being treated with ginkgo extract. After nine weeks, 59 percent of these test subjects rated their improvement in hearing from good to very good. Of the thirty-three people who initially reported having ringing in the ears (tinnitus), 36 percent said their symptoms were completely resolved, and 15 percent said they were substantially reduced.

Tinnitus

An estimated 50 million Americans suffer from some form of tinnitus (pronounced tĭn´-ĭ-tĭs), a medical term for a ringing in the ears. Most people with tinnitus report this as a constant, nonstop ringing noise, while others describe hearing an assortment of hissing, chirping, or clicking sounds. Tinnitus is not a disease, but is a very persistent disturbance that rarely lets up except for an occasional reduction in the loudness of the noise levels.

Tinnitus is most commonly caused by constant exposure to loud noises. Other conditions that can trigger tinnitus include ear, sinus, and respiratory infections, severe head trauma, some types of tumors, and wax build-up. Certain drugs, such as aspirin, birth control pills, quinine, and some antibiotics, can magnify the effects of tinnitus.

Ginkgo and Tinnitus

Although currently there is no cure or effective medical treatment for tinnitus, hearing aids and white noise audiotapes can offer some relief. But a systematic review of nineteen clinical studies on the subject found that ginkgo extract offered a significant reduction in tinnitus symptoms, particularly if the treatments got started soon after the symptoms were first detected.

In a 1986 double-blind study, French researchers treated 103 people for tinnitus with either 320 mg of ginkgo extract, or a placebo. While only 24.4 percent of those receiving the placebo showed improvement, 40 percent of those receiving the ginkgo reported marked relief from their symptoms.

The rest of the ginkgo group also derived varying degrees of benefits from it.

Vertigo and Dizziness

Like tinnitus, vertigo and dizziness are not diseases, but they are very unpleasant symptoms of underlying problems that affect balance. Vertigo is often described as a spinning or rotary motion. Some people say vertigo makes them feel as if they are spinning. Others say they are standing still, but the environment around them is rotating. Still others feel they are being pushed or pulled off balance.

Dizziness is similar to vertigo, but with added symptoms, such as disorientation, fuzzy vision, lightheadedness, nausea, sweating, and fainting.

Disruptions of Motion and Balance

Vertigo and dizziness can be symptoms of an underlying disorder affecting our vestibular system, the one responsible for helping us maintain our senses of motion and balance. It works by monitoring the direction and speed of our head movements and transmitting this information to specialized organs inside the ear before passing it on to different parts of our brain, mainly the cerebellum, for final processing. In the brain, this information on balance and motion is integrated with the sensory information received from our eyes, ears, legs, and arms to help it figure out our body's position in space.

Ginkgo can help control vertigo and dizziness, once again by promoting the flow of blood, this time to aid the brain in accurately receiving and evaluating sensory information.

Cerebellum
The part of the brain that coordinates movement so we can maintain balance, grasp objects accurately, and keep our eyes focused during motion, or while walking.

Motion and Balance Disorders and Ginkgo

The effects of ginkgo leaf extract on motion and balance (vestibular) disorders has been examined in animals. When researchers treated cats with ginkgo extract, their vestibular damage was reversed, and the cats had their balance completely restored. And, as little as four weeks of treatment with ginkgo extract improved the cochlear blood flow in rats and adult guinea pigs, and helped them recover from balance and motion disturbances.

These findings also apply in studies on humans. In one 1985 multi-center trial, seventy people with vertigo were given either 160 mg of ginkgo, or a placebo, daily for three months. In terms of intensity, frequency, and duration of the vertigo symptoms, the group treated with ginkgo extract showed a greater improvement than the placebo group. These improvements were noticed in as little as one month and they increased over the full three months of the trial. The outcome of this remarkable trial was that, by the end of the study, 47 percent of those treated with the ginkgo

extract were completely free of vertigo symptoms, while only 18 percent of those who received the placebos were symptom-free.

Based on the success of these studies, it seems worthwhile to consider taking ginkgo extract at the first sign of any problems you may have with balance or dizziness.

GINKGO'S OTHER HEALTH BENEFITS

In addition to its well-documented and clinically proven abilities to improve circulation and cognitive performance, researchers around the world continue to be impressed by the growing list of additional health properties being attributed to ginkgo.

In this section, we will briefly examine some recent studies on these other conditions that continue to impress researchers.

Ginkgo and Premenstrual Syndrome (PMS)

In 1931, scientists investigating problems of menstruation identified a group of symptoms that typically start a week or so prior to menstruation. They labeled the condition premenstrual tension (PMT), an umbrella term for the depression, extreme fatigue, and irritability that many women experienced during the premenstrual period. As research continued, it became evident that PMT was only part of a syndrome of more than 100 documented symptoms, so the name was changed to premenstrual syndrome (PMS). PMS affects up to 90 percent of all women at some point during their lives, some so severely that they cannot go about their daily tasks.

The most commonly reported symptoms of PMS are bloating, breast swelling or tenderness, cravings for sweets, depression, fatigue, headaches, irritability, loss of sex drive, and weight gain. Various treatments, including vitamins, minerals, and hormones, such as progesterone, have been shown to help some women cope with many symptoms of PMS.

Ginkgo and Fluid Retention

Fluid retention syndrome, medically referred to as cyclic edema, is a condition seen primarily in young women just before they menstruate. The symptoms include tissue swelling (edema) in the legs and abdomen after sitting or standing for periods of time, or heavy swelling of the face and eyelids when lying down, causing moderate discomfort. Other symptoms include aching, carpal tunnel syndrome, headaches, muscle and joint pains, and stiffness. The condition is thought to be caused by fluids leaking from the blood out into the surrounding tissues. It is often seen in existing premenstrual syndrome and it can worsen PMS symptoms.

In a 1993 French study, researchers discovered that ginkgo extract is highly effective in relieving the fluid retention associated with cyclic edema. Ten women with severe cases were treated with 160–200 mg of ginkgo extract daily for two months. Of the ten, three women showed a complete elimination of their swelling and, in fact, never experienced the problem again. The other participants improved significantly, and tests showed that the fluid leakage had been stopped completely.

Edema
Accumulation of fluid between the cells that leads to swelling. Edema is most often seen in the lower legs, the feet, and around the eyes.

In a continuation of this study, researchers treated five women who had even greater fluid retention with an intravenous infusion of 200–300 mg of ginkgo extract once a day. After five days, each of the women had lost between four and ten pounds of water weight.

Ginkgo and PMS Symptoms

A larger study confirmed the early findings of ginkgo's effects on fluid retention, showing that ginkgo extract was effective in relieving other symptoms commonly seen in PMS. French researchers conducted the trial with 165 women, eighteen to forty-five years old, who reported experiencing at least three consecutive cycles of discomfort related to PMS. The women were divided into two groups and given daily doses of either ginkgo extract, or a placebo. After two months, the ginkgo was found to be highly effective in treating their other PMS symptoms, particularly in relieving their breast symptoms and improving their moods.

Ginkgo and Depression

Statistics show that depression affects about 17 million Americans, with 25 percent of the population likely to suffer diagnosable depression during their lifetime. Prescription antidepressants are the conventional treatment, with their harmful side effects, and potential for overdose.

German researchers have investigated the effectiveness of ginkgo for treating people who are depressed. They treated forty people, aged fifty-one to seventy-eight, who were diagnosed with mild to moderate cerebral dysfunctions that were combined with episodes of depression. All of these people had failed to respond to conventional antidepressant medications. They continued to take their medications while also receiving either 80 mg of ginkgo three times a day or a placebo. In the ginkgo group, there was a 50 percent reduction in the severity of depression after four weeks, and a 68 percent reduction after eight weeks. Overall, these people were significantly more motivated, more optimistic, and happier. By contrast, those receiving the placebo showed a less than 10 percent improvement in their depression symptoms at both four and eight weeks.

As a result of the impressive effects ginkgo has on depression, the German Ministry of Health Committee for Herbal Remedies has approved the use of ginkgo extract for improving mood and mental processes.

Ginkgo and Radiation

Following the 1986 Chernobyl disaster in the Ukraine, researchers detected compounds that damaged chromosomes in the plasma of thirty people assigned to cleaning up and shutting down the Chernobyl nuclear plant after it malfunctioned. This genetic damage meant that the workers were at a greatly increased risk for developing cancer. Medical researchers gave the workers 40 mg of ginkgo, three times a day, in the hope that the same antioxidant effects that had preserved the surviving ginkgo tree at Hiroshima would reduce the dangerous compounds in the serum of the Chernobyl workers.

After eight weeks of treatment, the researchers reported that these dangerous compounds had been reduced significantly, to the same levels as people who had not been exposed to high levels of radiation. These levels were maintained for at least seven months after taking the herb. After seven months, researchers measured a return of the serum markers showing damage, suggesting that treatment with ginkgo needed to be extended, possibly for the life of the patients.

Ginkgo and Sunburn

Based on its powerful antioxidant properties and proven ability to protect the body against the ravages of high radiation exposure, it isn't surprising that ginkgo also protects against sunburn and prevents sun damage. This is because it increases circulation to the skin, which acts to protect and stabilize collagen, which, in turn, protects against the ravages of solar radiation from the sun. Experiments suggest that, once the skin has had sun damage, ginkgo extract can speed its recovery while helping to reduce the pain of sunburn.

Ginkgo and Hepatitis B

Hepatitis B (HBV) is a chronic liver infection that spreads from person to person through blood transfusions and sexual contact. HBV infection can cause severe liver disease, including liver failure (cirrhosis) and liver cancer. HBV affects one out of every twenty people living in the United States, and each year more than 5,000 people die from hepatitis-B-related liver disease.

Chinese researchers tested ginkgo, known to be a powerful anti-inflammatory, to see if it could help control the liver inflammation that occurs with chronic hepatitis infection. The researchers gave ginkgo to eighty-six patients with chronic, persistent and active HBV, with early fibrosis (scarring) confirmed by liver biopsy. After three months of

Fibrosis
Tissue scarring associated with the healing of wounds when excessive collagen has been produced.

treatment with ginkgo, the enzyme levels associated with liver fibrosis were significantly reduced, and all the patients showed signs of remission from their chronic infections. As a result of this study, it has been suggested that ginkgo extract is effective in arresting the development of liver scarring in chronic hepatitis.

Ginkgo and Asthma

For centuries, Chinese herbalists put ginkgo seeds in soups and other foods as a treatment for asthma and bronchitis. Ginkgo is a strong inhibitor of platelet-activating factor and might, therefore, have some value in the prevention or treatment of asthma. Platelet-activating factor (PAF) is a problem because it increases allergic inflammation and may trigger bronchial constriction, making breathing difficult.

Scientists at Shanghai Medical University used the lung tissues of guinea pigs to test the effectiveness of ginkgo extract in reducing the effects of PAF and histamine, a compound in the body that causes the inflammatory response. The results, published in 2000, showed that ginkgo improved the pulmonary functions and reduced the tendency for the lung tissues to contract under the influence of PAF and histamine. The researchers concluded that ginkgo was a promising treatment for bronchial asthma.

In a second, recent study, researchers in Kuwait tested the effects of a ginkgo extract on the blood cells of people with asthma. They found that, in addition to suppressing PAF, ginkgo acted as an anti-inflammatory agent that suppressed immune system antigens involved in triggering asthma attacks. These results led them to conclude that ginkgo extract may offer a novel therapeutic treatment for asthma.

HOW TO SELECT AND USE GINKGO

This chapter will help you understand what to look for when selecting ginkgo extract, including which form to purchase, what to look for on a label, and how to interpret what you read.

As with most herbs, ginkgo biloba can be purchased in dried leaf form (for homemade tea or tinctures), in capsules of leaf powder, and as a standardized extract in prepared tinctures, capsules, or tablets.

Standardized Ginkgo

When choosing a brand of ginkgo, we recommend that you read the label carefully to make sure you are getting a standardized extract. Unlike synthetic drugs, which contain a single compound, herbs often have a variety of active ingredients. We need to have a way of *standardizing* the product; that is, have a consistent, measured amount of product per unit dose, whether it's a capsule, a tablet, or a tincture. To achieve this, one active ingredient is selected as the marker.

As previously noted, in the case of ginkgo, Dr. Willmar Schwabe of the large German phytomedicine company, Schwabe GmbH, developed an extract of ginkgo leaves known as EGb 761, the one principally used in clinical trials worldwide. It contains 24 percent flavone glycosides and 6 percent terpene lactones. Most types of ginkgo extract sold today are in this standardized form that he developed.

Standardized ginkgo extract is also available in drop form, with 9.6 mg of flavone glycosides and 2.4 mg of terpene lactones per dose.

How Standardized Ginkgo Extracts Are Made

Making the standardized ginkgo begins when the leaves of the male plant are harvested in late summer or early fall. Several factors affect the potency of the ginkgo plant, including where the ginkgo leaves are grown, the conditions under which they are harvested, and the harvesting method used. The quality of the active components can vary by as much as 300 percent, depending upon the location, time of year, and harvesting method. Growers monitor the quality of the leaves and harvest them when the concentrations of active ingredients are at optimal levels. The leaves are dried to remove three-fourths of the water and are then pressed to prevent fermentation. It takes fifty pounds of leaves to yield one pound of finished extract. The final processing takes two weeks and involves twenty-seven steps as the active ingredients get isolated and standardized to arrive at the final extract.

Since plants grow naturally, their content of active, or marker, ingredients will always vary. To account for these variations and ensure a standardized product, the manufacturer will adjust the proportions in an individual mixture.

Tablets, Capsules, or Tea?

Tablets and capsules are made from measured amounts of ginkgo extract and are the most common and convenient forms. Gelatin or vegetable-based capsules filled with ginkgo extract come in a variety of sizes and strengths, so read the labels to ensure the proper dose. Tablets are powdered ginkgo extract, compressed into a solid pill, often with a variety of filler ingredients.

Ginkgo Tinctures, Teas, and Infusions

The liquid tinctures, teas, and infusions are absorbed more rapidly, but, by the same token, they may not last as long in your system. Many herbalists recommend these forms because the act of tasting the herb allows us to begin the process of allowing it to heal us. Perhaps, too, signals get sent to the appropriate parts of the body in preparation for healing.

Tinctures are liquid extracts of the herb that are not generally standardized, but do keep the vital components intact, preserved in a liquid base. To make a tincture, an herb is extracted by soaking it in alcohol. Usually one part of the herbal material is mixed with five or ten parts of liquid by weight. In the case of ginkgo, an alcohol base is used. For those who prefer not to taste the alcohol, we recommend that you put the tincture in warm water or tea for a few minutes, and let the alcohol evaporate. This will eliminate the taste of alcohol.

Teas are prepared from the whole herb, which is purchased in dried form from specialty herb shops and made into teas, decoctions, or infusions.

Chinese medicine often uses a decoction, which is made by boiling the dried herbs in water to extract the medicine and then reducing the liquid to concentrate the tea.

An infusion is like tea, but weaker. It is made using the same method you use to make tea from tea leaves or tea bags. You pour boiling water over the herb, let it steep, strain the liquid (or remove the tea bag), and then drink the mixture.

Note: Ginkgo is a bitter astringent. Ginkgo teas and infusions have a slightly sour flavor. They may require a sweetener to make the taste more palatable.

Determining the Correct Dose of Ginkgo

Most clinical studies conducted with standardized, guaranteed-potency ginkgo biloba extract (containing 24 percent flavone glycosides and 6 percent terpene lactones) recommend taking 40 mg, three times a day, with meals, for a total of 120 mg per day.

Clinical studies on treating intermittent claudication (leg cramps), tinnitus (ringing in the ears), and vertigo generally use a higher dose of the standardized extract, 160–320 mg daily, divided into two or three equal doses.

Clinical studies on treating more serious conditions, such as Alzheimer's disease, cerebral insufficiency, memory loss and depression, have used doses of 120 mg of ginkgo, taken one to three times a day with meals.

These recommendations are guidelines only, based on research and clinical use. Each person is different. We recommend that you start at the low end, watch for a response, including unwanted effects, and adjust the dose accordingly. Don't be concerned about getting the exact recommended dosage. If you have the (most common) 60 mg extract, you will, of course, be taking multiples of 60 (60, 120, 180, etc.); a 40 mg extract will be in multiples of 40 (80, 120, 160, etc.).

Note: Since ginkgo is rapidly absorbed by the body and has a half-life of about three hours, ginkgo is most effective if taken three times a day, with meals. Again, if that is impractical, simply adjust this to your own lifestyle, and take your daily amount in two doses instead.

Improvements with ginkgo are often gradual and subtle. It may take from four to eight weeks before effects are noticed. In some cases, results may take up to six months to appear.

Many health practitioners recommend ginkgo as an ongoing supplement, especially for those over age fifty. In cases involving serious conditions, you may want to review your condition after thirty days to see if you need to lower or increase your dosage, depending upon the results and your reasons for taking ginkgo in the first place. Be sure to read the safety cautions in the next section, as well.

Checking Labels—Reading Between the Lines

Most herbal products, including ginkgo biloba, are regulated as dietary supplements. In 1994, the FDA's Dietary Supplement Health and Education Act (known as DSHEA) set new guidelines with regard to quality, labeling, packaging, and marketing of supplements. It also sparked a surge of interest in herbal products. DSHEA allows manufacturers to make "statements of nutritional support for conventional vitamins and minerals," but since herbs aren't nutritional in the conventional sense, DSHEA allows them to make only what they call "structure and function claims."

The label can explain how a vitamin or herb affects the structure or function of the body. However, it cannot make therapeutic or prevention claims, such as "Treats headaches fast," or "Cures the common cold." A ginkgo biloba label can say, "helps support memory and cognitive functions," but it can't say, "it helps treat the symptoms associated with Alzheimer's disease," although this is one of many reasons people choose to use it. That would mention the condition and the treatment, and would be considered a drug claim.

Companies use verbal acrobatics in labeling products, so as not to fall over this line. You the consumer suffer from this, of course. Ideally, we should be allowed to label all supplements so you would know exactly what condition the product was for, and its possible side effects. Since the labels give insufficient information, you should use good resources, such as this one, to educate yourself.

Know Your Maker—Quality Control Counts

The Federal Drug Administration (FDA) has requested that supplement manufacturers follow specific standards, or Good Manufacturing Practices (GMPs). These are standards regarding quality control, which are essential. The product must also contain exactly what the label claims, in terms of the active ingredients, and any fillers, or other components. Of course, even herbal products can contain possible contaminants, such as bacteria, molds, and pesticides, so the manufacturing facility should follow high standards of cleanliness and processing procedures.

Trade organizations for the industry, such as the American Herbal Products Association (AHPA) and the National Nutritional Food Association (NNFA), are helping to enforce these quality standards for herbal products among their members. Their members agree to adhere to these high standards, and continue to work together to maintain them. In general, we recommend buying herbal products from a recognized manufacturer.

It is vital for manufacturers of herbal products to be responsible and maintain their high standards. Otherwise, the poor standards practiced by a few companies will taint the entire industry, and threaten our freedom to have these products available to us.

Another organization, the Council for Responsible Nutrition, continues to play a leading role in ensuring good manufacturing processes. It has worked on a political and public level to both educate and help shape appropriate legislation to allow continued freedom in our use of supplements.

When choosing a brand of ginkgo, we recommend looking at the label to see if the manufacturer follows specific standards or Good Manufacturing Practices (GMPs). Also, look for companies that commit their own resources to researching their products.

In addition to manufacturing procedures, there is the issue of fair work practices and intellectual property rights. Many herbs are grown in underdeveloped countries that can easily be exploited by Westerners. Basically, the manufacturers should have a partnership-oriented, rather than domination-type relationship, respecting native rights, ensuring that the farming is sustainable and renewable, and that the financial rewards are fair. With herbs, we are dealing with a gift of nature, and it would be a poor practice to show anything but the highest respect for the land, the people, and the environment from which they come.

GINKGO SAFETY AND CAUTIONS

Ginkgo is very safe. Extremely high doses of ginkgo have been given to animals without serious consequences. It has shown no toxicity to liver, kidneys, or new blood cell formation.

In all the clinical trials of ginkgo combined, involving a total of almost 10,000 people, the incidence of side effects produced by ginkgo extract was extremely small. Mainly there were a few cases of allergic skin reactions, dizziness, heartburn, nausea, and mild tension headaches. There were also a very few reports of an increased tendency for epistaxis—nosebleeds. This suggests that ginkgo's blood-thinning properties may increase the incidence of nose-

bleed in individuals prone to this problem, and they should check with their doctors prior to using ginkgo or combining it with other anticoagulant drugs.

Ginkgo and Pregnancy

Ginkgo appears to pose no danger to pregnant women or nursing mothers according to the current monograph of the German Commission E (equivalent to the United States Food and Drug Administration). However, this decision should be discussed with your health practitioner, as should any supplement or medication you take during pregnancy or while nursing.

Ginkgo and Overdose

While ginkgo is free of serious side effects, massive ginkgo overdoses have led to agitation, restlessness, and gastrointestinal distress.

Ginkgo and Drug Interactions

According to the Commission E Report, German medical authorities do not believe that ginkgo possesses many negative drug interactions. However, because of ginkgo's blood-thinning effects, due its ability to inhibit the platelet activation factor (PAF), authorities warn that it should not be combined with anticoagulants, or even aspirin.

For this same reason, we also recommend that you discontinue taking ginkgo at least two weeks prior to any surgical procedure.

Also, be sure to check with your physician before taking ginkgo if you are currently using any of the following medications:

1. Anticoagulants: Acetaminophen (Tylenol), aspirin, clopidogrel (Plavix), Dipyridamole (Persantine), Ticlopidine (Ticlid), and Warfarin (Coumadin).

2. MAO Inhibitors: Ginkgo may increase the effects of MAO inhibitors.

3. Thiazide diuretics: Ginkgo may increase blood pressure when used with thiazide diuretics.

Know When to Speak to Your Doctor

There are times when it's important to seek professional medical help—for example, in cases of deteriorating mental function, enlarged prostate, high blood pressure, liver ailments, or severe depression. All are potentially serious conditions and should be checked out before you embark on a self-treatment program with ginkgo.

In the best of all possible worlds, your doctor will be familiar with the use of ginkgo biloba, and will prescribe it as needed. We believe most doctors are motivated and curious to find the best, least harmful approaches to helping their patients. We therefore recommend that you take this book, or others like it, to your doctor to help inform him or her of the benefits of ginkgo biloba. Fortunately, those who seek complementary care tend to be the most likely to take responsibility for their own healing, and the least likely to expect the doctor to do or know it all. Sharing this knowledge can help you, your doctor, and his or her other patients.

CONCLUSION

Five thousand years ago, the legendary Chinese emperor Shen Nong, "wrested from Nature a knowledge of her opposing principles" to reveal the health-enhancing effects of ginkgo biloba, proclaiming that this gentle herb would allow one to follow the "Way of Long Life."

Today, Western researchers continue to add new and unexpected anti-aging and life-extending properties to an already impressive body of proven health benefits attributed to ginkgo.

First, acting as a potent antioxidant, ginkgo neutralizes free radicals to protect your cells and tissues, particularly those in your brain and your circulatory systems, the ones most prone to the ravages of aging. Second, ginkgo enhances the flow of blood in your arteries and capillaries to speed the delivery of life-giving nutrients and oxygen. And third, by inhibiting platelet activating factor (PAF), ginkgo keeps your blood from becoming sluggish, and prevents the formation of life-threatening blood clots.

Knowing about these essential properties helps you understand the wide array of important health benefits ginkgo offers you, including its ability to:

- Alleviate depression.

- Alleviate macular degeneration and improve visual acuity.

- Ameliorate intermittent claudication (leg pain due to poor blood flow when walking).

- Improve memory in both normal adults and those with Alzheimer's disease.

- Improve pulmonary function and relieve asthma.

- Improve sexual function and desire in both men and women.

- Inhibit platelet aggregation and the tendency for blood to clot abnormally.

- Reduce elevated blood pressure.

- Reduce or eliminate vertigo (dizziness and instability).

- Relieve angina pectoris due to coronary artery disease (atherosclerosis).

- Relieve PMS symptoms, including edema.

- Relieve tinnitus (ringing in the ears).

In the short space of this book, we've seen how clinical research has proven the safety and effectiveness of this ancient herb, demonstrating how ginkgo protects and strengthens our bodies in a variety of ways that can help us live longer and healthier lives.

We wish to close with the reminder that ginkgo is an important natural resource. With ginkgo, as with all herbs, we must incorporate an appreciation for the gift that nature offers us and, even as we enjoy the bounty of the harvest, be sure to replant and renew.

Remember to honor your Mother, the earth, and walk lightly on her surface as you follow your "Way of Long Life."

PART TEN

SAW PALMETTO & MEN'S HEALTH

MICHAEL JANSON, M.D.

Some dramatic changes have been taking place in Western medicine in the past few years, and you have the opportunity to benefit from some of these changes. Costs of health-care have been skyrocketing, and the government and insurance companies have tried to implement some form of control on the costs by managing the way doctors treat patients. At the same time, there has been an explosive growth in demand for treatments that are less invasive than surgery and less risky than prescription medications.

Why the changes? Consider that prescription medications are the fourth or fifth leading cause of death in the United States, with more than 100,000 people dying every year from their side effects, even when taken correctly. Heart bypass surgery is the ninth leading cause of death. Safe alternatives to drugs and surgery are available for almost every condition that plagues our society, but most doctors are only just beginning to learn about them. While still resistant to change, the medical profession is starting to recognize the benefits of natural treatments to complement or even replace some conventional medical care.

When I finished medical school in 1970, I knew very little about nutrition. Although I did learn the basic biochemistry of the individual nutrients, I did not have any training in how that related to good nutrition and dietary habits, or how the nutrients could be used as dietary supplements for treatment of different medical conditions. I also had no information about herbs and botanicals, which had been the mainstay of medicine in this country before this century, and still contribute greatly to medical therapy in many countries.

The German government, recognizing the popularity and importance of herbs in medicine, established a commission (commission E) to look into botanical medicine and establish some standards by which doctors could understand how to use herbs as part of their medical practices. In Germany and other countries, a large number of general practitioners use these herbs routinely, but they have still not been accepted in the United States. A small percentage of doctors here have been using these treatments—including vitamins, minerals, amino acids, essential oils, accessory nutrients, and botanicals—for many years with great success.

Often, these doctors have been the objects of ridicule among their peers. They have also been the objects of disciplinary action by their medical boards, which regulate the practice of medicine in every state. Public demand, fortunately, has been forcing a change in this policy, and creating a more congenial atmosphere for innovative physicians. Many states have now passed legislation protecting doctors from these medical board actions, and making sure that patients have access to alternatives to drugs and surgery. A movement is underway to change federal regulations to accomplish this on a nationwide scale, and everyone will benefit from these changes (except perhaps some drug companies).

In addition to beneficial foods, vitamins, minerals, essential fatty acids, and amino acids, herbs and botanicals are important contributors to this resurgence in natural health-care. One of the most valuable dietary supplements has been the botanical product derived from the berries of the saw palmetto tree. In addition to European doctors, physicians in the United States are recommending saw palmetto for the treatment of prostate disorders. This is based on its long history of use in folk medicine for the treatment of urinary tract disorders, and on the recent research supporting its value. The German commission, and even the United States Food and Drug Administration, have evaluated some of this information. The results of their investigations and their conclusions may surprise you.

The combination of research and clinical experience with saw palmetto gives you the opportunity to use this simple, safe, effective, and cost-effective dietary supplement to manage your prostate problems, and possibly avoid medication and surgery. However, saw palmetto is only a part of a complete program for prostate health, and prostate health is just one part of the overall picture of men's health. Functioning fully in every way, and maintaining that function for as long as possible as you age, is the end result of taking good care of yourself.

THE PROSTATE GLAND IN MEN'S HEALTH

Almost everyone has heard about the prostate gland, but you may not know what it is or how it is important in health. As men age, it is almost certain that they will become intimately familiar with the details of their prostate gland, and possibly have to deal with it as a health issue. The more you know about your prostate, the easier it will be to understand how to help yourself or help your doctor understand the treatments you prefer.

Prostate Anatomy and Function

Urethra
A canal that takes the urine from the bladder, past the prostate, and out through the penis. Semen is also discharged through it.

The prostate gland is a small organ found only in men that sits below and behind the bladder and above and in front of the rectum. It consists of a collection of ducts, fibrous tissue, glandular tissue, and muscle tissue, and it surrounds the urethra, which takes the urine from the bladder through the penis and out. The normal prostate is about the size of a walnut, weighs about two-thirds of an ounce (20 g), and produces prostatic fluids that combine with sperm from the testicles and other secretions to form semen. These fluids help sperm survive and improve their ability to travel (motility).

Prostate
A small organ in men that sits below and behind the bladder and produces prostatic fluids that help form semen.

The prostate also has some muscle fibers surrounding the urethra that help with urination. When they contract, they push urine out to aid in emptying the bladder. They also play a role during orgasm by pushing some of the prostate fluid and some of the sperm from the testicles into the urethra and out through the penis. Although it is very small, the strategic location of the prostate surrounding the urethra leads to far more health problems and medical care costs than would be predicted from its size alone.

Prostate Problems with Aging

One of the most common, and problematic, changes in the prostate results from its gradual enlargement with age (benign enlargement, not a cancer). This enlargement eventually leads to compression of the urethra and restriction of the urine flow. It is called benign prostatic hyperplasia (or hypertrophy—an older term that is still used), abbreviated as BPH. In addition to the direct obstruction that enlargement causes (the mechanical or static component of BPH), the muscles and nerves of the prostate, bladder outlet, and urethra can

Hyperplasia
Increased growth of cells of any kind, leading to enlargement of the organ. Also known as hypertrophy in reference to the prostate.

contribute further to the symptoms (the dynamic component).

Prostate problems are very common, indeed. More than 50 percent of men over age forty have enlarged prostate glands. By the time they reach eighty years old, 80 to 90 percent of men have an enlarged prostate. Although surgery to remove some of the prostate tissue is a common procedure for benign enlargement, it is not always necessary; only about 10 percent of men end up having prostate surgery at some time in their lives. According to a 1996 study, enlarged prostates lead to about $4 billion in healthcare expenditures.

There are also other possible problems with the prostate. It can be inflamed as a result of infection with bacteria, or even more frequently, with other organisms, leading to local aching, pain and burning on urination, testicular discomfort, and low back pain, as well as white blood cells in the prostatic secretions and urine. This prostate inflammation, or prostatitis, can be acute or chronic. It is even possible to see these symptoms with no signs of inflammation (no white blood cells in the prostatic secretions). In this situation, the symptoms are referred to as prostatodynia. These prostate ailments are not related to age, and are commonly seen in younger men.

The prostate is also subject to cellular changes that lead to cancer, the most common cancer in men. Prostate cancers are often undiagnosed, and only found in an autopsy when a man dies from other causes. As with many other cancers, diet may play a significant role in the development of prostate cancer.

The Symptoms of Prostate Enlargement

Benign prostatic hyperplasia (BPH) leads to a gradually increasing pinching of the urethra and obstruction of the urine flow. The early symptoms may simply start with reduction of the size and force of the urine stream. Young men with normal prostates have a peak urine flow of about two-thirds of an ounce (20 ml) per second or higher. This normally declines somewhat with age, but even more so with BPH. With mild BPH, the peak flow is reduced to approximately one-half ounce (15–20 ml) per second. With moderate prostate enlargement, the flow rate drops to between one-third and one-half ounce (10–15 ml) per second, and with severe BPH the peak rate is below one-third ounce (10 ml) per second. Severe obstruction of the urine flow can lead to serious kidney disease.

BPH
Benign prostatic hyperplasia (or hypertrophy). Enlargement of the prostate that leads to a pinching off of the urethra.

The urine flow may be difficult to start; a symptom called hesitancy. This delay in starting urination usually requires some pushing or straining in order to begin the urine flow. Because the bladder muscles help get the last bit of urine out, if there is an obstruction in your urethra, these muscles will have a harder time emptying your bladder completely (because they compensate for this by getting stronger, the symptoms of BPH may not appear early on). As a result of this difficulty, every time you urinate, some residual urine will be left in the bladder, which can give you the feeling that you have not finished emptying your bladder (another sign of prostate enlargement), and this constant feeling makes you want to urinate more frequently.

One of the most upsetting symptoms of BPH is frequent nighttime urination. Often, men with prostate enlargement may have to get up two, three, even six or more times at night to try to empty their bladder. This is obviously very disturbing to sleep, which is often already a problem for people as they get older. This nighttime urination is caused by a combination of urine left in the bladder, irritation of the urethra, and changes in the functioning of the kidneys.

Other Symptoms of Prostate Enlargement

The standard evaluation of a man with prostate enlargement includes estimating the severity of the problem. For example, being unable to hold in the urine or having difficulty postponing urination is called urgency—the sense that you have to go and can't wait. Sometimes there is interrupted stream, or intermittency where the urine flow will stop in the middle and the muscles have to strain to start again.

When there is very little urine in the bladder and the urge to urinate arises, this could be due to changes in the bladder, prostate, and urethra. With the prostate enlarged, the straining needed to start urinating, and the increased amount of work for the muscles of the bladder and prostate, there may be an irritation in the area of the bladder where the urethra starts, or in the part of the urethra that runs through the prostate. The irritation increases the sense of urgency and, therefore, the frequency of urination, but it is unrelated to the actual amount of urine present. This irritation of the urethra and the muscle spasms it causes in the bladder and prostate result in uncomfortable, sometimes painful urination, a symptom called dysuria.

Dysuria
Pain or discomfort on urination that results from irritation of the urethra and spasms of the bladder and prostate muscles.

Evaluating the Severity of Prostate Enlargement

In addition to physical examinations, for many years doctors have used a questionnaire called the Boyarsky Index where patients evaluate the level of nine symptoms on a scale from zero (not present) to three (most severe) for a maximum symptom score of twenty-seven. Another scale, the American Urological Association Symptom Index, uses six symptoms, rated from zero to five, plus the nighttime urinary frequency. In this scale, a score up to seven is mild, up to eighteen is moderate, and above nineteen is considered a severe prostate disorder (prostatism).

These, along with other scores and the examination, help evaluate the prostate symptoms, and are used to determine how much improvement there is with any treatment.

Finding out if You Have a Prostate Problem

Generally, symptoms appear early in the course of benign prostate enlargement, but they can vary a great deal. Even with moderate BPH, the symptoms may be minimal because the bladder muscle can grow to compensate for the obstruction. And the telltale symptoms of more frequent, more urgent, or nighttime urination may be caused by something else entirely, such as anxiety, caffeine consumption, or drinking large amounts of liquid.

After age forty, it's a good idea to have annual checkups to detect the presence or ongoing development of BPH. This normally includes a digital rectal examination (DRE), in which a doctor places a gloved finger in the rectum to evaluate the size and shape of the prostate gland. This exam does not always give the full picture, so other tests are also done, including one that measures the rate of flow of the urine, ultrasound studies, and magnetic resonance imaging (MRI).

Differentiating Benign Prostate Enlargement from Cancer

Benign enlargement is far more prevalent than cancer, but cancer is certainly common enough to be of concern. Cancers produce hard, rough, irregular lumps, or nodules, but with benign enlargement, the prostate is usually softer, smoother, and more even. This can vary, however—the cancer nodules could be buried deep within the prostate, for example, and the doctor's gloved finger would not be able to reach them so they would remain undetected in a physical examination.

There is also the prostate specific antigen test (PSA), which tests for a specific substance found in larger amounts in the blood of patients with prostate cancer. It is not foolproof in distinguishing prostate cancer from BPH or prostatitis, but it can help. The amount of the protein molecule PSA in the blood rises when prostate cells grow or are inflamed. Since cancer cells tend to grow more vigorously than other prostate cells, the level of PSA is likely to be much higher with prostate cancer than with other conditions. The PSA will, however, also be higher for a day or two after ejaculation, so it is important to give the doctor this information when taking this test.

Prostate Specific Antigen
A protein molecule produced by prostate cells and found in the blood. In increased levels, it may indicate prostate cancer.

Other Diagnostic Tests

Another test is an ultrasound of the prostate done through the rectum. Ultrasound tests are not dangerous. They are used all the time to evaluate hidden body structures and, in pregnancy, to evaluate the developing fetus. Sound waves are reflected off of tissue, and they give a picture of the prostate, which can indicate its size and the presence of lumps that can't be felt. This test is usually reserved for those who have had another positive test first.

Finally, a biopsy, where a tissue sample from a specific organ is taken, can be done on the prostate. It can be an open biopsy where a piece of tissue gets cut from the prostate, or it can be a needle biopsy, possible in this case because of the relatively easy access to the prostate gland through the rectum. With this kind of biopsy, a needle is inserted into the gland and a piece of tissue is taken for microscopic examination.

CONVENTIONAL MEDICAL TREATMENT OF THE PROSTATE

For many years, the only treatment for benign prostatic hyperplasia was to wait until the symptoms were intolerable, or the urinary retention created a more serious medical problem. If the prostate is enlarged but no symptoms appear, waiting is not a problem as sometimes the prostate does not enlarge further or cause symptoms. On the other hand, if it does progress enough for symptoms to appear, then a doctor would recommend treatment.

Surgical removal of the obstructive prostate tissue is common. Today, several surgical options are available. Doctors can do an open operation, from the outside, but this is not a common procedure for BPH, although it may be used for cancer or when there are massively enlarged glands. The prostate tissue can also be removed through a tube (cystoscope) placed into the urethra through the penis. This procedure, called a transurethral resection of the prostate (TURP), removes the tissue right where the urinary obstruction occurs, and can be quite effective.

However, even though TURP is still the main treatment for the more severe situations, there can be complications, as for example, a retrograde ejaculation where the semen is pushed into the bladder rather than out through the penis. Sexual dysfunction or impotence, seen in one out of every ten to twenty patients, is another complication, as is incontinence. Some men develop a urinary tract infection after the surgery, which requires antibiotics, and sometimes they have excessive bleeding that requires blood transfusions. In one out of five or ten patients, a repeat operation is often required if the symptoms return.

Other Treatments for BPH

Newer, minimally invasive treatments have been developed and are still being studied, but they seem very promising as far as surgical procedures go. Called minimally invasive because, although they use a catheter to enter the urethra, they do not cut the prostate tissue. For example, in the transurethral needle ablation (TUNA) procedure, a catheter is used to insert into the prostate small needles that transmit low-level radio waves that create heat and destroy some prostate cells. This has fewer complications than TURP, but it does not appear quite as effective in the long term.

Another treatment is called transurethral microwave therapy (TUMT), which uses microwaves, also to create heat and destroy prostate tissue. So far, TUMT appears to require repeat procedures sooner than other therapies, making it less effective in the long term than other treatments. While none of these newer treatments are as effective as TURP, they *are* safer, less invasive, and have fewer side effects. They also take less time, are less expensive, and can be done in a doctor's office, usually with very rapid recovery.

More recently, two other procedures have been evaluated. One of these is treatment with a transurethral ultrasound-guided laser-induced prostatectomy (TULIP) device. It also destroys some prostate tissue, using ultrasound to direct a laser beam at the prostate tissue. As with the above, it has fewer side effects than conventional surgery.

The other very promising treatment is called transurethral vaporization of the prostate (TUVP). In this method, the prostate tissue is rapidly vaporized with high heat. In one three-year follow-up of this treatment, published in the *British Journal of Urology International*, the relief from symptoms was equivalent to the results with TURP. However, the complication rate was also about the same in the two groups.

When considering treatment, it is well to appreciate that any procedure has some associated risks, and no one wants surgical procedures if they can avoid them. No doctor recommends such treatments unless the symptoms are significant, but even when they do recommend them, alternatives without the risks of surgery would often be adequate.

Nonsurgical Prostate Treatments

Until recently, most conventional physicians have not had any treatments to offer to patients with prostate enlargement other than to wait until the symptoms worsened and surgery was required. In the mid-1990s, a new medication called finasteride (trade name Proscar) was shown to help with prostate symptoms, but it was not nearly as effective as doctors (and especially patients) had hoped it would be. It also turned out to have undesirable side effects, among them a loss of libido, sexual dysfunction (inability to have or maintain an erection, or impotence), and abnormal ejaculation. There is also a risk of birth defects to a male fetus in a pregnant woman who has contact with the drug, through handling either the pill or the semen of a man taking it.

Because of these potential side effects and the drug's inadequate results, both doctors and patients would like to find other ways than finasteride to reduce BPH symptoms and delay or eliminate the need for surgery.

The Role of Enzymes and Hormones in BPH

Finasteride appears to work through its effects on hormones and an enzyme. Enzymes are protein molecules that act as catalysts—substances that make chemical reactions occur faster at body temperature. The rate of a reaction is determined by many factors, such as heat and the mixture of substances that are reacting. Because excessive heat might damage cells, enzyme catalysts help promote reactions at lower temperatures. Enzymes work with other substances, such as minerals and vitamins, to push these reactions. Many vitamins are called coenzymes because of their role in helping enzymes work.

Well-known examples of enzymes are the digestive enzymes, produced in the stomach and pancreas, which work with stomach acids to break down foods during digestion and help in their assimilation. Different kinds of enzymes also control the reactions that lead to the production of hormones and the reactions involved in the breakdown of hormones after they are used.

Hormones are regulatory substances produced by the endocrine glands. Unlike the output of other glands, such as sweat glands or salivary glands, they deliver their output directly into the bloodstream. Adrenaline (epinephrine), a well-known hormone, is produced by the adrenal glands in response to acute stress. Another hormone, cortisone, is produced by a different part of the adrenal glands. The pancreas produces insulin, a hormone that regulates blood sugar levels. The thyroid gland in the neck is another endocrine gland. Thyroid hormones regulate the metabolic rate, or how fast your body burns energy.

At the base of the brain is the master endocrine gland, the pituitary, which produces substances that regulate other glands. It also produces hormones that have direct effects on different bodily functions. For example, it regulates the amounts of testosterone produced in the testes of men, and the amounts of estrogens and progesterone produced in the ovaries of women. Referred to as the male and female sex hormones, there are, in fact, small amounts of each found in the other sex as well.

Finasteride's Effect on Hormones

The male sex hormones, or androgens, are primarily testosterone and a derivative called dihydrotestosterone (DHT) produced from testosterone with the help of an enzyme called 5-alpha reductase. Finasteride works by blocking this enzyme to reduce the production of DHT, which has been shown to promote prostate enlargement. Therefore, blocking its production helps reduce prostate symptoms.

The hormone relationship is not quite so clear, however. In dogs, the female hormone estradiol (a relatively strong member of the estrogen family of hormones) acts together with the DHT to increase prostate growth, and it may also do so in men. Another enzyme, aromatase, converts some of the circulating testosterone into estradiol, which may contribute more to prostate enlargement than DHT does. Finasteride does not directly influence the production of estradiol, but there is speculation that its blocking the production of DHT may lead to more estradiol production, which can worsen prostate symptoms, and may be one of the reasons finasteride does not work as well as we would like.

The Causes of Benign Prostatic Hyperplasia

We don't completely understand the cause of benign prostate enlargement. We do know that it happens with aging and requires the presence of male hormones, specifically DHT, derived from testosterone. Men who have had their testicles removed, and therefore have no testosterone production, do not develop benign prostatic hyperplasia. And, in dogs, we know that hormonal therapy, which increases DHT levels, leads to an enlargement of the prostate similar to BPH.

In addition, as men age, the level of the estrogen hormone estradiol increases. As we said, in dogs, estradiol works with DHT to induce prostate growth. If this happens in humans also, it might explain the increase in prostate size with aging because, as men age, their DHT level goes down, but their estradiol level goes up. Some researchers also suggest that the ratio of DHT to testosterone, which goes up with age, is more important than the absolute level of either one.

Lifestyle choices may play a role in the development of BPH, and improper nutrition may contribute not only to prostate enlargement, but also to prostate cancer. It is also possible that specific beneficial foods may contribute to the prevention of prostate enlargement.

Other Medical Treatments for BPH

Doctors may prescribe another drug that helps with the symptoms of prostate enlargement. This drug terazosin (Hytrin) has been used for high blood pressure because it relaxes the muscles of the blood vessels, allowing them to open and reduce the pressure in the circulation. Terazosin works to improve urine flow but does not affect the size of the prostate. Unfortunately, as with most medications,

Hormones
Regulatory substances produced by the endocrine glands that control numerous functions in the body.

Dihydro-testosterone (DHT)
A hormone derived from testosterone, the male sex hormone that is an apparent cause of benign prostate enlargement.

there are some potential side effects from terazosin. Because it is also a blood pressure medication, one major caution is that the first dose of terazosin may cause very low blood pressure and fainting in the first few days of taking it, or you could momentarily feel faint when you stand up quickly. It can also cause dizziness, fatigue, sleepiness, and sexual dysfunction as well as nasal congestion and a runny nose. If you also have high blood pressure, you may have other side effects, and if you are on other blood pressure medications, be sure to let your doctor know before taking terazosin.

Saw Palmetto: The Men's Herb

Dietary supplements, including herbs and botanicals, are becoming more popular as treatments for common medical conditions, partly because they usually have the advantage over drugs and surgery of being safer, more cost effective, and less invasive. In many cases, they are not only safer and less expensive, but they are also more effective than some drugs prescribed for the same conditions. There are supplements for the brain, digestion, the heart, the liver, and the skin, as well as for arthritis, diabetes, headaches, and many other conditions. Saw palmetto is one of the supplements that is not only cheaper, but more effective than the medications used for the prostate.

Saw Palmetto Compared to Drugs

It is likely that most men will have to consider dealing with their own prostate as they age. If it does become a problem for you, you have the choices listed above for treatment, or you may wish to choose an alternative that has numerous advantages over the drugs/surgery treatments used by conventional medicine. It is no secret that most people would prefer to avoid surgery if possible, especially men contemplating surgery on their prostate gland.

Based on the medical literature, my own use of it with my patients, and the experience of most of my colleagues in nutritional and botanical medicine, saw palmetto is a safe, effective alternative to these treatments. Even some urologists who have been disappointed with finasteride are recommending saw palmetto instead. It reduces the symptoms of prostate enlargement, and it also helps improve urinary tract function in a large percentage of men with benign prostatic hyperplasia (BPH). You might also consider taking saw palmetto as preventive medicine if you are in the age group at risk for BPH.

What Is Saw Palmetto?

The saw palmetto is a small palm tree eight to ten feet high that grows in the southeastern coastal states of North

Saw Palmetto
A small palm tree with red-brown berries that have been researched in Europe and the United States for treating disorders of the prostate gland.

America. The tree has large, fan-like leaves, and produces berries about the size of a grape that have a deep reddish-black to brown color. These berries have long been used for disorders of the urinary tract, especially by Native Americans. Saw palmetto is also known as Sabal serrulata, Serenoa repens, or by its trade name Permixon.

Recent European research on the oily, fat-soluble extracts of saw palmetto berries has shown their benefits in treating disorders of the prostate gland. Most of this research comes from France and Germany, where the use of botanical medicines is more accepted and better researched than in the United States. This is slowly changing, however, as North Americans have developed a strong interest in alternatives to drugs and surgery, and have opened their minds to nutrition and dietary supplements, including botanical medicines. Research is now being done in the United States, England, Scotland, Russia, Italy, and elsewhere.

Botanical Medicines

Botanical medicine is the use of any plant parts in treating or preventing illness. Doctors or other healers might use different parts of certain plants. Technically, herbs are the leafy or stem parts of the plant, but when used in medicinal treatments, the word "herb" often means botanical, referring to any part of the plant—the bark, fruit, leaf, rhizome, root, or stem. Many botanical medicines are at the root of our modern drugs, such as digitalis, for the heart, which comes from the leaf of the foxglove, or colchicine, for gout, from the bulb of the autumn crocus. And aspirin is a derivative of salicylic acid, a substance that comes from willow bark.

Botanical Medicine
Any therapeutic natural substance, commonly called an herb, derived from any part of a plant, usually with few or no toxic side effects.

The prescription medications that doctors commonly use for treatment of illness are often quite risky. Side effects are common, and can be serious, sometimes leading to hospitalization and even death. Even over-the-counter medications frequently have side effects, so it is no wonder people are looking for safer, more natural remedies for their health problems. Most of the time, botanical medicines are safer than more recently developed medicines, but that does not mean they are all without risk. Saw palmetto is a very safe herb, and is one of several natural treatments for prostate disorders.

Saw Palmetto and Prostate Treatment

For a number of years, practitioners who use nutrition and

botanical medicines have had several alternative treatments for prostate enlargement not commonly used by conventional medicine, especially in the United States. High doses of zinc, for example, have been shown to help with the symptoms of BPH, as have essential fatty acids and high doses of certain amino acids (amino acids are the building blocks of proteins) when taken as supplements.

As mentioned above, saw palmetto can have a profound effect in providing relief from the symptoms of BPH, even better than the results seen with finasteride, and without its troubling side effects. While saw palmetto may also act as an inhibitor of the enzyme 5-alpha reductase, thus reducing the DHT production thought to enlarge the prostate, it appears to have other physiological effects as well that make it superior to the medication. This is especially true because of its lack of side effects.

For example, saw palmetto extracts inhibit all of the testosterone, not just DHT, and unlike finasteride, which only acts on certain cells, the extracts work in all of the cells studied, helping to prevent prostate enlargement.

Studies on saw palmetto show that it improves both the rate and the volume of urine flow. It reduces the urgency and frequency of urination, including the number of urinations at night. Overall, about 90 percent of men report that it helps them with their symptoms compared to finasteride (which helps only about 50 percent of them, does not decrease nighttime urination, has minimal effect on urine flow, and has side effects!)

Other Effects of Saw Palmetto on the Prostate

Research shows there are other physiological effects of saw palmetto that help prostate symptoms, and may help other medical conditions as well. It can inhibit certain substances called prostanoids that lead to inflammation, irritation, and smooth muscle spasms, among other symptoms. Some of them promote inflammation while others decrease it, and any imbalance among the different types can lead to significant health problems.

These processes influence the symptoms of prostate enlargement, and saw palmetto can help reduce them, and minimize the irritation and spasm of the smooth muscles in the prostate and urethra that initiate the urgency and frequency of BPH. Research confirms that saw palmetto has these additional benefits for BPH, beyond its effect on DHT and the size of the prostate. So if you have prostate symptoms, you can get the benefits of both finasteride and terazosin from saw palmetto extracts without the risk of their side effects.

Saw Palmetto also Affects Estrogens

In addition to testosterone, men produce some female estrogen hormones (although less than women), just as women produce some testosterone. Receptors are the locations where the hormones bind to cells to have their ultimate effects, just as a key fits into a lock in order to turn it. You can influence the activity of a hormone without changing the amount that is produced if you change the number of receptors, or the ability of the hormone to attach to the receptor. Instead of inhibiting the production of the estrogen hormones, saw palmetto takes over the same receptor sites as the estrogen, and works on both kinds of these estrogen receptor sites to reduce the activity of estradiol, which otherwise increases the symptoms of BPH (not to mention its potential for increasing the risk of prostate cancer). So, saw palmetto reduces BPH symptoms that way also.

Estrogens
A group of hormones found in high amounts in women, and far lower amounts in men, that influence reproductive organs and other body functions.

Prostate Symptoms Vary from Time to Time

From hour to hour, or day to day, the intensity of prostate symptoms can vary, with stress contributing to the symptoms. For example, everyone has had the experience of having a strong urge to urinate, but before finding a bathroom the urge has diminished greatly or even disappeared. This is because the signals from the nerves of the urethra and bladder are variable. But stress can increase the sense of urgency, as can the sound of running water, or alcohol, caffeine, and any food sensitivities. Muscle spasms in the bladder, prostate, and urethra can also lead to a feeling of urgency and to more frequent urination. For these reasons, the urge to urinate can come and go, even when the amount of urine in the bladder is unchanged, and in spite of the size of the prostate.

In fact, in a large percentage of men, symptoms improve with no treatment, even though there is no change in the size of the prostate. Eventually, as the prostate enlarges with age, the symptoms will be more consistent, but in the meantime, this variation is common and expected.

PROSTATE RESEARCH: HOW IS IT DONE?

First, let me give you some information about medical research, so you can understand the studies on saw palmetto and drugs. Medical research varies greatly in quality and consistency, and for many reasons, any one study must be viewed with caution, especially if it is contrary to a number of other studies. The methods and design play a large role in determining the outcome, and the position of the authors strongly influences the interpretation and conclusions, and the way studies are reported. Even established journals may publish studies that are of inferior quality, but that does not mean the research is valueless. It may stimulate other studies and provide some good information, even if not all of it is valid.

Understanding the Placebo Effect

When doctors do medical research, they are always on the lookout for effects that may appear to be due to a treatment, but in reality are due to other factors. This is particularly the case when symptoms of an illness are variable and affected by stress or emotions. It is also an important consideration when the signs of an illness are subjective (reported by the patient) rather than objective (measured by a lab test or other equipment).

Symptoms are also affected by the expectations of the test subject and even the person administering the test, so medical researchers introduce controls to their studies to find out if the results are due to these expectations. *Placebo* comes from the Latin word meaning "to please"—the patients trying to please the doctor by reporting that their symptoms are better as a result of the doctor's treatment. The symptoms may actually be better, because we know that the brain has a strong influence on the healing process, but the symptoms may not be influenced by the treatment, which is what the study is trying to determine. This is what is meant by the placebo effect.

Placebo Effect
Any benefit that is due to a patient's expectation of improvement from a treatment, rather than from the specific treatment being administered.

Placebos in Practice

When doing a study, doctors will use a dummy pill, the placebo, in half the test subjects. The other half will get a real medicine that the doctors are trying to test. The placebo, formerly called a sugar pill, should look exactly like the real treatment, and is supposed to be completely inactive so the results of the study are not influenced by any physiological effect (sometimes the dummy pill unexpectedly turns out to be active, casting doubt on the results of the study). The group receiving the placebo is called the control group. The groups should be randomly selected (to avoid prejudice during selection) and carefully matched in every other way to increase the validity of the study.

The subjects in the study are not told what pill they are getting. If that is the only hidden information, it is called a single-blind study. If, in addition, those administering the pills do not know which group is receiving which pill (they are coded for later interpretation), it is called a "double-blind" study. In crossover studies, the groups are switched after a period of time, so the placebo group is given the real pill and the active-treatment group is given the placebo. (There are problems with some crossover studies because, if the active ingredients have long-lasting effects and the effects don't start right away, this confuses the outcome of the study.) Studies that test behavior or stress, instead of medication or some other substance, can also be conducted in a double-blind fashion, but they are more difficult to do.

Placebo-Controlled Studies Are Important for Prostate Research

Stress, the emotional state, or the person's expectations of the treatment's benefits often influence prostate symptoms. The dynamic component of these symptoms relates to spasms of the local muscles and irritation of the nerves and mucous membranes lining the bladder and urethra, and these dynamic symptoms are particularly influenced by the mind. Reactions, such as your hands sweating or becoming cold when you are nervous, are everyday evidence of the mind's influence on physical symptoms. Mind-body medicine, referring to harnessing the power of the mind to promote healing, is another bit of evidence showing how important your emotional and mental states are in any disease.

Studies designed to show that the effect of a particular treatment is due to the treatment itself, rather than the mind-body influence, need placebo controls in order for researchers to draw accurate conclusions. Although such controlled studies are not the only way to learn about the value of a treatment, establishment doctors do like to see them before accepting a treatment, especially one that is not typically part of conventional medicine. Fortunately, many nutritional and herbal treatments have controlled studies to support their value. Saw palmetto has been researched in a number of double-blind, placebo-controlled studies, many of them from France, Germany, and Italy.

Research on Saw Palmetto and Prostate Symptoms

Quite a few of the studies showing how saw palmetto works have been published in recognized medical journals. There are human studies, animal studies, and studies of cells in laboratories, the latter designed to show how a substance works—show which biochemical and hormonal actions explain the results when the substance is given to a person. Skeptical scientists like to have some understanding of how something might work to show whether it really does work. Of course, this is not always possible. Many beneficial treatments are valuable, even though we have little understanding of their mechanisms. For many years, medical science did not have an explanation of how aspirin worked, but this did not stop doctors from recommending it. Many treatments today are in a similar situation. Cholesterol-lowering drugs, for example, have actions that are too quick to be related only to their effect on cholesterol. Researchers are now trying to find out if this is due to their effects on platelets or inflammation, or some other action.

Studies in cells have shown some of the actions of saw palmetto. Although we are not sure if the effects we see in cells in the lab are the ones responsible for the actual results when people take saw palmetto, it is likely that they are related.

Specific Studies and Their Results

The earliest study that I can find, from 1969, is a description of a substance in saw palmetto that has an estrogenlike effect. Fourteen years later, in 1983, a cell study showed that saw palmetto extract affected the testosterone receptors in rat prostate cells.

The first human study I could find was done in Germany in 1979. Seventy-four men were treated with an extract of *Sabal serrulata* (another name for saw palmetto). In this study they showed that, although the objective measurements of the prostate and urine flow did not change, every patient reported a reduction of their symptoms.

Another early human study was done by a French team in 1984. These researchers also reported the favorable results of a double-blind study using saw palmetto in 110 patients with BPH. A number of other studies since have shown similar results. One in Spain, in 1992, compared saw palmetto with a drug similar to terazosin, and both substances were found to be about equally effective.

A 1995 study done in Italy showed that saw palmetto was beneficial, but not quite as effective as another drug similar to terazosin. This is important for doctors and the public to know, because if they have a choice, most people would prefer to take a natural substance that is almost as effective and has fewer side effects, especially if it is less expensive. If it turns out the natural treatment doesn't control the symptoms, the person can always then take the medication.

Other Studies and United States Research

A New Zealand study showed saw palmetto and finasteride were similarly effective. The test subjects all had significant improvement in nighttime urination, daytime frequency of urination, and peak urine flow rates. In two large uncontrolled trials, about 90 percent of those studied reported that their symptoms were much better within three months after starting saw palmetto.

Some American doctors only trust studies done in the United States, not a reasonable prejudice because studies done in Italy, Germany, France, Spain, and elsewhere are just as valid as those done in the United States. Although most studies have been done abroad, in 1998 there was a study done in Chicago to evaluate saw palmetto for its effectiveness in treating prostate enlargement. After six months, they found that about half the people reported they had at least a 50 percent improvement in symptoms.

The FDA Evaluation of Saw Palmetto Research

The United States Food and Drug Administration (FDA) evaluated saw palmetto research in response to a request by one company that wanted to make a health claim for the effectiveness of their product on the label. Interestingly, this FDA evaluation came shortly after the prescription drug finasteride was approved. A number of the studies mentioned above were submitted for the FDA review. In their analysis, the FDA looked at these and published their conclusions in *Food Drug Cosmetic Law Reports*. After noting that the saw palmetto extract appeared to be safe, they evaluated nighttime urination frequency, urinary output, and residual urine, as well as the patients' reports on improvement of their discomfort while urinating. They reported that the urine-flow rate increased and the residual volume (the amount left in the bladder after urination) decreased, as did the nighttime urinations. They also noted that more than 92 percent of the patients reported that their symptoms were better.

These changes, the FDA admitted, were statistically significant. However, they went on to say that they did not consider these improvements to be clinically significant because the symptoms were not completely cured, even though in every case they were better than the already-approved drug. Over 90 percent of the patients reported they were better with saw palmetto, while only 50 percent did so with finasteride. The urine flow improved 50 percent with saw palmetto, compared to only 22 percent with finasteride. With saw palmetto, residual urine volume went down compared to no change with finasteride. *The Physicians' Desk Reference*, a guide to drugs that every physician uses, states that most patients report at least a 30 percent improvement with finasteride. This is *less* than in any of the studies I have seen with saw palmetto.

The FDA Conclusions: Did They Approve Saw Palmetto Claims?

In spite of their favorable review of the effects of saw palmetto, the FDA has not yet approved the use of saw palmetto for the prostate, but this has to be understood in context. It would be very unusual for the FDA to approve any natural substance in the treatment of medical conditions. Their official role is to assure the safety and promote the development of new drugs. In spite of that, many drugs that reach the market are neither safe nor effective, and are eventually pulled from the market (examples are thalidomide, Fen-phen, and Baycol), usually after they have done damage.

Drug companies pour enormous amounts of money into research and development to meet the standards of the FDA. But this is not a guarantee of safety or effectiveness. Most natural products on the market today have a long history of safety, but do not have the expensive studies that meet the FDA standards. This is because natural products cannot be patented, so the drug companies have no incentive to spend the money to meet those standards.

The FDA has an apparent bias against natural products like saw palmetto. Even when they do meet the standards, the FDA seems to find some excuse not to approve them. As mentioned above, the FDA found that saw palmetto produced better results than the prostate drug that they had already approved, but they still did not approve label claims for saw palmetto. The fact that the FDA has not approved saw palmetto says more about them than about this remarkable supplement, and in no way detracts from its value.

Doctors Recommend Saw Palmetto

Along with many of my medical colleagues, I regularly recommend the use of saw palmetto, but most doctors here are unfamiliar with herbal or nutritional medicine, and do not recommend it. This is beginning to change, however, as increasing numbers of urologists are starting to suggest it. Naturopaths and nutritionists, of course, have an interest in alternatives to drugs and surgery, and they regularly recommend saw palmetto for prostate enlargement.

In America, conventional doctors are often opposed to using herbal treatments or other dietary supplements, and doctors who do start using such treatments are no longer considered conventional, but this is not true in many other countries. In Germany, for example, about half of the primary doctors routinely use these treatments. And in Italy in 1991, herbal treatments represented almost 10 percent of all prescriptions for prostate enlargement.

As increasing numbers of doctors are dissatisfied with the available drug treatments, and as their patients continue to demand more natural remedies, the number of conventional doctors who begin to use saw palmetto and other natural treatments will expand even further.

Natural Treatments May Take Time to Work

Saw palmetto takes some time to be effective in relieving the symptoms of prostate enlargement. Many people are used to medications having an instant effect to help with medical conditions, but this is not usually true for natural remedies. In the first few weeks of treatment, terazosin and similar drugs have been shown to be somewhat better at providing relief than saw palmetto, but longer studies show that saw palmetto eventually catches up with and surpasses these drugs.

Although some will report symptom relief sooner, typically you need to take saw palmetto for one to three months before significant results can be expected. In some studies, it appears that results are even better if those studied continue taking the saw palmetto for six months or more. In the Chicago study, one-fifth of the men were better after two months, one-third were better after four months, and nearly half were better after six months. Since they ended the study at that point, we don't know if any of the men would have had even further improvement with longer treatment. Of course, for those who do not respond adequately, it may help to take a larger dose, which might speed up and enhance the response.

Clinical Experience with Saw Palmetto

I have been treating my patients with saw palmetto for a number of years now. In my experience, patients usually tell me their symptoms have improved within two to three months, but sometimes sooner, even within a week or two. Occasionally, they tell me their symptoms persist. For them, it either takes much longer to see improvement, or they need a higher dose.

Very few fail to respond, at least to some extent, to saw palmetto, especially if they are given higher doses. For those few who don't, or for those with a more advanced disease, I recommend additional supplements, as you will see later. I have been very impressed with the success of this treatment. There have not been any serious side effects from it, in fact, almost no side effects at all. I myself am taking saw palmetto preventively as I approach sixty, even though I have never had any symptoms of prostate enlargement and have no evidence of it.

GUIDELINES FOR BUYING AND USING SAW PALMETTO

Just learning about a supplement is not enough if you really want to use it for your health. You really need to know how to take it, what the precautions are, if any, what dose to use, and how it is available. You also need to know what to look for in products, so you are sure to get what will be most effective for you. I always give my patients specific instructions, and you need the same information.

Proper Dosing of Saw Palmetto

The typical recommended dose for most men with prostatic enlargement is 160 mg twice a day of the standardized extract, which contains 85 to 95 percent sterols and fatty acids. Most saw palmetto research is done with this daily dose of 320 mg, but if this is not effective, some men might benefit from higher doses. Responses are always variable with any medical treatment, especially natural substances. We have to be prepared to make adjustments for individuals.

I had one eighty-seven-year-old man who was taking 320 mg of saw palmetto daily, and he reported it gave him only minimal, sporadic success in relieving his symptoms. Before giving up, after almost three years of disappointment, he decided to double his usual dose for a while. To his delight, after just one month, he reported back that his symptoms were almost completely controlled. From having to get up and urinate three to four times a night, he now only has to get up once, or sometimes not at all. Needless to say, he is staying on the 320 mg, twice-a-day dosage.

Timing the Doses of Saw Palmetto

Unlike some supplements, there is no special time that will make saw palmetto more or less effective. The most convenient times to take dietary supplements are with your breakfast and dinner. Since supplements are basically foods, taking them with meals usually helps to avoid any digestive upset that might occur with concentrated food products. Also, since there are usually some oils in foods, these may help absorb the fatty substances in saw palmetto.

Although you could take your entire daily dose at once, I usually recommend dividing the dose in two. Taking it more than twice a day, however, often results in forgetting the other doses, and any supplement you don't take is going to be totally ineffective. If you don't eat breakfast (although it is a good idea to do so), you can take saw palmetto with lunch and dinner, along with your other supplements, or you can take it all in the evening. It's your choice; just don't forget to take it.

Available Forms of Saw Palmetto

As with many botanical and herbal treatments, a number of preparations are available. There are whole berries, powders made from whole berries, liquid extracts, such as concentrates, standardized extracts, and tinctures. Almost any of the preparations will have some benefit, as long as they honestly contain what is claimed on the label. However, the dose needed to be effective may vary greatly from one brand to another, and from one form to another.

Tinctures are extracts in a base of alcohol. You usually take a dropperful or two twice a day, unless otherwise instructed on the label. Some liquid extracts are in a glycerin base for people who prefer to avoid any alcohol. Liquid extracts can be effective if you take enough for your needs.

The dose of the berry powders will exceed the one for the extracts, and the most effective form is the standardized extract. Both the powders and the standardized extracts are available in either tablets or capsules. Some people find capsules easier to swallow, but manufacturers can fit more of the raw material into a tablet because it is compressed, and therefore smaller than the comparable dose in a capsule. Most of the time I have seen them in capsules. Read the dose carefully, as some products contain less than the usual 160 mg per pill. There are a number of these products on the market, and you just have to find what works for you.

Standardized Herbal Extracts

As our knowledge of botanical medicines advances, we are learning to identify the active substances in them that are therapeutic. We are able to research botanicals more easily if we can be sure that the amount of the active substance is consistent from batch to batch. Standardization means that the presumed active principles are always present in the same amount. Most of the standardized extracts have fairly reliable amounts of all the potential active components. In addition, it is a good idea to choose products that have at least some of the whole herb in them.

Most of the recent research on botanical medicines has been done with standardized extracts because they are the most reliable scientifically based herbs. Remember, however, that before there were standardized extracts, herbs had been used therapeutically for many centuries, and simple herbal preparations are still of value. Still, if you want the most reliable form of an herb, it is probably best to choose the standardized extracts as they have the known amounts of active components.

Getting the Right Product

If a product contains the standardized extract, it should say so on the label. It should also specify that it is standardized to contain 85 to 95 percent liposterols right on the ingredient label. If it simply says "extract" or "concentrate," or any other wording, it is probably not the standardized extract. This does not mean you may not get some value from it, only that it has not been as extensively researched. Most pills on the market contain 120 or 160 mg, so you can take two or three to get the recommended amount.

It is also a good idea to look at the price of a few products (making sure that the doses are comparable). Occasionally, a product will be misbranded, and will not contain what the label says, but this is not the usual situation. As the supplement industry has matured, only a few disreputable companies may be cutting corners and charging less for their inferior products. If you compare prices for different high-quality brands at several health food stores and mail-order sources, you should have some idea of the usual price range for saw palmetto (as well as for any other health product you buy). If a product is far above or below the average price, be suspicious—on the high end, that you're not receiving value for your money, and on the low end, that you're not getting the right product. Good quality brands do, of course, go on special sale at a very good price from time to time, but that is usually a temporary deal.

> **Standardized Extract**
> *An herbal medicine that contains specific amounts of active components based on the current state of research.*

Taking Saw Palmetto: How Long?

If saw palmetto is working, you will probably have to continue taking it indefinitely. Prostate enlargement is a progressive condition that generally worsens with age, and if you stop taking the treatment, the condition will gradually return. For some of the symptoms, the effect of saw palmetto is short term, and they may come back within a short time if you stop taking the supplement.

We don't really have any long-term studies to show what happens after someone improves with saw palmetto, then stops taking it, but we know from anecdotal experience that the hormonal changes from saw palmetto continue for only a short time after stopping the treatment. So basically, since there are no side effects to saw palmetto, it's a good idea to continue taking it in order to maintain your prostate health and control the symptoms of BPH.

Tolerance to the Effects of Saw Palmetto

In studies lasting up to twelve months, it was found that the benefits of taking saw palmetto do not decline if you continue taking it for the long term. The improvement in symptoms is maintained, and you do not develop a tolerance to it, meaning that the dose you need to maintain the benefits does not have to be increased. In fact, it appears that at the same dosage, the benefits continue to *increase* for the entire duration of the longer studies.

Although I have not seen any studies longer than one year, from the available research, my own clinical experience, and that of my colleagues, it seems the effects of saw palmetto last well beyond the duration of the longest studies.

Side Effects from Saw Palmetto

As previously stated, there are almost no side effects from saw palmetto, even in the higher doses. Of course, any substance, even water, given in extremely large quantities may have some negative effects, so it is probably best not to take more than twice the recommended amount. Approximately 5 percent of those studied have reported side effects, such as minor indigestion that does not last, but they're not usually enough for them to stop taking saw palmetto. In my own practice, only a few have reported digestive upset, and it was never clear that this was related to saw palmetto.

Saw palmetto has no contraindications (medical language for special medical situations in which you should not take a substance). There are also no known negative interactions with drugs or other dietary supplements. In fact, other dietary supplements and natural treatments may help relieve the symptoms of prostate enlargement, and these often enhance the action of the saw palmetto.

I have not seen any studies on people taking saw palmetto along with either terazosin (Hytrin) or finasteride (Proscar). Most of the time, people take either the drug or the natural supplement, and it is probably best to choose between them, although harmful side effects are still unlikely, even if you combine saw palmetto with either of these drugs.

Saw Palmetto for Younger Men

Since saw palmetto has no contraindications, no significant side effects, and no known negative interactions with drugs or other dietary supplements, you should have no reason to worry about taking it, no matter how old you are. If you are under forty, I see no need to take saw palmetto unless there is some specific reason for it. If there is, you can rest assured that it will not interfere with your stamina or endurance, and it will not affect your exercise program. The same holds true for older people.

Saw Palmetto and Side Benefits

As with many herbs and dietary supplements, there may be some unexpected effects. Unlike drugs, however, where the side effects are almost invariably negative, with vitamins, minerals, flavonoids, fatty acids, and other dietary supplements, there are often side benefits—unexpected effects that are beneficial. But this is not always the case, so if you have an unexpected negative reaction, you should stop taking any supplement and consult a doctor, preferably one knowledgeable about alternative and complementary medicine. You may only need to stop for a while, then start again, to learn that the negative reactions were unrelated to the supplement.

With saw palmetto, you may see other benefits for the urinary tract, or experience its historical usefulness in treating inflammation and respiratory symptoms, and its effectiveness as a mild sedative. Women have also taken it successfully for bladder and urinary tract health.

Saw Palmetto and Drugs

Saw palmetto, as we said, has no contraindications, and will not interfere with sleeping pills, anxiety medications, or other drugs. It may even help them work. One of the reasons older men have problems sleeping at night is that their enlarged prostate wakes them up frequently to urinate. For them, one of the benefits of taking saw palmetto is that it reduces this frequency, which in itself may lead to better sleep and reduce the need for sleeping pills.

If the medication is prescribed, it is not a good idea to stop taking it without first checking with your healthcare professional. Although medications are sometimes prescribed for more than one reason, sleeping pills are usually just for sleep, and if your sleeping does improve after taking saw palmetto, you might consider asking if you can reduce your medication. Doctors sometimes tell their patients that a pill is to help them sleep when it is really for something else and the doctor hopes it will also help sleep. For example, drugs that improve the function of your heart may also make it easier to sleep, so just be sure you know what you are taking, and why, before making any changes.

Taking Saw Palmetto without BPH

Research studies have not examined the question of whether saw palmetto is valuable as a preventive for prostate problems, but its action to reduce both DHT and estrogen hormone levels would seem to indicate its usefulness in prevention. And since you will not incur any risk by taking saw palmetto, it is probably a good idea to consider using it as preventive medicine. It doesn't cost very much, so that should not be an obstacle, and, again, there are no significant side effects.

The high numbers of men who end up with enlarged prostates argues in favor of doing everything possible to keep this from happening. This is especially true of men over age fifty, so starting to take saw palmetto in your forties is not unreasonable. As I said, I take small doses of saw palmetto regularly for prevention, and have done so for the past six years.

Proscar Risks Are Not Seen with Saw Palmetto

The drug finasteride (Proscar) has a history of possible problems for women who have any contact with its active ingredient, even if they are not taking the drug themselves. For example, a woman who gets pregnant while her partner is taking finasteride, or who comes into contact with the contents of the pills, may absorb enough of the drug herself to lead to birth defects in the urinary or genital organs of male fetuses. This may have given some people of childbearing age concern about this drug.

If a pregnant woman has contact with saw palmetto, however, there does not appear to be any risk to male offspring. Its beneficial effects on the hormones and enzymes do not seem to translate to side effects, even during pregnancy. There is no evidence of any side effects directly to the woman who contacts either finasteride or saw palmetto.

Saw Palmetto for Women

All the research I have seen on saw palmetto is for its value with prostate symptoms. However, there is also a history of its use in treating urinary tract disorders in both men and women. Saw palmetto has anti-inflammatory properties, which might help with painful urination and other symptoms of cystitis and urethritis (urinary tract infections). Since it is not an antibiotic, it would only help the symptoms, not eliminate a bacterial infection. (There are other herbs that might help with the infection: echinacea by enhancing immune function, or cranberry by preventing bacteria from attaching to the bladder lining.) For serious infections, of course, antibiotics may be necessary.

Saw palmetto may also help women with painful menstrual periods by relieving the spasms and cramps that often accompany their periods. Although these effects are not well documented, it could be that saw palmetto's beneficial effects on estrogen and testosterone hormones might contribute to these reported benefits.

OTHER STEPS TO A HEALTHY PROSTATE

As beneficial as it is, saw palmetto is only one of many dietary supplements that may help the prostate, and it is only part of a comprehensive program for prostate health. A complete program must also consider diet, lifestyle issues, and prevention of other prostate disorders besides benign enlargement, such as cancer.

Pygeum Africanum for Prostate

Pygeum africanum, an extract of an African tree bark, is another natural treatment for the prostate. It is a botanical supplement that helps relieve prostate symptoms and has research to prove it. In one study, although there were no changes in hormone levels in the blood of those who took pygeum, all of the evaluations showed improvement in the urinary symptoms and a reduction in the swelling of the prostate around the urethra. In another study done jointly in Austria, France, and Germany, the researchers found similar results, with highly significant improvement in BPH symptoms—the number of nighttime urinations, the residual urine volume, and the urine-flow rates all improved. And, as in the other studies, there were very few side effects, and these only minor.

In yet another study, with a placebo control, the researchers showed that, although many of the men improved with the placebo, there were significantly more that did well with the pygeum extract. The improvements were seen in the ease of starting urination, the frequency of nighttime urinations, and the sensation of incomplete emptying of the bladder.

Similar to other natural remedies for the prostate, all the pygeum studies indicate only a few minor side effects, although some experienced digestive upset. A comparison of saw palmetto and pygeum in one study showed that both were effective, but saw palmetto was somewhat better. The usual dose of Pygeum africanum is 25–50 mg of the standardized extract taken twice a day.

Pygeum Africanum
A botanical extract from an African tree bark that helps reduce the symptoms of BPH. It works well in combination with other herbs and nutrients.

Combining Saw Palmetto and Pygeum

In the natural treatment of prostate enlargement, it is common to combine supplements that complement each other because, unlike many medications, nutrition and dietary supplements work well together and the results are even enhanced when taken in combination. Because nutrients work together in all cells, it is a good idea to combine different treatments unless there is a known negative interaction. There are no negative interactions when you take saw palmetto and pygeum together. Conversely, in most medical treatments, doctors and their patients are looking for some sort of magic bullet that will, all by itself, cure a problem with few, minor side effects. Unfortunately though, with most drugs, this is far from the typical result, and, unlike supplements, combining drugs can lead to serious adverse reactions.

Although there are only a few studies where several natural treatments are combined, they have mostly shown that different supplements enhance the actions of the others. The health food stores have several combinations of herbs and nutrients that help the prostate, and if taken in combination, it may be possible that a lower dose of each of the combined supplements will help the prostate.

Other Herbs for the Prostate

At least one other herb has been helpful with prostate symptoms. Studies with extract of the stinging nettle plant (also called common nettle) have shown that it reduces prostate symptoms. Nettle may work by reducing the ability of DHT to bind to the sites where it is active, which results in less activity of this hormone, even though its amount remains unchanged.

In studies where it is combined with pygeum or saw palmetto, nettle extracts appear to enhance the action of each one. Although stinging nettles get their name from the stinging hairs on their stems and the leaves that cause a skin rash when you rub up against them, the extracts do not have any irritant effect. Nettle has been used as a food and a tea, and cooking eliminates its irritant properties. In fact, nettle extract has an anti-inflammatory effect, and among its other beneficial actions, it reduces allergy symptoms. The typical dose of nettle is 150–300 mg of standardized extract taken twice a day, but for allergies, a dose of 300 mg every three to four hours is sometimes recommended.

Other Natural Prostate Treatments

For many years, before saw palmetto or pygeum were commonly available as therapeutic supplements, nutritionally oriented doctors used other natural remedies for prostate enlargement with some success. One of the most widely used supplements for the prostate has historically been high doses of the trace mineral zinc. Zinc is important for many different body functions, such as antioxidant activity, immunity, the sense of taste and smell, wound healing, and managing the common cold. Some studies have shown that zinc lozenges can reduce the respiratory symptoms of a cold and cut short the duration of colds.

Zinc is particularly important for the normal functioning of the prostate. The prostate gland is very rich in zinc, with far more of it than any other organ in the body. It influences the hormones in the prostate, and, like saw palmetto, it can reduce the activity of the enzyme 5-alpha reductase, which promotes prostate enlargement. Small amounts of zinc are necessary for the activity of this enzyme, but higher levels appear to inhibit it.

It is also known that zinc levels are low in those who have either benign enlargement of the prostate or prostate cancer. In the past, physicians have recommended zinc in doses up to 150 mg per day for prostate enlargement. Recently, however, recommendations are to take 30–60 mg zinc *with* copper, to avoid an imbalance, as high doses of zinc can reduce the absorption of copper. Such high doses can also lower the good HDL cholesterol, which is not good. For this reason, I recommend the lower, but adequate, doses of zinc, along with the other effective treatments. In the context of a comprehensive program, this lower dose appears to be enough.

More Supplements for the Prostate

Numerous dietary supplements help the prostate, partly because they have either a direct effect on the prostate tissues, an indirect effect on hormone balance, or effects on other nutrients. For example, vitamin B$_6$, or pyridoxine, can help with the absorption of zinc, so the lower levels of zinc in the diet or in supplements may be more effective. Pyridoxine also helps to reduce the production of prolactin, a hormone produced in the pituitary gland, which stimulates milk production in lactating women. Prolactin also has an effect on the prostate because it promotes DHT production and, as a consequence, can stimulate the growth of prostate tissue. Reducing prolactin levels can help reduce the overgrowth of prostate tissue. Typical doses of pyridoxine are in the range of 50–200 mg per day. Very high doses, in excess of 500–2,000 mg, have been associated with peripheral neuropathy, a neurological disorder that includes loss of sensation, numbness, and tingling of the extremities, so it is wise to stay away from the highest doses.

Magnesium may be very important for symptoms of prostate enlargement, particularly the symptoms in the smooth muscles of the bladder, prostate tissue, and urethra. Magnesium helps to relax these involuntary muscles (those out of our conscious control). It is also important to take magnesium when you are taking extra vitamin B$_6$, because it helps to balance this nutrient. Typical doses of magnesium are from 300–1,000 mg daily. Magnesium aspartate, one of many forms found in any health food store, is one of the best-absorbed forms of this mineral. Magnesium is also very important for heart health and for the maintenance of normal blood pressure.

Similar to beta-carotene, lycopene is a red pigment in the carotenoid family of antioxidant nutrients that is found in pink grapefruit, tomatoes, and watermelon. High amounts of it in the diet or in supplements can protect the prostate from developing cancer, or can help in the treatment of prostate cancer if it does develop. Typical doses of a lycopene supplement range from 5–15 mg daily.

An herbal combination called PC-SPES has been shown to help reverse prostate cancer. It is a mixture that contains saw palmetto among a number of other less well-known herbs, and both research and my experience confirm that it is effective. Although it does have some side effects, such as breast enlargement and tenderness, it can clearly lower the PSA levels. When taking PC-SPES, I advise supervision by a nutritionally oriented practitioner. In 2001, some batches of PC-SPES were shown to contain hormones that were not on the label, and it has been removed from the market while further evaluations are done.

Amino Acids and Prostate Health

Amino acids are the building blocks of proteins. They get their name from a nitrogen-hydrogen combination called an amine, or amino group. There are eight essential amino acids, essential meaning the kind you must get in your diet because your body cannot manufacture them.

Amino Acids
The building blocks of proteins. They get their name from a nitrogen-hydrogen combination called an amine, or amino group.

Generally, people get enough of the amino acids they need from the protein they eat. Most Americans, in fact, get too much protein, especially animal protein, so they have an abundance of amino acids. The amino acids from the diet go into manufacturing the different proteins of the body, or they are burned for energy, and any excess is converted to fat.

Some amino acids are also used for other purposes, such as providing the base molecule for the manufacture of hormones or nerve transmitters that carry the nerve signal from one nerve in a chain to the next one. Serotonin, for example, is a nerve transmitter derived from the amino acid tryptophan, and the hormone for the thyroid is derived from tyrosine, another amino acid.

Several reports suggest the value of certain amino acids in the treatment of prostate enlargement. The amino acids alanine, glutamic acid, and glycine were shown to reduce prostate symptoms in 70 to 90 percent (depending on which symptom was being evaluated) of the subjects in a study.

When amino acids are used for treatment, you cannot depend on getting them from food sources because other the amino acids present in protein drown out the therapeutic ones. To get the therapeutic levels, you need to take supplements. The recommended daily amounts vary from 50–200 mg for alanine, 200–1,000 mg for glutamic acid, and 200–400 mg for glycine.

Fats and the Prostate

Depending on the types, and the balance in your diet and supplements, fats and oils can play a very important role in either maintaining prostate health or causing prostate problems. It is well known that too much fat or the wrong kind of fat in the diet is hazardous to your health in many ways. It is especially a problem when they are animal fats, or if the oils are hydrogenated (such as in margarine and shortening), or heavily processed (such as commercial vegetable oils).

Heating any oils during cooking increases the damage by oxidizing them and creating dangerous byproducts. Although polyunsaturated oils were heavily promoted for a time, they are exactly the ones that have the greatest likelihood of being oxidized by heat and light, and they increase the risk of cancer in many organs. When consuming any polyunsaturated oils, it is important to choose those that are minimally processed and not heated (look for labels that say cold-pressed). It is also important to take extra antioxidant nutrients, such as vitamins E and C, when you consume these oils.

Most people have too much fat in their diets, but not enough of the essential fatty acids (those that are required in the diet). Essential fatty acids influence hormone activity, immunity, inflammation, platelets, and smooth muscle action. In the right amounts, they are specifically valuable for prostate health. According to studies, men with BPH are deficient in essential fatty acids, and supplementing with them can help. I often recommend a combination of unrefined flaxseed oil for the omega-3 oils (one of the two essential fatty acids), and evening primrose oil or borage oil for gamma-linolenic acid (GLA), the source for the omega-6 oils (the other essential fatty acid).

The dose of flaxseed oil is one to two tablespoons per day, and the dose of GLA is 240 mg (the equivalent of one borage oil capsule, or six evening primrose oil capsules). Certain fish, such as salmon and sardines, also contain an omega-3 oil called EPA. This oil is also available as a supplement in capsules or from cod liver oil. I recommend wild fish rather than farmed fish as much as possible, as the essential fatty acid composition is likely to be better. Alaskan salmon is always wild, as Alaska does not permit fish farming.

Essential Fatty Acids
Beneficial dietary oils omega-3 and omega-6, called essential because they are required in the diet.

Dietary Habits and Prostate Health

As with almost every disease, lifestyle choices play a role in the prevention and treatment of prostate disorders. This is especially true for preventing prostate cancer, but may also play an important role in prostate enlargement.

Try to choose a diet rich in vegetables, fresh fruits, whole grains, seeds, nuts, and beans. The more colorful the vegetable or fruit, the more likely it is to contain healthful nutrients. Eating meat has been shown to dramatically increase your risk of getting prostate cancer, and a vegetarian diet is healthier in many ways than one that includes meat. Also, avoid adding much oil of any kind to the diet. Although olive oil may not cause a problem, other oils and fats may be a serious risk, and it is no accident that, in places where the fat intake is low, there is also a low incidence of prostate cancer. (Black Africans who are native have a low incidence of prostate cancer and a low-fat diet, while African-Americans have a high incidence of prostate cancer and a high fat intake.) The foods I have recommended here provide a diet that is high in fiber, low in fat, and rich in phytonutrients and flavonoids, all of which are protective.

Read ingredient labels carefully and avoid foods that contain added sugar and artificial or synthetic additives, such as colors, flavorings, preservatives, and sweeteners. These do nothing to enhance health, and are usually present only in heavily processed foods that you don't need in your diet anyway.

Avoid caffeine and alcohol as much as possible. Caffeine has been associated with fibrocystic breast disease, and since the breast contains glandular and fibrous tissue like the prostate, it is possible that caffeine may also cause problems for the prostate. It is also a diuretic, and increases the frequency of urination, which is already a problem for men with BPH. Alcohol affects the hormones that play a role in prostate enlargement, and it is best to keep alcohol intake low. Liver damage from excess alcohol consumption leads to increases in estrogen levels, because the liver is the organ that breaks down these hormones, and if it is damaged, it cannot do its job properly.

Specific Foods to Prevent Prostate Cancer

Several specific foods are even more beneficial than the general guidelines above. Include some soybean products in your diet, such as soymilk or tofu. Natural hormonelike isoflavone substances in soy (called phytoestrogens) help to prevent cancer of the prostate and many other organs. If you think you don't like tofu, you may be surprised to learn that it is commonly used in fried rice dishes in Chinese restaurants where it is disguised by the other ingredients. Most people find they do like it if it is prepared correctly. Other forms of soy products are tempeh, a fermented soybean cake common in Indonesia, and soy protein powders that can be added to fruit smoothies, other blender drinks, or even vegetable stews. However, avoid the highly processed soy-derived products such as texturized vegetable protein (TVP) and the many imitation foods made from it, including some vegetable broths and imitation chicken and meat.

Whole grains have also been shown to decrease cancer risks. In population studies, those who have the highest intake of whole grains have a lower incidence of cancer for almost every cancer studied, including prostate. This means it is important to include whole grains in the diet, such as barley, brown rice, corn, millet, oatmeal, rye, whole wheat, and several others. On the other hand, refined grains, such as white flour products, are associated with increasing risks of disease, including cancer and heart disease, so it is best to avoid them altogether.

Nutrients That Help the Prostate

As previously mentioned, lycopene is in the carotene family of vitamins (beta-carotene is the best-known carotenoid, being the orange color found in carrots, but there are many other nutritious carotenoids). Lycopene is found in pink grapefruit, tomatoes, and watermelon, and it is also available as a supplement. Research shows that tomatoes can reduce the risk of prostate cancer, probably because of the lycopene they contain. We know that men whose diets are high in lycopene have a lower chance of getting prostate cancer than men with lower levels of lycopene intake. Any tomato product is beneficial, from fresh tomatoes, to tomato sauce, to tomato juice, with the highest amounts of lycopene found in tomatoes that have been concentrated by cooking. You can also take 5–15 mg lycopene supplements to make sure you get enough.

Garlic contains a number of substances that are protective. Whether taken as a food or a supplement, it is associated with a lower chance of getting prostate cancer. Garlic is widely available in a deodorized supplement for those who don't like garlic, or don't wish to smell of it every day. (I personally like it a lot, I eat it often, and it is a common ingredient in many of the ethnic foods I enjoy.) Supplements of deodorized garlic contain about 500 mg of concentrated extract. You might take two to four of these a day if you are not eating garlic regularly.

Selenium is a trace mineral that protects against many cancers. It works with vitamins C and E as a free radical scavenger. Selenium is low in the diets of most people, mainly because of selenium-depleted soil, but it is readily available as an inexpensive supplement. Typical supplemental doses range from 100-400 mcg (micrograms) a day (a microgram is one thousandth of a milligram).

Lifestyle Habits and Prostate Health

As with almost any health issue, it is important to get regular exercise, such as bicycling, jogging, skating, skiing, walking, or using exercising machines—ski machines, stair machines, and treadmills are examples. Exercise stimulates our immunity and eliminates toxins. There are specific exercises that help urinary control. Known as Kegel exercises, they consist of contracting the muscles around the rectal area as though you are trying to stop urination or a bowel movement, and doing them many times a day may help in bladder control.

Regular exercise reduces prostate symptoms. Try to do at least thirty minutes of exercise most days. When people ask me if they have to exercise every day, I ask them, "How often does a gorilla exercise?" The answer, of course, is every time they want to eat or play, which is more than once a day. This may be too much to fit into your schedule (gorillas don't have to sit at a desk and work), but there is consensus that exercising at least four to six times a week is beneficial. It has even been associated with a decreased risk of cancer and heart disease. (And, as another peripheral benefit, recent findings suggest that exercise contributes to weight loss more than any diet.)

If you have not been doing exercise regularly, start with just ten or fifteen minutes of walking and increase your time by a few minutes a week. It is easy to determine how fast to go, because you should not get out of breath during the exercise, but you should work up a sweat by the time you get to thirty minutes. You don't need a formal exercise program if you keep very active by gardening, mowing the lawn, walking or bicycling on your errands, and taking stairs instead of elevators when possible. However, most people tend to miss out on exercise unless they make specific exercise a part of their routines.

Other Lifestyle Habits in Prostate Health

The placebo effect demonstrates that our emotional state, thought processes, and expectations are components of most illnesses. They lead to both the feeling of improvement and an actual measurable improvement, but if they can influence illness for the better, they can also be involved in causing, or worsening, symptoms. Stress is particularly damaging. It increases general health risks in many ways, including its role in increasing the output of the adrenal hormones, the metabolism, and the damaging oxidation byproducts. Practicing a stress-reduction technique can be very helpful in reducing cancer risks, and with health in general.

Five or six times a day, you should try to do some breathing exercises, stretching, or yoga, or simply close your eyes and imagine your favorite place for about three or four minutes. You might consider reading about meditation, or getting some help learning how to do it. Whatever relaxation method works for you is fine.

Finally, I can't say enough about the dangers of tobacco smoke, even the secondhand smoke that most of us find hard to avoid. It is probably one of the most dangerous substances we humans expose ourselves to voluntarily. It leads to many cancers, and puts an enormous burden on our normal protective mechanisms. Smoking also appears to increase the risk of developing BPH. Avoid it!

SEXUAL FUNCTION AND MEN'S HEALTH

Healthy sexual functioning is a pleasure that can be enjoyed until very late in life. However, many unhealthy habits and practices can adversely influence the ability to maintain this function. Although many men equate the prostate with their sexual functioning, an enlarged prostate (BPH) doesn't need to affect your sexual function at all. Sexual dysfunction, or erectile dysfunction (a better term than impotence), is a significant issue for men as they age, but it is not necessarily related to problems with the prostate. Good nutrition, hormonal balance, physical fitness, and stress can all contribute to your normal sexual functioning, and they are all in your control.

BPH and Sex Drive

Benign prostatic hyperplasia does not affect your libido (sex drive), your ability to have an erection, or your ability to have normal orgasms and ejaculations. If you are taking saw palmetto for your enlarged prostate symptoms, it not only has no harmful side effects in relation to sexual functioning, it has even been used to enhance libido and potency.

If you have an infection or an inflammation of the prostate (prostatitis) that leads to painful or uncomfortable urination, it may temporarily decrease your desire or sexual function. This should clear up after proper treatment of the infection. While being treated, it is a good idea to take dietary supplements that may help reduce the inflammation and speed your recovery from the infection.

Early prostate cancer is also not a problem, but in the later stages, or after treatment with surgery, radiation, or drugs, there can sometimes be interference with sexual functioning. Depending on the treatment, however, this is often not a permanent problem. Even if you have surgery to remove your prostate, it is still possible to have an active sex life. Although this is not always the case, you should be aware that the prostate is not essential to the desire or the ability to have sex.

Remember that prostate enlargement is extremely widespread, and it should not interfere with your sexual pleasure. There are many natural treatments available to help you avoid the side effects of drugs and surgery, and they all can help you feel good about yourself, in spite of having an enlarged prostate, or even prostate cancer. Sexual activity, in fact, is probably helpful in maintaining the health of the prostate.

Lifestyle and Sexual Functioning

A number of lifestyle choices play a role in healthy sexuality. Alcohol consumption, lack of exercise, obesity, and poor nutrition in general can decrease both your libido and your sexual functioning. The diet I recommended earlier for the healthy prostate is the same diet I recommend here for optimum sexual functioning: one that is high in vegetables, fruits, whole grains, beans, seeds, nuts, fish, and organic eggs. Losing weight (and 75 percent of Americans are overweight) requires you to avoid fatty or fried foods, hydrogenated oils, processed foods containing artificial ingredients, sugar, and white flour, as well as overeating any foods. These choices are also good for your overall health.

Regular consumption of alcohol, beyond a small amount, can lead to a deterioration in your sexual function, probably due in part to its effects on your hormones and your liver. Too much alcohol at any one time can have an immediate negative effect on the ability to achieve and maintain an erection. The evidence that red wine may be good for your heart is still controversial (heart disease is still the leading cause of death in France), and, so far, there is no reliable evidence that a healthy non-drinker in middle age should take up drinking to improve health.

Many studies have shown that exercise helps your health. You don't have to be a competitive athlete to benefit, and you don't have to exhaust yourself to be healthy. A simple plan of regular, repetitive motion, such as bicycling, jogging, rollerblading, skiing, swimming, using exercise machines, or just plain walking, is beneficial. If you do twenty to forty minutes of repetitive-motion exercise four to five times a week, you will be in shape in no time. You can exercise without getting out of breath, but do try to work up a sweat. This simple guideline should keep you at aerobic levels of exercise. If there is no exercise you love, get an exercise machine and work out while watching the news or reading a magazine.

Exercise will give you more energy, improve your digestion and elimination, your psychological well-being, and your sleep. If you can add some muscle-building exercise, such as elastic resistance bands or light weights, it would further improve your health. Increasing your muscle mass improves your insulin regulation and your sugar metabolism and, by burning calories, your ability to control your weight. Doing this for fifteen to twenty minutes three times a week would be a good start.

Health Conditions and Sexuality

If you have hardening of the arteries (atherosclerosis), and you have problems with erectile dysfunction, this could be due to poor circulation through the arteries to the penis. With the standard American diet (SAD), plaque in the arteries starts in the teen years, and without changing your diet, this will build up over the years, leading to a closure of your arteries, and contributing to the problem. It also leads to heart disease, another contributor to sexual dysfunction.

Diabetes, increasingly prevalent now, leads to two problems that play a role in sexual functioning: it increases hard-

ening of the arteries, and it causes diabetic peripheral neuropathy, which is a decreased ability of the long nerves to carry impulses. This problem leads to numbness and tingling, and a loss of sensitivity in the nerves that is essential to normal erections.

Other health conditions, such as chronic back pain, a low thyroid, neurological diseases, or psychiatric disorders, can also lead to sexual dysfunction. It is essential that you get a complete medical evaluation is to find out whether atherosclerosis, diabetes, or any of these conditions are part of the problem.

Supplements Help Sexual Function

While many supplements can contribute to general health, and the management of back pain, diabetes, heart disease, neuropathy, and psychiatric disorders, some specific supplements may be helpful with erectile dysfunction.

Normal erections require the presence of nitric oxide, a substance made by the cells lining the arteries that is essential for the muscles of the blood vessels to relax and open up the blood flow. In fact, nitric oxide was called the endothelial-derived relaxing factor before it was chemically identified. This blood flow is necessary for engorgement of the penile erectile tissue. The cells make nitric oxide from the amino acid L-arginine, and taking supplements of L-arginine has been helpful with erectile dysfunction. The typical dose of L-arginine is 2,000–8,000 mg at one time, shortly before sexual activity. It may also help to take it regularly, in a dose of 1,000–2,000 mg daily. L-arginine should be balanced with some extra L-lysine, as some experts believe that an excess of arginine makes a person more prone to the development of herpes viruses.

Another supplement that helps with blood flow through the small blood vessels is ginkgo biloba. Ginkgo extract contains protective antioxidant flavonoids that also help circulation by inhibiting the platelet activity that can slow circulation. It also contains substances called terpenes that increase circulation and protect the nervous system. These benefits of ginkgo for the nervous tissue and circulation may make it beneficial for erectile dysfunction. The usual dose is 120–240 mg per day of the standardized extract containing 24 percent flavones and 6 percent terpene compounds.

The herb yohimbe has been successfully used in the treatment of erectile dysfunction. Its active component is yohimbine, an indole alkaloid that dilates blood vessels. Since yohimbe does have potential side effects, such as anxiety, increased blood pressure, and a rapid heart rate, it is a good idea to consult with a nutritionally oriented practitioner before taking this herb. And, if you have kidney or liver disease, you should avoid taking yohimbe. The typical dose is 15–30 mg of the standardized extract.

Taking chromium supplements in relatively high doses

enhances the action of insulin, and can help with sugar control in diabetes. Research shows that those with type II diabetes who take 1,000 mcg of chromium per day can reduce their blood sugars to normal 50 percent of the time, and in 90 percent of the cases, they can help people come off their medications. Chromium also helps control lipids in the blood.

Another supplement that helps people with diabetes is alpha-lipoic acid. This is an antioxidant that works in both the water- and lipid-based tissues, and it is particularly good for the nerves and the brain. Doses from 100–300 mg daily can help control blood sugars and 1,000 mg daily is helpful for peripheral neuropathy.

HEART DISEASE AND MEN'S HEALTH

Although heart disease due to atherosclerosis (hardening of the arteries) is the leading cause of death for both men and women, it is often thought of as a men's disease. Perhaps this is because, prior to menopause, it is much less common in women. (When all age groups are tested, heart disease is the leading killer of women.) In developed countries, heart disease starts in youth, largely because of diet, and later, because of the diet combined with the sedentary lifestyle that most people lead. Heart disease is almost always the result of lifestyle choices that can be changed with a little education, effort, and motivation.

Atherosclerotic Heart Disease and Lifestyle

Atherosclerotic (also called arteriosclerotic) diseases result from a buildup of plaque (fatty, fibrous, calcified deposits) in the arterial wall, which reduces and eventually blocks the blood flow to the vital organs. The damage to the arteries results from free radical injury and inflammation, both of which can be related to lifestyle choices. Common symptoms of heart disease include chest tightness or pain, which may be felt in the left arm, the back, or the jaw, shortness of breath, and fatigue. The chest symptoms may also be perceived as a sensation of pressure, like an elephant sitting on your chest, as heartburn, or simply as indigestion. Some of the recent tests to predict the risks of heart disease are related to inflammation.

Atherosclerosis
The gradual buildup of plaque in the arterial wall, which reduces, and eventually blocks, the flow of blood to the vital organs.

The lifestyle modifications that are the most important for helping to prevent and treat heart disease are dietary changes and exercise, with stress management and dietary supplements also playing vital roles in reducing the problem. Heart disease is not simply genetic. When we see that American teenagers between the ages of fifteen and nine-

teen already have plaque in their arteries, we cannot blame it on genetics. It is almost certainly related to their diets and their lack of exercise. In the Korean War, doctors examined young American soldiers who died of trauma, and they already had plaque in their arteries, while the young Koreans did not. But when Koreans move to the United States and eat the Western diet, they too develop the same arterial diseases. As fast foods and heavily processed fatty and sugary foods spread around the world, we see in their wake preventable increases in diabetes, heart disease, hypertension, obesity, and other degenerative diseases.

Diet Changes for Better Health

This diet is the same one I recommended above for the prostate and for sexual function. Cut down on artificial flavors, colors, preservatives, and sweeteners, processed foods, white flour, and sugar, all of which are junk, not food. Reduce animal products in the diet, except for fish, which is beneficial because of the essential fatty acids they contain. Meat, chicken, and dairy products, especially fatty ones, contribute to increased mortality from heart disease and cancer. In fact, mortality from all diseases is lower in vegetarians than non-vegetarians. Eat more fresh vegetables, fruits, whole grains, beans, seeds, and nuts. Numerous scientific studies come to this same conclusion, and they come from the evaluation of many different populations all over the world.

There are any number of fad diets that claim to be helpful in losing weight. They may lead to weight loss because they reduce caloric intake, but they are not healthful diets. The so-called value of the high-protein and high-fat diets is not supported by the medical literature. Just the opposite, in fact, because they are associated with more arthritis, cancer, diabetes, gallstones, gout, heart disease, and osteoporosis. These diets have little fiber, an important dietary component, and they are low in protective phytochemicals and bioflavonoids (healthful plant pigments).

If you eat dairy products, choose low-fat, organic sources, and try to eat only organic eggs, preferably those from chickens fed omega-3 oils, if these are available. Although I used to recommend mainly salmon, the farming of fish is now widespread, and not many fish farms use natural methods. As a result, the good essential fatty acid composition of the fish is altered. The growth hormone that is used to double the growth rate of the fish is untested for its health effects, and both infections and the use of antibiotics in fish farming are increasing. In order to avoid these problems, I now suggest sardines (water packed) as the preferred source, or Alaskan salmon (Alaska does not permit fish farming). You don't need much animal product in the diet, but I believe it is beneficial to have some, and small amounts of fish, low-fat organic yogurt, or organic eggs are the best sources.

Exercise for the Heart

Please review the exercise program described above. It is critically important for both prevention and treatment of heart disease. Of course, if you already have heart disease, you must pay attention to the intensity of your exercise, so you don't develop symptoms, such as chest pain or tightness, lightheadedness, palpitations, or shortness of breath.

Supplements for Preventing Heart Disease

I always recommend starting with a high-potency, multivitamin/mineral combination. This should give you the B-complex (50–100 mg), some vitamins C and E, calcium and magnesium (500 mg each), and trace minerals. However, no multivitamin preparation has everything you need in adequate doses, so you do need to take some extra supplements for greater protection.

For example, take extra vitamins C and E. They act as potent antioxidants, protecting the blood vessels from free-radical damage. These vitamins also help to lower cholesterol while raising the good HDL cholesterol. I usually recommend about 4,000 mg of vitamin C and 400 IU of vitamin E. If your multiple has this amount of E, then it may be enough until you are over age forty, when you might want to take an extra 400–800 IU. I advise using only the natural d-alpha tocopherol (as opposed to dl-alpha), plus the mixed tocopherols (beta, gamma, and delta, and especially the gamma, which is being increasingly studied for its benefits).

Selenium is a trace mineral that is associated with less heart disease (and less cancer). Along with other antioxidants, it works as a component of the enzyme glutathione peroxidase, which boosts the activity of vitamin E. Usually 200–400 mcg per day is a good dose. The same daily 200–400 mcg dose of chromium contributes to preventing heart disease because chromium helps control blood sugar (diabetes is a risk factor for heart disease), and it promotes normal blood fat and cholesterol. Folic acid and vitamin B_{12} help to lower homocysteine levels, and homocysteine, an amino acid in the blood, has been found to damage arteries and lead to increased atherosclerosis. While many supplements are useful in preventing heart disease, some of them are particularly important for treatment if you already have heart disease.

Coenzyme Q_{10} and Heart Disease

Coenzyme Q_{10} (CoQ_{10}) is essential for the production of energy in the membranes of the tiny mitochondria engines in every cell. It is needed for the conversion of fatty acids to the energy molecule called ATP. CoQ_{10} is especially abundant in heart muscle, and it is an excellent antioxidant. Some studies have found it to be about four times more potent than vitamin E. CoQ_{10} supplements can help alleviate angina, arrhythmias, congestive heart failure, high

blood pressure, and shortness of breath. CoQ_{10} also increases exercise tolerance. Side benefits of taking CoQ_{10} are antioxidant protection from the free-radical damage associated with aging, improved immunity, and increased energy levels in general.

Antioxidants
Protective substances that prevent damage to cells, membranes, molecules, and tissues from excessive exposure to hazardous molecules called free radicals.

Although CoQ_{10} is not really a vitamin because your body makes it, the amount your body makes declines with age and illness. The typical dose for treatment of heart disease is 100–400 mg daily, depending on the severity of the problem. For prevention, I think it is a good idea to take 50–100 mg a day, especially if you are over age forty, if you have any other illness, or if you have a family history of heart disease.

L-Carnitine and Heart Disease

Another supplement that helps the heart is L-carnitine. This derivative of amino acids is essential for transporting fatty acids across the membranes of the mitochondria where they are used for energy production (because of this, it works well with CoQ_{10}, and they are commonly taken together). When there is pain due to a lack of oxygen in the heart muscle (angina), the level of L-carnitine drops dramatically, and the heart muscle switches to glucose metabolism instead of fat. As a result, more lactic acid is produced, and this makes the pain worse. If there is enough L-carnitine available in advance, the pain is lessened, and the likelihood of damage to the heart is reduced. Although you normally produce L-carnitine, as with some other essential substances, the production declines with age. Supplements of L-carnitine are typically in the range of 500–1,000 mg twice a day. Some athletes take even more to enhance their stamina.

Botanical Supplements for the Heart

Garlic has been used for millennia, not only as a culinary delight, but also as a therapeutic dietary supplement. It helps the heart in many ways. It reduces your blood pressure, which is a risk factor for the development of heart disease. Garlic supplements also reduce the adhesiveness (stickiness) of platelets, reducing the possibility of excessive clotting inside the blood vessels.

Garlic reduces total cholesterol levels while increasing the good HDL cholesterol, so it helps in both prevention and treatment. As a free radical scavenger, garlic helps prevent the oxidative reactions that promote atherosclerosis. It appears to protect the enzymes in the cells lining the arteries. These are the cells that produce nitric oxide, the molecule essential for relaxation of the blood vessels, and garlic appears to promote the production of this vital substance. Additionally, garlic acts as an antibiotic and antiviral substance, it can enhance immunity, and it can reduce the incidence of some cancers, all without side effects.

I recommend eating garlic as part of the diet, and supplementing for treatment. The usual dose of garlic is 500–1,500 mg twice a day. If you use deodorized garlic, you can take your garlic every day without fear of being ostracized socially.

Hawthorn berry is a valuable herb that has been used for centuries for the heart. Its active components include several flavonoid pigments, and it improves the strength of the heart muscle, and relaxes the blood vessels, allowing for improved blood flow. Hawthorn berry supplements can improve exercise capacity, and can mildly reduce elevated blood pressure in people with congestive heart failure. The usual dose of standardized hawthorn extract is 250–500 mg twice a day.

I mentioned ginkgo biloba earlier for the circulation benefits it provides. Those same effects make it useful in heart disease, and it is commonly taken in the same doses, 60–120 mg of standardized extract, twice a day.

Amino Acids for Heart Disease

L-taurine, an amino acid, helps to increase the strength of the heart muscle and reduces the overactivity of the fibers that conduct the impulse for the heartbeat. For people with congestive heart failure, L-taurine supplements are safe and effective additions to their treatment, and they may also reduce arrhythmias. In animal studies, taurine has been shown to be helpful in controlling blood pressure. The typical dose is 500–1,000 mg twice a day.

Earlier I mentioned L-arginine as a precursor to nitric oxide, the blood-vessel relaxant. For this same reason, it is helpful in heart disease. In doses of 1,000–6,000 mg daily, it improves angina, heart failure, hypertension, and immune function, as well as sexual function.

L-lysine reduces the tendency of blood-lipid components to stick to artery walls and release deposits of damaging lipoprotein(a). The usual dose is about 1,500 mg daily for treatment.

Relaxation and the Heart

Putting together a complete program for prevention or treatment must include more than diet, exercise, and supplements. Stress management is also an important therapy for almost any health condition, including cancer, heart disease, and sexual functioning. I always recommend some form of relaxation for all my heart patients, and there are many that work well. I would also recommend that you practice breathing exercises, laughter, various forms of meditation, and visualization to reduce your stress responses. Norman Cousins, the author of *Anatomy of an Illness*, also wrote *The Healing Heart* about his recovery from a serious heart attack, using laughter and other health-

ful practices, and emphasizing the powerful role that our minds play in healing.

I also recommend that you look into chelation therapy for heart disease. This is a very safe intravenous treatment with a synthetic amino acid that binds with calcium and heavy metals, such as lead, and removes them from the body. Chelation therapy has been done since the 1950s, but it remains controversial. In spite of this, the number of doctors who are doing chelation is increasing. Doctors in the American College for Advancement in Medicine usually administer this therapy, and you can find a doctor in your area by looking at their website, www.acam.org.

CONCLUSION

Prostate health is only one of the issues that men face as they age, and most of them can be influenced by diet and lifestyle. Saw palmetto is a part of a comprehensive program to take care of your prostate. Similar health programs can prevent and treat sexual dysfunction and heart disease, the leading cause of death in the United States and other Western countries, and they not only help with the prostate, sexual functioning, and heart disease, but also with almost any health problem, in the process giving you some measure of control over your own care.

Your own practitioner may be very willing to participate with you in this kind of care, because many of them are becoming aware of their patients' interest in more natural remedies, and increasing numbers of them are beginning to get trained in complementary and alternative medicine. If your doctor is unwilling to consider using saw palmetto or other dietary supplements, perhaps you should give him or her a copy of this book, or go to another practitioner who is more versed in alternative/complementary methods.

No matter what your health problems, consider all the options and make informed decisions about the kind of care that you want. If you can't find a doctor who will work with you in this form of treatment, you can call the American College for Advancement in Medicine (ACAM) at 1-800-532-3688 to locate a doctor in your area who is open to innovative treatments. You can also look them up online at www.acam.org.

Using natural remedies as part of your comprehensive healthcare program for both treatment and prevention is a positive step in the changing healthcare picture. As more conventional doctors become aware of these treatments and add them to their medical skills, you will find it easier to get the medical help you want. Today, the American population is doing this more than ever before, and you would do well to join them. It will help you, your family, and anyone who learns from your example.

PART ELEVEN

NUTRITION FOR WOMEN'S HEALTH

LAUREL VUKOVIC, MSW

Women are different from men in more ways than meet the eye. The most fundamental difference can probably be summed up in one word: hormones. The same hormones that give a woman her feminine characteristics and enable her to create a child are also the cause of many of the health problems that are unique to women.

From the time a young girl's body begins to prepare for menstruation, through pregnancy, menopause, and the years beyond, a woman's body and emotions are influenced by her shifting hormones. Women have special needs to consider, needs that have not always been taken into account by conventional medicine and researchers. It's only in recent years that researchers have started realizing that, although men and women share some physiological traits, women are different, and need to be treated as such.

For example, although drinking alcohol may have some positive health benefits, such as lowering cholesterol levels, it also appears to increase a woman's risk of breast cancer. And while, for many years, women were thought to be virtually exempt from cardiovascular disease, it's now clear that women, after menopause, have an equal, and possibly greater, risk of heart disease than men.

There is still a great deal to learn about women's health, and researchers are attempting at this moment to find the keys to PMS, menopause, osteoporosis, breast cancer, and heart disease. Information revealing the latest findings about women's health appears almost daily in newspapers and magazines, and much of it can be confusing and even contradictory.

What we do know for certain is that diet and lifestyle play a central role in health. It's never too early to begin to eat well, exercise, and adopt healthful habits that will help prevent degenerative diseases such as cancer, heart disease, and osteoporosis. In fact, research shows that risk factors for these diseases begin as early as the teen years, because lifestyle habits have a cumulative effect. However, no matter what your current age or level of health, it's never too late to upgrade your diet and lifestyle to enhance your well-being.

By reading this part of this book, you're taking a significant step toward improving your health and well-being. Perhaps you're suffering from one of the common ailments that affect women, such as menstrual cramps or PMS. If you're pregnant, you might be looking for information about how you can best care for yourself and your baby. Or you may be entering menopause, and wondering how you can smoothly navigate this significant life transition.

In the pages ahead, you'll discover clear and concise information that will help you to be as healthy as possible at every stage of life. You'll find specific recommendations for common problems associated with menstruation, suggestions for a healthy pregnancy, and guidance for the menopausal years. You'll also find comprehensive information about how you can avoid cancer, heart disease, and osteoporosis. At the end of this part is a section that will help you choose, and get the most out of, dietary supplements.

Read through this part from start to finish if you want an overall guide to health care throughout a woman's life. If you have a particular health concern, turn right to that section. By following the suggestions you find in these pages, you can begin today to improve your health.

MENSTRUATION AND MENSTRUAL DIFFICULTIES

The onset of menstruation is a significant physiological and emotional event in a young girl's life, and will likely be a monthly occurrence for approximately forty years. The subtle but powerful hormonal shifts that regulate the menstrual cycle can cause a variety of problems, ranging from cramps to endometriosis. In this section, you'll learn the most important factors for supporting healthy reproductive function, and you'll discover natural remedies for relieving common problems associated with menstruation.

The Basics of Menstruation

In the United States, most girls generally begin menstruating at about the age of twelve. But it's also perfectly normal if a girl begins to menstruate as early as age ten, or as late as age seventeen. The onset of menstruation seems to be dependent upon a girl having a sufficient amount of body fat, which is related to estrogen production. Girls who exercise regularly and strenuously, such as athletes or dancers, may begin menstruating later, as may those who diet excessively.

Each month, beginning at puberty, a woman's body prepares for possible pregnancy. The female reproductive organs consist of the ovaries, fallopian tubes, and uterus. The fallopian tubes connect the ovaries to the uterus, and are the channel through which eggs stored in the ovaries travel to the uterus. At birth, an infant girl's ovaries hold the thousands of eggs that will be released during her fertile years.

In the first phase of the menstrual cycle, the endometrium, or lining of the uterus, builds up layers of extra blood and tissue. Midway through the cycle, a ripened egg is released from an ovary. The egg passes through the fallopian tube, and if it is fertilized by sperm, the egg attaches to the wall of the thickened uterus, where it begins the process of developing into a baby. Most of the time, however, the egg is not fertilized and it simply dissolves. The extra blood and tissue built up by the uterus is shed and leaves the body through the vagina. This process continues each month until pregnancy occurs, or until ovulation ceases at menopause.

> **Endometrium**
> The lining of the uterus, which builds up extra layers of tissue in the first phase of the menstrual cycle.

The average menstrual cycle is generally about twenty-eight days, but some women menstruate every twenty-one days, and some menstruate every forty-five days. The average menstrual period lasts from three to five days, but anywhere from two to seven days is also considered normal. The amount of bleeding during menstruation varies between women, too, and is the result of how much blood and tissue have been built up in the uterus. The menstrual cycle is controlled by the hormonal interplay of the hypothalamus, the pituitary gland, and the ovaries, which produce the primary female hormones, estrogen and progesterone. Estrogen governs the first half of the menstrual cycle; following ovulation, estrogen levels subside and progesterone levels increase.

A woman's menstrual cycle is governed by this intricate dance of hormones, and hormonal production is significantly affected by diet, emotions, and lifestyle. Let's look at some of the most common problems related to the menstrual cycle.

Menstrual Cramps

More than half of all women experience menstrual cramps (medically known as dysmenorrhea) to some degree. Cramping generally occurs in the pelvic area, but it's also common for the pain to radiate into the low back and down into the legs. For some women, cramps merely cause mild discomfort, but for others, menstrual cramps can be painfully severe and incapacitating. Severe menstrual cramps often cause associated symptoms, such as diarrhea, low-back pain, and nausea.

The Cause of Cramps

Although menstrual cramps can be caused by a medical problem, such as endometriosis, a pelvic infection, or uterine fibroids, in the vast majority of cases, cramps are not the result of any physiological disorder. Cramps are often simply the result of the uterus working to expel menstrual blood and tissue. Hormonelike substances called series-2 prostaglandins can also trigger cramps. These inflammatory substances constrict blood vessels, inhibiting the flow of blood to the uterus and causing cramping. Blood-calcium levels also usually fall just prior to menstruation, and low levels of calcium can contribute to cramps, as can hypothyroidism (an underactive thyroid).

> **Dysmenorrhea**
> The medical term for menstrual cramps, which most commonly occur in the pelvic area and affect more than half of all women.

While series-2 prostaglandins are prime troublemakers in menstrual cramps, another type—called series-1 prostaglandins—has beneficial pain-relieving and hormone-balancing benefits.

Series-1 prostaglandins are made from linolenic acid (omega-3 fatty acids) and series-2 prostaglandins are derived from linoleic acid (omega-6 fatty acids). What you eat has a direct effect on which type of prostaglandins are dominant in your body. Omega-3 fatty acids are found in cold-water fish, such as mackerel, salmon, and sardines, and in flaxseeds and walnuts. Omega-6 fatty acids are found in grains, meats, seeds, and vegetable oils. Because omega-6 fatty acids are so abundant in the typical diet and omega-3 fatty acids are so scarce, most women get far more linoleic acid than linolenic acid. To add to the problem, hydrogenated oils and the foods containing them (such as most chips, cookies, crackers, and processed foods) also stimulate the production of inflammatory series-2 prostaglandins. It's easy to understand how an excess of series-2 prostaglandins can arise.

> **Prostaglandins**
> Hormonelike substances. Some have beneficial pain-relieving effects, others have inflammatory properties that can trigger cramps.

Strategies for Easing Cramps

To increase the levels of series-1 prostaglandins, eat foods that are good sources of omega-3 fatty acids frequently. Try to eat at least two servings of cold-water fish per week, as well as a small handful of raw walnuts, or a tablespoon of freshly ground flaxseed several times a week. You might also consider supplementing your diet with one tablespoon of cold-pressed flaxseed oil daily. Taking supplements of gamma-linolenic acid (GLA), another essential fatty acid, can also help to balance prostaglandin production. GLA is found in black currant oil, borage oil, and evening primrose oil. Take enough capsules to equal 240 mg of GLA daily.

Eating foods rich in calcium and magnesium is another dietary strategy for helping to prevent menstrual cramps. Both of these essential minerals have a natural relaxing effect on the body. Dark leafy greens, legumes, nuts, and seeds are good sources of both calcium and magnesium. Taking a daily supplement of 1,000 mg of calcium and 400 mg of magnesium will boost your intake into an optimal range.

Regular exercise—at least thirty minutes five times a week—will also help to relieve menstrual cramps. Both aerobic exercise, such as brisk walking, and stretching exercises, such as yoga, increase circulation to the pelvic organs and help to relieve the emotional and physical tension that exacerbates menstrual cramps.

An excellent herbal remedy for easing menstrual cramps is cramp bark (*Viburnum opulus*). It contains natural compounds that help to relax the uterus. Take one-half to one teaspoon of liquid extract, or two capsules three to four times daily, as needed.

Sometimes, the simplest remedy can provide immediate relief from cramping. Give yourself some time out from your daily activities, and rest with your feet up and a hot water bottle over your abdomen for at least half an hour.

Supplements for Relieving Menstrual Cramps

- Calcium: 1,000 milligrams daily

- Magnesium: 400 milligrams daily

- Flaxseed oil: 1 tablespoon daily

- GLA: 240 milligrams daily

- Cramp bark (as needed): 1/2 to 1 teaspoon liquid extract or 2 capsules three to four times daily

Premenstrual Syndrome

During their reproductive years, most women will experience, to at least some degree, premenstrual syndrome (PMS). Abdominal bloating, backache, breast tenderness, digestive disturbances, fatigue, headache, insomnia, joint pain, mood swings, and water retention are just some of the many ways that shifts in hormones affect a woman's body and mind.

The Causes of PMS

PMS most commonly occurs during the week to ten days prior to the onset of menstruation. Some women, however, are plagued by PMS symptoms throughout most of the month.

Although the precise cause of PMS has not been determined, PMS symptoms appear to be caused by an excess of estrogen in relation to progesterone, and by increased levels of the inflammatory series-2 prostaglandins. Symptoms may also be related to the dip in calcium and magnesium levels that occurs prior to menstruation. For some women, premenstrual symptoms are mild and insignificant. For others, however, PMS can be debilitating, both physically and emotionally. While there is still much to learn about PMS, it is clear that diet and exercise play an important role in the onset and severity of symptoms.

The Role of Diet in PMS

What you eat on a daily basis determines how well your body processes hormones. Through your dietary choices, you can help your body eliminate excess estrogen, reduce problem-causing prostaglandins while enhancing the production of beneficial prostaglandins, and improve hormonal balance.

A high-fiber diet that is rich in fruits, vegetables, legumes, and whole grains, helps your body eliminate excess estrogen. Nurturing a healthy population of intestinal flora also aids the intestinal tract in its job of excreting estrogen, and a diet rich in complex carbohydrates, such as fruits, vegetables, and whole grains, encourages the growth of these beneficial flora. To replenish healthy bacteria in the intestinal tract, you can also take supplements of probiotic bacteria such as *Lactobacillus acidophilus* and *Bifidobacterium bifidum*. Take a supplement that supplies at least five billion live bacteria daily.

Probiotic Bacteria
Beneficial bacteria, such as Lactobacillus acidophilus *and* Bifidobacterium bifidum, *that aid in digestion and elimination and help to keep the intestinal tract healthy.*

Curtailing your intake of hydrogenated and partially hydrogenated fats, polyunsaturated vegetable oils, and saturated fat also helps to lower estrogen levels and decreases the production of inflammatory prostaglandins. As much as possible, don't eat meat or dairy foods that have been produced with hormones, and avoid toxins, such as pesticides and fungicides, which have estrogenic activity.

If you suffer from PMS, it's best to stay away from all sources of caffeine, including coffee, tea, chocolate, and caffeinated soft drinks. Even the small amounts of caffeine found in decaffeinated coffee or tea can trigger PMS symptoms. To prevent mood and energy swings, eat small, frequent meals that are high in protein and low in sugar.

To improve hormonal balance and encourage the production of beneficial prostaglandins, eat foods rich in omega-3 fatty acids, such as salmon, sardines, walnuts, and flaxseed oil. Aim for three servings of fish per week, and a small handful of walnuts or one tablespoon of ground flaxseeds or flaxseed oil daily. In addition, take 240 mg daily of gamma-linolenic acid (GLA), found in black currant, borage seed, and evening primrose oils.

Soy foods, such as soy milk, tempeh, and tofu, are excellent sources of plant estrogens, which also help to regulate estrogen levels. Consume one serving of soy daily: four ounces of tempeh or tofu, or one cup of soy milk.

Supplements for PMS

To help your body metabolize estrogen more efficiently, take a high-potency B-complex vitamin daily. Vitamin B_6 is particularly important here because it supports the liver in its job of breaking down estrogen, and also helps to alleviate premenstrual bloating and mood swings.

Lipotropic Agents
Nutrients that enhance the liver's function of metabolizing and detoxifying estrogen by improving fat metabolism and promoting bile flow.

In addition, you can support optimal liver function (the liver plays a critical role in metabolizing and detoxifying estrogen) by taking a supplement that contains the lipotropic agents choline, methionine and/or cysteine. Take 1,000 mg of choline and 500 mg of methionine or cysteine every day.

Other useful supplements include calcium and magnesium. A recent study of 466 women at St. Luke's-Roosevelt Hospital in New York showed that calcium supplements effectively relieve PMS symptoms such as mood swings, pain, and water retention. The women, aged eighteen to forty-five, were randomly divided into two groups. Half were given 1,200 mg of calcium daily, and the rest were given a placebo. After three months, those taking the calcium supplement reported a 48 percent reduction in symptoms, compared with those in the control group who reported only a 30 percent reduction in symptoms.

Magnesium is necessary for your liver to metabolize estrogen, and it's also needed to stabilize blood sugar levels. In addition, low levels of magnesium contribute to fluid retention. If you have a strong craving for chocolate premenstrually, it may be your body telling you that you need magnesium. Chocolate is rich in magnesium, but it's not the best way to get this nutrient because the caffeine and sugar in chocolate tend to make PMS symptoms worse. Instead, try eating magnesium-rich foods, such as legumes, nuts, and seeds, and take 400–600 mg of magnesium daily.

Vitamin E is important for relieving breast tenderness, which is a common symptom associated with PMS. Take 400–800 IU of vitamin E daily.

Endorphins
The body's natural mood-elevating chemicals. They can be increased by exercising.

In addition to a healthful diet and supplements, exercise is essential for relieving PMS. Regular exercise, at least thirty minutes a day, helps regulate hormone levels and stimulates the production of endorphins, the body's natural mood-elevating chemicals. In addition,

exercise helps to ease the emotional tension that is often a component of PMS.

Herbal Help for PMS

Herbs can help regulate hormonal balance and can also ease the symptoms of PMS. Perhaps the most important is chasteberry (*Vitex agnus-castus*), which has been used since the time of Hippocrates to tone and regulate the reproductive system. Chasteberry improves the functioning of the pituitary gland, which is responsible for regulating the production of progesterone. By increasing the production of progesterone, chasteberry helps to bring hormones into a more favorable balance.

In a 1994 German study of 550 women with PMS and menstrual disorders, 32 percent of the participants showed improvement within the first four weeks after taking chasteberry. By the end of the third menstrual cycle, 84 percent of the women demonstrated an improvement in symptoms. For best results, chasteberry should be taken over a long period of time—at least six months. Take one-half teaspoon of liquid extract, or one capsule up to three times a day.

St. John's wort (*Hypericum perforatum*) is helpful for the depression, insomnia, irritability, and mood swings that commonly occur in PMS.

A study of nineteen women at the University of Exeter in the United Kingdom showed that two-thirds of these women found significant relief when taking St. John's wort. They were given 900 mg of the herb daily for two complete menstrual cycles, and reported that their PMS-related symptoms of anxiety, confusion, crying, depression, and nervous tension were diminished by more than half.

Supplements for PMS

- Calcium: 1,000 mg daily
- Magnesium: 400–600 mg daily
- Vitamin-B complex: 50–100 mg daily
- Vitamin E: 400–800 IU daily
- Flaxseed oil: 1 tablespoon daily
- GLA (black currant seed, borage seed, or evening primrose oil): 240 mg daily
- Lipotrophic formula: 1,000 mg choline and 500 mg methionine and/or cysteine daily
- Probiotic formula: 5–10 billion viable *Lactobacillus acidophilus* and *Bifidobacterium bifidum* daily
- Chasteberry: $1/2$ teaspoon liquid extract or one 500–600 mg capsule one to three times daily
- St. John's wort (as needed): 300 mg three times daily

Cervical Dysplasia

Cervical dysplasia is the medical term used to describe

abnormal cell growth in the cervix, which is the entrance to the uterus. Although cervical dysplasia is considered to be a precancerous condition, it is easily treatable and reversible when it is discovered early.

Understanding Cervical Dysplasia

Abnormal cell growth is diagnosed through a Pap smear, which is a routine gynecological exam. Cells taken from the cervix are examined and graded on a scale of one to four, with higher numbers indicating greater cell abnormality. If you have stage-2 dysplasia, your doctor will probably simply want to monitor your condition. Many times, stage-2 dysplasia heals with no need for medical intervention. If you have stage-3 or stage-4 dysplasia, you should be treated by a physician. In any case, you can use the information in this section to reduce your risk of further cell abnormalities.

Risk factors for cervical dysplasia include birth control pills, cigarette smoking, exposure to the genital herpes virus or venereal warts, multiple sexual partners, and sexual activity before the age of eighteen. In addition, cervical dysplasia has been strongly linked to an insufficient intake of the B-complex vitamins, especially folic acid.

If you have been diagnosed with cervical dysplasia, it is important to rule out a vaginal infection, which could be the underlying reason for cell abnormalities. If a vaginal infection is the cause, treating it will resolve the condition.

Dietary Factors in Cervical Dysplasia

The incidence of cervical dysplasia and cervical cancer is clearly associated with deficiencies of a variety of nutrients. Studies of women suffering from cervical dysplasia show that they have insufficient blood levels of antioxidants and folic acid.

Folic acid, a B-complex vitamin, is especially important for preventing and reversing cervical dysplasia. Dark leafy greens are an excellent source of this nutrient. Eat at least one generous serving of collards, kale, spinach, or other dark leafy greens daily. In addition, take a B-complex supplement that contains 400 mcg of folic acid. If you have been diagnosed with cervical dysplasia, take 10 mg of folic acid daily for up to three months, along with a high-potency B-complex supplement.

If you have cervical dysplasia, eating a diet rich in fresh fruits and vegetables, and supplementing with antioxidants is essential for protecting cells and preventing abnormal cell growth. As a general daily antioxidant supplement, take 25,000 IU of beta-carotene with mixed carotenoids, 500 mg of vitamin C, 200 mcg of selenium, and 400 IU of vitamin E.

Supplements for Cervical Dysplasia

- B-complex: 50–100 milligrams daily
- Folic acid: 400 mcg daily; 10 mg daily for three months if cervical dysplasia is present

- Beta-carotene: 25,000 IU with mixed carotenoids
- Selenium: 200 mcg daily
- Vitamin C: 500 mg daily
- Vitamin E: 400 IU daily

Uterine Fibroids

Almost half of all women develop uterine fibroids, a benign growth of muscle tissue in the uterus. Fibroids can be as tiny as the head of a pin, or as large as a grapefruit, and it's not uncommon for a woman to have multiple fibroid growths in her uterus.

Understanding Uterine Fibroids

Although fibroids often present no symptoms, they can cause heavy menstrual bleeding, irregular menstrual periods, and pelvic discomfort. Fibroids are not associated with a higher incidence of uterine cancer, but they are one of the primary reasons for hysterectomies. Many times, a woman can live with fibroids for years without problems. However, the fluctuating hormones that occur during the perimenopausal years often trigger the increased growth of existing fibroids, and can exacerbate their symptoms.

Perimenopause
The months or years of hormonal fluctuations prior to menopause.

More serious symptoms of fibroids include anemia brought on by heavy menstrual bleeding, or discomfort of the bladder or bowel if the fibroid puts pressure on the bladder or intestines. Unless a fibroid growth is causing undue discomfort, or becomes a health risk, it's safe to simply leave it alone. In the vast majority of cases, fibroids shrink dramatically after menopause. Meanwhile, there are ways you can ease your symptoms and perhaps even reduce the size of your fibroids.

Dietary Help for Fibroids

If you have been diagnosed with fibroids, the most important thing you can do is decrease your body's production of estrogen. Avoid all animal products (such as dairy products, eggs, poultry, and meat) that have been grown or treated with hormones or drugs. Also stay away from foods treated with herbicides and pesticides because these substances have hormonal effects in the body. Hydrogenated fats and saturated fats also stimulate the production of estrogen.

A fiber-rich diet will help your body eliminate excess estrogen. Fresh fruits and vegetables, legumes, and whole grains are excellent sources of dietary fiber. Include soy products such as tempeh and tofu in your diet as often as possible—every day, if you can. Soy helps to naturally regulate estrogen levels.

In addition to dietary changes, daily aerobic exercise, such as bicycling or brisk walking, is essential for bringing hormones into balance.

Natural Therapies for Fibroids

To help your body metabolize estrogen more efficiently, take a high-potency B-complex vitamin daily. In addition, you can help your liver function at its best (the liver plays a critical role in metabolizing and detoxifying estrogen) by taking a supplement that contains the lipotropic agents choline, methionine and/or cysteine. Take 1,000 mg of choline and 500 mg of methionine or cysteine daily.

Nurturing a healthy population of intestinal flora also helps the body to eliminate excess estrogen. A diet rich in complex carbohydrates, such as fruits, vegetables, and whole grains, helps to feed beneficial flora, and supplements of probiotic bacteria such as *Lactobacillus acidophilus* and *Bifidobacterium bifidum* replenish healthy bacteria in the intestinal tract. Take a supplement that supplies at least five billion live bacteria daily.

An herb that can help to reduce fibroid growth is chasteberry. It stimulates the production of progesterone, which creates a more favorable balance of hormones and lessens the effect of estrogen on the body. For best results, take chasteberry for at least six months. Take one-half teaspoon of liquid extract or one capsule three times daily.

Supplements for Uterine Fibroids

- B-complex: 50–100 milligrams daily

- Chasteberry: $\frac{1}{2}$ teaspoon liquid extract or one 500–600 mg capsule three times daily

- Lipotrophic formula: 1,000 mg choline and 500 mg methionine and/or cysteine daily

- Probiotic formula: 5–10 billion viable *Lactobacillus acidophilus* and *Bifidobacterium bifidum* daily

PREGNANCY AND BIRTH

Pregnancy and birth are generally wonderful events in a woman's life. At the same time, pregnancy brings challenges as a woman's body undergoes the task of creating a life and preparing for birth. In this section, you'll learn about diet, supplements, and lifestyle factors that will keep you and your growing baby healthy. You'll also find suggestions for the common problems that plague pregnant women, such as morning sickness and constipation.

Preparing for Pregnancy

Paying attention to your health is always important, but it's doubly so when you're pregnant. If you're of childbearing age and considering having a child, it's best to plan ahead for a healthy pregnancy. During your nine months of pregnancy, your body will go through many changes as the baby develops. Pregnancy places great demands on a woman's body, and your baby is completely dependent upon you to provide what it needs to grow healthy and strong.

The first trimester is the most critical stage in your baby's development, because this is the time that major organs are being formed. Your nutritional needs during pregnancy are different than usual, and it's necessary to pay close attention to your diet to make sure you are supplying your baby with everything it needs. A healthy diet is also vital for your well-being, because the baby draws nutrients from you and can leave you depleted if your diet is inadequate. In addition to providing all the necessary nutrients for your baby, it's essential to avoid all substances that can harm your baby, such as alcohol, drugs (other than those prescribed by your doctor), and smoking.

During the first three months, many women experience uncomfortable symptoms such as fatigue, mood swings, and nausea. In later stages of pregnancy, as the baby grows larger, you may suffer from backaches, constipation, difficulties sleeping, and needing to go to the bathroom frequently. Although unpleasant, it can be helpful to know that these discomforts are normal, and are related to shifting hormones and your body's adjusting to the growing baby. It's important to listen to your body, to give yourself time to rest, and to nurture yourself as much as possible.

Throughout your pregnancy, you should stay in close touch with your healthcare practitioner, who can offer guidance for your particular needs.

A Healthy Diet for Pregnancy

What you eat during pregnancy is vital for your health and the well-being of your baby. Your diet should be centered on nutrient-dense foods such as fresh fruits and vegetables, high-quality proteins, and whole grains. You should figure on gaining about twenty-five to thirty-five extra pounds during pregnancy. While you don't want to pile on unnecessary pounds, pregnancy is not the time to diet.

Certain nutrients, particularly calcium, folic acid, and iron, are especially essential during pregnancy. Folic acid, a member of the B-complex vitamin family, is required for the formation of a healthy brain and spinal cord. A deficiency of this nutrient during pregnancy has been clearly linked to two serious birth defects: spina bifida, a defect of the spinal column that can cause paralysis and mental retardation, and anencephaly, a defect where the baby does not develop a brain and is stillborn or dies shortly after birth.

Folic acid is found abundantly in dark leafy green vegetables, dried beans, peas, and citrus fruits, but few women get enough from dietary sources. Taking a supplement that provides 400 mcg of folic acid is critical for protecting your baby. Because the fetus needs folic acid within the first few weeks of development, you should be taking supplements of folic acid all the time, not just while you're pregnant. Folic acid has many other health benefits as well, such as preventing cervical-cell abnormalities, so it's a good idea to take it regularly throughout your life, anyway.

Iron is also necessary for you and your baby, and ensures the production of healthy, oxygen-carrying red blood cells. A deficiency of iron causes anemia, a frequent reason for excessive fatigue during pregnancy. Anemia can increase a pregnant woman's susceptibility to infections, and make it more difficult for her body to cope with excessive bleeding during childbirth.

Many foods are high in iron, including dark green leafy vegetables, dried beans, dried fruits, nuts, seeds, chicken, salmon, shellfish, and red meat. But iron is not easily assimilated. And some foods, especially caffeine, milk, and bran, inhibit iron absorption. You can enhance iron's absorption by eating foods high in vitamin C at the same time that you eat iron-rich foods. Because getting enough iron is tricky, and low iron levels are so common among pregnant women, most women need supplements of it during pregnancy. Your doctor can perform a simple blood test and will tell you if you need supplemental iron.

Adequate calcium intake is essential for a woman throughout her life, and pregnancy is no exception. During pregnancy, the baby needs calcium for making bones and teeth. If your calcium intake is less than optimal, the baby will draw on the calcium stored in your bones, leaving you at risk for osteoporosis later in life. During pregnancy, you need to consume enough calcium for both you and your baby. The recommended amount of calcium for a pregnant woman is 1,200 mg per day.

Many foods are good sources of calcium, including cheeses, milk, yogurt, and dark leafy greens. Milk and yogurt contain about 300 mg of calcium per cup, so four one-cup servings per day will provide you with your ration of calcium. But many women either don't like milk or don't digest it easily. Alternative sources of calcium include dark leafy greens, with one cup of cooked collards weighing in at 300 mg of calcium and one cup of cooked kale at 200 mg. However, it's unlikely that you'll eat four to six cups of cooked greens. To obtain sufficient calcium, you may need calcium supplements. It's best to consult your health practitioner for advice.

Be sure to eat a wide variety of fresh vegetables and fruits while you're pregnant. They are excellent sources of protective antioxidants, especially dark green leafy vegetables and deep yellow and orange fruits and vegetables. A number of studies have linked insufficient intake of antioxidants to preeclampsia, a serious condition that causes fluid retention, headaches, and high blood pressure. If preeclampsia is not treated, it can progress to eclampsia, which can result in convulsions, coma, and death. This is another good reason to take a well-balanced prenatal multivitamin and mineral during pregnancy.

Fluid intake is also important while you are pregnant, because your blood volume greatly increases to accommodate your growing baby. Keeping your fluid intake up can also help ward off constipation. Drink at least eight glasses of water daily.

Other Lifestyle Suggestions for Pregnancy

While you are pregnant, it's essential that you completely avoid alcoholic beverages, including wine and beer. Drinking alcohol can cause fetal alcohol syndrome, a significant and completely preventable cause of birth defects and mental retardation. You should also avoid or limit your consumption of caffeine, which can cause insomnia, nervousness, and dehydration. Excessive amounts of caffeine may also result in low-birth-weight babies. Coffee is not the only offender: tea, cola, chocolate, cocoa, and some over-the-counter drugs, including pain relievers and allergy medicines, are also significant sources of caffeine.

If you smoke, you must stop, not only for your own health, but also for the health of your baby. Smoking puts your baby at risk for a low birth weight, and smokers are in danger of having premature or stillborn babies. Babies born to mothers who smoke during pregnancy are more susceptible to asthma and respiratory infections, and are at higher risk of sudden infant death syndrome (SIDS). Because breathing second-hand smoke is also unhealthy, you should avoid being around people who smoke.

While you are pregnant, you should also avoid x-rays, which expose the baby to radiation and can cause birth defects. And hot tubs and saunas are not appropriate during pregnancy because they can raise core body temperature, which may harm the developing baby. Soaking in a warm bath is fine, though, and can be wonderfully relaxing. Just make sure that the temperature is not excessively hot.

Exercise is an indispensable ingredient for optimal well-being, and pregnancy is no exception. A 1998 study published in the *American Journal of Public Health* reported that women who engaged in regular vigorous exercise were more likely to carry their babies to full term than those who didn't exercise, or who exercised less. Exercise maintains muscle and cardiovascular fitness, improves sleep, relieves tension, and enhances mood. Obviously, you shouldn't participate in contact sports or those that involve a risk of falling, such as downhill skiing.

The best exercises during pregnancy are brisk walking, prenatal aerobics classes, riding a stationary bicycle, and swimming. Prenatal yoga classes are excellent for stretching and relaxation. Exercise is appropriate for the majority of pregnant women, but you should check with your healthcare practitioner before starting an exercise program.

Common Problems during Pregnancy

Pregnancy is often fraught with minor, but annoying maladies, such as morning sickness, constipation, and frequent urination. Morning sickness is somewhat of a misnomer, because nausea and vomiting can occur at any time during the day. Nausea plagues the majority of women during the first trimester, and, for some women, it persists throughout the entire nine months. The hormonal changes of pregnancy are a likely cause of morning sickness, but recent theories also suggest that nausea is your body's way of protecting your baby from foods that may be harmful.

To ease symptoms of nausea, pay attention to what your body is telling you. Don't eat foods that you find unappealing, or that upset your stomach. You'll probably find that your tastes change during pregnancy, and the best thing to do is to follow your intuition. You may find it helpful to eat frequent, smaller meals and drink less fluid with meals. Many women also find that starchy carbohydrates, such as crackers, help to ease nausea.

Ginger (*Zingiber officinale*) has been proven in numerous research studies to effectively relieve nausea, and it's safe to use during pregnancy. In a study reported in the *European Journal of Obstetrics & Gynecology*, ginger was shown to be more effective than a placebo for easing the nausea and vomiting of severe morning sickness. Drink up to three cups of ginger tea daily (it's best to sip $1/4$ to $1/2$ cup of tea at a time) or take up to 250 mg in capsules up to four times a day.

Almost half of all pregnant women suffer from constipation. Hormonal changes relax the muscle tone of the large intestine, which slows the passage of food through the digestive tract. Iron supplements, which are commonly prescribed to treat anemia, can also be the culprit. Drinking plenty of water, eating a fiber-rich diet, and exercising daily are often enough to cure constipation. A daily ration of stewed prunes is another time-honored way of encouraging sluggish bowels to move.

For extra help, you can take a fiber supplement, such as those made from psyllium, to provide additional bulk. Be sure to drink plenty of additional water when taking a fiber supplement to avoid creating constipation. During pregnancy, you should never resort to stimulant laxatives (such as those made from senna or cascara sagrada) because of the risk of causing uterine contractions.

While your intestines may be slowing down during pregnancy, your kidneys and bladder are doing the opposite, and you will probably experience an increased need to urinate, even when your bladder is almost empty. During pregnancy, your kidneys step up their activity, and as the baby grows, it puts pressure on your bladder. It's important to urinate as often as you feel the need, and to keep drinking plenty of fluids—at least eight glasses of water daily—to prevent bladder infections. If you have pain, burning, or difficulty urinating, consult your health practitioner right away. An untreated bladder infection can spread to the kidneys and be life-threatening.

To help prevent bladder infections, drink sixteen ounces of unsweetened cranberry juice daily. Cranberry juice helps to foil infection by making the walls of the bladder slippery, which keeps bacteria from attaching to the bladder walls and multiplying. You can also take capsules of cranberry extract; follow the directions on the label.

If you come down with any kind of infection during pregnancy, echinacea (*Echinacea spp.*) is an excellent herb to help support your immune function. Echinacea is effective for treating bladder infections, colds and respiratory infections, sinus infections, and other common illnesses. A recent study reported in the *Archives of Internal Medicine* showed that echinacea is safe during pregnancy. In general, take one-half teaspoon of echinacea extract four times a day for up to ten days. If you contract any type of infection during pregnancy, consult your healthcare practitioner for advice.

Supplements for Pregnancy

Consult your doctor before taking any supplements during pregnancy.

A prenatal multivitamin and mineral daily, which should contain:

- Antioxidants: (beta-carotene and mixed carotenoids, vitamin E, vitamin C)
- Calcium: 1,200 mg daily (less if dietary sources are sufficient)
- Folic acid: 400 mcg daily
- Iron: 15–30 mg daily

For morning sickness:

- Ginger: three cups tea; or 250 mg in capsules up to four times daily

For constipation:

- Fiber supplement: 1–3 tablespoons daily

For colds and other infections:

- Echinacea: $1/2$ teaspoon extract four times daily for up to ten days

MENOPAUSE

The menopausal years are a time of great change for a woman, and affect all levels of her physical and emotional well-being. Most women experience at least some of the symptoms that are commonly associated with menopause, such as forgetfulness, heart palpitations, hot flashes, joint pain, mood swings, sleep disturbances, urinary tract infections, and vaginal dryness. At this time in life, it becomes more important than ever before to pay attention to your health.

The Challenges of Menopause

The hormonal changes that a woman experiences in the years surrounding menopause are powerful. The conventional medical approach to menopause is to prescribe hormone therapy (HRT), both for symptom relief and for preventing cardiovascular disease and osteoporosis in postmenopausal women. The combination of estrogen and progesterone is often effective for relieving depression, hot flashes, and vaginal dryness, and it also has been thought to offer some protection from cardiovascular disease and osteoporosis, although the benefit of HRT for heart disease has recently been called into question.

Many women object to taking synthetic hormones because of unpleasant side effects, such as acne, breast soreness, headaches, and nausea. More dangerously, conventional hormone replacement therapy puts a woman at greater risk for blood clots, breast cancer, gallbladder disease, and high blood pressure. There are natural hormones available that have a far lower risk of side effects, and these hormones can be formulated in the precise combination that your body requires. If you are interested in natural hormone replacement therapy, consult a naturopathic doctor, or one who practices a holistic approach.

There's no doubt that the considerable hormonal shifts taking place in your body at this time are responsible for the symptoms of menopause. But you can greatly influence your passage through menopause in a positive way, and lessen your symptoms by eating well, getting regular exercise and plenty of rest, using nutritional supplements and herbs to help regulate your hormones, and taking time for yourself. First, it's helpful to understand what is taking place in your changing body.

Understanding Menopause

Menopause is the cessation of menstruation, and is marked by the final menstrual period. But menopause actually encompasses the years prior to menopause when your hormones begin to shift in preparation for menopause (a stage referred to as perimenopause) and the year or two following the final menstrual cycle.

By the time most women reach their mid-forties, ovulation becomes erratic and the ovaries slow down their production of both estrogen and progesterone. One of the first signs of decreased hormone levels is erratic menstrual cycles. Most women find that their menstrual periods are initially more frequent and heavier, and then, as they move toward menopause, their cycles become lighter and further

apart. Skipping a month or two, and then resuming menstruation is also common.

It's significant to note that your ovaries are responsible for producing not only estrogen and progesterone, but also for making other hormones called androgens, such as testosterone and DHEA. Although the ovaries do not produce estrogen or progesterone after menopause, they do continue producing androgens. Androgens are also made by other organs and glands, primarily the adrenal glands. These hormones are necessary for muscle tone, sex drive, and overall well-being. In addition, androgens are converted by fat cells into small amounts of estrogen, which helps to keep you healthy.

Androgens *Hormones produced by the adrenal glands that are essential for muscle tone, sex drive, and overall well-being.*

Your adrenal glands become extremely important in the menopausal years. When your ovaries slow down and eventually stop making hormones, your adrenal glands fill in the gap by taking over the production of hormones. Although the amount they produce is small in comparison to the amount once generated by the ovaries, they make enough to ease the transition through menopause and keep you vital for the rest of your life.

The Key to Vitality

Unfortunately, many women enter the menopausal years with less-than-optimal adrenal function. One of the roles of the adrenal glands is to help the body respond to physical and emotional stressors. But our bodies were not meant to be continually bombarded with the level of tension that is typical of modern life, and the adrenals become exhausted trying to maintain balance under conditions of recurring stress. As a result, the adrenal glands are overworked, and by the time most women reach menopause, their adrenals are not up to the task of generating sufficient hormones to maintain health and vitality.

Common symptoms of adrenal depletion include depression, fatigue, hypoglycemia, insomnia, lowered immunity, and poor concentration. With care, however, you can rebuild the health of your adrenal glands. Any steps you can take to reduce stress in your life will help to ease the demands on your adrenals. Rest and sufficient sleep are also essential. And it is advisable to avoid caffeine and refined sugars, which provide a temporary boost of energy, but further deplete your adrenals.

One of the most significant dietary changes you can make is to cut down on sodium and eat at least seven servings of fresh vegetables and fruits daily. This will help restore a healthy balance of potassium and sodium, which supports adrenal health. In addition, eat frequent small meals with plenty of high-quality proteins, such as chicken, eggs, and fish, and take a high-potency multivitamin and mineral supplement daily. The B-complex vitamins, vitamin

C, magnesium, and zinc are especially important for adrenal health. Take 50–100 mg of B-complex, 500 mg of vitamin C, 400 mg of magnesium, and 25 mg of zinc daily.

An Herbal Energy Tonic

Siberian ginseng (*Eleutherococcus senticosus*) is an excellent herb for helping to rebuild adrenal health. For centuries, it has been used in traditional Chinese medicine to enhance energy and vitality, and is prescribed as a longevity tonic. In the former Soviet Union, Siberian ginseng was studied extensively and the Soviet scientists noted its ability to help the body adapt to physical and emotional stressors. Siberian ginseng is approved by the German Commission E (a regulatory agency similar to the Food and Drug Administration) for the treatment of fatigue and debility.

To obtain its full benefits, the herb must be taken for two to three months, and it can be taken indefinitely. Although Siberian ginseng is very safe, taking higher-than-recommended doses can cause anxiety, insomnia, and irritability. If you don't feel a noticeable difference in energy within a couple of months, you may be taking an inferior product. Buy from reputable herb companies, or look for extracts standardized for eleutherosides, which are considered to be the active ingredient. Take one gram of powdered root, $1/2$ teaspoon of fluid extract, or 100 mg of standardized extract two times daily.

Dietary Guidelines for Menopause

At midlife, the foods you choose to eat (and those you avoid) have a significant effect on how your body adapts to the changes of menopause. Your diet also influences your health and well-being in the years to come. It's essential at menopause to pay close attention to your diet, and to choose foods that are concentrated sources of health-supporting nutrients.

Phytoestrogens
Plant compounds with weak estrogen properties that can help balance estrogen levels in the body.

Certain foods have a profound effect on hormone levels, particularly foods that are rich in phytoestrogens. Phytoestrogens are plant compounds with weak estrogenic properties—they're approximately fifty times weaker than estrogen. But these compounds are similar enough to estrogen that they are able to attach to receptor sites in the body that are normally occupied by estrogen.

If you have an excess of estrogen (which causes such menopausal symptoms as hot flashes), phytoestrogens help to reduce estrogen levels. If, on the other hand, you are at risk for osteoporosis (low estrogen is a contributing factor), phytoestrogens help to protect you by providing some estrogenic activity.

Many foods are rich in phytoestrogens, and it makes sense to include several servings of these helpful foods in your daily diet. Apples, celery, flaxseeds, legumes, nuts, and whole grains are all good sources of phytoestrogens. Of special value during menopause are soybeans and the products made from them, such as soymilk, tempeh, and tofu. Researchers believe the reason Japanese women have an easier time during menopause, and a significantly lower rate of breast cancer than American women, is their high consumption of soy products. Soy is a rich source of phytoestrogens called isoflavones, which are available in supplement form.

But it's best to include soy in your diet in the form of foods, such as soymilk, tempeh, or tofu, instead of using supplements of concentrated isoflavones. Although a daily serving (one cup of soymilk or one-half cup of tempeh or tofu) of soy foods is protective for your health, no one is certain of the effects of large doses of concentrated isoflavones. Some researchers have expressed concern that high doses of isoflavones may contribute to estrogen-dependent cancers, such as certain forms of breast cancer.

Isoflavones
A type of phytoestrogen (plant estrogen) that occurs abundantly in soy and can be of benefit to women.

Essential fatty acids are also important during the menopausal years. Foods rich in omega-3 fatty acids help to keep hair, skin, and vaginal tissues healthy, and they aid in hormonal balance. Good sources of omega-3 fats are cold-water fish, such as salmon and sardines, and flaxseeds and walnuts. During menopause, it's a good idea to supplement your diet with one tablespoon of flaxseed oil daily to ensure sufficient amounts of omega-3 essential fatty acids. Vitamin E is also helpful for keeping vaginal tissues healthy; take 400–800 IU daily.

Herbal Help for Menopause

Women have traditionally relied on herbs to help ease the transition through menopause. As mentioned previously, Siberian ginseng helps to build vitality and strengthen the adrenal glands. Other herbs that are helpful for balancing hormones include chasteberry and black cohosh (*Cimicifuga racemosa*). Chasteberry increases progesterone levels by enhancing the activity of the pituitary gland, and is particularly effective for women who suffer from PMS-like symptoms associated with menopause.

Black cohosh has estrogenic-like activity, and helps ease such menopausal symptoms as depression, headaches, heart palpitations, hot flashes, irritability, night sweats, and vaginal atrophy. In at least twenty clinical studies, black cohosh has been shown to be as effective as synthetic estrogen for relieving menopausal symptoms. Symptom relief is not immediate, but black cohosh is far safer than synthetic hormones and has no toxicity or harmful side effects, other than occasional minor stomach upset. In a German multicenter study of 629 women, 80 percent of the women reported improvement of their symptoms within six to eight weeks.

Clinical studies have generally used extracts of black cohosh standardized for triterpenes, with the typical dosage equal to 4 mg of triterpenes daily. Black cohosh can also be taken as a liquid extract, approximately 1/2 teaspoon twice daily, or one 500–600 mg capsule of the powdered herb three times a day.

Supplements for Menopause

- High-potency multivitamin and mineral supplement, supplying:
  - B-complex: 50–100 mg daily
  - Vitamin C: 500 mg daily
  - Vitamin E: 400–800 IU daily
  - Calcium: 1,200 mg daily
  - Magnesium: 400 mg daily
  - Zinc: 25 mg daily
- Flaxseed oil: 1 tablespoon daily
- Black cohosh: approximately $1/2$ teaspoon liquid extract, or one 500–600 mg capsule of the powdered herb, two to three times daily
- Chasteberry: $1/2$ teaspoon liquid extract or one 500–600 mg capsule three times daily
- Siberian ginseng: one gram powdered root, $1/2$ teaspoon fluid extract, or 100 mg standardized extract two times daily

PREVENTING OSTEOPOROSIS

One out of every four postmenopausal women will be faced with a diagnosis of osteoporosis, and more than 45,000 women will die this year from injuries related to weakened bones, such as fractures of the hip and spine. Equally tragic is the crippling loss of mobility that occurs with osteoporosis. There are a number of specific risk factors that predispose a woman to osteoporosis, including heredity. But while you can't control your genetic heritage, you can control the other risk factors that contribute to bone loss.

Osteoporosis: Risk Factors for Women

- Excessive alcohol or caffeine intake
- High phosphorus intake
- High protein or sodium diet
- Lack of vitamin D

- Low calcium intake
- Menopause
- Sedentary lifestyle
- Smoking
- Thin build, particularly for those of Northern European or Asian descent

The Basics of Bone Health

Bones are dense, hard structures, but they are continually in the process of being broken down and recreated. Your bones are a storehouse for calcium in your body, a mineral that is vital for a variety of essential body processes. Calcium reserves are drawn upon to keep bones and teeth strong, to regulate heartbeat and muscle contractions, to transmit nerve impulses, and to aid in blood clotting.

Childhood and early adulthood are critical times for building healthy bone. Ideally, young women will have optimal nutrition and plenty of exercise to help them build a strong bone structure that will carry them into their later years. Unfortunately, many young women diet excessively, don't get enough exercise, and don't obtain sufficient amounts of nutrients for maximum bone strength. By the time a woman reaches thirty, her bones have achieved their greatest density; after the age of about thirty-five, more bone is being withdrawn than replaced.

At menopause, bone loss escalates when levels of estrogen decline, because estrogen plays an important role in regulating the ability of the bones to absorb calcium. But it's not all hormonally driven. A poor diet and a sedentary lifestyle greatly intensify the process of bone loss, and it's these factors that make or break bone strength. If your diet is rich in calcium and other necessary bone-building nutrients, and if you exercise regularly, your body will deposit calcium into your bones and your bones will grow stronger.

Factors in Bone Loss

Factors that accelerate bone loss include dieting, nutrient deficiencies, smoking, and excess alcohol, caffeine, phosphorus, protein, and sodium. Dieting, or trying to be too thin, is harmful to bone health at any age. Low-calorie diets are often deficient in calcium and other essential nutrients, and the body tries to make up for the lack by taking calcium from the bones to perform necessary metabolic functions. In addition, if you are very thin, you are at higher risk for osteoporosis because fat reserves in the hips and thighs are essential for the production of estrogen after menopause.

In general, the habits that are harmful to your general health are also harmful to your bones. Smokers are at greater risk for osteoporosis than non-smokers: they tend to go through menopause (which decreases levels of estrogen) earlier and smoking suppresses the activity of the parathyroid glands, which are responsible for regulating calcium levels. Excessive amounts of alcohol, caffeine, or sodium increase the amount of calcium that is lost in the urine, and this weakens the bones.

Too much protein can also leach calcium from the bones. Although your body needs the amino acids in proteins to make bone from calcium, too much protein creates an acidic condition in the blood that must be neutralized—and calcium is used in this process. It's best to limit your protein intake to no more than about eight ounces per day, and to choose vegetable proteins, such as tempeh and tofu, as well as animal proteins. While you don't have to become a vegetarian to avoid osteoporosis, it's worthwhile to note that research has shown that women who eat a balanced vegetarian diet have the least incidence of osteoporosis, while women who eat a diet high in meat sustain the highest rate of bone loss.

An often overlooked factor in osteoporosis is the mineral phosphorus. Phosphorus is necessary for building bone, and we need about twice as much calcium as phosphorus for optimal calcium absorption. But if more phosphorus than calcium is consumed, a bone-dissolving hormone is secreted to maintain the proper calcium-to-phosphorus ratio in the bloodstream. Unfortunately, our diets are not only lacking in sufficient calcium, but they are loaded with phosphorus—dairy products, meats, nuts, poultry, seafood, seeds, and whole grains contain significant amounts of phosphorus. Many processed foods, such as baked goods, also contain phosphorus, and carbonated soft drinks contain large amounts of phosphoric acid. When the numbers are tallied, most women take in four times as much phosphorus as calcium.

To decrease the risk of osteoporosis, conventional doctors tend to rely on drug therapy, often prescribing hormone replacement therapy (HRT). But HRT is not appropriate for women who have a history of breast or uterine cancer, cardiovascular disease, diabetes, gallbladder disease, liver disease, or migraine headaches. Bone-building drugs such as Fosamax (alendronate sodium) are also commonly prescribed to slow the rate of bone loss. However, these drugs can cause serious digestive problems, including constipation, diarrhea, nausea, severe heartburn, stomach pain, and even ulceration of the esophagus. It takes more effort to build bone with diet and lifestyle changes, but the only side effects are positive ones that enhance your overall well-being.

Dietary Recommendations for Strong Bones

When you think of eating for strong bones, the first thing that probably comes to mind is milk. But although milk is a good source of calcium, and calcium is an essential nutrient for bone health, simply drinking milk is not going to protect your bones. In fact, researchers who evaluated the dietary intake of 78,000 women over a twelve-year period (part of the long-term Harvard Nurses' Health Study) found that those women who had a higher intake of calcium from dairy foods did not have a decreased risk of bone fractures. Despite what the dairy industry would have you believe, the truth is that strong bones are not only related to how much calcium you are getting from your diet, but are also dependent upon how well you are absorbing calcium. To prevent osteoporosis, you need to supply your body with all the essential nutrients for strong bones, avoid foods that contribute to bone loss, and optimize your digestion to aid in the absorption of nutrients, including calcium.

In addition to calcium, the nutrients that are essential for building bone include magnesium, vitamins D and K, zinc, and the trace minerals boron, copper, and manganese. Eating a varied diet, including at least seven servings a day of fresh fruits and vegetables, is the best way to obtain most of these nutrients. For additional insurance, you should also take a high-potency multivitamin and mineral supplement that includes trace minerals.

Dairy products are good sources of calcium, but there are some problems associated with them. Dairy foods are high in phosphorus and protein, both of which can contribute to bone loss if there are excessive amounts in the diet. In addition, many women are lactose intolerant, and experience abdominal cramps, bloating, and diarrhea when they eat dairy foods. Fermented dairy products, such as yogurt, are generally better tolerated because they contain beneficial bacteria that aid in digestion. But there's no reason to rely primarily on dairy to meet your calcium requirements. There are many other calcium-rich foods to choose from, including almonds, broccoli, canned salmon or sardines with bones, dark leafy green vegetables (such as collards, kale, and mustard greens), and tofu processed with calcium.

Dark leafy green vegetables are not only rich in calcium, but they are also an excellent source of vitamin K, a nutrient that is critical for bone formation and for regulating levels of calcium in the blood. About half the vitamin K you need is produced by helpful bacteria in the intestinal tract. You can optimize your body's production of vitamin K by maintaining a healthy population of friendly bacteria in your intestinal tract, and eating yogurt that contains live acidophilus cultures is a good way to do this. You can also obtain beneficial intestinal flora through supplements. Take supplements that supply at least 5–10 billion viable *Lactobacillus acidophilus* and *Bifidobacterium bifidum* daily for at least one month.

Soy foods are especially helpful for protecting against bone loss. Tofu can be an excellent source of calcium if it is

> **Lactobacillus Acidophilus and Bifidobacterium Bifidum**
> Beneficial flora, called probiotics, that are found in the intestinal tract and aid in digestion and assimilation.

processed with calcium, but more importantly, soy foods are rich in isoflavones, natural compounds that have estrogenic effects and help to build bone. But while studies have shown that soy isoflavones help to increase bone density and slow the rate of bone loss, concentrated supplements of isoflavones may not be helpful, and can be harmful. A 2001 study published in the *Journal of the American Medical Association* showed that ipriflavone, a commonly prescribed isoflavone supplement, did not prevent bone loss and, in addition, lowered white blood cell counts.

Instead of turning to concentrated supplements, it seems prudent to rely on whole foods, such as soymilk, tempeh, and tofu to get your protective ration of isoflavones. For bone health, eat one or two servings of soy daily (one cup of soymilk, or four ounces of tempeh or tofu equals one serving).

Supplements for Strong Bones

To insure that you're getting enough calcium, it's a good idea to take a calcium supplement in addition to eating calcium-rich foods. There are many different forms of calcium available, but calcium citrate is probably the most easily absorbable form. It's important to avoid supplements made from bone meal, dolomite, and oyster shell. They are poorly absorbed, and are likely to be contaminated with lead, which is highly toxic and accumulates in the body. If you eat at least two or three servings of calcium-rich foods daily, a supplemental dosage of 1,000 mg of calcium is sufficient. If you don't get enough calcium in your diet, then aim for 1,500 mg daily. For best absorption, take calcium supplements with meals, and don't take more than 500 mg at a time.

Magnesium is another nutrient necessary for bone strength. It's found in a variety of foods, such as leafy greens, legumes, nuts, seeds, and whole grains. But there are many factors that deplete magnesium, including alcohol, and emotional and physical stress. And many women don't eat sufficient amounts of magnesium-rich foods. To provide adequate levels of magnesium, take 600 mg of magnesium daily in an easily absorbable form, such as aspartate, citrate, gluconate, or lactate.

Getting enough calcium in your diet is only part of the strategy for maintaining healthy bones. You also need to ensure that you're absorbing the calcium you ingest. Vitamin D aids the absorption of calcium in the gastrointestinal tract, and it also helps to maintain adequate levels of calcium in the blood for building bone. Your body makes vitamin D, but it needs sunlight to do so. When your skin is exposed to sunlight, a cholesterol compound in your skin is transformed into vitamin D. But many women get little or no sun exposure, and clothing, glass, smog, and sunscreens all block the rays that produce vitamin D. Only a few foods contain vitamin D—primarily butter, eggs, and fortified milk—all things that many women may not regularly eat.

The best way to get this essential vitamin is through moderate sun exposure; about fifteen minutes in direct early morning or late afternoon sunlight three days a week is sufficient. It's also a good idea to take a supplement of 400 IU of vitamin D daily, which is the amount that is found in most multivitamins. While you want to be certain that you're getting enough, vitamin D is not something that you want to get too much of because an excess can contribute to heart disease, kidney damage, and tissue calcification.

The Importance of Exercise

No matter how healthful your diet is, exercise is a necessity for building and maintaining strong bones. A sedentary lifestyle is clearly linked to osteoporosis, and studies have shown that as little as one week of bed rest weakens bones. But the good news is that bones become stronger when they are stressed by moderate weight-bearing activity. When you engage in weight-bearing exercise, a mild electrical charge is generated in your body that causes more calcium to be deposited in the bones. If your dietary intake of calcium is adequate, then your body has calcium available to fortify your bones.

It's important to realize that not all exercise is helpful for strengthening bones. For exercise to be beneficial, it has to stress your bones to trigger the necessary electrical charge. Weight-bearing exercises, such as walking, dancing, and strenuous yoga are excellent. Make sure to also include activities that involve your upper body, such as gardening, rowing, and cross-country skiing. If you find it challenging to regularly engage in physical activities that involve both lower and upper body exercises, try a simple exercise program that uses hand-held weights, or join a gym that has weight-training equipment.

To keep your bones strong, you should engage in at least thirty minutes of weight-bearing exercise five times per week. Even if you have been diagnosed with osteoporosis, you should be exercising regularly. Weight-bearing exercise can slow down the rate of bone loss, and it can help to build stronger bones.

Exercising throughout your life is essential for remaining strong and vital into old age. People often become frail and weak, not because of aging, but because they have stopped using their bodies. When muscles weaken, coordination usually deteriorates as well. The stronger you are and the more confident you are in your body, the less likely you are to have an accident such as a fall.

Supplements for Preventing Osteoporosis

- High-potency multivitamin and mineral supplement daily that includes:

  - Calcium: 1,000–1,500 mg daily

  - Magnesium: 600 mg daily

- Vitamin D: 400 IU daily
- Probiotic formula: 5–10 billion viable *Lactobacillus acidophilus* and *Bifidobacterium bifidum* daily (to promote vitamin K)

PREVENTING CANCER

According to the American Cancer Society, approximately one-third of all women will be stricken with cancer at some time in life. Because there are at least 200 different types of cancer, it's unlikely that there will ever be one single drug or vaccine that will offer protection from this dreaded disease. But even though cancer appears in so many forms and can be so challenging to treat, cancer cells have a lot in common with one another—they all begin when something in normal cell replication goes awry. And many of the reasons that cells replicate abnormally and become cancerous are within our control.

Researchers estimate that one-third of all cancer deaths in the U.S. are related to dietary factors, and another third are caused by cigarette smoking. Clearly, these are factors over which you have influence. Our bodies have marvelous built-in mechanisms for searching out and destroying cells that have gone astray. By supporting your body's natural processes of healing, and by avoiding the toxins that contribute to the formation of mutant cells, you can do a great deal to protect yourself from cancer.

How Cancer Arises

It's important to understand that your body is perfectly equipped to handle cancerous cells. Your cells are constantly replicating—approximately 10 million cells are replaced every second in your body. With so much activity, it's not uncommon for a cell to occasionally turn out a faulty reproduction.

Free Radical
A harmful molecule produced by the body and pollutants. Free radicals have one electron too few or one too many, making them highly unstable.

In addition, cells are continually bombarded by substances that can damage DNA, which is the cellular blueprint for cell reproduction. Cellular injury is often caused by free radicals, which are unstable molecules created as a result of normal metabolic processes, and by environmental factors, such as exposure to cigarette smoke, excessive sunlight, pesticides, and pollution.

When abnormal cells arise, they must be destroyed to keep them from creating additional flawed cells. The job of finding and destroying deviant cells falls to the immune system, where specialized white blood cells hunt for abnormal cells, and eradicate them before they have the opportunity to reproduce. In addition, any cell that begins to multiply uncontrollably is programmed to self-destruct.

Most of the time, these built-in methods of protection are sufficient to prevent the development of cancer. But sometimes, the immune system loses its ability to recognize and destroy cancerous cells, and defective cells can multiply out-of-control. The immune system can also be overwhelmed by large amounts of abnormal cells and not be able to provide adequate protection. Enhancing the ability of your immune system to defend you against the development of cancer is critical.

How to Strengthen Your Immune System

Your immune system is an intricate network of glands, organs, and specialized cells that work together to protect your well-being. The essential components of the immune system include an extensive arrangement of lymph nodes scattered throughout the body, bone marrow, the spleen, the thymus gland, and a variety of white blood cells and other blood elements. It's a complex and magnificient structure, and one that scientists are still learning about. One thing is certain: Your immune system is your first line of defense against cancer, and strengthening your immunity requires a holistic approach that includes diet, exercise, supplements, and a healthy lifestyle. Let's take a closer look at these factors.

One of the primary causes of depressed immunity is a diet lacking in sufficient nutrients. Adequate amounts of protein are necessary for proper immune function, but too much protein can impair immunity. The optimal amount for a healthy immune system is approximately eight ounces of chicken, eggs, fish, tofu, turkey, or other high-quality proteins daily. Avoid commercially produced meats and dairy foods because they often contain residues of antibiotics, which are harmful to the immune system. In addition to protein, eat a wide variety of fresh fruits and vegetables, legumes, nuts, seeds, and whole grains to provide your immune system with an array of vitamins, minerals, and trace nutrients. As much as possible, eat organic foods to avoid the toxic chemicals that are found in commercially produced foods.

What you avoid eating also plays a critical role in the health of your immune system. A diet high in hydrogenated oils, polyunsaturated oils, and saturated fats impairs the functioning of your immune system. And sugar and other concentrated sweeteners can significantly hinder your immune system's capabilities. Studies have shown that even one serving of a sugary food can inhibit immune function for several hours.

Exercise helps to strengthen your immune system in several ways. Approximately thirty to forty-five minutes of moderate exercise, such as brisk walking, has been proven to increase immune activity, relieve stress, and improve lymphatic circulation, all of which enhance immunity. Studies have shown that women who exercise at least four hours a week have a significantly lower risk of breast cancer than women who do not exercise. This may be because exercise helps to regulate estrogen levels. Exercise also boosts mood, which has a positive effect on immune function.

But despite all of the benefits attributed to exercise, it is possible to overdo it. Extremely stressful exercise, such as training for a marathon, has been shown to deplete the immune response. If you are involved in a very strenuous exercise program, you should be careful to get enough rest, allow your body sufficient time to recover after training, and take supplements and herbs that support your immune system.

Getting enough sleep is also essential for keeping your immune system strong. In order to function properly, your body and your immune system need a minimum of seven hours of sleep every night. During sleep, powerful immune-enhancing compounds are released. If you are sleep-deprived, all aspects of your immunity are impaired, and you are more likely to succumb to a virus or other infection. Chronic sleep-deprivation can significantly affect your immune system's ability to protect you from cancer. In our fast-paced world, it's often challenging to make time for sufficient rest and relaxation. But failing to provide your body with time for restoration and rejuvenation creates a state of chronic physical and emotional stress that is one of the primary causes of immune weakness.

A number of research studies have proven that emotional stress has a measurable effect on immunity. During times of stress, adrenal hormones that suppress immune function are released. Living in a continual state of stress wears down your immune system and leaves you much more susceptible to everything from the common cold to cancer. While a stress-filled life that negatively affects your physical and emotional well-being is often accepted as normal, it's certainly not a healthy way to live.

Learning to manage stress is one of the most powerful steps you can take to support your immune system and your overall health. It's important to find ways of relieving stress that are effective for you. Exercise can be a great stress-reliever, as can breathing exercises, meditation, prayer, and yoga. Cultivating close relationships with friends and family also plays a role in building a strong immune system because having people with whom you can share your deepest feelings and concerns is a tremendous stress-reliever and enhances overall well-being.

The Importance of Avoiding Toxins

No matter how committed you are to a healthful diet and lifestyle, we are all exposed to a large number of potentially carcinogenic toxins on a daily basis.

Some of these toxins are environmental pollutants, some are diet-related, and some arise internally as byproducts of natural metabolic processes. These toxins trigger the formation of free radicals, which damage healthy cells and can result in cancerous changes. It's impossible to completely avoid contact with toxic substances, because you don't have control over environmental pollutants, nor can you stop the metabolic processes of your body that generate toxins. But you can limit your exposure to toxic substances as much as possible, and you can decrease your body's production of toxins through diet and supplements.

Researchers are finding that many chemicals in the environment, such as hormones in dairy products and meats, pesticides, and pollutants, have estrogenlike activity. These chemicals are referred to as hormonal disrupters, or xenoestrogens, and are suspected of playing a role in hormonally triggered cancers, such as breast cancer and uterine cancer.

Some plastics can also be hormonal disrupters, especially the plastic wrap used by most supermarkets for wrapping cheese, fish, poultry, and meat. It contains a chemical known as DEHA, which readily migrates into food. To be safe, avoid buying foods wrapped in plastic, and never microwave foods in plastic wrap or plastic containers.

Other actions you can take to decrease your exposure to toxins include avoiding unnecessary exposure to radiation, choosing natural alternatives to chemical household and garden products, drinking filtered water, and eating organic foods. Of course, it's absolutely essential to avoid tobacco smoke, which accounts for one-third of all cancer deaths. It's also a good idea to limit your alcohol intake to no more than one drink per day. If you are at high risk for breast cancer, it's probably best to refrain completely from drinking alcohol. Some research indicates that even small amounts of alcohol are associated with an increased incidence of breast cancer.

Prevent Cancer with Fruits and Vegetables

As previously discussed, eating a diet rich in protective nutrients is vitally important for healthy immune functioning. Because diet is targeted as being responsible for one-third of all cancers, it makes sense to understand, as much as possible, how to safeguard your health through nutrition. One of the most important dietary changes you can make is to increase the amount of fresh fruits and vegetables that you eat. Fresh fruits and vegetables are the richest sources of antioxidants, which help to neutralize free radical damage. In addition, they contain other protective phytochemicals, such as flavonoids and carotenoids.

Try to eat at least seven servings of fresh fruits and vegetables every day, and preferably strive for ten servings. A

Carcinogen
A toxic substance in the environment, in our diet, or as a byproduct of normal metabolic processes in our bodies, that causes cancer.

Xenoestrogen
A chemical toxin that acts like estrogen and disrupts hormonal activity in the body.

Phytochemicals
Compounds in plants, such as flavonoids and carotenoids, that have protective, disease-preventing properties.

serving is one-half cup of a vegetable, one cup of leafy greens, one average-size piece of fruit, one-half cup of fruit, or six ounces of fresh fruit or vegetable juice. To get a wide range of protective nutrients, vary the fruits and vegetables you eat and choose those that have the deepest, richest colors—for example, choose dark green leafy romaine or red lettuce over pale iceberg lettuce and dark purple grapes over green grapes. A variety of color in your choices will provide a variety of beneficial nutrients.

Certain vegetables and fruits contain special protective compounds, and it's worthwhile to include these foods in your diet as often as possible. Broccoli, cabbage, cauliflower, collards, kale, and other members of the cruciferous

Glutathione
A powerful detoxifying and antioxidant compound made by the body and found in some foods, including those in the cruciferous vegetable family.

family are rich in beneficial sulfur compounds called indoles; cruciferous vegetables also enhance the production of glutathione, which helps to neutralize carcinogens. Garlic, onions, scallions, and other members of the allium family improve immune activity and increase the levels of the enzymes that break down carcinogens.

Foods rich in vitamin C and beta-carotene have potent antioxidant activity. Broccoli, citrus fruits, red peppers, and strawberries are good sources of vitamin C. Dark leafy green vegetables and deep yellow-orange fruits and vegetables, such as apricots, cantaloupe, carrots, and sweet potatoes, are high in beta-carotene, which may help to reverse precancerous changes in cells.

Eating a variety of fruits and vegetables ensures that you are providing your cells with a comprehensive array of cancer-fighting phytonutrients, such as ellagic acid, limonene, and lycopene. Apples, grapes, raspberries, and strawberries contain ellagic acid; lemons, limes, and oranges are rich in limonene; and carrots, red peppers, tomatoes, and watermelon are good sources of lycopene.

Other Dietary Suggestions for Cancer Prevention

Because experts estimate that at least one-third of all cancers are directly related to diet, it makes sense to eat as healthfully as possible. In addition to eating generous amounts of fruits and vegetables, the most important dietary steps you can take to prevent cancer are to choose healthful fats, including omega-3 fatty acids, consume plenty of fiber, drink green tea, and eat soy foods daily.

Current research indicates that the *type* of fat you eat is much more important than the *amount* of fat in your diet. Hydrogenated oils, polyunsaturated oils, and saturated fats have all been associated with an increased risk of cancer.

These types of fats have been found to generate large numbers of cell-damaging free radicals; they also create chemicals in the intestinal tract that are converted by bacteria into harmful types of estrogen involved in breast and reproductive cancers.

Worst of all are hydrogenated or partially hydrogenated oils; they contain trans-fatty acids, a particularly harmful fat to your cells. Trans-fatty acids are created during a chemical process known as hydrogenation during which oils are made solid or semi-solid at room temperature. Hydrogenated and partially hydrogenated fats are found in many margarines, vegetable shortenings, and baked goods and processed foods made with these fats. Polyunsaturated oils, such as corn, safflower, soybean, and sunflower oils, are highly susceptible to oxidation (which creates cell-damaging free radicals) when exposed to air, heat, and light. It is impossible to keep these oils from turning rancid in your kitchen, and most of the time, they have already started to oxidize before they leave the store shelves. Saturated fats are found in large amounts in full-fat dairy products, poultry skin, red meat, and tropical oils, such as coconut and palm oils. It's best to minimize these foods in your diet.

Now for the good news about fats. Certain types of fats, especially olive oil and omega-3 fats, are beneficial for your health and help protect against cancer. Olive oil is a monounsaturated fat that makes your cell membranes more resistant to the destructive effects of free radicals. In large population studies of Mediterranean cultures, a high intake of olive oil has been associated with their remarkably low rates of cancer. The premium type is extra-virgin olive oil. It's made from the first pressing of olives, has the best flavor, and contains the most protective nutrients.

Omega-3 fats, found in cold-water fish, flaxseed, and walnuts, also help to protect cell membranes and inhibit the development of cancerous cells. In a recent study in Tours, France, reported in the *International Journal of Cancer*, 241 women with breast cancer and 88 women with benign breast disease had samples of breast tissue taken during surgery; the fatty tissue was then examined for omega-3 fatty acid content (the body stores omega-3 fats and other fats in fatty tissues, such as breast tissue). The researchers found that those women with higher levels of omega-3 fats in their tissues had a significantly lower incidence of breast cancer. Omega-3 fats have also been shown to be protective against other types of cancers.

Lignans
A type of phyto-estrogen, found in flaxseeds, that helps protect against breast cancer and other cancers.

To saturate your cells with these beneficial fatty acids, eat two to three servings of cold-water fish, such as salmon and sardines, weekly; a small handful of walnuts several times a week; and take one tablespoon of flaxseed oil, or one tablespoon of freshly ground flaxseeds daily. Ground flaxseeds and specially processed flaxseed oil are rich sources of lignans, compounds that help to inhibit the growth of estrogen-related cancers.

Never heat or cook with flaxseed oil, but instead, add it to salad dressings, or pour it onto baked potatoes, pasta, vegetables, or other dishes.

Soy foods are extremely beneficial in helping to prevent cancer. Soybeans contain compounds called protease inhibitors, which block the action of enzymes that stimulate tumor growth.

The anticancer substances found in soy foods work to block cancer in several ways. They inhibit the development of blood vessels that feed tumors and make them grow, they speed up the death of cancer cells, and they help break down carcinogens in the body. Soy foods are especially helpful for women. They contain a natural plant estrogen called genistein, which blocks estrogen from causing cancerous changes in hormone-sensitive tissues, such as the breasts. To reap the cancer-protective benefits of soybeans, consume four ounces of soy foods, such as tempeh or tofu, or one cup of soy milk daily.

Protease Inhibitor

Plant compounds found in soybeans that block the action of enzymes that stimulate tumor growth.

Few women obtain sufficient dietary fiber, and yet fiber is essential for preventing cancer. A fiber-rich diet helps move waste products efficiently through the intestinal tract, and keeps toxins from lingering in the body. Fiber has the additional benefit of helping to reduce levels of harmful estrogen because it binds to this estrogen in the intestinal tract and prevents it from being reabsorbed into the bloodstream. For optimal protection, eat between twenty-five and thirty-five grams of fiber daily. Some of the best sources of fiber include fruits, legumes, and vegetables. If your diet falls short of providing sufficient fiber, you can increase your intake with fiber supplements made from flaxseeds, guar gum, pectin, and psyllium seed husks. Take between one and three tablespoons daily.

Green tea helps protect against cancer in more than one way. It contains compounds called polyphenols, which are potent antioxidants that prevent free radicals from damaging healthy cells.

These compounds all support the body's efforts to eliminate carcinogens, improve the cells' resistance to cancer-causing substances, and help prevent cancer cells from multiplying. Researchers believe that one compelling reason the Japanese have a significantly lower incidence of cancer is their daily habit of drinking green tea. To obtain the protective benefits of green tea, drink at least three cups daily. Since green tea has a subtle flavor that can quickly turn bitter if it is steeped for too long, to get the best flavor, you should bring water

Polyphenols

Potent antioxidants, found abundantly in green tea, that prevent free radicals from damaging healthy cells.

to a boil, let it cool slightly before pouring it over the tea, then steep it no longer than three minutes. If you prefer, you can use a standardized extract of green tea. Take approximately 400 mg daily of an extract standardized to 90 percent polyphenols.

Supplements for Preventing Cancer

Dietary supplements provide a concentrated source of nutrients that help strengthen your immune system and protect your cells from cancer-causing substances. For starters, it's a good idea to take a high-potency multivitamin and mineral supplement to provide your immune system with the nutrients it needs to function optimally. The supplement should contain 50 mg of B-vitamin complex, including 400 mcg of folic acid, which helps prevent cervical dysplasia, a potential precursor to uterine cancer. It should also contain 400 IU of vitamin D because a clear relationship has been established between a deficiency of vitamin D and breast cancer.

Make sure that your multivitamin supplement supplies a variety of antioxidants, including beta-carotene and mixed carotenoids (25,000 IU), vitamin C (500 mg), vitamin E (400–800 IU), selenium (200 mcg), and zinc (25 mg). If your multivitamin and mineral falls short of these recommendations, take additional supplements to fill the gap. In addition, CoQ_{10} has potent antioxidant properties. Take 30–60 mg daily.

Herbal Help for Immune Support

Herbs can be valuable allies in protecting your immune system and helping ward off cancer. Some of the most potent protective herbs are found in Chinese medicine, which has a long tradition of using herbs to strengthen immunity.

Astragalus (*Astragalus membranaceous*) is a fibrous root that has proven effective for increasing immune activity, and is also prescribed for restoring immune function in people who have undergone radiation or chemotherapy. Maitake (*Grifola frondosa*), reishi (*Ganoderma lucidum*), and shiitake (*Lentinula edodes*) are all mushrooms with powerful immune-enhancing properties; they also inhibit the growth of cancer. All these herbs are available as extracts, or in capsules, and can be taken long-term for immune enhancement. Follow the manufacturer's dosage recommendations.

Supplements for Cancer Prevention

- High-potency multivitamin and mineral supplement daily that includes:
  - Beta-carotene with mixed carotenoids: 25,000 IU daily
  - Folic acid: 400 mcg daily
  - Selenium: 200 mcg daily
  - Vitamin C: 500–1,000 mg daily

- Vitamin D: 400 IU daily

- Vitamin E: 400–800 IU daily

- Zinc: 25 mg daily

- CoQ_{10}: 30–60 mg daily

- Flaxseed oil with lignans: 1 tablespoon daily

- Astragalus, maitake, reishi, or shiitake, for immune support: follow label instructions for dosages

- Green tea: three cups daily, or 400 mg of a standardized extract

PREVENTING HEART DISEASE

Many people still have the misconception that heart disease is something that happens primarily to men. It's true that women are fortunate in having the natural heart-protective effects of estrogen prior to menopause. Estrogen helps to keep coronary arteries flexible, and also plays an important role in keeping cholesterol levels low. But during and after menopause, when estrogen levels naturally decline, the risk of heart disease for women increases dramatically. After menopause, women are more likely than men to be stricken with heart disease. In fact, cardiovascular disease is the leading cause of death for women, affecting one out of every three women over the age of sixty-five.

Recent studies have shown that hormone replacement therapy, which was long thought to provide cardiovascular protection for post-menopausal women, does not help to prevent heart disease, and is probably a bad idea for women who have a prior history of heart disease. A four-year study of 2,763 postmenopausal women with a history of heart disease, reported in the *Journal of the American Medical Association* in 1998, revealed that hormone replacement therapy *increased* cardiac risk during the first year of use. As a result, the American Heart Association recently recommended against hormone replacement therapy for the prevention of heart disease by women with a history of cardiovascular disease. As for healthy post-menopausal women, the association says there is insufficient evidence to indicate that hormone replacement therapy prevents heart disease.

Fortunately, with the proper diet, exercise, and supplements, there is a great deal else you can do to keep your cardiovascular system healthy.

Heart Disease: Risk Factors for Women

- A family history of heart disease

- A high total cholesterol, high triglycerides, and a low HDL cholesterol

- A sedentary lifestyle

- Being over age sixty-five

- Being more than 20 percent over ideal weight

- Cigarette smoking

- Diabetes

- Entering menopause before age forty-five

- Having excess weight in the abdomen

- High blood pressure

- High levels of homocysteine

- High levels of stress

The Causes of Heart Disease

Heart attacks and strokes are the most common cardiovascular diseases. The primary contributing factors are atherosclerosis (a thickening and hardening of the arteries) and high blood pressure. Atherosclerosis occurs when the lining of an artery is injured by free radicals, unstable molecules that occur naturally in the body or can be initiated by exposure to environmental toxins, stress, or a virus. The body attempts to repair the damage, and in the process, cholesterol, other fats, and cellular debris all accumulate in the arteries and roughen the artery walls with plaque, at which point platelets and other compounds in the blood can stick to their surface and form a clot. The disease often progresses silently until arterial blockage causes a heart attack or stroke.

Atherosclerosis *A thickening and hardening of the arteries, which can lead to heart attacks and strokes.*

Although it would seem that lowering cholesterol levels is the most critical step for preventing atherosclerosis, it's not the only factor in the development of heart disease. High cholesterol levels can play a role in atherosclerosis, but not all people with high cholesterol have clogged arteries, and people with atherosclerosis can have cholesterol levels in the normal range.

However, conventional medical practitioners tend to focus on cholesterol, and usually prescribe cholesterol-lowering drugs. While these drugs do help to decrease cholesterol levels, they can have unpleasant and even dangerous side effects, including possible liver damage. A better approach is to focus on lowering your cholesterol naturally and protecting your arteries from free radical damage, at the same time identifying and reducing other risk factors.

Understanding Cholesterol

Cholesterol is a waxy, fatlike substance that is found in every cell of your body. Even if you were to eat a no-cholesterol diet, your body would still manufacture it, because cholesterol is essential for the production of bile, cell membranes, hormones, and vitamin D. Cholesterol only becomes a problem when too much of it accumulates in your bloodstream or arteries. Factors that contribute to this unhealthy buildup include a lack of dietary nutrients essential to the normal metabolism of cholesterol, poor liver function, or a sedentary lifestyle.

It's important to note that not all cholesterol is implicated in cardiovascular disease. A type of cholesterol called HDL (high-density lipoproteins) actually helps protect your arteries, and you want as much of this beneficial cholesterol as possible in your bloodstream. But for cardiovascular health, you want low levels of LDL cholesterol (low-density lipoproteins) and low levels of triglycerides (another type of blood fat).

Here's how cholesterol operates in your body: It is carried in your blood on molecules called lipoproteins. Low-density lipoproteins (LDL) transport cholesterol and triglycerides from your liver to your cells. While it's circulating through your bloodstream, cholesterol can accumulate on artery walls. High-density lipoproteins (HDL) pick up this cholesterol from the arteries and return it to the liver, where it is metabolized and eliminated.

Lipoproteins
Molecules in the bloodstream that transport cholesterol and trigylcerides to and from your liver and your cells.

Although high levels of LDL cholesterol and triglycerides are clearly associated with an increased risk of cardiovascular disease, people who have high levels of HDL cholesterol tend to have a low risk of clogged arteries. On the other hand, if your HDL levels are too low, you are at risk for cardiovascular disease, even if you have a low level of total cholesterol. For cardiovascular health, you should focus on lowering your LDL cholesterol and triglycerides while raising your HDL cholesterol. It's not as complicated as it sounds. Many of the lifestyle and dietary suggestions that lower harmful cholesterol also boost helpful cholesterol.

For optimal cardiovascular protection, your total cholesterol should be less than 200 mg/dl, your LDL no higher than 130 (preferably closer to 100), your triglycerides less than 150 mg/dl, and your HDL greater than 35. More important than the individual numbers in your cholesterol profile, however, is the ratio of your HDL cholesterol to your total cholesterol, and also the ratio of your LDL to HDL. This tells you how effectively your liver is metabolizing and eliminating cholesterol. The ideal ratio of total cholesterol to HDL is below 3.5, and the ratio of LDL to HDL should be no higher than 2.5.

Managing Blood Pressure

High blood pressure (also called hypertension) is the most common type of cardiovascular disease. A blood pressure reading of more than 140/90 puts you in the category of having hypertension, and greatly increases your risk of heart disease and stroke. The vast majority of the time, there is no physiological cause of high blood pressure. However, there are a number of factors that contribute to elevated blood pressure, principally a diet high in sodium or low in calcium, magnesium, and potassium, excessive alcohol intake, overweight—and stress.

Although doctors often prescribe drugs for controlling blood pressure, drugs can cause such side effects as dizziness and fatigue, and can increase levels of harmful cholesterol and triglycerides. It's far better to avoid drugs and adopt lifestyle changes, such as eating a healthful diet, exercising regularly, managing stress, and taking nutritional supplements and herbs. If you have hypertension, it's essential that you monitor your blood pressure regularly to make sure it is within a healthy range.

Other Risk Factors in Heart Disease

Although high cholesterol is generally regarded as the primary cause of cardiovascular disease, there are two other factors—homocysteine and fibrinogen—that should also be considered. Homocysteine, a byproduct of the metabolism of the amino acid methionine, is usually neutralized by your body into harmless compounds. But if you are deficient in folic acid, vitamin B_6, or vitamin B_{12}, homocysteine levels can increase to dangerous levels in the blood. Homocysteine damages arteries, increases the risk of blood clots, and promotes the buildup of cholesterol in arteries.

Homocysteine
A byproduct of amino-acid metabolism that can be a risk factor in heart disease if there are high levels of it in the blood.

You can generally obtain an adequate supply of B-vitamins by taking a B-complex supplement that supplies 400 mcg of folic acid, 50 mg of B_6, and 400 mcg of B_{12}. Some people, however, are genetically predisposed to high levels of homocysteine, and may have much greater requirements for B-vitamins than the recommended standard amounts. If you have high levels of homocysteine in your blood, you should work with your health practitioner to determine the correct dosages of B-complex supplements.

Fibrinogen is another factor that plays a role in cardiovascular disease. A blood protein, fibrinogen makes blood platelets sticky and is necessary for blood clotting. But, if you have too much fibrinogen in your blood, it becomes sticky and you run the risk of forming blood clots.

Causes of excess fibrinogen include high levels of LDL cholesterol, high blood-sugar levels, obesity, smoking, stress, and synthetic estrogen in birth control pills and hormone replacement therapy. You can keep your fibrinogen levels under control by eating foods, such as garlic and omega-3 fatty acids (found in flaxseeds, salmon, and walnuts), that help keep blood

Fibrinogen
A blood protein that makes blood platelets sticky and promotes blood clotting. Too much fibrinogen can cause dangerous blood clots.

platelets from becoming overly sticky. Regular exercise also helps to keep fibrinogen in a healthy range.

A Heart-Healthy Diet

Your diet is a powerful tool in keeping your heart and circulatory system healthy. Through diet, you can decrease your LDL cholesterol and triglycerides, increase your levels of beneficial HDL cholesterol, and lower your blood pressure. To make the transition to a heart-healthy diet, make sure you are including plenty of fresh fruits and vegetables, fish, green tea, healthy fats (such as olive oil), legumes, nuts, oats, and soy foods in your daily diet. In addition, it is essential to avoid trans-fatty acids completely, limit your intake of refined foods, salt, and sugar, and reduce saturated fats. Here's the rationale behind these suggestions.

Fresh fruits and vegetables are rich sources of antioxidants, which help to prevent free radicals from damaging your heart and arteries, and aid in keeping blood pressure low. Fruits and vegetables are also high in potassium, which is essential for keeping blood pressure in a favorable range. A deficiency of potassium causes cells to retain too much sodium, which increases fluid retention and raises blood pressure. Researchers at the Heart, Lung, and Blood Institute (part of the National Institutes of Health) have developed a diet based on a large-scale research study that identified dietary factors affecting blood pressure. Their recommendations—which have been shown to lower blood pressure as effectively as prescription drugs—emphasize eating eight to ten servings of fruits and vegetables daily.

That's not as daunting as it may seem, when you consider that a serving is one piece of fruit, one-half cup of vegetables, or one cup of leafy greens. A glass of orange juice and blueberries with breakfast, carrot sticks for a snack, a salad, or a bowl of vegetable soup for lunch, a stir-fry with a generous amount of vegetables for dinner, and a fresh fruit bowl for dessert easily meet the goal.

Fresh fruits and vegetables also supply soluble fiber, which helps to sweep excess cholesterol out of the body. Apples, carrots, and citrus fruits are especially good sources, and legumes and some grains (barley and oatmeal) are loaded with this helpful type of fiber. Try to eat between twenty-five and thirty-five grams of fiber daily, with an emphasis on foods rich in soluble fiber.

Fish (especially fish high in omega-3 fatty acids, such as salmon and sardines), raw nuts (such as almonds and walnuts), and healthy fats (such as extra-virgin olive oil) keep arteries flexible, promote the production of beneficial HDL cholesterol, and help to lower blood pressure. Eat at least two servings of omega-3-rich fish weekly, a small handful of nuts, and a tablespoon or more of olive oil daily. Flaxseed oil is also a good source of omega-3 fatty acids and is beneficial for lowering cholesterol. Take one tablespoon daily.

Soy foods, such as soymilk, tempeh, and tofu, have been shown to help lower cholesterol levels. Eat at least one serving of these foods every day. And green tea is a good source of protective antioxidants called polyphenols that help to lower cholesterol and prevent the oxidation of cholesterol. For optimal protection, drink three cups of green tea daily. To prevent bitterness, steep green tea for no more than three minutes. If you are highly sensitive to caffeine, try a decaffeinated variety.

Eliminating certain foods from your diet is also critical for your cardiovascular health. Saturated fats (the most concentrated sources are full-fat dairy products and red meat) and trans-fats (found in partially hydrogenated oils) increase cholesterol levels. In addition, trans-fats raise LDL cholesterol and decrease beneficial HDL cholesterol. It's also best to avoid polyunsaturated oils, such as corn, safflower, and soy oil. When these oils are heated or exposed to light, they quickly become rancid and form compounds that are damaging to the arteries.

In recent years, sugar has been identified as a prime suspect in the development of cardiovascular disease. Eating excessive amounts of sugary foods and refined carbohydrates triggers the production of insulin, a hormone that is secreted by the pancreas and regulates how your cells use sugar. If your cells are subjected to frequent overdoses of sugar and simple carbohydrates, they can lose their ability to respond appropriately to insulin. The result is that the pancreas continues to produce insulin, and elevated levels of insulin raise cholesterol and triglyceride levels and increase blood pressure. To prevent insulin resistance, avoid sugars (which can be disguised as concentrated fruit juice sweeteners, corn syrup, fructose, glucose, honey, lactose, maltose, maple syrup, and sucrose) and refined carbohydrates.

Because sodium may be a factor in hypertension, it's important to cut back on excess salt. Too much sodium can cause water retention, which swells blood volume and increases blood pressure. Reducing your sodium intake is simple if you avoid processed foods, which generally contain large amounts of salt or related sodium compounds, such as monosodium glutamate. In addition, avoid obvious sources of excess sodium, such as chips and salted pretzels. When cooking, you can usually cut in half the amount of salt called for in recipes, and you won't even notice the difference.

Supplements for Cardiovascular Health

A variety of supplements, including herbs, can help keep your heart and cardiovascular system healthy. Antioxidants, such as beta-carotene and other carotenoids, grapeseed extract, selenium, vitamin C, and vitamin E, all help to prevent artery damage caused by free radicals. Grapeseed extract is a rich source of natural compounds, called proanthocyanidins, which have powerful antioxidant properties. These compounds improve circulation, inhibit the oxidation of LDL cholesterol, prevent the clumping of blood platelets that can lead to clots, prevent damage to the arteries, and strengthen the blood vessel walls. Take 50 mg daily as a preventive dose, or 150 mg daily if you have high cholesterol or heart disease.

Proanthocyanidins *Natural compounds, found abundantly in grapeseed extract, that have powerful antioxidant properties and help protect the cardiovascular system.*

Coenzyme Q_{10} is one of the most important supplements you can take to protect your cardiovascular system. It is an enzyme that is vital for the production of energy within the cells, and it is found in especially high concentrations in the heart. CoQ_{10} has antioxidant activity, helps to prevent LDL cholesterol from oxidizing, and improves heart function. As a protective dose, take 30–60 mg of CoQ_{10} once a day. If you have cardiovascular disease, take up to 240 mg daily, divided into two equal doses. For best absorption, take CoQ_{10} in gel capsules with a meal that contains some fat.

The B-complex vitamins (especially folic acid, B_6, and B_{12}) help to prevent dangerous levels of homocysteine from accumulating. For most women, taking a B-complex supplement that provides 400 mcg of folic acid, 50 mg of B_6, and 400 mcg of B_{12} will control homocysteine levels. But if you have high levels of homocysteine, you may need larger amounts of these B-vitamins. Consult your healthcare practitioner to determine the appropriate dosage.

Magnesium works in a variety of ways to improve cardiovascular health. It dilates the coronary arteries, which improves blood flow to the heart, increases beneficial HDL cholesterol, prevents blood platelets from clumping together, and stabilizes heart rhythm. Take 400–600 mg of magnesium daily.

If you are postmenopausal, you shouldn't be eating iron-fortified foods or taking multivitamin supplements that contain iron. Iron can accumulate in your body, promoting free radicals that oxidize cholesterol and damage arteries.

Niacin Therapy for High Cholesterol

Niacin (vitamin B_3) has been recognized for more than fifty years as an effective treatment for lowering cholesterol levels. Not only does niacin decrease total cholesterol, but it also lowers triglycerides and fibrinogen levels, and at the same time increases the levels of beneficial HDL cholesterol. In a 1994 clinical study published in the *Annals of Internal Medicine*, researchers compared niacin and the cholesterol-lowering drug lovastatin. After twenty-six weeks of therapy, patients taking lovastatin had a 32 percent decrease in LDL cholesterol, while those taking niacin had a 23 percent decrease. However, those taking niacin had a 33 percent *increase* in HDL cholesterol, while those taking lovastatin had only a 7 percent increase. Niacin compared reasonably

well to drug therapy for decreasing LDL cholesterol, but was clearly the winner for increasing beneficial HDL cholesterol.

Large doses of niacin are necessary for lowering cholesterol, and although the therapy is generally safe, it does cause a harmless flushing of the chest and face. To prevent this reaction, take inositol hexaniacinate, 500 mg two to three times a day. Do not take sustained-release niacin supplements, because they can be toxic to the liver. If you have diabetes, do not take large amounts of niacin without the supervision of your doctor, because niacin can affect blood-sugar levels.

If you want to use niacin to improve your cholesterol profile, your should have your cholesterol and liver enzymes monitored. Positive results are usually seen in about two months, but may take six months or more, especially for cholesterol levels above 300 mg/dl. When your cholesterol levels go below 200 mg/dl, you can gradually discontinue the niacin and have your cholesterol level checked after two months. If necessary, resume taking niacin until your cholesterol has stabilized at a level below 200 mg/dl.

Herbs for Your Heart

Herbs play a valuable role in a holistic approach to cardiovascular health. Some herbs can be used as tonics to keep your heart and arteries healthy, while others are specific remedies for such problems as high cholesterol and hypertension.

One of the best herbs for your cardiovascular system is one that you probably have in your kitchen. Garlic (*Allium sativum*) is not only a delicious addition to meals, but has significant effects on cholesterol profiles and blood pressure. When taken regularly, garlic increases beneficial HDL cholesterol, lowers blood pressure, lowers LDL cholesterol and triglycerides, prevents the oxidation of cholesterol that causes artery damage, and reduces the risk of blood clots. Both raw and cooked garlic are beneficial, but raw garlic has more powerful properties. To reap the beneficial effects of garlic, consume one or two cloves per day. If you can't tolerate fresh garlic, take a standardized extract that provides a daily dose of at least 10 mg of alliin (recognized as the active ingredient), which is equal to approximately one clove of fresh garlic.

Flavonoids *Powerful antioxidant compounds that help protect cells from free radical damage.*

Hawthorn (*Crataegus oxycantha*) has been used in Europe for centuries as a cardiovascular tonic. Hawthorn contains flavonoids (antioxidant compounds) that increase blood flow to the heart, reduce blood pressure, and strengthen and steady the heartbeat. Hawthorn also helps to lower blood pressure, and protects the arteries against free radical damage.

As a protective tonic, hawthorn can be made into a pleasant-tasting tea by pouring one cup of boiling water over two teaspoons of the berries and steeping them for fifteen minutes. Drink two cups daily. If you have cardiovascular disease, take one teaspoon of liquid extract or 120–240 mg of a standardized extract three times daily. The best results are obtained with long-term use. However, if you are taking medication for any type of cardiovascular disease, check with your healthcare professional before taking hawthorn, because it can magnify the effects of cardiovascular drugs.

Guggulipid (*Commiphora mukul*) is an Ayurvedic herb that is used in the treatment of high cholesterol and atherosclerosis. It improves the ability of the liver to process cholesterol, and helps to lower LDL cholesterol while increasing beneficial HDL cholesterol. In clinical studies, guggulipid has been shown to be as effective as pharmaceutical drugs for lowering cholesterol. Guggulipid is generally standardized to contain 2.5 percent guggulsterones. Take 25 mg of guggulsterones three times a day for at least four weeks. Guggulipid is safe, but should not be used during pregnancy because it may stimulate uterine bleeding.

The Importance of Lifestyle

While an appropriate diet and supplements can go a long way toward protecting your cardiovascular system, there's no doubt that other lifestyle factors also play a prominent role in the health of your heart and arteries. Regular exercise, managing stress, and avoiding exposure to toxins are also critical for optimal cardiovascular health.

Your heart is a muscle and needs the stimulus of regular aerobic exercise to be strong and healthy. Exercise also improves circulation, keeps blood pressure low, helps to decrease cholesterol and triglycerides while increasing HDL cholesterol, and is a great stress-reliever. Plan for at least thirty minutes of aerobic exercise five days a week.

Emotional stress can wreak havoc on your heart and cardiovascular system, and addressing the stressors in your life is essential for preventing cardiovascular disease. When you are stressed, adrenaline and other hormones that increase blood pressure and heart rate are released into your bloodstream. Chronic or prolonged stress causes elevated cholesterol, free-radical damage, and high blood pressure. Learning to manage stress is one of the most helpful things you can do to protect your heart and arteries. Deep breathing exercises, meditation, and yoga are all proven ways of reducing stress. For best results, choose a technique of stress management that appeals to you and practice it daily.

Reducing your exposure to environmental toxins is another important factor in preventing cardiovascular disease. Household and garden chemicals, over-the-counter and prescription drugs, and tobacco smoke are all toxins that trigger the production of free radicals that damage arteries. You can decrease your exposure to environmental toxins by avoiding tobacco smoke, buying organic foods, drinking filtered water, using herbs and natural remedies instead of pharmaceutical drugs, and using natural household and garden products.

Supplements for Cardiovascular Health

- B-complex: 50–100 mg daily, containing at least:
  - B_6: 50 mg
  - B_{12}: 400 mcg
  - Folic acid: 400 mcg
- Beta-carotene with mixed carotenoids: 25,000 IU daily
- Vitamin C: 500 mg daily
- Vitamin E: 400 IU daily
- Selenium: 200 mcg daily
- Magnesium: 400–600 mg daily
- CoQ_{10}: 30–60 mg daily (up to 240 mg if you have cardiovascular disease)
- Grapeseed extract: 50–150 mg daily
- Flaxseed oil: 1 tablespoon daily
- Garlic: 1 clove, or 10 mg alliin daily
- Hawthorn: 2 cups tea daily (1 teaspoon fluid extract or 120–240 mg standardized extract three times daily if you have cardiovascular disease)
- Guggulipid: 25 mg gugglesterones (if you have high cholesterol)

HOW TO BUY AND USE NUTRITIONAL SUPPLEMENTS

It seems that new research appears almost daily regarding the benefits of dietary nutrients, supplements, and herbs and their role in maintaining health. There's no question that dietary supplements make an important contribution to optimal well-being. But choosing between the vast array of products available can be confusing. In reading this book, you've learned about the supplements that are best suited to your particular needs. Now, you need information that will enable you to buy and use supplements with confidence.

Determining Your Supplement Needs

First, it's important to address the question of whether you need to take supplements at all. Unless you live in a pristine environment, eat a perfectly balanced organic diet, get just the right amount of exercise and rest, and are under no stress, then the answer is yes—supplements are a good idea. We live in a world that has a greater number of chemical toxins than ever before in history, and the quality of our air, soil, and water has been seriously compromised. In general, the nutrient content of most foods is diminished because we're not getting food fresh from the garden—instead, it's transported across the country, and sometimes across the world, losing nutrients in the process.

Most of us don't consume even the meager five servings a day of fruits and vegetables recommended by the government for preventing disease. That's far below the recommendations of experts who suggest that, for optimal health, we should be eating approximately nine to ten servings of fruits and vegetables daily. While it's essential to plan for a healthy diet, the reality is that most of us fall short, at least some of the time. This is where dietary supplements can insure that you're providing your body with the nutrients it needs to function optimally and stay healthy.

A good foundation for a supplement program is a well-rounded high-potency multivitamin and mineral. A well-balanced multiple will provide most of the basic nutrients you need. You can then fill in any gaps with additional supplements, and add specific herbs and nutrients that fit your particular needs. It's important, however, to realize that supplements are not a substitute for a healthful diet and lifestyle. No amount of supplements can make up for insufficient sleep, a lack of exercise, a poor diet, or such habits as cigarette smoking or excessive alcohol intake. But by following the dietary and lifestyle suggestions in this book, and taking the recommended supplements, you can be assured that you are taking the right steps to provide your body with all that it needs for optimal health and well-being.

Because people vary somewhat in their nutritional needs, it's necessary to realize that the guidelines this book, or anywhere else, are merely guidelines. The recommendations here are based on the latest research and are safe when taken in the suggested dosages. But you may have greater or lesser needs for certain nutrients, depending on your age, your biochemistry, your genetic heritage, your diet and lifestyle, and your current state of health. To determine what is optimal for you, it's best to work with a health practitioner who is skilled in prescribing dietary supplements.

How to Take Supplements

Taking supplements properly involves more than just gulping them down with a glass of water. Most supplements are assimilated best when taken with, or just after, a meal. This is especially true for supplements that are better absorbed with a meal containing some fat, such as vitamins A, D, E, and CoQ_{10}. A bit of protein also aids in the absorption of minerals. And taking supplements with meals helps prevent the digestive upset that can occasionally occur if you take supplements on an empty stomach. If you are taking liquid herbal supplements, however, they seem to be best absorbed on an empty stomach. Take them a few minutes before a meal, and dilute the dosage with a small amount of water or juice to make them more palatable.

If you can remember to do so, it's also best to divide up supplement dosages so that you're taking them two or three times a day instead of all at once. This provides your body with a consistent supply of nutrients throughout the day, improves absorption, and minimizes the amount that is excreted. For example, with some nutrients, such as calcium, your body can't absorb more than about 500 mg at a time.

Don't err on the side of thinking that more is better. That's not necessarily true, and in the case of certain nutrients, such as vitamins A or D, taking too much can actually be harmful. Even in the case of antioxidants, which are invaluable for protecting cells against damage, taking too much of them can be counterproductive and cause fatigue. Stick with the amounts recommended in this book, or consult your health practitioner if you think you would benefit from larger dosages of any of the supplements recommended here.

Some supplements, such as herbal products, tend to vary greatly in potency. If you're uncertain about how much you should take, it's safe to follow the manufacturer's recommendations on the label. It's also wise to continue educating yourself about your health. There are many excellent books that can guide you in making appropriate choices, including those listed in the References section of this book.

Buying and Storing Supplements

Shelves of natural foods stores, supermarkets, and drug stores are typically stocked with hundreds of nutritional and herbal supplements. If you go into the store knowing what you're looking for, you're ahead of the game. You shouldn't depend on a store clerk to provide you with supplement prescriptions. Although some may be well-educated in the use of supplements, it's best if you have some understanding about which supplements are appropriate for your needs and goals. There are many wonderful resources available, written by leading health experts who can guide you in the right direction. When in doubt, you should consult your healthcare practitioner for advice.

When choosing between various brands of supplements, you'll invariably see a wide variation in price. More expensive is not necessarily better, but just as with most other things in life, there is usually a correlation between price and quality. In other words, you generally get what you pay for. Higher quality products are usually made without artificial colors, preservatives, or sugar.

As far as the question of natural versus synthetic, in most cases, it doesn't really make a difference. Most nutrients have to go through a significant amount of processing to condense them into a capsule or tablet. But one nutrient that should always be taken in the natural form is vitamin E because the synthetic form is not effective. Natural vitamin E is identified as d-alpha tocopherol (preferably formulated with mixed tocopherols) and synthetic vitamin E is listed on labels as dl-alpha tocopherol.

It's also important to buy supplements in a form that appeals to you. Some people have trouble swallowing large vitamin tablets. Hard tablets can also be difficult to digest, and your body may not break them down efficiently. Capsules of powdered supplements or softgel capsules are usually easier to digest.

To maintain potency, store your supplements in a cool, dark place, such as a kitchen cabinet away from the stove. Don't keep them in the bathroom because high levels of humidity also affect potency. Most supplements should not be refrigerated, either, with the exception of gel capsules of oil-based supplements, such as vitamin E, CoQ_{10}, and evening primrose oil.

To reap the maximum benefits from nutritional supplements, you need to take them consistently. Obviously, if the supplements are just sitting in your kitchen cabinet, they're not doing you any good! To help remember to take your supplements, establish a specific time (for example, always take them immediately after meals). It usually takes a month or two to obtain the benefits of nutritional supplements, and for many herbs, it can take three months or more.

It's important to give dietary supplements time to have an effect. But it's equally important to periodically review the supplements you are taking to make sure they are meeting your needs. At least every six months, inventory the supplements you are taking and review your reasons for taking them. You can then update your supplement program, eliminating those which are no longer a necessity, and adding those that are in line with your current needs.

CONCLUSION

You now have a good understanding of the special health needs you have as a woman, and the role that hormones play in your well-being. From the teenage years through the postmenopausal years, hormones have a significant effect on your emotional and physical health.

As you've discovered, your diet and lifestyle have a great deal to do with how smoothly your hormones perform. A diet that contains excessive alcohol, caffeine, or sugar, and unhealthful fats throws your body off-balance. Equally important to your well-being is your ability to manage stress, how much you exercise, and whether or not you get sufficient sleep and rest.

There's no question that how you live on a daily basis determines the state of your health now and in the years to come. New research emerges almost daily that links diet, exercise, and lifestyle to disease-prevention and longevity. This book contains the most up-to-date information to help you achieve optimal health. At the most basic level, adequate sleep, a nutritious diet, regular exercise, and stress-management skills are the foundation of health. In addition, the supplements recommended in this book provide you with the assurance that you are doing everything possible to provide your body with all that it needs for health, healing, and the prevention of disease.

In reading this book, you've taken an important step toward improving your health and well-being. Be patient with yourself as you make changes in your diet and lifestyle. Small, consistent steps are generally the most successful way to integrate new behaviors. As you begin to feel the positive benefits of caring for yourself in new ways, you'll find subsequent changes easier to make.

I wish you good health in your journey.

PART TWELVE

SPORTS NUTRITION SUPPLEMENTS

DAVE TUTTLE

During the past decade, there has been an explosion of new sports-nutrition products. From meal-replacement powders to esoteric nutrients like ecdysterone and methoxyisoflavone, supplement companies are offering an unprecedented number of products that can build muscle, reduce recovery time, and enhance sports performance.

This has been a double-edged sword for consumers. On one hand, some of these new offerings are among the most powerful and effective nutrients ever sold. On the other hand, the vast numbers of available products can be confusing for even the most advanced athlete. Which products are the real winners, and which are also-rans? Since money doesn't grow on trees, how can you make the best choices for your particular sports needs and budget? This part of the *User's Guide to Nutritional Supplements* will answer these questions.

Some of the nutrients discussed in this book are probably familiar to you, such as protein powders and creatine. But do you know the best times to take these nutrients, and which of the available forms works best? By the time you finish this guide, you will have a comprehensive knowledge of these supplements, allowing you to use them to peak advantage in advancing your sports progress.

Other products are so new that you may not have heard about them yet. With fancy names like ipriflavone and phosphatidylserine, these complex molecules certainly sound like they should work. And many of them do. This guide will reveal the current state of research into these new kids on the block. Some have impressive bodies of scientific investigation behind them, while others have only animal studies to support their use. This part of the *User's Guide to Nutritional Supplements* will tell it like it is, helping you to make decisions regarding your own purchases in this ever-changing field. This will include information on dosages, the need for on and off cycles to maintain effectiveness, and much more.

Everyone wants to get the biggest bang for their supplement bucks. You may have been disappointed that certain products didn't live up to their advertisers' claims, and as a result, you may be hesitant to sample new products.

But you can't progress in your sports endeavors without trying new things. This part of the *User's Guide to Nutritional Supplements* will provide you with the unbiased information you need to make the right choices.

PROTEIN SUPPLEMENTS AND MEAL-REPLACEMENT POWDERS

It is hard to overemphasize the importance of protein in an athlete's diet. While there are numerous supplements that enhance protein synthesis, you can't synthesize new muscle proteins without adequate raw material—the amino acids in dietary protein. Training at a high intensity and then depriving your body of the protein it needs is like hitting your head against a wall. Nothing beneficial will result, and you could damage your hard-earned muscle growth in the process.

While it is theoretically possible to eat enough meat, fish, poultry, and dairy products to get the protein you need, most athletes find it difficult to do so. It takes time to fix meals and even more time to eat them and clean the dishes. This has led many busy men and women to get part of their protein requirements from protein powders and meal-replacement powders (MRPs).

Essential Building Blocks

Protein is an essential nutrient for all people, but especially for athletes. There is some protein in every single cell of the human body. Brain cells, for example, are 10 percent protein while red blood cells and muscle cells contain as much as 20 percent protein. All in all, protein makes up nearly 15 percent of your body weight, more than any other substance except water.

These body proteins have a wide range of functions, including tissue growth and development. Two protein-based filaments inside the muscle fiber, known as actin and myosin, are responsible for all muscle contraction. Tendons, ligaments, hair, skin, and nails are specialized kinds of structural proteins. Proteins are even needed to form most hormones, including insulin and growth hormone.

The body manufactures all of these different proteins from amino acids.

Amino Acid
A component of dietary protein that contains nitrogen and other elements. The human body requires twenty amino acids to function properly.

The adult body can normally produce twelve of these amino acids on its own, hence the term "nonessential" amino acids. They are alanine, arginine, asparagine, aspartic acid, cysteine, glutamine, glutamic acid, glycine, histidine, proline, serine, and tryptophan. The other eight amino acids are called "essential" because they must be supplied by the diet. They are isoleucine, leucine, and valine (the branched-chain amino acids) plus lysine, methionine, phenylalanine, threonine, and tryptophan.

When your body has enough amino acids, you have a positive nitrogen balance. This means that you have sufficient nitrogen to support all of your body's needs with enough left over to permit muscle growth. Inadequate protein consumption relative to your needs results in a negative nitrogen balance.

Your Daily Protein Requirement

Kilogram
A measurement in the metric system. A kilogram is equal to 1,000 milligrams or 2.2 pounds.

One of the main questions that athletes ask is how much protein they should consume. The United States Government has established a recommended intake of 0.8 grams per kilogram (g/kg) of body weight per day. That's equal to 0.36 grams per pound (g/lb). While some nutritionists maintain that this is a liberal allowance that provides enough protein for active individuals, recent research shows otherwise.

A number of studies, including several by Dr. Peter Lemon of the University of Western Ontario, show that most strength athletes need 1.7–1.8 g/kg (about 0.8 g/lb). Endurance athletes need a bit less: 1.2–1.4 g/kg (about 0.6 g/lb). These figures are based on total body weight. (Although body fat does not require protein, it is easier for athletes to compute their protein needs based on total body weight.)

The foregoing requirements are for athletes who train three to four times per week. If you exercise more than this or train at a very high level of intensity, your protein requirement could be as high as 2.5 g/kg (1.1 g/lb) according to some researchers. For simplicity, try to maintain a daily intake of 1 g of protein per pound of body weight.

You need to eat an adequate amount of protein every day, even on the days you don't exercise. The body uses protein continuously to provide the raw materials for muscle growth, repair, and maintenance. However, only so much protein can be stored inside the muscle cells and in the blood and organs. So, if you consume too much protein at once, your body may eventually convert the excess into carbohydrate or fat.

At the same time, there is no scientific evidence to support the frequently heard idea that the body can assimilate only 35 g of protein at once. You can eat more than this amount per meal if you like, but it's better to spread out your protein consumption over three or four small meals to maintain relatively constant amino-acid levels throughout the day.

You can wind up with a negative nitrogen balance even at these recommended protein levels if you do not also consume enough carbohydrates. This can occur during the carbohydrate-depletion diets that are sometimes used prior to competitions with weight classes. It often occurs during long-distance marathon racing, too, as long-distance running dramatically depletes the body of carbohydrates.

When your body needs energy and does not have sufficient carbohydrates to meet its needs, it converts the protein in the liver and in the muscles into energy. This can result in a loss in muscle mass, as the body literally eats away at itself to get the nutrients it needs. Hardly what an athlete wants!

Protein Powders to the Rescue

It can be difficult to get enough protein from whole foods. Fortunately, a wide variety of protein supplements is now available. Soy, milk and egg, and whey powders each have their own special advantages. They also come in a wide variety of flavors to keep things interesting.

Soy powders are usually made from soy isolate, which is 99 percent protein. Because it is a vegetable protein, soy is low in methionine, although it is higher in glutamine than whey. Soy is also high in branched-chain amino acids and arginine, each of which is important for muscle growth. However, some of the plant chemicals in soy exert a mild estrogenic effect, which can reduce muscle definition, so male athletes should not consume large amounts of soy.

Milk and egg powders are protein blends. Originally made from powdered milk, they now contain a variety of milk components. As cheese is produced, the milk divides into two main products: a solid portion called *casein* and a liquid known as *whey*. Milk and egg powders combine various amounts of these fractions, usually adding some egg white (also called albumin) to the mix.

Scientists have learned that casein and whey have their own unique characteristics. Casein is assimilated relatively slowly, so it provides a steadier flow of amino acids to the bloodstream. This allows it to significantly reduce protein breakdown. Casein also has larger amounts of the amino acids that can be used for energy during exercise. However, because casein contains lactose, it can cause gastrointestinal distress in individuals who lack the enzyme lactase, which breaks down lactose. Whey, on the other hand, is assimilated very quickly, so it boosts protein synthesis much more than casein.

Whey: The Market Leader

Most of the protein powders on the market today are whey powders. In the early nineties, scientists developed a number of systems, including ion-exchange and microfiltration, to distill whey into a high-quality product that is nearly fat- and lactose-free. These systems use cool temperatures that preserve the taste and natural configurations of the amino acids.

Whey has the highest bioavailability of any protein. It dissolves easily in water, allowing the athlete to mix a protein drink on the run. While whey has less glutamine, arginine, and phenylalanine than either casein or soy, its ability to dramatically increase protein synthesis has made it a favorite of athletes. Whey also has immune-enhancing properties due to its ability to increase levels of the antioxidant glutathione.

Bioavailability
A measure of how much of an orally consumed nutrient actually passes through the intestinal tract wall so it can be utilized by the body.

Whey isolate is the purest form of whey. It has less moisture and lactose than whey concentrate, so gram for gram you get more protein for your money than with whey concentrate. However, whey isolate costs more than whey concentrate, so there is a trade-off. Whey products that use the old high-temperature process cost less but are not as effective because the proteins are denatured aznd less biologically active.

Remember that these supplements are not intended to replace the protein in your regular meals. Their value lies in giving you an easy way to get additional protein when your meals do not provide enough to meet your daily requirement. They can therefore help you to achieve the goals you have set for your sport.

Meal Replacements Offer Convenient Nutrition

Numerous studies have shown that the best way to build muscle and lose fat at the same time is to eat five or six small meals spread throughout the day. Such a division of food intake provides a steady stream of protein, promoting maximum growth. Each meal has a thermic effect as well, which boosts your metabolic rate and minimizes the amount that is stored as fat. Moreover, dividing your carb intake into smaller portions helps to restore your muscle glycogen without fat accumulation.

Glycogen
The storage form of glucose (blood sugar). Found primarily in the liver and muscle fibers, it is one-third glucose and two-thirds water.

But who has the time and energy to prepare and eat five or six meals from whole foods each day? Not most athletes, to be sure. With their work, training, family, and other obligations, athletes need a convenient way to get nourishment on the run, and meal-replacement powders (MRPs) provide the answer to their needs.

These powders are usually high in protein, moderately high in carbohydrates, and low in fat. Most can be mixed with water in a shaker to form a flavorful drink, although some need to be prepared with a blender. Several of them become very thick (due to the guar gum and other thickeners that they contain), while others have the consistency of chocolate milk. They are artificially sweetened and therefore have a low sugar content, even when they contain substantial amounts of carbs.

Many Different Ingredients

A survey of the MRPs currently on the market shows that the protein content ranges from 25–52 g per serving with anywhere from 9–28 g of carbs. Fat content is always very low—no more than 4.5 g. Based on the total number of calories per single-serving packet, the macronutrient ratio of these MRPs ranges from 52 to 73 percent protein, from 19 to 41 percent carbohydrate, and from 0 to 14 percent fat. Total caloric value varies from 170–340 calories per serving.

The main protein in most MRPs is whey—usually whey concentrate but sometimes a blend of whey isolate, concentrate, and hydrolysate. Some products combine whey with casein and egg albumin to provide a more slowly assimilated blend of amino acids. A number of products also include protein-based growth factors and bioactive peptides, such as casomorphins, immunoglobulins, glyco-macropeptides, IGF-1, and lactoferrin, which help to promote muscle growth and repair while providing support for your immune system.

The carbohydrate content usually comes from maltodextrin, brown-rice complex, fructooligosaccharides, fructose, corn-syrup solids, and/or sucrose. Fat sources consist of medium-chain triglycerides, borage oil, flaxseed oil, coconut oil, sunflower oil, and/or sometimes partially hydrogenated oils.

Many manufacturers also add a variety of sports-related nutrients to their formulations. Some of the more common nutrients are chromium, glutamine, taurine, tyrosine, creatine monohydrate, branched-chain amino acids, hydroxymethylbutyrate (HMB), and alpha-ketoglutarate. Fat burners and blockers are occasionally included as well, such as hydroxycitric acid (HCA), lecithin, choline, inositol, carnitine, and chitosan. MRPs are also fortified with vitamins and minerals, ranging from 33 to 100 percent of the recommended daily value per serving.

There are many flavors available, so there is no reason to get bored with your MRP. In addition to the standard chocolate, vanilla, and strawberry, the selection includes orange, wild berry, chocolate peanut butter, and even a variety pack of tropical flavors.

Picking the Best Product for You

With so much diversity, you need to carefully select the product that is right for you. Figure out your total daily protein requirement and subtract the amount you obtain from whole-food sources. The remainder is what you need to get from a protein supplement or MRP.

As far as carbs are concerned, your daily requirement depends on your metabolism and energy expenditure. Most athletes require 2–3 g of carbs per pound of body weight. Do the math and determine how many carbs you need each day. Then divide the total between MRPs and dietary carbs such as oatmeal, whole-grain breads, pasta, legumes, and potatoes.

Even if you are extremely busy, you should try to get at least half of your carb intake from whole food. While the carbs in MRPs tend to be fairly low on the glycemic index, they contain virtually no fiber—an important part of a balanced diet. The fat content of MRPs and protein powders is so low that it should not impact your waistline.

When used appropriately, these powders can help you to achieve your sports objectives. They provide the nutrients you need for muscle growth without excessive calories, allowing you to control your body-fat level as you pursue peak performance. MRPs and protein powders are tailor-made for the fast-paced, active lifestyle of athletes, so be sure to include them in your dietary regimen.

CREATINE

Of all the sports supplements available, none has been more extensively studied than creatine. This white, odorless powder burst onto the sports scene in the mid-nineties and transformed the supplement industry in the process. Initially, only creatine monohydrate was available, but soon creatine citrate followed, along with effervescent creatine, liquid creatine, creatine-transport drinks, and even creatine candy.

It has been nearly a decade since creatine first appeared, which means it has outlasted the usual two- or three-year window for a supplement fad. Why? Because creatine works for most everyone in a wide variety of sports. It increases energy and strength, which translates into more muscle mass and greater performance for athletes—particularly those in sports that involve short bursts of maximal intensity.

Your Three Energy Pathways

Creatine is an essential player in one of the three primary energy systems used for muscle contraction. It exists in two different forms within the muscle fiber: as free (chemically unbound) creatine and as creatine phosphate (CP). This latter form of creatine makes up two-thirds of your total creatine supply.

When your muscles contract, the initial fuel for this movement is a compound called adenosine triphosphate (ATP).

ATP releases one of its phosphate molecules to provide energy for muscle contraction and other functions. Once ATP releases a phosphate molecule, it becomes a different compound called ADP (adenosine diphosphate). Unfortunately, there is only enough ATP to provide energy for about ten seconds, so for this energy system to continue, more ATP must be produced.

Creatine phosphate (CP) comes to the rescue by giving up its phosphate molecule to ADP, recreating ATP. This ATP can then be "burned" again as fuel for more muscle contraction. The bottom line is that your ability to regenerate ATP largely depends on your supply of creatine. The more creatine you have in your muscles, the more ATP you can remake.

This greater ATP resynthesis keeps your body from relying as much on another energy pathway called glycolysis, which has lactic acid as a byproduct. This acid irritates the muscle fiber, causing pain. Eventually lactic-acid levels rise so high that they interfere with the biochemical reactions needed for muscle contraction. So, if you have less lactic acid in your muscles, you can train longer and gain strength, power, and muscle size. You also don't get tired as quickly.

In less than a minute, your demands for energy exceed the limits of the ATP-CP pathway, and you start to produce energy through glycolysis. If you train long enough at a high enough intensity, you will get so much lactic acid in your muscles that you will have to temporarily stop working out. Anyone who has given his or her all in the gym or on the playing field knows this feeling.

The third energy pathway is the aerobic pathway. It can be utilized only when adequate oxygen is available. This occurs when the sports activity involves less than maximal effort, even though you can get tired if you do enough of it. Submaximal activities, such as jogging, treadmill walking, and of course "aerobics" classes primarily use this energy pathway, which does not involve creatine.

A Natural Nutrient

Creatine is naturally present in your body at a level of around 0.75 g per pound of body weight. Approximately 95 percent of the total supply is found in the skeletal muscles. The remaining 5 percent is scattered throughout the rest of the body, with the highest concentrations in the heart, brain, and testes. (Sperm is chock-full of creatine!)

The body gets its creatine from two sources: food and its own internal production. Creatine is found in moderate amounts in most meats and fish, which are, after all, skeletal muscles. Good sources of dietary creatine include beef, chicken, turkey, tuna, cod, salmon, and pork. Tiny amounts are found in milk and even cranberries. Unfortunately, cooking destroys part of the creatine that exists in these foods.

The body can also make creatine using the three amino

acids arginine, glycine, and methionine as raw material. This production occurs in the liver, pancreas, and kidneys. The body will manufacture only so much on its own, however. If you want to maximize the creatine stores in your muscles, you need to take a creatine supplement.

Please note that the creatine on store shelves is synthesized in a factory from chemicals. No one grinds up meat to get creatine. This manufacturing process can produce modest amounts of impurities if the factory owner is not careful. (The Chinese creatine available a few years ago was notorious for its impurity levels.)

To make sure that you get minimal impurities in your creatine monohydrate, use a brand that says "Creapure" on the label. These brands are made with a patented technology. Creatine is very affordable nowadays, so it is silly to put impurities in your body just to save a couple of bucks.

Mountains of Research

Unlike some supplements that have only rat or test-tube studies to support their use, creatine has been the subject of hundreds of published clinical trials. Most of these studies involved athletes, giving us an unprecedented level of certainty about creatine's benefits.

There has been so much research on creatine that you could write a book about it. In fact, I did—with Ray Sahelian, M.D., called *Creatine: Nature's Muscle Builder* (Avery Publishing, 1999). Check out this book if you want to learn the many details of this exciting supplement.

Virtually all of the available research has been done with creatine monohydrate, a powder with a neutral taste that is stable until put in water. Creatine monohydrate in moderate amounts is easily absorbed in the intestinal tract and raises blood levels of creatine within an hour.

Once in the muscle cell, creatine remains there for up to a month. Creatine can occasionally be converted in the body to creatinine, a harmless but useless substance that is filtered by the kidneys and excreted in urine. Creatinine is also produced when creatine remains in water for extended periods.

Not everyone benefits from creatine supplementation. One study found that up to 30 percent of users are nonresponders. It is not known why this occurs, but it is thought to relate to the amount of creatine you store naturally. While the average concentration in muscle tissue is 125 mmol (millimoles per liter), normal creatine levels can range from 100–160 mmol. If your muscles are already at or near this maximum concentration, you may not experience an increase in strength or sports performance. The only way to tell is to try creatine and find out for yourself.

The Athletes Who Benefit Most

Because creatine is involved in the energy pathway used for bursts of explosive power, it should not be surprising that athletes in sports relying heavily on this pathway derive the greatest benefits. This includes bodybuilders, powerlifters, wrestlers, short-distance track and field athletes, and football and hockey players.

Studies at the Karolinska Institute in Sweden found that a dose of 20 g of creatine monohydrate per day produced an average 5 percent increase in peak torque (a measure of force production) and similar gains in the amount of work performed. The subjects also gained an average of 2.4 pounds of body weight during the one-month experiment.

A study at three Texan research institutions found significant increases in strength from creatine monohydrate. The male volunteers, who regularly trained with weights, got stronger and more muscular from a regimen of 20 g of creatine per day for twenty-eight days. After four weeks, the amount of weight they could lift for one repetition (1-RM) rose by 8.2 kg (more than eighteen pounds), and the number of reps they could do at 70 percent 1-RM rose from eleven to fifteen. They also gained an average of 3.7 pounds of body weight with only a 0.2 pound increase in body fat. That means that 95 percent of the gain was muscle mass!

So many studies have been performed with athletes that it is impossible to list them all in this short book. Suffice it to say that any athlete who relies strictly on strength and power will benefit from creatine use. The only times when creatine is not recommended is when other factors influence performance, such as body weight.

For a bodybuilder, more weight is great—as long as it's lean muscle. Ditto for wrestlers, powerlifters, and other strength athletes. But if you are a marathon runner, the increased body weight may slow you down, even if you are stronger. For this reason, marathon runners and triathletes should sample creatine in the off-season to see what trade-offs they experience. The increased muscle mass could also prove counterproductive for swimmers and martial artists, although the greater power and speed would be beneficial. Again, an off-season trial is recommended.

Creatine Monohydrate versus Creatine Citrate

Creatine monohydrate is a molecule of creatine attached to one molecule of water (*mono* means "one"), while creatine citrate has a molecule of creatine and a molecule of citrate. The creatine is identical in both cases, but the carrier molecule changes the total package somewhat.

Gram for gram, creatine monohydrate has more creatine than creatine citrate. Creatine monohydrate is about 60 percent creatine, while creatine citrate is only 40 percent creatine. This means you need to take a bit more creatine citrate to get the same effects, so be sure to look at the label to see what creatine you are getting.

While no published research has compared the performance benefits of monohydrate with citrate directly, an

Italian study found that the absorption rates of both forms are about the same. Also, please note that some manufacturers list the amount of creatine in the product instead of the total with the carrier molecule attached, so check the label. You may be getting more creatine than you thought at first glance.

One supposed advantage of creatine citrate is that it does not cause "bloating." The argument is that your body takes in added water with creatine monohydrate, which can boost the amount of water in your skin. But even if the hydrate molecule is assimilated, the amount you consume is unlikely to cause noticeable bloating.

A 5-g dose of creatine monohydrate has 2 g of water, so you would be taking in one ounce (28 g) of water every two weeks. That's peanuts compared with the amount you drink. Also, there is virtually no creatine in the skin, so the bloating would not occur there. Rather, it would take place inside your muscle cells—precisely where you want it.

It is true that creatine monohydrate increases water levels inside the muscle cell. This is one of the reasons why it works, because higher intramuscular water levels boost protein synthesis and muscle growth. Since creatine citrate is effective, it probably does the same thing. However, there is so little research on creatine citrate that much remains unknown at this point.

Creatine-Transport Powders Boost Uptake

In 1996, a study at Queens Medical Centre in Nottingham, England, compared creatine retention in twenty-two healthy men. Researchers divided the men into four groups. Group A took 5 g of creatine, Groups B and C consumed 5 g of creatine with 93 g of simple sugar (creatine-carb mixture), and Group D took an inert substance technically called a placebo. All groups took their supplements four times per day. In addition, Group C rode stationary bikes for an hour each day, while the other groups did not exercise.

The researchers found that the creatine-carb mixture boosted total muscle-creatine levels 24 percent by day three, while creatine alone produced only a 14 percent increase. Furthermore, although exercise normally increases creatine retention, the added carbs were so effective that there was no difference between the creatine levels in Groups B and C.

This study led to the introduction of several creatine-transport powders. All of these supplements include simple sugars (usually dextrose but sometimes maltose or maltodextrin) in varying amounts along with other ingredients that have anabolic properties, such as the amino acids taurine and glutamine. They come in lemon-lime, orange, grape, and fruit-punch flavors.

Some products have nutrients that may further boost creatine uptake and retention. The antioxidant alpha-lipoic acid has been shown to increase insulin sensitivity in people with diabetes. Since insulin is involved in creatine uptake, alpha-lipoic acid may therefore help deliver creatine to the muscle cells.

Arginine increases blood flow to the penis, which is why it is included in "male health" products. Logically, it should increase blood flow to other muscles as well, permitting more nutrients (including creatine) to be transported. However, no studies have been published that specifically show enhanced creatine uptake from alpha-lipoic acid or arginine. On the other hand, a recent study did show increased uptake with D-pinitol, a nutrient found in pine wood and legumes.

Another study compared pure carbs with a 50/50 protein-carb blend and found that creatine uptake was the same in both cases. As a result, you can add protein powder to your creatine-transport drink without any reduction in benefit. Given the need for amino acids before and after your workout, this is a very good idea.

Effervescent Creatine: The Fizz That Builds Muscle

Recently, numerous effervescent creatine powders have been introduced. When combined with water, these powders provide an effective dose of creatine in a bubbly, flavorful beverage. A well-designed effervescent creatine increases the solubility of creatine, so less is left in the glass and more can reach the bloodstream and muscle cells.

Although some brands use creatine monohydrate, most effervescent creatine is made with creatine citrate. Sometimes, citric and/or ascorbic acid are also added to the mix. The addition of these acidic ingredients lowers the pH of the drink, which has been shown to increase the amount of creatine that dissolves in water.

Sodium carbonate and/or bicarbonate combines with the citric and/or ascorbic acid to produce the effervescence, while various sweeteners, such as dextrose, fructose, stevia, aspartame, and acesulfame-K, reduce the extreme tartness of the creatine citrate. Natural sweeteners, particularly dextrose, help to increase the uptake of creatine, although, of course, the artificial sweeteners do not. Effervescent creatine is available in four flavors: orange, grape, fruit punch, and berry.

It's funny how things change as our knowledge expands. When creatine was first introduced, the locker-room talk was that you shouldn't mix it with orange juice because it would neutralize the effect. Now we know that the opposite is true: Not only does the acid in orange juice not neutralize it, it can actually enhance its solubility.

Effervescent creatine is a lot more enjoyable than downing creatine with water. This taste advantage is a big reason why these powders are so popular. However, there is no published evidence that effervescent creatine citrate increases the amount of creatine that makes it to the bloodstream compared with an equivalent amount of creatine monohydrate. Hopefully, future research will clarify this question.

Liquid Creatine: Revolutionary Discovery or Hoax?

Liquid creatine is the most controversial form of creatine on the market. While creatine monohydrate and creatine citrate are very stable compounds in dry form, nearly all scientists believe that they begin to degrade when dissolved in water. They wind up largely as creatinine, a harmless substance that is also the natural byproduct of creatine metabolism. Unfortunately, creatinine has zero anabolic properties.

This process begins after several hours, so there is no reason to be concerned when you mix creatine or an effervescent formulation with water and drink it immediately. However, it does become an issue when the creatine is packaged in liquid form.

Liquid-creatine products contain ample amounts of creatine when they leave the factory. However, the products sit at a distributor for some time before being shipped to stores. They then spend time on store shelves before eventually being purchased. How much active ingredient is still there for the consumer is a topic of much debate.

"We've tried all sorts of ways to stabilize creatine in solution," says Joan Dean, a representative for SKW, the leading German manufacturer of creatine monohydrate. "We have one of the best laboratories in the world, and it can't be done."

Yet, billion-dollar, multinational corporations do not have a monopoly on wisdom and invention. Perhaps there is a Thomas Edison of creatine out there who has unlocked the mystery of stabilizing creatine in liquid. This revolutionary discovery would certainly make it more convenient to use creatine by eliminating the need to mix it with water or other liquid before taking it.

However, there is no peer-reviewed research on the content of liquid creatine purchased by athletes, and independent lab results put the creatine content at around 10 percent of the amount on the label. Also, no study has been performed comparing the anabolic potential of liquid creatine with the powdered forms.

Given the millions of dollars that are spent advertising liquid creatine each year, one would think that Mr. Edison would want to spend the $20,000 needed to do a clinical trial verifying its benefits. Alas, this has not occurred. You can draw your own conclusions.

Dosage Recommendations

Traditionally, athletes took 20–30 g per day for five to seven days (know as a loading phase), followed by 4–7 g daily (maintenance phase). This was based on early research that showed it was an effective way to maximize muscle-creatine concentrations. And it is highly effective—as long as you can handle the possible side effects.

While the body can easily assimilate small amounts of creatine, if you take too much, you can overload your intestines and suffer the consequences, including gas and diarrhea. If you can't wait a month to get the full effects of creatine, then do a loading phase but stay close to a bathroom until you see how your body responds. (Some people have no problem at all with loading.)

However, if you don't mind waiting a month or don't want to take a chance with side effects, simply start with the old-style maintenance phase. Studies have shown that this dosage is perfectly capable of giving you all that creatine has to offer in thirty days without the downside.

The 4–7 g recommendation is valid for creatine monohydrate and citrate, regardless of the delivery system. Athletes who train intensely should aim for 7 g per day, while weekend warriors need only 4 g. Also, because creatine stores are related to muscle mass, larger athletes need more creatine to make the greatest gains.

Some athletes believe that doing on and off cycles with creatine is a must, while others say they experience no benefit. If you decide to give your body a "break," remember that it takes a full four weeks after you stop supplementing for creatine levels to return to normal. Cycling one day on/one day off or even one week on/one week off is therefore pointless.

Also, since there is a maximum creatine concentration in muscle tissue, once you get there, you can't exceed this physiological limit with cycling or anything else. Cycling will allow you to feel the great pump you felt when you first started taking creatine, but only because you lost its benefits during the time off. It's your choice.

Creatine is a relatively inexpensive supplement with an excellent cost-benefit ratio. Its effectiveness has been verified beyond a shadow of a doubt, as has its safety. (Rumors about cramping and dehydration have proved unfounded.) If you haven't given creatine a try, you definitely should.

GLUTAMINE AND OTHER SECRETAGOGUES

Growth hormone (GH) is one of the most important hormones for the athlete. While testosterone gets most of the attention, GH does much of the work in increasing your strength and muscle mass. GH has a major role in muscle growth and retention due to its ability to promote cell division and proliferation throughout the body. It enhances protein synthesis and nitrogen retention, and stimulates the liver to produce various growth factors. GH also promotes the growth of the bones and connective tissues, as well as enhancing the rate of healing. It even reduces body-fat levels by raising your metabolic rate and increasing the use of fats as an energy source.

Because of these many roles, you can't train and perform at your peak unless you have an ample supply of GH. Teenagers and young adults tend to have enough, which is part of the reason they grow so quickly. Older individuals have less and less each year. While bioengineered GH is available, it requires a prescription, which can be obtained only if you are extremely deficient in this hormone. This has led supplement manufacturers to develop a number of GH boosters, known as *secretagogues*, to help you increase your supply of this essential hormone.

This section discusses the most common secretagogues for growth hormone. Some, like glutamine and arginine, are amino acids, while others are brain chemicals or precursors to these chemicals. All help your pituitary gland to release more GH.

Glutamine: An Important Amino Acid

Scientists have known about glutamine for decades, but it was written off as "just" an amino acid for many years. Since the body can produce glutamine under normal conditions from other amino acids, glutamine has been called a nonessential amino acid—even though it has many essential roles in the body. However, when you are sick or under a great deal of stress, recent research has shown that these supplies of glutamine can be insufficient to meet all your body's needs.

Due to their increased activity levels and metabolic requirements, athletes can develop relative deficiencies of glutamine that can hold back their training progress. In these situations, glutamine supplementation can remove a limiting factor and help the athlete to achieve his or her optimal performance.

Glutamine is the most abundant amino acid in the human body. The majority of this glutamine is stored within the skeletal muscles, although significant amounts are also found in the blood, lungs, liver, and brain. The cells of the immune system use glutamine for fuel (most of the body's cells use glucose). In addition, glutamine provides fuel for the mucosal cells of the intestinal wall, which helps to promote the maximum assimilation of vital nutrients for athletic activity.

Because it has a nitrogen atom to spare, glutamine is able to transport nitrogen around the body. This "shuttle" activity helps it to neutralize the lactic acid that builds up during exercise. The greater the availability of glutamine, the quicker this lactic acid can be neutralized. This can allow exercise to resume sooner and may even permit higher strength levels during your workout. Glutamine also acts as a nitrogen precursor for several coenzymes and the phosphate molecules that muscles use for energy production.

This amino acid plays a role in the maintenance of protein balance in muscle by increasing protein synthesis and reducing protein breakdown. The more glutamine in the muscle cells, the higher the rate of protein synthesis. This is because glutamine increases the amount of fluid inside the muscle cell, which is a powerful anabolic signal for the building of new proteins. This volumization is similar to (but not as strong as) that produced by creatine.

A Proven Growth-Hormone Booster

A study at Louisiana State University found that oral glutamine supplementation had a dramatic impact on growth-hormone secretion. Nine healthy volunteers aged thirty-two to sixty-four consumed 2 g of glutamine over a twenty-minute period that started forty-five minutes after a light breakfast. During the next ninety minutes, blood samples were measured every half-hour for plasma GH and the level of bicarbonate, which is a salt that can reduce acid levels in the body.

The researchers found that GH levels rose 430 percent above baseline levels after ninety minutes. There was a dramatic rise in bicarbonate concentration as well, which could help neutralize the lactic acid produced during a workout.

To stimulate your GH secretion, you should consume 2 to 3 g of glutamine with a glass of water several times per day. Tomas Welbourne, the author of this study, notes that high blood-sugar levels prevent glutamine from promoting GH release, so be sure to take it at least one hour after a meal or one hour before your next one.

Also, Welbourne recommends that you don't exceed a 3-g dose, because greater amounts could be counterproductive for GH production. Larger dosages, however, have proved effective for immune enhancement.

Glutamine Enhances Immunity

Strenuous exercise taxes your immune system. There is a higher incidence of infections and cold symptoms after a bout of intense exercise. Researchers at the University of Oxford found that there is a decrease in the plasma level of glutamine in endurance athletes after a marathon. This reduction continues for one hour, then slowly returns to normal sixteen hours after the event.

During this period, there is also a drop in the number of lymphocytes (white blood cells), which are dependent on glutamine for optimal growth. The decline in lymphocyte count, along with other negative changes in the immune system, is considered by many researchers to be the cause of the increased frequency of illness among athletes.

Here again, glutamine can help. Researchers at Oxford and the Free University of Brussels found a correlation between oral glutamine consumption and the absence of illness in trained athletes. They measured the levels of infection in more than 200 runners and rowers. Middle-distance runners had the lowest infection rate, while the rowers and full- or ultra-marathon runners had the highest levels.

The researchers then gave a total of 5 g of glutamine to half of these athletes while the others drank a placebo. Half of the dosage was taken right after the exercise bout and the remainder was consumed two hours after exercise. The results were dramatic. Only 19 percent of the athletes using glutamine reported infections during the next seven days, while 51 percent of the athletes on the placebo came down with a cold or similar infection. Given how frustrated athletes get when they are forced to take time off, supplementation with glutamine is great health insurance.

Best Supplementation Regimen

Even though the body produces 50–120 g of glutamine on its own each day, supplementation has been shown to provide additional benefits. While part of your dose winds up being metabolized by the mucosal cells of the small intestine, it is still beneficial because the body uses this external source instead of getting the glutamine it needs from your muscles (the main storage area for this amino acid).

You can minimize this drain on your muscle stores by taking 5 g of glutamine right before your workout. This will help to reduce lactic-acid concentrations during exercise as well. You should also take 5 g after your workout to speed up your recovery. While these larger doses may not stimulate GH production, they will help to keep your body in a positive glutamine balance and minimize any negative impact from your training. This by itself may help the pituitary gland to release more GH on its own. To maximize glutamine's benefits, take an additional 2 to 3 g between meals to bump up your GH level.

Arginine Has Many Important Functions

Arginine is another amino acid that is considered nonessential because the body can normally produce enough of it. However, as with glutamine, dietary deprivation, trauma, severe stress, and other conditions can create arginine deficiencies.

This amino acid has a variety of vital functions. It is used for the synthesis of many proteins and is the only source for a chemical group used by the body to manufacture creatine. (Lysine and methionine provide the other chemical raw materials.) It promotes wound healing and is found in large amounts in semen.

Arginine is involved in the regulation of nitric oxide. Elevated levels of nitric oxide dilate the arteries and increase blood flow. This boosts the volume of nutrients delivered to the target tissues, which is why some supplement companies include arginine in their creatine-transport drinks or other products.

Arginine is also required for the detoxification of ammonia, which is formed during the metabolism of amino acids, nucleic acids, and other substrates that contain nitrogen. Since the average body produces 3–4 g of ammonia each day, adequate arginine intake is clearly important.

How to Get a GH Release

Arginine is found in relatively high quantities in chicken, turkey, and nuts. However, supplementation is needed to get an increase in growth-hormone levels. Some researchers have reported positive effects from as little as 5–10 g of arginine per day, although most studies have used larger dosages (up to 30 g). The amino acid has normally been taken right before bedtime on an empty stomach so it can increase the amount of GH released during sleep, which is when the body secretes the greatest amount of this hormone. Why you need to take more arginine than glutamine to get results is not clear at this point.

A study at the Rome Medical Clinic in Italy found that a combination of arginine and lysine dramatically increased GH levels at a much smaller dose. The test subjects took 1,200 mg of arginine pyroglutamate and 1,200 mg of lysine hydrochloride. Within ninety minutes of taking this supplement, GH levels rose 700 percent above baseline levels. Eight hours later, GH levels were still elevated by as much as 300 percent. These dosage levels are more in line with those required for GH release with glutamine. Apparently, the combination with lysine and/or the form of arginine used made the difference.

Arginine is usually a very safe amino acid. However, if you have herpes simplex or suffer from schizophrenia, you should avoid using arginine, since it could worsen your condition. Choose a different secretagogue instead.

Other Effective Secretagogues

Many researchers believe that you can boost GH levels by increasing the concentrations of the neurotransmitters acetylcholine and dopamine.

Like most hormones, the levels of these neurotransmitters decrease as you get older. A precursor to acetylcholine, alpha-glycerylphosphorylcholine, has been shown to stimulate GH secretion by reducing the amount of somatostatin (GH-inhibiting hormone) that is released.

L-dopa, an amino acid that the brain uses to make dopamine, is an effective secretagogue. Made popular by Durk Pearson and Sandy Shaw in their bestseller *Life Extension*, L-dopa was reported to increase GH output at a dose of 500 mg per day. L-dopa is produced naturally by the body through the oxidation of the amino acid tyrosine. Available as a prescription drug, L-dopa is also found in the herb *Mucuna pruriens* and in fava beans. *Bacopa monniera* is sometimes added to these neu-

Secretagogue
An amino acid or other substance that stimulates a gland of your body to secrete a particular hormone.

rotransmitter-based formulas because the bacosides it contains help to repair damaged neurons.

A study at Walsh University gave a single dose of a botanical supplement containing 666 mg of *Mucuna pruriens*, 100 mg of alpha glycerylphosphorylcholine, and 50 mg of *Bacopa monniera* to five young men thirty minutes before performing six sets of squats. The researchers found that total GH levels were 19.8 percent higher during the sixty-minute recovery period, while peak GH levels increased nearly 90 percent.

Another way to stimulate your GH release is to use homeopathic products. Homeopathy is a branch of medicine that uses highly diluted concentrations of certain substances to trigger a response by the body. In this case, it is believed that a small amount of GH will cause the pituitary gland to secrete more GH.

Homeopathy has many followers, but the FDA is not one of them. It considers such diluted doses to be useless (although harmless), and therefore permits real growth hormone to be sold over the counter as long as the amount of GH in the pill is small enough. There is little research on these products, so you'll need to experiment and see what results you get for yourself.

With the increasing recognition of growth hormone's many contributions to sports performance, more and more athletes are using GH secretagogues. They can be valuable additions to your supplement regimen, but don't go overboard with them. The pituitary gland and the brain are complex organs with many feedback loops, so stick with the manufacturers' recommendations. That way you can get all of the benefits of this vital hormone.

VITAMINS AND MINERALS

Athletes need to be sure that they consume sufficient vitamins and minerals. These micronutrients play vital roles in muscle development, energy production, and many other essential functions. While they are often taken for granted, vitamins and minerals enable you to perform at your peak.

Your micronutrient requirements go up as the intensity of your training increases, so you want to be sure you get enough. At the same time, taking more than you need is expensive and does not provide any additional sports benefit.

This section is limited to the role of vitamins and minerals in enhancing your performance as an athlete. While these nutrients can provide many additional health benefits, these topics are outside the scope of this book. For a detailed look at the micronutrients, check out Part One of this book.

Vitamins Are Needed for Chemical Reactions

There are currently thirteen vitamins that are recognized as essential for humans: vitamin A (retinol), B$_1$ (thiamin), B$_2$ (riboflavin), B$_3$ (niacin), B$_6$ (pyridoxine), B$_{12}$ (cobalamin), pantothenic acid, folic acid, biotin, C, D, E, and K. Even though your body's requirements for these nutrients are small compared with the macronutrients (protein, carbs, and fat), a deficiency of any one of them can lead to illness and disease.

> **Vitamins**
> *Nutrients that are required for many different chemical reactions within the body. They help regulate the chain of metabolic reactions that controls tissue synthesis, the release of energy in food, and other functions.*

Without the right vitamins, essential chemical reactions cannot take place at the proper rates, impacting your body's metabolic processes. Some vitamins also act as antioxidants, helping to protect you from potentially cancer-causing compounds called free radicals.

There are two types of vitamins: fat-soluble and water-soluble. The fat-soluble vitamins (A, D, E, and K) can be dissolved only in fat. A small amount of fat must therefore be included in the diet so that these vitamins can be assimilated and used by the body. Fat-soluble vitamins that are not immediately needed are stored in the fat tissues for later use, so deficiencies of fat-soluble vitamins are relatively rare.

In fact, because these vitamins remain in the system for so long, athletes who take extremely high amounts of fat-soluble vitamins can actually develop toxic levels in their bodies. For this reason, care should be taken when consuming fat-soluble vitamin supplements.

The water-soluble vitamins (B-complex vitamins and vitamin C) act as coenzymes. They combine with small protein molecules to form active enzymes. These vitamins dissolve in water but not in fat. As a result, they cannot be stored to any great degree by the body. Water-soluble vitamin supplies that are not immediately needed are likely to be excreted in the urine. It is therefore necessary to eat foods and supplements that contain these vitamins on a regular basis to prevent deficiencies.

Minerals Build a Strong Body

Minerals are also required for sports performance. There are twenty-two minerals that are currently recognized as essential: calcium, phosphorus, sulfur, potassium, chlorine, sodium, magnesium, iron, fluorine, zinc, copper, selenium, iodine, chromium, cobalt, silicon, vanadium, tin, nickel, manganese, molybdenum, and lead.

While vitamins are able to facilitate chemical reactions in the body without actually becoming part of them, minerals usually become incorporated within the body's physical and chemical structures. Minerals are found in the body's enzymes and hormones, too. They regulate the acid-base balance of the body, help control cellular metabolism, and stimulate various reactions that allow energy to be released from the foods we eat.

Minerals have been divided into two groups, known as major minerals and trace minerals, depending on the quantity of the mineral you need. Individual minerals also vary in the degree to which the body absorbs them. This variation, called bioavailability, can range from as low as 5 percent for manganese to 30 to 40 percent for calcium and magnesium. The bioavailability of a mineral is taken into consideration when the daily value for that mineral is established.

It should be noted that the levels of toxicity for minerals are much lower than they are for vitamins. This is because minerals are metals, so they should be treated with a great deal of respect. Taking too many minerals can definitely harm your health without giving you any performance benefit in return.

Daily Requirements for Athletes

Athletes tend to eat relatively large quantities of good food. This dietary intake should provide a substantial portion of your total vitamin and mineral requirements. In some cases, it may supply all of an athlete's needs for a particular micronutrient. Also, bear in mind that vitamins have the ability to be used over and over in metabolic reactions, so there is not a direct correlation between activity levels and vitamin needs. Still, many athletes require additional micronutrients to perform at their best. This can be achieved by taking a multivitamin/multimineral supplement that contains the daily value for each micronutrient once or twice a day depending on how nutritious your meals are.

There are four micronutrients that are particularly important for muscle growth and sports performance: vitamin C, vitamin E, calcium, and magnesium. Several studies have shown sports benefits from these nutrients at levels significantly greater than the daily value, so you should take extra amounts of them in addition to your multivitamin/ multimineral supplement.

Vitamins C and E Fight Free Radicals

Vitamin C is well known for its ability to help strengthen the immune system. This antioxidant vitamin can also help neutralize potentially damaging free radicals, which have been connected with a number of diseases. Researchers at the University of Cape Town, South Africa, gave 600 mg of the vitamin to the participants of a ninety-kilometer race. They found that supplementation significantly reduced the incidence of common cold symptoms during this acute physical stress.

Other placebo-controlled studies have shown that 1–2 g of vitamin C per day can decrease the severity of common cold symptoms. Therefore, in order to keep your immune system in peak condition, you should consume 1–2 g of vitamin C each day. Citrus fruits, tomatoes, green peppers, and green leafy vegetables contain good amounts of this vitamin. If you do not get enough from your diet, inexpensive tablets are available.

Vitamin E is another antioxidant vitamin. It is fat-soluble and is found primarily in cell membranes. Vitamin E helps to prevent free radical damage in the muscles and bloodstream. It protects the red blood cells as well, and plays an essential role in cellular respiration in cardiac and skeletal muscle, which increases endurance and stamina.

Vitamin E also reduces the membrane disruption that occurs in exercised muscles due to increased free radical production. A placebo-controlled study at Pennsylvania State University gave 1,200 IU of vitamin E to six weight-trained males for two weeks. The men were then asked to perform a vigorous whole-body workout after a two-day rest period. Vitamin E supplementation significantly reduced the muscle damage created by this workout program.

You should consume 600–1,200 IU of vitamin E per day. Good food sources include grains, green leafy vegetables and seeds. Many oils contain vitamin E as well, but you may prefer to take a supplement to keep your calorie count down.

Calcium Builds Strong Bones and Muscles

Calcium is the most abundant mineral in the human body. It assists in regulating the heartbeat and helps to build and maintain the bones and teeth. Calcium reduces lactic-acid concentrations in the blood during and after exercise. It is also essential for muscle contraction.

When a muscle fiber is stimulated to contract, calcium binds to one of the protein-based filaments deep inside the muscle cell, and, in effect, turns it on. When the nerve impulse to the muscle fiber is removed, the calcium ions move back to their storage location, which stops the contraction of the muscle.

In order to ensure an adequate calcium supply, you should consume 7 mg of calcium per pound of body weight (16 mg/kg). Good food sources of calcium include nonfat milk and yogurt, mozzarella cheese, broccoli, and green leafy vegetables. If you don't get enough from your diet, you should buy calcium carbonate or calcium citrate tablets to make up the difference. These forms of calcium are more bioavailable than the less expensive bone-meal or oyster-shell products.

Magnesium Activates Many Enzymes

Magnesium helps to control carbohydrate synthesis and is an essential activator of many enzyme systems. It counteracts the stimulatory effect of calcium in the muscle fibers and helps to prevent muscle cramps. A study at the University of North Dakota found that it enhances oxygen delivery to working muscles in trained subjects. Magnesium supplementation has also been shown to reduce the level of hormones that can produce a loss of muscle tissue.

Despite its importance, the body contains less than an ounce (20 g) of magnesium, 27 percent of which is found in muscle. You should consume 3.5 mg of magnesium per pound of body weight (8 mg/kg). There are not many good food sources of magnesium except for cod, snapper, and some other seafood. Whole grains and vegetables contain small amounts. Fortunately, magnesium tablets are relatively inexpensive.

By providing your body with a balanced spectrum of micronutrients, you ensure that no vitamin or mineral becomes a limiting factor in your muscle growth. Given the moderate expense involved, you should make sure that you get enough vitamins and minerals every day.

ECDYSTERONE

During the Cold War, there were plenty of rumors about the "secret" training techniques of athletes in the former Soviet Union. Depending on who was doing the telling, they were all jacked up on anabolic steroids, subjected to bizarre training programs, underwent psychological brainwashing, or all of the above. Lost in the hysteria was the use by Soviet athletes of benign, but effective, natural substances like ecdysterone and related ecdysteroids.

An Adaptogen That Works

The Russians who dominated the USSR have been big believers in the power of herbs for a long time. While scoffed at by American researchers who think that only refined pharmaceuticals hold any value, the Russians have experimented with herbs for decades. Their main focus has been on adaptogenic herbs, which are plants that have the ability to restore optimal function in athletes who are depleted because of their training.

Adaptogen
An herb that has a variable effect depending on your physical condition. The further you are from an optimal state, the more benefit you receive.

The concept of adaptogens can be difficult for Americans to understand, but it is well recognized in Asia and even in Europe, where herbs play a much greater role in medicine than in this country. If you are in prime condition already, you may not see much of a change from using adaptogenic herbs. However, if you are overtrained or depleted in some way, as athletes often are, you may see a significant change for the better.

Once the Iron Curtain fell, Westerners learned about the effectiveness of *Rhaponticum carthamoides*, also known as *Leuzea carthamoides*. This herb is a perennial that grows in Central Asia. Long recognized as a rejuvenator and metabolic stimulant in local folklore, scientists discovered that it contains a high concentration of ecdysteroids, especially 20-hydroxyecdysone (20-E).

Ecdysteroids Are Widespread

There are about 200 members in the ecdysteroid family, all of which are chemically related to 20-E. These ecdysteroids are widespread in plants and even in insects. In fact, ecdysteroids are the steroid hormones of invertebrates, functioning much as testosterone does in man. Ecdysteroids regulate many biochemical and physiological processes in insects, including maturation and reproduction.

The role of ecdysteroids in plants is still unclear, although they are thought to help protect the plant from insect damage. Concentrations are highest in the parts of the plant that are most important to its survival. In many species, 20-E is the most common ecdysteroid, and it is considered to be the most biologically active of these compounds.

A review of thousands of plant species has revealed that *Rhaponticum carthamoides* has the highest proportion of 20-E of any plant studied. However, *Pfaffia paniculata*, an herb found in the Brazilian rain forest, also contains 20-E in moderate amounts. This has led to a debate about whether the extracts of these plants provide the same benefits.

While the absence of research on *Pfaffia paniculata* makes it difficult to make a categorical statement, bear in mind that the other ecdysteroids in an herbal extract likely play a role in its effectiveness. Since nearly all of the available research is on *Rhaponticum carthamoides*, it is your best bet at this time as a source of 20-E.

Among vegetables, spinach has the highest concentration of 20-E. Could this be the real reason that Popeye has such big arms?

Numerous Anabolic Properties

Because of their many plant sources, ecdysteroids are commonly found in humans in low concentrations. They pass through the acidic conditions of the stomach without apparent changes to their structure and are easily assimilated. Maximum levels in the blood occur thirty minutes to two hours after they are consumed, depending on whether food is eaten along with the ecdysteroids.

A Half-Life
A measure of how long it takes for half of a substance to be degraded and eliminated by the body.

They are eliminated relatively quickly from the blood. Ecdysone, a fairly common ecdysteroid, has a half-life of four hours, while 20-E has a half-life of nine hours.

This suggests that you should take ecdysteroids several times per day to maintain high blood levels. Studies in mice indicate that the bioavailability is around 50 percent—fairly high for an herb.

Ecdysteroids have a number of anabolic properties. Several studies have shown a rise in protein synthesis with ecdysterone administration. A Japanese study found a 51 percent increase in protein levels when mice were given orally 5 mg of ecdysteroids per kilogram of body weight. The increase in protein levels peaked two to four hours after ecdysterone administration. These results were confirmed by two Russian studies.

In all cases, the changes were largely due to an increase in ribosomal activity. Ribosomes are cellular proteins that hook amino acids together to form new proteins. Also detected was a greater amount of messenger ribonucleic acid, which the body uses as a template for protein synthesis.

Remember that your body can create new muscle proteins only if sufficient raw material is available. Therefore, be sure to eat plenty of dietary protein each day (at least 1 g per pound of body weight). This will provide an adequate supply of amino acids, which your ribosomes can then incorporate into new muscle proteins. And, of course, give it your all in the gym.

More Advantages for Athletes

Training is hard work, and if you do it right, it will drain you of energy. Increases in work capacity are therefore very helpful. The longer you can work out, the more likely you are to accomplish your sports goals.

Several Russian studies have found enhanced work capacity with ecdysteroids. A study with mice found that a *Rhaponticum carthamoides* extract increased swimming time by 22 percent, while the length of time the mice could run before exhaustion rose by 32 percent. A twenty-day study of forty-four athletes found a similar increase in working capacity, which was measured on a bicycle ergometer (a tool used to measure work performance). Unfortunately, information regarding the dosages used in these studies is not available.

Most athletes are interested in gaining muscular size and strength, and several studies suggest that ecdysterone can help. A study performed at the Czech Academy of Sciences found that 20-E was effective in increasing the growth rate of Japanese quail. These animals, which grow quickly anyway, packed on 7 percent more body mass than the control group in only four weeks when given 20 mg of 20-E per kilogram of body weight. This occurred despite the fact that the 20-E group ate less, indicating that this ecdysterone may increase the efficiency of food assimilation.

These studies show that ecdysteroids can be effective anabolic agents. Even better, toxicological studies show that ecdysteroids are very safe. Because they do not operate through hormonal pathways, ecdysteroids cannot cause the negative effects produced by anabolic steroids. This makes them a much better choice for long-term use.

Other Health-Related Benefits

Ecdysteroids have other benefits as well. A study published in *Eksperimentalnaia i Klinicheskaia Farmakologiia* found that ecdysterone enhanced the sex function and behavioral characteristics of rats, especially in the first few days. The scientists, who gave the rats 5 mg of ecdysterone per kilogram of body weight each day for ten days, also found that it increased copulative function and improved the quality of their sperm.

Other experiments have shown that ecdysteroids have antioxidant properties, reducing the oxidation of LDL cholesterol (the so-called "bad" cholesterol) in both test-tube and animal studies. Ecdysteroids have also stimulated immune function in mice at a dosage of 5–20 mg/kg (milligrams per kilogram). In addition, a study on sixty Soviet cadets and forty-seven sailors found increased appetite and an improved mental state from an ecdysteroid extract. These studies support the traditional use of *Rhaponticum carthamoides* as a rejuvenator.

With such an extensive array of benefits, it is no wonder that ecdysterone and related ecdysteroids have become part of the supplement regimen of many athletes. They promote protein synthesis, boost work capacity, and increase muscle mass. As with all herbs, be sure to consider the dosages given in the studies and take the same amounts. And for maximum effect, choose an extract with a high concentration of 20-E. When used appropriately, ecdysteroids can be a valuable addition to your training program.

GINSENG AND ASTRAGALUS

Ginseng is one of the most popular herbs in the world, while astragalus is relatively unknown in Western countries. Both of these herbs have important benefits for the athlete, ranging from increased endurance and strength to enhanced immune function. Like *Rhaponticum carthamoides*, ginseng and astragalus work through nonhormonal pathways, so they can be used for extended periods. But it takes a while for you to see noticeable effects.

Ginseng has been the subject of a wide variety of research experiments in Western countries, both in animals and in humans. The results of these studies are all over the board for reasons that are discussed in this chapter. Nearly all of the experiments with astragalus have been done in China, where the herb is even more popular than ginseng. The bottom line from these studies is that ginseng and astragalus will help you perform better in your sport—provided that you take enough of a standardized extract for a long enough time.

The Many Types of Ginseng

While ginseng is often considered a single plant, there are

actually three to nine types of ginseng depending on who's counting. The three most popular ginsengs are *Panax ginseng* (Chinese or Korean ginseng), *Panax quinquefolius* (American ginseng), and *Eleutherococcus senticosus* (Siberian ginseng). Virtually all of the research in humans has been done with *Panax ginseng*, which is the most stimulating of the ginseng varieties.

The other plants that are similar to these ginsengs are *Panax pseudoginseng* (Tienqi ginseng), *Panax japonica* (Japanese ginseng), *Codonopsis pilosula* (False ginseng), *Pseudostellaria heterophylla* (Prince's ginseng), *Angelica sinensis* (dong quai), and *Glehnia littoralis* (glehnia root). As you can tell from the botanical names, several of these "ginsengs" aren't even in the same plant family as the Panax varieties.

Be sure to look at the label on your ginseng supplement to see which herb it contains. The non-Panax ginsengs are much weaker than the real thing, so you could be paying for a cheap imitation. If the supplement does not specify which ginseng it contains, choose a different product.

The King of Herbs

Panax ginseng has been revered in China as the King of Herbs for centuries. It is said to replenish the *qi*, or life force, of the body through a number of mechanisms. *Panax ginseng* works with the body to help restore balance. Chinese practitioners use it as a tonic to increase physical strength and energy and to promote the proper functioning of the body's organs. They also use it to treat fatigue.

Panax ginseng builds stamina and endurance by enhancing the body's ability to adapt to stress, and it was used extensively in former Soviet countries as a way to boost strength and athletic performance. (Siberian ginseng and *Rhaponticum carthamoides* were also used for these purposes.)

VO_{2max}
A measure of aerobic fitness. It measures the maximum volume of oxygen (O_2) that your lungs can hold.

A number of animal studies have confirmed these benefits. A placebo-controlled study at the University of Alberta with rats not accustomed to exercise found a significant increase in VO_{2max} after four days of ginseng saponin injections.

Ginseng treatment also significantly increased the amount of free fatty acids in the blood and preserved glucose levels during exercise. These alterations are favorable for the athlete, as they allow you to burn more fat and keep you from "hitting the wall" due to low glucose levels. The end result in greater exercise endurance.

A study published in *Ethnopharmacology* gave 100 mg/kg of an aqueous ginseng extract to mice orally for seven days. *Panax ginseng* produced a significant increase in swimming time compared with the control group. There was also an increase in body weight and in the mass of the *levator ani muscle*, the muscle that forms the floor of the pelvic cavity. (This was the only muscle studied.) In addition, an experiment at Toyama Medical and Pharmaceutical University with aged rats found that 8 g/kg per day of extract given orally for twelve days increased their performance in learning their way through a maze.

Proven Effectiveness in Humans

These animal studies, and most of the others before them, showed that *Panax ginseng* was effective in enhancing performance in rodents. Logically, scientists would then turn to human studies using the same relative amounts of ginseng to determine the effects in humans. However, in most cases this did not occur.

The animal studies that give the herb orally used a minimum of 100 mg per kilogram of body weight. The average human weighs 80 kg (176 lb). This means that an equivalent dose for a human would be 8,000 mg (or 8 g, a bit less than a third of an ounce). Yet most of the human studies used 200 mg of standardized extract (usually 4 percent ginsenosides), or 2.5 mg/kg. Surprise, surprise, these studies showed that ginseng didn't work! Whether these researchers were excessively conservative, out to show that the herbs didn't work, or simply clueless is unknown.

When appropriate levels of *Panax ginseng* are given for long enough periods, they consistently show the effectiveness of this herb. A six-week placebo-controlled study published in *International Clinical Nutrition Review* gave 1,000 mg of ginseng root powder per day to fifteen men and fifteen women. Compared with the placebo, *Panax ginseng* significantly improved VO_{2max}. The heart rate of the test subjects was six beats per minute lower for the six minutes after exercise, suggesting improved recovery from the workout. Even better, pectoral strength increased by 22 percent, while quadriceps strength rose 18 percent. There was, however, no significant increase in grip strength.

A Danish study gave 400 mg of standardized extract to 112 healthy volunteers for eight to nine weeks. The researchers noted faster reaction times among the participants. Also, an abstract presented at the XXIII FIMS World Congress of Sports Medicine Abstracts noted improved endurance, VO_{2max}, post-exercise recovery, and simple reaction time in a study of 214 individuals. Unfortunately, the length of this study and the dosage given to the volunteers were not reported.

The Other Ginsengs

There has not been as much research into the benefits of the other ginsengs. *Panax quinquefolius* (American ginseng) is used as a tonic and natural stress reducer. According to practitioners of traditional Chinese medicine, it also helps to build *qi*, or life force, although it is less stimulatory than *Panax ginseng*. American ginseng promotes strength by increasing immunity through several mechanisms.

Curiously, American ginseng is more popular in China than in this country. Most of the American crop is exported to Asia, where *Panax quinquefolius* has a reputation as an aphrodisiac. American ginseng is sometimes combined with *Panax ginseng* to produce an herbal blend that can boost energy levels while still relieving stress.

Siberian ginseng (*Eleutherococcus senticosus*) is not even from the same plant family as the Panax varieties. However, it does have some of the same stimulating and tonic effects as the other ginsengs. Like *Rhaponticum carthamoides*, it is native to Russia and has been used for generations to boost the strength and stamina of that country's athletes.

A study at two Japanese universities gave 300 mg per day of Siberian ginseng extract to six males to determine its effect on work capacity. This single-blind, cross-over study found significant increases in total work and time to exhaustion compared with the placebo group following eight days of supplementation. The researchers concluded that the improvements were due to changes in the participants' metabolisms, noting that VO_{2max} also increased.

No study to date has compared the benefits of *Panax ginseng* with American or Siberian ginseng. Also, there is virtually no research on the other types of ginseng. For now, you should avoid them. Stick with the proven winners.

Tips for Using Ginseng

Numerous studies have confirmed that ginseng can be of major benefit to athletes. Anything that increases your strength and aerobic potential while enhancing recovery and mental alertness will translate into significant gains in sports performance. However, you need to bear in mind that ginseng is an herb, not a prescription drug. As a result, you need to take a relatively large amount to get the results you want (although less than the dose for creatine or glutamine).

Always use a standardized root extract. Avoid products that are simply root powder and those that say only ginseng. If root is not specified, the manufacturer has probably substituted the less expensive (and less beneficial) leaves and branches of the plant. The root is where the highest concentrations of the active ingredients are found, so don't go simply by the milligrams per capsule. Buy the real thing.

The most beneficial chemicals in the plants are glycosylated steroidal saponins, usually referred to as ginsenosides. Thirteen different ginsenosides have been isolated so far, and each has specific properties. The most prevalent in *Panax ginseng* and *Panax quinquefolius* are R_b, R_c, and R_g, although their concentrations within these two herbs vary.

Because these ginsenosides interact with one another,

herbal specialists recommend that a whole-root extract be used instead of a brand that only has a particular ginsenoside. Besides, at this point, we don't know enough about the properties of each one to be that precise. This remains a topic for future research.

How to Maximize Ginseng's Benefits

All extracts are standardized for total ginsenosides, so go for the strongest one you can get. The products currently on the market have a wide range of ginsenoside content. The most well-known product has 4 percent ginsenosides, although you can buy products with up to 10 percent ginsenosides. If the label does not mention the ginsenoside content, pick another brand. The manufacturer is not keeping you in the dark to save ink on the label, if you catch my drift.

Ideally, the extract will also include standardization for polysaccharides. This is because there are beneficial components in ginseng other than ginsenosides. Aim for a product that has 10 percent polysaccharides.

While the precise dosage depends on the percentage of ginsenosides and polysaccharides, you should consume a minimum of 500 mg of extract per day. Begin at this level and increase it to 750 mg and then 1,000 mg per day as needed. It is best to give your body time to adjust to this herbal extract. Also, take it for a minimum of three months before deciding whether you want to continue it for the long term. It takes time to achieve ginseng's benefits.

Astragalus: The Immune Booster

While largely unknown in Western countries, *Astragalus membranaceus* has been used for thousands of years in traditional Chinese medicine as part of the Fu Zheng therapy to enhance natural defense mechanisms.

Chinese herbalists have utilized astragalus to treat every type of fatigue and exhaustion. The herb is said to stabilize the exterior of the body and increase its resistance to disease by increasing the circulation of *wei qi*, or protective life force, on the body's surface. This enhances immune function and boosts the body's ability to adapt to stress.

What difference does this make for the athlete? Exercise is inherently stressful. The body is forced to perform intensely, which can reduce your resistance. Many an athlete has caught a cold or the flu because he or she trained so much that his or her body was susceptible to any bug that passed by. By fortifying your immune system, you can help to prevent these frustrating and strength-depleting episodes with illness.

Researchers have undertaken numerous experiments with astragalus to confirm its benefits using the tools of modern science. It has been shown to have a very strong antioxidant effect. The herb also stimulates the production of white blood cells, stem cells, macrophages, and lymphocytes, helping the immune system to hold off invading organisms and accelerating healing. Astragalus also helps to protect the liver from toxins, and it has even been shown to increase sperm motility.

A study in the *Japanese Journal of Hygiene* gave mice 200 mg/kg of astragalus per day. They were then forced to run at a rapid rate for sixty minutes five times per day for twelve weeks. The scientists found that astragalus intensified the functioning of their host defense systems, allowing them to tolerate the exercise regimen better.

Astragalus has many active components. Most are plant chemicals called astragalosides, seven of which have been isolated. Astragalus is also a natural source of methoxy-isoflavone, which is discussed later. Each of these nutrients has a specific role, so you want to get a whole extract of the root. Various polysaccharides in astragalus have immune-stimulating properties as well.

As with ginseng, the astragalus products on the market have a wide variety of strengths. Only buy astragalus extracts, preferably water-based ones. Avoid products that just contain root powder. Aim for a flavonoid content of at least 1 percent and a polysaccharide content of 20 percent or more. This will ensure that you get an effective level of the active ingredients.

Synergy between Ginseng and Astragalus

Astragalus is frequently combined with ginseng in traditional Chinese medicine because of its synergistic actions with that herb. While ginseng stimulates the body's "aggressive" energy levels, astragalus strengthens the body's "defensive" energies, promoting a balance that gives you vitality without the jitters produced by most stimulants.

A recent study at Wichita State University examined the impact of a patented supplement that combines creatine with two forms of ginseng and astragalus (U.S. patent). Forty-four volunteers were divided into three groups. One group received a placebo, another took 3 g of creatine per day, and a third took 3 g of creatine plus 1,500 mg of an herbal extract that was 50 percent astragalus, 30 percent *Panax ginseng*, and 20 percent *Panax quinquefolius*. The test subjects trained with weights for forty minutes three times per week for twelve weeks.

"The creatine/herbal blend produced statistically significant strength increases compared to placebo on all six exercises measured," noted lead researcher Dr. Michael Rogers. On the bench press, the subjects using this blend had strength increases that were three times greater than did those who took creatine alone. Vigor, as measured by the standardized Profile of Mood States, rose 18.9 percent. There were also dramatic increases in immune function.

These findings confirm that ginseng and astragalus are powerful herbs, especially when taken together. For maximum benefit, use a product that contains a single extract made from these herbs in the 50/30/20 ratio. This proven formulation will promote the greatest gains in your strength and sports performance.

PHOSPHATIDYLSERINE

Physical exercise produces hormonal changes both during and after your workout. These hormones have a variety of impacts on the muscles and other tissues. Some of them are positive, helping the body to recuperate from the stresses of training. Others are negative, potentially keeping your body from recovering as quickly as you would like.

One of the hormones that can be negative is cortisol. Researchers have now found that phosphatidylserine (PS) can reduce cortisol levels, possibly promoting quicker recovery and growth.

Cortisol
Cortisol is a hormone produced by the adrenal gland. It stimulates protein breakdown and can lead to a negative nitrogen balance when present in high concentrations over prolonged periods.

Athletes try to reduce cortisol secretion because it suppresses the rate of protein formation and stimulates protein breakdown in tissues other than the liver. However, cortisol has other vital functions. It supports the action of hormones such as growth hormone and glucagon (which counteracts insulin and restores blood-sugar concentrations to normal levels). Cortisol also accelerates the release of stored fat and its use for energy, and even acts as an anti-inflammatory agent.

This means that the body often produces cortisol for a reason. As Thomas Fahey, Ph.D., professor of physical education at California State University, Chico, notes, "Suppressing cortisol levels a little bit is good because of its role in curbing protein synthesis. But you would never want to shut off its production entirely. It's there for a purpose!"

Benefits of This Essential Nutrient

Phosphatidylserine is an essential nutrient in our cells. It is one of a number of fat-based molecules that help to hold the cell membrane together. PS is particularly plentiful in nerve cells. Studies have shown that PS helps these cells to communicate with other cells by promoting the accumulation, storage, and release of neurotransmitters such as dopamine. This allows it to improve memory. PS also helps to transport nutrients into the cell and assists in the removal of waste products.

Scientists first looked at PS's ability to reduce cortisol levels with oral supplementation. A study at the University of Naples, Italy, gave 400 mg and 800 mg of PS to eight healthy males who performed an exercise protocol on a bicycle ergometer. The researchers found that 400 mg pf PS reduced cortisol levels in the blood by 16 percent, while 800 mg lowered cortisol concentrations by 25 percent.

Fahey and his associates conducted the second study. In this double-blind, crossover study, ten trained weightlifters were given 800 mg of PS per day and then put through a vigorous whole-body workout four times per week that was intentionally designed to overtrain them. Each athlete received PS for two weeks, then repeated the workout program for another two weeks with the placebo after a three-week period in which no supplement was taken. Blood samples were taken fifteen minutes after their last workout on these two regimens and twenty-three hours after those workouts to see what the effects of overtraining were on their cortisol levels.

The study found that PS reduced postexercise cortisol levels by 20 percent. Exit interviews showed that the persons on PS "felt better" and had less muscle soreness. However, no differences in cortisol levels were found twenty-three hours after exercise. Apparently, the body is able to return cortisol levels to normal during this timeframe without supplemental PS.

Many Unknowns at This Point

These studies clearly show that PS can reduce cortisol levels when administered orally. However, we still don't know if cortisol production is a limiting factor in recuperation and muscle growth. "Science moves forward in small steps," notes Fahey. "First, we establish the correlation between cortisol and exercise, and then we investigate the implications of these findings."

So while researchers feel confident that PS reduces cortisol levels, they still don't know whether supplementation with PS will permit faster recovery or improve sports performance.

PS is found in only trace amounts in most foods. While the body is able to produce PS on its own, it must go through reactions that require a substantial amount of energy. This makes supplementation a better option.

Recommended Dosage and Side Effects

Phosphatidylserine is usually sold in 500-mg capsules or tablets containing a combination of PS and other phospholipids. Usually, about half of the total amount is PS. The standard dosage is two to three capsules per day, which would provide a daily dosage of PS approximately equal to the dose found effective in the clinical studies.

When PS is taken orally, it is rapidly absorbed. However, the single dosage of pure PS should be kept to around 250 mg for a couple of reasons. One, it's expensive. Two, in rare instances, dosages greater than this have been reported to cause nausea. This effect is minimized when PS is consumed with food. Also, don't take it right before going to bed, as the neurotransmitters it helps to release may make

it harder for you to fall asleep. There do not appear to be any other side effects when taken at the recommended dosages.

In the future, PS may be considered a major anticatabolic nutrient. Until additional studies are completed, however, you'll need to do your own experiment and see what benefits you receive.

METHOXYISOFLAVONE AND IPRIFLAVONE

In the last few years, a large number of products have been introduced that contain methoxyisoflavone and ipriflavone. Judging from the sales of these products, athletes seem to find them very effective. Unfortunately, these nutrients are so new that there isn't a lot of research on them, so you'll need to try them for yourself and see what improvements you get.

There Are Many Methoxyisoflavones

Flavones are naturally occurring substances found in fruits and vegetables. They have been shown to have a variety of positive health benefits when included in the diet, such as a decreased risk of various cancers. This has led scientists to look for the mechanisms behind these improvements.

Two test-tube studies have shown that biochanin A (5,7-dihydroxy-4-methoxyisoflavone) inhibits the activity of the enzyme aromatase, which converts testosterone to estrogen. While not the strongest reducer of aromatase levels out there, it does have a statistically significant level of activity. Another test-tube study showed that biochanin A mildly inhibits the 5-alpha-reductase enzyme. This enzyme converts testosterone to dihydrotestosterone, the form of the hormone largely responsible for the prostate problems most men experience later in life.

While soy is a good source of biochanin A, a study at the Institute of Endocrinology in Prague, Czech Republic, found that beer also contains this isoflavone, along with another called formononetin (7-hydroxy-4-methoxyisoflavone). It's good to know that there are some beneficial nutrients in beer, but don't drink more because of it. Beer isn't exactly the breakfast of champions!

As you can see, there is more than one methoxyisoflavone. (I'll skip the rest of the list.) However, the one that supplement manufacturers include in their formulations is 5-methyl-7-methoxyisoflavone—not biochanin A. This is important because claims are sometimes made for products using research on similar, but not identical, isoflavones.

The 5-methyl-7 Patent

The 5-methyl-7 form of methoxyisoflavone was first developed in Hungary, and a Budapest company received U.S. patent 4,163,746 for its efforts in 1979. This patent gave the company exclusive control over the invention until the mid-nineties, which is why methoxy products only started appearing on the market a few years ago.

In their patent application, the inventors stated that 5-methyl-7 increased the retention of calcium and phosphorous to a significant degree. In fact, one of the early uses for this compound and a related isoflavone called ipriflavone was as a treatment for osteoporosis. The inventors also noted that 5-methyl-7 increased nitrogen retention, which would lead to greater protein synthesis and consequent muscle growth. Unfortunately, the extent to which it enhanced protein synthesis was not revealed.

The patent did include the results of two studies on chickens. After five weeks, 5-methyl-7 increased the total body weight of chickens by 8 percent, while the weight of uncastrated cocks rose by 8.7 percent. These increases were primarily meat (muscle) and not fat.

No human studies were performed for this patent, much less studies with athletes. The inventors suggested, however, that an appropriate dose for humans would be 100 mg two or three times per day.

Good News about Ipriflavone

So where did all the claims you hear for methoxyisoflavone come from? From an earlier patent on ipriflavone (7-iso-propoxyisoflavone) by the same inventors. Like 5-methyl-7, ipriflavone is a synthetic isoflavone that does not work through hormonal pathways. Animal studies suggest that it has several benefits for athletes.

The inventors gave 5 mg of ipriflavone per kilogram of body weight to rats for forty-five days. The rats were then forced to swim daily until exhaustion with a weight attached to their legs. At the end of the experiment, the ipriflavone-treated animals were able to swim an additional thirty-three minutes (an increase of 39 percent) compared with the controls. A second study found significant (but unspecified) increases in protein synthesis when rats were given 30 mg per kilogram of body weight for three weeks.

Another experiment with rats found that 5 mg of ipriflavone per kilogram of body weight partially suppressed the effect of cortisone, which can be converted into the hormone cortisol. High levels of cortisol can produce a loss of muscle tissue—the opposite of what you want. This mechanism could be partly responsible for the anabolic actions of this nutrient.

A fourth study gave 20 mg of ipriflavone per kilogram of feed to various farm animals for one to four months. It found increases in body weight ranging from 12 percent in guinea pigs to 20 percent in poultry and rabbits. Testing showed that most of the weight gain was meat (muscle) and not fat.

Hopefully, results of this magnitude will be achieved in healthy human subjects. However, the only human study included was on ten hospital patients suffering from pathological thinness. In this case, a dose of 150 mg three times per day produced an average weight increase of 2–3 kg. The length of the study was not provided.

Ipriflavone has been shown to be a very effective treatment for osteoporosis in more than 150 published studies on animals and humans. Because it does not have a direct estrogenic effect, ipriflavone is able to increase bone-mineral density in older women without the problems that estrogen replacement therapy can have, in part by increasing calcium absorption. Ipriflavone reduces osteoporosis in men, too. That's great news, particularly if you're getting on in years.

The Great Unknown

Since most athletes do not suffer from catabolic disorders, they should be able to make greater gains in muscle mass than weakened hospital patients do. Unfortunately, a MEDLINE data search revealed that no studies on the sports benefits of ipriflavone or 5-methyl-7-methoxyisoflavone have been published to date.

Now that the performance benefits of creatine have been established beyond a shadow of a doubt, it would be nice if researchers redirected their efforts to the study of these exciting isoflavones. Only then will we know for sure how effective they are in helping you achieve your sports goals.

RIBOSE

In order to achieve peak performance, your muscle cells need to provide the maximum amount of energy for muscular contraction. They can do this only when they have ample supplies of a chemical compound called ATP, also known as the "energy currency."

Earlier, you learned that creatine is able to increase the resynthesis of ATP, which is the main reason why it is so effective for boosting strength. But under conditions of heavy training, creatine cannot resynthesize ATP fast enough, and energy molecules escape from the muscle cell. If you train again before your body is able to replenish its ATP stores, your strength and energy levels will suffer. Fortunately, studies show that ribose can speed up this restoration process.

A Powerful Simple Sugar

In healthy individuals, the cells of the body contain ample amounts of ATP at rest. These ATP levels are tightly regulated, and there is no way to increase them beyond their maximum concentrations in the cell. Exercise draws upon these supplies for muscle contraction, temporarily reducing the amount available by up to 30 percent.

When oxygen is available in the cell, ATP resynthesis occurs rapidly. However, when there is a temporary shortage of oxygen (anaerobic conditions), the restoration is much slower. After an extremely intense workout, it can take up to four days for ATP levels to return to normal. During this period of time, your strength and performance will be less than optimal due to the lack of energy resources.

The time lag in ATP recovery occurs primarily because there is not enough of a compound called PRPP.

While PRPP can be made from glucose (blood sugar), it is a relatively slow process. Supplemental ribose has been found to quickly increase PRPP levels.

Ribose is a sugar that is found in all living cells. It is the carbohydrate backbone for RNA (ribonucleic acid) and DNA (deoxyribonucleic acid). These nucleic acids contain the information needed for cells to grow, divide, and carry out their normal functions.

PRPP

PRPP, or 5-phosphoribosyl-1-pyrophosphate, is a naturally occurring metabolite that the body uses to restore levels of ATP after exercise or other physical exertion.

Ribose can be converted into an energy molecule known as pyruvate, which allows ATP to be produced in the presence of oxygen. Another function of ribose is the formation of cyclic nucleotides, compounds that help regulate the activity of calcium and other electrolytes (minerals that conduct electricity) in the cell. These nucleotides control the contraction of your heart and skeletal muscles.

While ribose is found in meat and vegetables, you can't get enough from these sources to boost your sports performance. Supplementation is therefore required. "When you consume ribose, it is converted to PRPP through a metabolic pathway that is much quicker than the body's usual slow conversion of glucose," says Tim Ziegenfuss, Ph.D., CSCS. "This increases the supplies of PRPP and dramatically speeds up the restoration of ATP, both by salvaging the breakdown products of ATP metabolism and by helping to produce more ATP from scratch."

Increases in Strength and Performance

A study at Ball State University found that ribose increased power output. Sixteen male athletes took 10 g of ribose or a dextrose placebo two times per day for a three-day loading phase. They did not exercise during these three days. The athletes then performed five days of high-intensity exercise, consisting each day of two bouts of ten-second sprints on a cycle fifteen times in a row with only fifty seconds of rest between each sprint. After the five days, they rested for sixty-five hours but continued to take the ribose or placebo.

The group that took ribose had an increase in average power output of 4.2 percent during the training period, compared with only 0.6 percent for the placebo group. Also, the ribose group felt less fatigued, although the differences were not statistically significant. Even better, the levels of ATP and a similar compound called ADP returned to normal in the ribose group by the end of the sixty-five-hour recovery period, while the placebo group was still 23 percent below pre-exercise levels.

A similar study at Eastern Michigan University found increases in power of up to 10 percent with a dosage of 10 g per day. "This study confirmed that ribose supplementation can improve explosive anaerobic performance during intense training," says Dr. Ziegenfuss, a researcher in the study.

A study with twenty bodybuilders was performed at the University of Delaware. The athletes in this four-week double-blind study took 5 g of ribose or dextrose placebo twice daily. They then performed ten sets of bench presses per day using a three-day-on/one-day-off training cycle. Ribose supplementation increased their one-rep max by 3.2 percent, while the total number of repetitions they could perform rose by 19.6 percent.

Safe and Effective

The athletes who participated in these experiments experienced no side effects, indicating that ribose is a safe supplement. Because it is a simple sugar, this is hardly surprising. However, you should not take more than 20 g per day, as diarrhea and slight decreases in blood glucose levels have been experienced at higher levels.

In fact, a study at the University of Missouri found that the greatest amount of ATP salvaging per gram of ribose occurred at relatively low doses of ribose (up to 5 g). While larger amounts provided greater benefits, the rate of increase declined, suggesting that the body is prepared to handle only so much ribose at a time.

So stick with 5-g doses (a rounded teaspoon), taking it two to four times per day as needed. The best times to take ribose are before and after your workout. This will allow maximum ATP concentrations during the period when your body needs them the most.

As to ribose's effectiveness, this depends on your sport and type of training. Studies have shown that if you work out frequently at a high level of intensity, ribose will provide benefits. Competitive athletes in sports requiring short bursts of maximal work, such as track and field, powerlifting, and bodybuilding, will likely gain the most. However, if you are a weekend athlete or don't do a large volume of intense training, chances are that you won't experience any change from supplementation.

Weekend athletes have five days to recover, so their bodies can restore ATP levels without the help of ribose. And if you aren't hardcore with your training, you probably won't overtax your ATP levels to begin with. But if you frequently exercise with gung-ho intensity, give ribose a try. You may find that it gives you more energy when you work out.

MSM

If you are serious about your training, you have no doubt experienced delayed-onset muscle soreness as well as occasional tendonitis. This muscle soreness is caused by the microcellular damage that can occur from the stresses of your training program. At the microscopic level, the protein filaments that permit muscle contraction lose some of their integrity. Structural damage can also occur in tendons and ligaments.

Some scientists speculate that the lactic acid produced during your sets irritates these injured muscle tissues as well, further increasing the damage. The soreness can begin within hours and often continues for several days after your workout.

MSM supplementation can dramatically reduce this muscle soreness. This white, crystalline powder, technically known as methylsulfonylmethane, is also effective at reducing inflammation, so it can help your "tennis elbow." It inhibits pain impulses along nerve fibers, dilates blood vessels, and increases blood flow, which could reduce the amount of irritating lactic acid inside the muscle cell. Yet, how it actually does these things remains a mystery.

Sulfur Is an Essential Nutrient

It is widely assumed that MSM works because it is a bioavailable source of sulfur. (One-third of the MSM molecule is sulfur by weight.) Sulfur is found in virtually all body tissues, particularly the red blood cells, muscle, skin, hair, and nails. It is also involved in a number of endocrine and neurotransmitter functions.

Sulfur provides raw material for many enzymes and for compounds that protect against toxicity and free-radical damage. Sulfur is the eighth most abundant element in the human body, comprising 0.25 to 0.5 percent of your body weight. Despite these facts, there is no RDA for this vital mineral.

Sulfur is contained in four amino acids: the essential amino acid methionine and the nonessential cysteine, cystine, and taurine. Nutritionists have historically assumed that if you eat enough protein, you will get enough sulfur. However, these are the same people who think that you don't have to take vitamins if you eat right.

Less Soreness Means More Growth

Many athletes report that their soreness drops by as much as 40 percent when they take MSM. Some note that they don't have to use the railing anymore to climb stairs the day after their leg workout! Even better, the apparent decrease in microcellular damage lessens the amount of repair work needed inside the muscle fiber, giving your body more time to build new muscle tissue. Strength levels often increase, permitting more intense workouts. This can lead to greater muscle mass over time, provided of course that you eat right and don't overtrain.

There is little published research on MSM. We do know that it is a metabolite of DMSO, which has been the subject of thousands of studies over the past forty-five years. (About 15 percent of the DMSO molecule metabolizes into MSM in the body.) Logically, if there were a problem with 15 percent of this molecule, we would know it by now.

One unpublished study by Ronald Lawrence, M.D., president of the American Medical Athletic Association and coauthor of *The Miracle of MSM: The Natural Solution for Pain* (Penguin Putnam, 1999), found dramatic improvements in the frequency of connective-tissue injuries with MSM supplementation. The volunteers took 750 mg of MSM or placebo three times per day for four weeks along with standard chiropractic treatment. Even though the subjects in the MSM group were nearly a decade older on average, they experienced significantly less pain and tenderness than the placebo group. They also needed to make 40 percent fewer visits to the chiropractor for assistance.

The Most Effective Dosage

Although your body contains tiny amounts of MSM naturally (about 2 parts per million) from food sources such as milk, vegetables, coffee, and tea, you need to supplement in order to get enough MSM to help your workouts. MSM comes in crystal form, tablets, and capsules. The crystals are much less expensive, but you may find the bitter taste to be intolerable.

If you decide to try crystals, buy a small container. Drink it with juice or other strong-flavored liquid to mask the taste. A level teaspoon of crystals contains 5 g of MSM. Uncoated tablets are easier to take, but swallow quickly. Capsules, of course, do not have an unpleasant taste, but they are more expensive. The decision is yours.

Begin your supplementation at a dose of 1 g per day before your workout. Some athletes who have taken too much too quickly have experienced headaches. It is better to give your body time to adjust to the higher MSM levels. After a week, start taking one dose before your workout and another dose afterward. This will ensure the greatest concentration of MSM during your training session and the postworkout recovery phase. If you still experience soreness, increase each dose to 2 g.

On the days that you don't work out, a single dose is sufficient. Taking it with meals will reduce the likelihood of any gastrointestinal upset. Also, some athletes say that it increases their energy level. If you notice this, don't take it before bedtime, as it may keep you awake. Other benign side effects include smoother skin and stronger nails.

A Few Precautions

MSM is a very safe nutrient. In fact, a study performed at one of the world's leading toxicology centers in Italy found that it is less toxic than table salt. Still, there are big holes in our knowledge of MSM. Therefore, a few precautions are in order.

Clinical observations indicate that MSM has an aspirin-like effect on platelet aggregation, which results in thinner blood. "If you are taking high doses of aspirin or other blood-thinning medications, consult with your physician before taking MSM," says Lawrence. "Also, MSM may interfere with the accuracy of a test for liver damage that measures enzyme levels, so inform your doctor if you are supplementing with this nutrient." In addition, approximately 1 percent of users experience a rash, particularly in warmer climates. If this occurs, reducing the dosage usually eliminates the problem.

More and more athletes are discovering that MSM reduces the muscle soreness and tendonitis that they get from their workouts. This often leads to greater muscle growth and a new enthusiasm at the gym. So give MSM a try. It could eliminate a nutrient deficiency that has been holding back your training progress.

CAFFEINE, EPHEDRINE, AND OTHER DIET AIDS

One of the benefits of participating in sports is that the increased activity level boosts your daily caloric expenditure, helping to reduce body-fat levels. Whether it's lifting weights or playing volleyball on the beach, an active lifestyle helps to reveal your six-pack abs and lean musculature. However, unless you're a marathon runner or triathlete, chances are that you won't burn enough calories to have a physique as defined as you would like.

This reality has led supplement manufacturers to sell a wide variety of diet aids. Most have thermogenic properties.

Other products suppress your appetite, boost fat oxidation, or stimulate the release of thyroid hormones. A few of these supplements can even improve your sports performance.

Thermogenic
A nutrient that increases your heat production and metabolic rate so you burn more calories each day.

Caffeine: An Ancient Stimulant

Caffeine is a traditional part of virtually every culture on Earth. Whether it's consumed in the form of coffee, tea, yerba mate, guarana, or cola drinks, nearly everyone has experienced the uplifting sensation of caffeine. Most of us take this stimulating drug daily. Recently, caffeine has been added to a variety of sports drinks, gels, and even bottled waters for its energizing effects.

The caffeine content of a 12-ounce can of cola ranges from 35–46 mg, while black tea has 45–70 mg per 8-ounce cup depending on the strength. Green tea averages 25 mg per cup. The amount of caffeine in coffee varies even more. A cup of traditional American drip coffee can have as little as 130 mg, while the same amount of espresso has 400 mg.

Bear in mind that coffee, tea, and similar plants contain a variety of natural chemicals in addition to caffeine. Some of these may counteract caffeine's effect, so if your goal is to increase performance or lose body fat, you should consume a supplement with caffeine instead of drinking huge amounts of coffee. It's great for waking up in the morning, but keep it at that.

Caffeine is rapidly absorbed by the body and remains in circulation for more than seven hours. Plasma concentrations reach a peak one hour after it is consumed. It is then slowly metabolized, with a half-life of four to six hours. There is a large variation among individuals in the response to a given caffeine dose. For some, a small amount can cause jitters and sleeplessness, while others can consume large doses without any negative effects. The precise reasons for this variation are unknown, although it is widely recognized that people can build up a tolerance to caffeine.

Another concern with caffeine is its diuretic effect. Clearly, caffeine increases urine output during the first four hours after you consume it. However, the change is not as great as some people believe. Regular-strength coffee increases urine volume by about 10 percent compared with an equal amount of water, while a large dose of caffeine (8.7 mg per kilogram of body weight) was shown to boost output by 30.6 percent. To prevent dehydration, which can reduce performance even if it is so slight that you don't feel thirsty, be sure to drink at least four liters of water per day and more if you participate in prolonged physical activity.

Proven Sports Benefits

Caffeine is a proven performance enhancer. A wide range of studies has shown that it increases endurance, speed, and power in a variety of sports. There is also evidence that caffeine boosts strength. Some of these studies used a standard 250-mg dose, which was administered to all subjects regardless of weight. Other studies gave the participants a fixed amount per kilogram of body weight. This latter procedure is much more precise, because caffeine makes its way into—and has effects in—many different body tissues.

A study by researchers at RMIT University in Australia and the University of Otago in New Zealand compared the effects of 6 mg/kg and 9 mg/kg of caffeine on performance during a 2,000-meter rowing exercise. Eight competitive oarsmen completed the rowing tests on different days. Compared with the results without caffeine, there was an average reduction in rowing time of 1.2 percent and an increase in mean power of 2.7 percent. There was no significant difference between the two dosage levels, suggesting that more is not always better with caffeine.

Caffeine also helps swimmers. A study published in the *Canadian Journal of Applied Physiology* found significant reductions in swim times. Time to completion for the 500-meter race dropped by seven seconds when 6 mg/kg of caffeine was consumed, while the improvement for the 1,500-meter race was twenty-three seconds. Similar benefits have been noted in studies with cyclists. A study involving soldiers at training camp even showed that it moderately increased the time to exhaustion during intense drills.

Caffeine has also been shown to boost strength levels. A study at York University in Toronto found that 5 mg/kg increased maximum lifting weight by 3.5 percent, while the time to fatigue for exercise performed at 50 percent of the one-rep max rose by 26 percent. This suggests that caffeine has a localized effect within the muscle fibers.

These and other studies show that caffeine can improve sports performance at doses between 3 and 6 mg/kg. This is important because caffeine use is limited at the Olympics and other major sports events. You may have been under the impression that caffeine was prohibited at the Olympics, but this is an overstatement.

The International Olympic Committee (IOC) has set a limit of 12 mcg of caffeine per milliliter of urine. Yet most people would have to take an acute dose of 9 mg/kg to get close to 12 mcg per milliliter. Clearly, you can get a performance benefit from caffeine and still pass your IOC drug test. Remember, however, that not everyone gets the same urinary concentration from a given dose of caffeine. For unknown reasons, some athletes excrete more than others do. Most people are safe at 6 mg/kg, but if you are competing at the elite level, you might want to test your levels beforehand to be sure.

Athletes are sometimes told that the sports benefits of caffeine will occur only if they avoid regular use of caffeine and caffeinated beverages. Research has shown this to be false, however. Comparative studies have revealed no difference in performance between regular users and abstainers. (The drug clears your system within forty-eight hours.) So if you want a cup of Joe in the morning, go right ahead.

How Caffeine Works

There are a number of theories about how caffeine improves performance. Traditionally, it was felt that caffeine works by increasing free fatty-acid levels. This provides an additional source of fuel that "spares" the glycogen stores. While it is true that some (but not all) studies show a rise in fatty acids, lactate levels also go up, indicating an increase in the use of blood glucose and glycogen for fuel. So little sparing may actually be going on.

Besides, the availability of substrates such as fat and carbohydrate is rarely a limit on performance for exercise lasting less than sixty minutes. If you are a marathon runner or triathlete, caffeine may actually help you to maintain your performance longer by increasing the time before you use up your glycogen stores (also called "hitting the wall"). But it is unlikely that this mechanism explains the benefits for athletes who do short-term, intense exercise, such as weightlifters and sprinters.

Adrenaline
Adrenaline is a hormone released during stressful situations. Often called the "fight or flight" hormone, it binds to the receptors in many tissues and increases alertness, allowing athletes to function at a higher performance level.

Recent studies suggest that an important mechanism of action for caffeine is increasing adrenaline levels.

Caffeine has also been shown to stimulate uptake of potassium into muscle cells. Since the loss of potassium is partly responsible for muscle fatigue, this mechanism results in prolonged activation in the motor units of the muscle fibers and greater force production. Caffeine changes the ionic balance within muscle tissue, as well.

There is no question that caffeine is an important ergogenic aid. But can it help you to lose body fat? Don't count on it. Several studies have looked at caffeine doses ranging from 100–600 mg per day. While caffeine had a mild thermogenic effect and slightly increased fat burning, the differences were not statistically significant compared with the placebo. The increased adrenaline level may reduce your appetite somewhat, but that's about all. Yet, when you combine caffeine with ephedrine, it's a different story.

Ephedrine Boosts Performance

Ephedrine is a natural chemical found in the *Ephedra sinica* plant, from which it gets its name. Also known as ma huang, this plant has a long history of usage in Asian countries for the treatment of asthma and other bronchial conditions. A related chemical, pseudoephedrine, is also found in the plant and is an ingredient in many cold and flu remedies.

Ephedrine is a stimulant that works on the receptors in the central nervous system. It has been shown to increase the level of dopamine, which is a precursor to both epinephrine and norepinephrine, both vital neurotransmitters. Dopamine is also an important neurotransmitter around the hypothalamus, an area of the brain that is important for body arousal. Unlike caffeine, which exerts many of its benefits in muscle tissue, ephedrine appears to work primarily on the central nervous system.

Several studies have looked at ephedrine's role in improving sports performance. It appears that significant gains can be achieved only when you take at least 1 mg per kilogram of body weight. Less than that is not effective.

For example, a study at Victoria Hospital and the University of Western Ontario gave 24 mg of ephedrine to twenty-one young males who then performed an extensive battery of tests designed to measure everything from muscle strength, endurance, and power to lung function, VO_{2max}, and recovery time. About the only thing that ephedrine did was increase the average heart rate. A similar study with 120 mg of pseudoephedrine showed no benefit during one hour of high-intensity exercise, although it should be noted the pseudoephedrine is only a third as strong as ephedrine.

On the other hand, studies at the Defense and Civil Institute of Environmental Medicine in Toronto showed positive results. Unlike the debate about doping in athletic events, no one has a problem with giving ephedrine to soldiers if it can increase their fighting potential. When 1 mg/kg was given to sixteen healthy males, there was a significant increase in power output during the first fifteen seconds of a thirty-second test that measures anaerobic power. Another study by this institute found that the same amount of ephedrine increased the time to exhaustion on a set of military drills by 19 percent.

The King of Thermogenics

Ephedrine is an effective fat burner on its own. Renowned weight-loss expert Arne Astrup, M.D., and his associates performed a study at the University of Copenhagen and two Danish hospitals. Five young females were given 20 mg of ephedrine three times per day one hour before meals and were told to continue eating normally. Even though there was no dieting involved, the women lost an average of 2.5 kilograms of body weight after four weeks and 5.5 kilograms after twelve weeks. They also held on to their lean muscle, while their body-fat percentage dropped by 3.5 percent after four weeks and 5.2 percent after twelve weeks. Two months after the experiment stopped, they had only gained back 0.5 kilograms. The only side effect was a mild rise in blood pressure at the start of the experiment.

When ephedrine is combined with caffeine, the effects are even greater. This combination has been extensively studied, but space limitations do not allow a detailed listing of the many studies that have showed benefits. All of this research, however, supports the effectiveness of the E/C stack (combination of ephedrine and caffeine) and demonstrates the moderate level of side effects that occur when you take specific dosages.

Two studies by the same Danish researchers indicate the extent of the benefits. In both studies, the participants took a supplement with 20 mg of ephedrine and 200 mg of caffeine three times per day. They also followed a low-calorie diet. In the first study, the test subjects lost 16.2 percent of their body weight in twenty-four weeks, significantly more than the 13.4 percent loss by the placebo group. The second study confirmed that most of this loss was body fat. In that eight-week study, the E/C group lost 10.1 kg, compared with only 8.4 kg with the placebo. But the E/C group lost twice as much fat (9.0 kg versus 4.5 kg) and much less fat-free mass (1.1 kg versus 3.9 kg). Only mild side effects, such as upset stomach and jitteriness, were reported in some individuals.

While the mechanisms are still not known, it is thought that caffeine has a "permissive" action on ephedrine, lowering the amount needed to achieve its physiological effects. In other words, caffeine potentiates ephedrine's effect. The E/C studies that showed the greatest benefits used a 10:1 ratio of caffeine to ephedrine, so be sure to use a supplement that contains this ratio.

Some products contain natural plant extracts as the sources for these nutrients. Guarana, for example, is a source of caffeine. If the product uses an extract, look for the amount of the active ingredient on the label. It is the active ingredients that must be in a 10:1 ratio—not the amount of extract, which can come in varying concentrations.

Some thermogenic supplements add aspirin or willowbark extract to the basic E/C combination. (Willow bark is a natural source of salicin, which is similar to the acetylsalicylic acid in aspirin.) These ingredients are said to further increase the effects of the E/C stack by helping to raise the body's set point for temperature regulation and keeping the body from reregulating itself. This would boost the basal metabolic rate and help to burn more body fat. However, this may not always be the case.

"While a study with obese mice showed that aspirin contributed to energy expenditure, one human study showed no improvement compared to ephedrine and caffeine alone, and another found significant benefits only in obese individuals," notes Will Brink, author of the e-book *Diet Supplements Revealed* (www.aboutsupplements.com). "So aspirin may not provide a benefit in athletes. Studies still need to be performed in these individuals."

A number of studies have been published in which entire over-the-counter products with caffeine, ephedrine, aspirin or willow bark, and other ingredients were tested and found to be effective compared with a placebo. However, since additional substances were involved, the role of the aspirin or willow bark cannot be established. Only time will tell the precise role of salicin or acetylsalicylic acid in athletes.

Be Aware of Possible Side Effects

The studies on ephedrine and caffeine reported very few side effects with the use of these stimulants in healthy subjects. There were occasional reports of headaches, irritability, anxiety, and tremors. These effects were most frequent during the first week or two of supplementation, after which the study participants seemed to get accustomed to the stimulation.

However, there is a wide variability in how an individual responds to these plant chemicals. Some people, for example, can drink coffee all day and fall asleep easily, while others wind up staring at the ceiling if they have coffee for lunch. Start out with a half-dose to see how you respond to these strong stimulants, and never exceed the recommended dosage.

Some studies have reported a mild increase in heart rate or blood pressure, especially at the start of the study. As a result, if you have high blood pressure, you should not take these stimulants. If your blood pressure is high-normal, bear in mind that caffeine and ephedrine could push you into the high range. If you are in this category, you should ideally measure your blood pressure before you begin supplementation and then again a month later to see if any change has taken place.

Also, do not use caffeine or ephedrine if you are pregnant or breast-feeding, elderly, under age eighteen, or chronically ill. Talk to your doctor before using these stimulants if you are taking any prescription or over-the-counter medication, including but not limited to antidepressants, stimulants, allergy medications, and drugs for cardiovascular conditions.

Skip your afternoon dose if you have trouble sleeping, and discontinue use entirely if you feel any dizziness, nausea, anxiety, headaches, or heart palpitations. You can still lose weight through a sensible diet and exercise regimen. It will take a while longer, but that's better than worsening a medical condition.

More Thermogenic Options

Caffeine is found in a variety of plants, and extracts of these plants are sometimes included in thermogenic supplements. Guarana (*Paullinia cupana*) is a shrub that is native to Brazil. It contains caffeine and traces of related alkaloids, as do kola nut, yerba mate, and various teas. These extracts may be added to thermogenic products instead of, or in addition to, the usual caffeine from coffee.

While these herbs and plants may be advertised as "natural" alternatives to the caffeine in coffee, don't be misled. Coffee is also a natural plant grown in mountainous regions around the world. Quite simply, caffeine is caffeine. Your body neither knows nor cares what plant it came from. However, because the caffeine content of these plants varies, be sure to check for the amount of caffeine in the extract. That is what should be in the 10:1 ratio with ephedrine.

Citrus aurantium, also called bitter orange, contains synephrine, a compound that is similar to ephedrine.

Although not as strong as ephedrine, it increases metabolic activity and boosts thermogenesis. It does not suppress appetite, however. Because *Citrus aurantium* produces fewer side effects, it is a good choice if you find that you are sensitive to ephedrine.

Sida cordifolia is another source of ephedrine, but it is not found in high concentrations in the plant. Be sure to check the strength of the *Sida cordifolia* extract you are considering using. Norephedrine, another cousin to ephedrine, has a stimulating effect similar to these two compounds. These products are normally part of a combination weight-loss product and are rarely sold separately.

Carnitine and HCA Boost Fat Oxidation

You can also lose body fat by increasing the rate at which you oxidize the fats, or lipids, in your bloodstream. Hydroxycitric acid (HCA) and carnitine have been shown to assist in this process. The enzyme that regulates fatty-acid oxidation is carnitine palmitoyl transferase-1 (CPT-1). It transports fat into the mitochondria (energy factory) of the cell for oxidation. When you supplement with carnitine, you increase the supply of the main raw material needed to activate CPT-1, which can boost the amount of fat oxidation that takes place. Take 1–3 g of carnitine per day to maximize this process.

HCA is an acid that comes from the rind of *Garcinia cambogia.* This grapefruit-sized fruit, also known as Malabar tamarind, has been used as a condiment for thousands of years in India. Scientists now know that HCA inhibits the action of citrate lyase, an enzyme that reduces the level of lipid oxidation in the body. By putting the handcuffs on citrate lyase, you increase the body's propensity to burn fats while decreasing the utilization of carbohydrates. This has the effect of keeping more carbs in the liver, which is where your hunger receptors are located. End result: less hunger.

HCA works best in combination with carnitine, since this allows you to alter the oxidation equation on both sides. Take 2–6 g of HCA per day at the same time you take your carnitine. Some diet supplements contain both nutrients.

Guggulsterones and Thyroid Boosters

The thyroid gland plays a pivotal role in regulating your metabolism. It releases hormones that increase the rate at which your cells release energy from carbohydrates, while promoting protein synthesis and the utilization of fatty acids. If your thyroid does not release as many of these hormones as the average person, you are said to have a "slow metabolism." On the other hand, if the thyroid gland releases too much of these hormones, you could end up with a catabolic condition known as muscle wasting.

Guggulsterones are the active ingredients in guggul lipids, which are fatty substances that are extracted from the herb *Commiphora mukul.* For centuries, practitioners of the traditional Ayurvedic system of medicine have recommended this Indian plant for weight loss. It appears to promote the production of thyroid hormones, helping to counteract the usual slowing of the metabolic rate during a diet. While there is little Western research on this nutrient, it has been shown to reduce cholesterol levels by lowering the amount of LDL (the "bad" cholesterol), so you may get a double benefit.

Coleus forskohili is another thyroid booster. The active ingredient in the plant, called forskolin, has been shown to increase the efficiency of T3, an important thyroid hormone. "Coleus enhances T3 efficiency by increasing the level of cyclic AMP, which is a gatekeeper for energy regulation," says Dallas Clouatre, Ph.D., author of *Anti-Fat Nutrients* (Pax, 1997). "This results in a greater metabolic expenditure and will help to reduce body-fat levels as long as your diet and exercise regimens are appropriate."

Other Diet Supplements

A number of other products are sold as weight-loss enhancers. One is alpha-lipoic acid (ALA). In people with diabetes, ALA increases insulin sensitivity, which is the body's ability to respond to a rise in blood glucose. The theory is that higher insulin levels will shunt more of the glucose into the muscle cells, so it won't be stored as body fat. While this may be true, there is no published evidence to date that it occurs in healthy athletes. ALA is a strong antioxidant, however.

Chromium is a mineral that helps insulin bind to its receptor sites. It is also involved in the metabolism of glucose for energy. A deficiency of chromium can lead to increased fat storage, fatigue, sugar cravings, and mood swings, all of which are counterproductive to your weight-loss goals. The average American diet does not provide enough chromium for a sedentary person, much less an athlete. For this reason, you should supplement with 200 mcg of chromium picolinate per day and eat plenty of chromium-rich whole-grain cereals.

Tyrosine is an amino acid that plays an important role in human metabolism. It is the precursor to stimulatory neurotransmitters such as epinephrine, norepinephrine, dopamine, and some of the thyroid hormones. While there is no published evidence that tyrosine works on its own as a weight-loss agent, several studies have shown that it increases the benefits of caffeine/ephedrine products, in part by helping to curb appetite. Tyrosine also appears to reduce stress and fatigue, so you can more easily stick to your diet. If your weight-loss supplement does not include tyrosine, try taking 500 mg of tyrosine along with it. You may find that this amino acid enhances its effectiveness.

With the wide variety of weight-loss products available, it's easy to get confused. Most, however, contain various combinations of the nutrients mentioned in this chapter. Because individual sensitivities vary, always start with a small dose and work your way up. You've wanted to lose weight for some time now—another week or two won't make a big difference. And be sure to control your food intake and exercise regularly. Diet supplements are a lot more effective when you give them a helping hand!

SPORTS DRINKS

Not that long ago, the category of sports drinks had one entry: Gatorade. Originally developed for the Gators football team at the University of Florida, Gatorade became a household word with the once-revolutionary concept that water is not the best thing to drink during exercise.

When studies confirmed that drinks with electrolytes and simple carbohydrates improved sports performance, a new market segment was born. It has since grown to a billion-dollar industry with a large number of entries and an ever-expanding variety of flavors. While it is not possible in this short book to review them all, this chapter will discuss the five main types of sports drinks available for consumers. Depending on your sport and recovery goals, all of these drinks may be appropriate for you at one time or another.

Low-Carb Drinks Reduce Fatigue

The earliest sports drinks were all low-carb drinks. These Gatorade competitors are designed to be consumed before and during exercise. They provide a relatively low amount of simple carbs that helps to maintain your blood-sugar levels during exercise. This carbohydrate usually comes from sucrose, glucose, glucose polymers, fructose, or high-fructose corn syrup.

These drinks are around 6 to 8 percent carbs, so they are predominantly water. This makes them valuable sources of fluids to replace the water lost through perspiration and breathing. The low carb level also maximizes fluid absorption while minimizing stomach upset during exercise.

Low-carb drinks also contain the electrolytes sodium and potassium. This helps to restore the appropriate levels of these minerals, which are lost during training. Another advantage of sodium is that it increases thirst, encouraging the appropriate consumption of fluids to keep your body fully hydrated.

The drinks are equally beneficial for strength and endurance athletes, who need to maintain their energy levels during exercise. Since most forms of sustained exercise primarily use glucose and glycogen for energy, providing small amounts of carbs can help to prevent a loss of training intensity.

Don't go overboard drinking low-carb drinks. They are intended to be sipped in small amounts, not guzzled a bottle at a time. If you overdo it, you could experience gastric distress. Too many carbs right before or during exercise also reduces the beneficial hormonal responses to exercise. In moderation, however, low-carb drinks can reduce fatigue and promote maximal performance.

High-Carb Drinks Promote Glycogen Resynthesis

High-carb drinks contain two to four times as many carbs as the low-carb versions. They should not be used during exercise, because they can upset your stomach if consumed too quickly and can reduce desirable elevations in testosterone and growth hormone. However, after exercise they provide a convenient way to get the carbs you need right after your workout to maximize glycogen resynthesis.

Studies have shown that your first meal after a workout should be an easily digestible meal such as a sports drink or meal-replacement drink. These drinks are assimilated quicker than a meal from whole food, allowing you to start the rebuilding process as soon as possible. This can help to minimize muscle breakdown as well.

One of the advantages of high-carb drinks is that they can be mixed with creatine to form an impromptu creatine-transport drink. They can also be used to increase total calorie count if you are on a weight-gain diet. Some brands contain electrolytes, vitamin C, and chromium and other minerals, while others are pure carb beverages.

High-carb drinks are made from the same simple sugars used for the low-carb drinks, with possibly some maltodextrin or other complex carbohydrate added. This makes them beneficial after a workout when your primary objective is rebuilding your glycogen stores. However, you shouldn't live on simple sugars. Use these drinks as postworkout beverages, and eat mainly complex carbohydrates the rest of the day.

Protein Drinks Provide Essential Amino Acids

Protein drinks are an easy way to get the high-quality protein you need to recover and build muscle. These beverages can be put in a gym bag or briefcase, allowing you to get essential amino acids right after your workout or when you are on the run and don't have access to a blender to mix a regular protein shake.

These drinks are usually made from whey protein, although some contain casein and/or soy as well. The amount of protein varies with the size of the container, although most provide between 20 and 45 g. Some drinks have additional ingredients, ranging from vitamins and minerals to nutrients that may increase uptake and delivery of amino acids to the muscle cells. Others provide added glutamine or branched-chain amino acids. Most have very little carbs and fat.

Many of the products in this category are ready-to-drink beverages, but some of them come in powdered form. While these powder drinks have the disadvantage that you need to fill the bottles with cold water, they do provide a mess-free, premeasured dose of protein powder. They are also much lighter than the liquid drinks. This could be an advantage depending on the number that you are carrying.

Recovery Drinks Combine Carbs and Protein

Recovery drinks were originally designed as postworkout beverages, but new research at the University of Texas shows that they can also boost performance when taken during exercise. These drinks usually contain 10–15 g of protein and 15–35 g of carbs with little or no fat. A few have higher carb levels. Since your body needs both carbs and protein to maximize recovery, these combination drinks can be very beneficial.

"There is some evidence that protein helps the uptake of carbs, even during exercise," notes Edmund Burke, Ph.D., author of *Optimal Muscle Recovery* (Avery Publishing, 1999). "Research has shown that a sports drink with carbs and protein improves the fuel efficiency and recovery of muscle even better than a drink that only has carbohydrates."

The study at the University of Texas used a 4:1 ratio of carbs to protein. Scientists found that this amount of protein provided essential amino acids without negatively impacting fluid and carbohydrate replenishment. Too much protein, the researchers warned, could reduce these benefits, so you should try to maintain this ratio during the two hours after your workout. This would require the intake of more carbs than the amount contained in most recovery drinks.

Even with the macronutrients in these drinks, they have substantial amounts of water. This makes it easier to rehydrate after a workout. Also, since intense training decreases appetite, these drinks offer a convenient and flavorful way to get the nutrients you need to recover and increase your strength.

Fat-Burner Drinks Help You Lose Weight

These drinks contain no protein and virtually no carbs. What they do have are fat-burning nutrients such as ephedra, caffeine, guarana, white willow bark, hydroxycitric acid, and carnitine. While these supplements are also available in capsule form, consuming them in a drink gives you a flavorful beverage with water (which is especially important while you are dieting).

All of these nutrients are stable in water, so there is no loss of potency as occurs with creatine. You pay more for the nutrients when they are in sports drinks instead of pills, but there is a convenience factor involved as well as a taste advantage.

If you are sensitive to stimulants or only want to take a small amount of them, consuming a drink may give you all of the assistance you need to shed unwanted pounds. However, because fat-burners can cause side effects in some individuals, please read the section "Caffeine, Ephedrine, and Other Diet Aids" before taking these nutrients.

CONCLUSION

Every athlete wants to reach his or her goal as soon as possible. Nowadays, that means you have to eat right, train hard, and take a variety of sports nutrients to ensure your progress. These supplements can increase your strength and muscle size, enhance endurance, and keep your immune system strong, making them essential tools in your training regimen.

This guide has given you a good understanding of the leading sports nutrients in the marketplace. Armed with this knowledge, you can now make the best purchases for your own needs. You can tailor your supplement program to match your sport and intensity level, while keeping your expenses down to a minimum.

At the same time, never lose track of the fact that sports excellence does not come in a bottle. Sports nutrients are meant to supplement a healthy diet with plenty of protein, carbs, and healthy fats. They cannot make up for poor workouts, either, so don't use them as a crutch. Stick to a focused exercise regimen that provides plenty of training stimuli along with sufficient time for rest and recuperation.

When you give it your all at the gym or on the playing field, you'll find that these valuable nutrients will return the favor by giving you the maximum benefits they have to offer. Best of luck on your sports progress!

SELECTED REFERENCES

VITAMINS & MINERALS

Anderson, RA. Chromium, glucose intolerance and diabetes. *J Am Coll Nutr*, 1998; 17(6):548–555.

Badmaev, V, Prakash, S, Majeed, M. Vanadium: a review of its potential role in the fight against diabetes. *J Altern Complement Med*, 1999; 5(3):273–291.

Burton, GW, Traber, MG, Acuff, RV, et al. Human plasma and tissue a-tocopherol concentrations in response to supplementation with deuterated natural and synthetic vitamin E. *American Journal of Clinical Nutrition*, 1998; 67: 669–684.

Bohmer, H, Muller, H, Resch, KL. Calcium supplementation with calcium-rich mineral waters: a systematic review and meta-analysis of its bioavailability. *Osteoporosis Int*, 2000; 11(11):938–943.

Cathcart, RF. Vitamin C, titrating to bowel tolerance, anascorbemia, and acute induced scurvy. *Medical Hypotheses*, 1981; 7:1359–1376.

Clark, LC, Dalkin, B, Krongrad, A, et al. Decreased incidence of prostate cancer with selenium supplementation: results of a double-blind cancer prevention trial. *Br J Urol*, 1998; 81(5):730–734.

Crawford, V, Scheckenbach, R, Preuss, HG. Effects of niacinbound chromium supplementation on body composition in overweight African-American women. *Diabetes Obes Metab*, 1999; 1(6):331–337.

Douglas, RM, Chalker, EB, Treacy, B. Vitamin C for preventing and treating the common cold. *Cochrane Database Syst Rev*, 2000; 2:CD000980.

Eberlein-Kinig, B, Placzek, M, Pryzybill, B. Protective effect against sunburn of combined systemic ascorbic acid (vitamin C) and d-a-tocopherol (vitamin E). *Journal of the American Academy of Dermatology*, 1998:45–48.

Hoeger, WW, Harris, C, Long, EM, et al. Four-week supplementation with a natural dietary compound produces favorable changes in body composition. *Adv Ther*, 1998; 15(5):305–314.

Jacques, PF, Taylor, A, Hankinson, SF, et al. Long-term vitamin C supplement use and prevalence of early age-related lens opacities. *American Journal of Clinical Nutrition*, 1997; 66:911–916.

Jialal, I, Traber, M, Deveraj, S. Is there a vitamin E paradox? *Current Opinion in Lipidology*, 2001; 12:49–53.

Keniston, RC, Nathan, PA, Leklem, JE, et al. Vitamin B6, vitamin C, and carpal tunnel syndrome. *Journal of Occupational and Environmental Medicine*, 1997; 949–959.

LéCone, J, Delhinger, V, Maes, D, et al. *Revue Du Rhumatisme* (English edition), 1997; 64:428–431.

Milam, SB, Zardeneta, G, Schmitz, JP. Oxidative stress and degenerative temporomandibular joint disease: a proposed hypothesis. *Journal of Oral and Maxillofacial Surgery*, 1998; 56:214–222.

Mocchegiani, E, Muzzioli, M, Giacconi, R. Zinc and immunoresistance to infection in aging: new biological tools. *Trends Pharmacol Sci*, 2000; 21(6):205–208.

Nelson, HK, Shi, Q, Van Dael, P, et al. Host nutritional selenium status as a driving force for influenza virus mutations. *FASEB Journal*, 2001; 15:1481–1483.

Packer, L. Oxidants, antioxidant nutrients and the athlete. *Journal of Sports Sciences*, 1997; 15:353–363.

Reddy, VN, Giblin, FJ, Lin, L-R, et al. The effect of aqueous humor ascorbate on ultraviolet-B-induced DNA damage in lens epithelium. *Investigative Ophthalmology and Visual Science*, 1998; 39:344–350.

Robinson, K, Arheart, K, Refsum, H, et al. Low circulating folate and vitamin B_6 concentrations. *Circulation*, 1998; 97: 437–443.

Rouault, TA. Iron on the brain. *Nature Genetics*, 2001: 299–300.

Sazawal, S, Black, RE, Jalla, S, et al. Zinc supplementation reduces the incidence of acute lower respiratory infections in infants and preschool children: a double-blind, controlled study. *Pediatrics*, 1998; 102:1–5.

Scott, R, MacPherson, A, Yates, RW, et al. The effect of oral selenium supplementation on human sperm motility. *Br J Urol*, 1998; (1):76–80.

Simon, JA, Grady, D, Snabes, MC, et al. Ascorbic acid supplement use and the prevalence of gallbladder disease. *Journal of Clinical Epidemiology*, 1998; 51: 257–265.

Stephens, NG, Parsons, A, Schofield, PM, et al. Randomised controlled trial of vitamin E in patients with coronary disease: Cambridge Heart Antioxidant Study (CHAOS), *Lancet*, 1996:781–786.

Wang, HX, Wahlin, A, Basun, H, et al. Vitamin B_{12} and folate in relation to the development of Alzheimer's disease. *Neurology*, 2001; 56:1188–1194.

VITAMIN E

Boaz, M, Smetana, S, Weinstein, T, et al. Secondary prevention with antioxidants of cardiovascular disease in endstage renal disease (SPACE): randomised placebo-controlled trial. *Lancet*, 2000; 356:1213–1218.

Bursell, SE, Clermont, C, Aiello, LP, et al. High-dose vitamin E supplementation normalizes retinal blood flow and creatinine clearance in patients with type I diabetes. *Diabetes Care*, 1999; 22: 1245–1251.

Burton, GW, Traber, MG, Acuff, RV, et al. Human plasma and tissue a-tocopherol concentrations in response to supplementation with deuterated natural and synthetic vitamin E. *American Journal of Clinical Nutrition*, 1998; 67:669–684.

Eberlein-König, B, Placzek, M, Pryzybilla, B. Protective effect against sunburn of combined systemic ascorbic acid (vitamin C) and d-a-tocopherol (vitamin E). *Journal of the American Academy of Dermatology*, 1998; 38:45–48.

Engelen, W, Keenoy, BM, Vertommen, J, De Leeuw, I. Effects of long-term supplementation with moderate pharmacologic doses of vitamin E are saturable and reversible in patients with type I diabetes. *American Journal of Clinical Nutrition*, 2000; 72(5)1142–1149.

Grundman, M. Vitamin E and Alzheimer disease: the basis for additional clinical trials. *American Journal of Clinical Nutrition*, 2000; 71: 630S–636S.

Heinonen, OP, Albanes, D, Virtano, J, et al. Prostate cancer and supplementation with a-tocopherol and b-carotene: incidence and mortality in a controlled trial. *Journal of the National Cancer Institute*, 1998; 90:440–446.

Ishi, K, et al. Prevention of mammary tumorigenesis in acatalasemic mice by vitamin E supplementation. *Japanese Journal of Cancer Research*, 1996; 87:680–684.

Jialal, I, Traber, M, Deveraj, S. Is there a vitamin E paradox? *Current Opinion in Lipidology*, 2001; 12:49–53.

Katz, DL, Hawaz, H, Boukhalil, J, et al. Acute effects of oats and vitamin E on endothelial responses to ingested fat. *American Journal of Preventive Medicine*, 2001; 20:124–129.

Kaul, N, Devaraj, S, Jialal, I. Alpha-tocopherol and atherosclerosis. *Experimental Biology and Medicine*, 2001; 226(1):5–12.

Kodama, H, Yamaguchi, R, Fukuda, J, et al. Increased oxidative deoxyribonucleic acid damage in the spermatozoa of infertile male patients. *Fertility and Sterility*, 1997; 68:519–524.

Meydani, S, Meydani, M, et al. Vitamin E supplementation and in vivo immune response in healthy elderly subjects. *Journal of the American Medical Association*, 1997; 27:1380–1386.

Miller, JW. Vitamin E and memory: is it vascular protection? *Nutrition Reviews*, 2000; 58:109–111.

Packer, L. Oxidants, antioxidant nutrients and the athlete. *Journal of Sports Sciences*, 1997; 15: 353–363.

Plotnick, GD, Corretti, MC, Vogel, RA. Effect of antioxidant vitamins on the transient impairment of endothelium-dependent brachial artery vasoactivity following a single high-fat meal. *JAMA*, 1997; 278:1682–1686.

Poulin, JE, Cover, C, Gustafson, MR, Kay, MB. Vitamin E prevents oxidative modification of brain and lymphocyte band 3 proteins during aging. *Proceedings of the National Academy of Sciences*, 1996; 93:5600–3.

Qureshi, AA, Salser, WA, Parmar, R, Emeson, EE. Novel tocotrienols of rice bran inhibit atherosclerotic lesions in C57BL/6 ApoE-deficient mice. *Journal of Nutrition*, 2001; 131(10):2606–2618.

Rimm, EB, et al. Vitamin E consumption and the risk of coronary heart disease in men. *New England Journal of Medicine*, 1993; 328:1450–1456.

Sano, M, Ernesto, C, Thomas, RG, et al. A controlled trial of selegiline, alpha-tocopherol, or both as treatment for Alzheimer's disease. *The New England Journal of Medicine*, 1997; 336: 1216–1222.

Seth, RK, Kharb, S. Protective function of alpha-tocopherol against the process of cataractogenesis in humans. *Annals of Nutrition and Metabolism*, 1999; 43:286–289.

Stampfer, MJ, et al. Vitamin E consumption and the risk of coronary heart disease in women. *New England Journal of Medicine*, 1993; 328: 1444–1449.

Stephens, NG, Parsons, A, Schofield, PM, et al. Randomised controlled trial of vitamin E in patients with coronary disease: Cambridge Heart Antioxidant Study (CHAOS). *Lancet*, 1996; 347: 781–786.

Verlangieri, A. Effects of a-tocopherol supplementation on experimentally induced primate atherosclerosis. *Journal of American College of Nutrition*, 1992; 11:130–137.

VITAMIN C

Cameron E, Pauling L. Supplemental ascorbate in the supportive treatment of cancer: Prolongation of survival times in terminal human cancer. *Proceedings of the National Academy of Science, USA*, 1976; 73(10):3685–3689.

Carr AC, Frei B. Toward a new recommended dietary allowance for vitamin C based on antioxidant and health effects in humans. *American Journal of Clinical Nutrition*, 1999;69(6):1086–1107.

Cheng Y, Willett WC, Schwartz J, et al. Relation of nutrition to bone lead and blood lead levels in middle-aged to elderly men. The Normative Aging Study. *American Journal of Epidemiology*, 1998; 147(12):1162–1174.

DeRitter E. Physiologic availability of dehydro-L-ascorbic acid and palmitoyl-L-ascorbic acid. *Science*, 1951;113:628–631.

Duffy SJ, Gokce N, Holbrook M, et al. Treatment of hypertension with ascorbic acid. *Lancet*, 1999;354 (9195): 2048–2049.

Food and Nutrition Board, Institute of Medicine. Vitamin C. Dietary Reference Intakes for Vitamin C, Vitamin E, Selenium, and Carotenoids. Washington D.C.: National Academy Press; 2000:95–185.

Gokce N, Keaney JF, Jr., Frei B, et al. Long-term ascorbic acid administration reverses endothelial vasomotor dysfunction in patients with coronary artery disease. *Circulation*, 1999; 99 (25):3234–3240.

Hemila H. Vitamin C intake and susceptibility to the common cold. *British Journal of Nutrition*, 1997; 77(1):59–72.

Jacques PF, Chylack LT, Jr., Hankinson SE, et al. Long-term nutrient intake and early age-related nuclear lens opacities. *Archives of Ophthalmology*, 2001; 119(7):1009–1019.

Khaw KT, Bingham S, Welch A, et al. Relation between plasma ascorbic acid and mortality in men and women in EPIC-Norfolk prospective study: A prospective population study. *European Prospective Investigation into Cancer and Nutrition*. *Lancet*, 2001;357(9257):657–663.

Kromhout D. Essential micronutrients in relation to carcinogenesis. *American Journal of Clinical Nutrition*, 1987;45(5 Suppl):1361–1367.

Lee SH, Oe T, Blair IA. Vitamin C-induced decomposition of lipid hydroperoxides to endogenous genotoxins. *Science*, 2001;292(5524):2083–2086.

Levine M, Rumsey SC, Daruwala R, Park JB, Wang Y. Criteria and recommendations for vitamin C intake. *Journal of the American Medical Association*, 1999; 281(15):1415–1423.

Michels KB, Holmberg L, Bergkvist L, Ljung H, Bruce A, Wolk A. Dietary antioxidant vitamins, retinol, and breast cancer incidence in a cohort of Swedish women. *International Journal of Cancer*, 2001;91(4): 563–567.

Moertel CG, Fleming TR, Creagan ET, Rubin J, O'Connell MJ, Ames MM. High-dose vitamin C versus placebo in the treatment of patients with advanced cancer who have had no prior chemotherapy. A randomized double-blind comparison. *New England Journal of Medicine*, 1985;312(3):137–141.

Padayatty SJ, Levine M. Reevaluation of ascorbate in cancer treatment: Emerging evidence, open minds and serendipity. *Journal of the American College of Nutrition*, 2000;19(4):423–425.

Sauberlich, HE. A history of scurvy and vitamin C. In Packer, L. and Fuchs, J. Eds. *Vitamin C in Health and Disease*. New York: Marcel Decker Inc., 1997: pp. 1–24.

Simon JA, Hudes ES. Relationship of ascorbic acid to blood lead levels. *Journal of the American Medical Association*, 1999;281(24):2289–2293.

Simon JA, Hudes ES. Serum ascorbic acid and gallbladder disease prevalence among US adults: The Third National Health and Nutrition Examination Survey (NHANES III). *Archives of Internal Medicine*, 2000;160(7):931–936.

Steinmetz KA, Potter JD. Vegetables, fruit, and cancer prevention: a review. *Journal of the American Dietetic Association*, 1996;96(10):1027–1039.

Weinstein M, Babyn P, Zlotkin S. An orange a day keeps the doctor away: Scurvy in the year 2000. *Pediatrics*, 2001; 108(3): E55.

Will JC, Byers T. Does diabetes mellitus increase the requirement for vitamin C? *Nutrition Review*, 1996; 54(7):193–202.

Will JC, Ford ES, Bowman BA. Serum vitamin C concentrations and diabetes: Findings from the Third National Health and Nutrition Examination Survey, 1988–1994. *American Journal of Clinical Nutrition*, 1999;70(1):49–52.

Yokoyama T, Date C, Kokubo Y, Yoshiike N, Matsumura Y, Tanaka H. Serum vitamin C concentration was inversely associated with subsequent 20-year incidence of stroke in a Japanese rural community. The Shibata Study. *Stroke*, 2000;31(10): 2287–2294.

COENZYME Q$_{10}$

Baggio, E, et al. Italian multicenter study on safety and efficacy of coenzyme Q$_{10}$. *The Molecular Aspects of Medicine*, 1994; 15:S287–S294.

Blasi, MA, Bovina, C, Carella, G, et al. Does coenzyme Q$_{10}$ play a role in opposing oxidative stress in patients with age-related macular degeneration? *Ophthalmologica*, 2001; 215(1):51–54.

Bliznakov, E, Casey, A, Premuzic, E. Coenzyme Q: Stimulants of the phagocytic activity in rats and immune response in mice. *Experientia*, 1970; 26:953–54.

Folkers, K, Brown, R, Judy, W, et al. Survival of cancer patients on therapy with coenzyme Q_{10}. *Biochemical and Biophysical Research Communication*, April 15, 1993; 192(1):241–245.

Folkers, K, Langsjoen, P, Willis, R, et al. Lovastatin decreases coenzyme Q levels in humans. *Proceedings of the National Academy of Sciences*, 1990; 87:8931–8934.

Folkers, K, Wolaniuk, J, Simonsen, R, et al. Biochemical rationale and the cardiac response of patients with muscle disease to therapy with coenzyme Q_{10}. *Proceedings of the National Academy of Sciences*, 1985; 82: 4513–4516.

Hoppe, U. Coenzyme Q_{10}: a cutaneous antioxidant and energizer. Presented at the First Conference of the International Coenzyme Q_{10} Association, 1998.

Iwamoto, Y, Watanabe, T, Okamoto, H, et al. Clinical effect of coenzyme Q_{10} on periodontal disease. In: Folkers, K, Yamamura, Y, (eds) *Biomedical and Clinical Aspects of Coenzyme Q_{10}*, Elsevier, Amsterdam, 1981; vol.3:109–119.

Langsjoen, P, Langsjoen, PH, Treatment of essential hypertension with coenzyme Q_{10}. *Molecular Aspects of Medicine*, 1994; 15supplement:S265–S272.

Langsjoen, PH, Langsjoen, AM. Overview of the use of CoQ_{10} in cardiovascular disease. *Biofactors*, 1999; 9 (2–4):273–284.

Linnane, AW, Marzuki, S, Ozawa, T, et al. Mitochondrial DNA mutations as an important contributor to ageing and degenerative diseases. *Lancet*, 1989; 1(8639): 642–645.

Linnane, A W, et al. Cellular redox activity of coenzyme Q_{10}: Effect of CoQ_{10} supplementation on human skeletal muscle. In press: *Free-Radical Research*, 2002.

Lockwood, K, Moesgaard, S, Folkers, K. Partial and complete regression of breast cancer in patients in relation to dosage of coenzyme Q_{10}. *Biochemical and Biophysical Research Communications*, 1994; 199(3): 1504–1508.

Lockwood, K, Moesgaard, S, Yamamoto, T, et al. Progress on therapy of breast cancer with vitamin Q_{10} and the regression of metastases. *Biochemical and Biophysical Research Communications*, 1995; 212:172–177.

Luft, R. The development of mitochondrial medicine. *Biochimica et Biophysica Acta*, May 24, 1995; 1271:1–6.

Mazzio, E, Huber, J, Darling, S, et al. Effect of antioxidants on L-glutamate and N-methyl-4-phenylpyridinium ion-induced neurotoxicity in PC12 cells. *Neurotoxicology*, April 2001; 22(2)283–8.

Musumeci, O, Hirano, M, DiMauro, S, et al. Familial cerebellar ataxia with muscle coenzyme Q_{10} deficiency. *Neurology*, April 2001; 56(7):849–855.

Pepe, S, Lyon, W, Rosenfeldt, FL, et al. Improved outcomes in coronary artery bypass graft surgery with preoperative coenzyme Q_{10} therapy: A randomized, double-blind placebo-controlled Trial. Presented at the 2001 American Heart Association Scientific Sessions Conference in Anaheim, CA.

Thomas, SR, Witting, PK, Stocker, R. A role for reduced coenzyme Q in atherosclerosis? *Biofactors*, 1999; 9 (2–4):207-224.

CALCIUM & MAGNESIUM

Abraham, GE. The calcium controversy. *The Journal of Applied Nutrition*, Fall 1982; 34(2).

Abraham, GE, and Flechas, JD. Management of fibromyalgia: Rationale for the use of magnesium and malic acid. *Journal of Nutritional Medicine*, 1992; 3: 49–59.

Briscoe, AM, and Ragan, C. Effect of magnesium on calcium metabolism in man. *American Journal of Clinical Nutrition*, Nov. 1966.

Brown, SE. Osteoporosis: Sorting fact from fallacy. *The Network News, National Women's Health Network*, July/August 1988.

Bushinsky, DA, Monk, RD. Calcium. *The Lancet*, July 25, 1998; 352: 306–311.

Cumming RG, Cummings SR, et al. Calcium intake and fracture risk: Results from the first study of osteoporotic fractures. *Epidemiology* 1997; 145: 926.

Durlach, J., Ed. First International Symposium on Magnesium Deficiency in Human Pathology, Paris, Springer, Verlag, 1971; 11.

Feskanich, D, Willett, WC, Stampfer, MJ, Colditz, GA. Milk, dietary calcium, and bone fracture risk in women: A 12-year prospective study. *American Journal of Public Health*, 1997; 87 (6): 992–997.

Heaney, RP, Recker, RR, and Weaver, CM. Absorbability of calcium sources: The limited role of solubility. *Calcified Tissue International*, 1990; 46.

Hornyak, M., et al. Magnesium therapy for periodic leg movements-related insomnia and restless legs syndrome: An open pilot study. *Sleep*, Aug. 1, 1998; 21(5).

Hudson, Tori, N.D. *Women's Encyclopedia of Natural Medicine*. Los Angeles: Keats Publishing, 1999.

Levenson, DI, and Bockman, RS. A review of calcium preparations. *Nutrition Reviews*, 1994; 52(7).

Lipkin, M, and Newmark, H. Effect of added dietary calcium on colonic epithelial-cell proliferation in subjects at high risk for familial colonic cancer. *The New England Journal of Medicine*, Nov. 28, 1985; 1381–1384.

McLaren-Howard, J, et al. Hormone replacement therapy and osteoporosis: Bone enzymes and nutrient imbalances. *The Journal of Nutritional and Environmental Medicine*, 1998; 8.

McLean, RM. Magnesium and its therapeutic uses: A review. *The American Journal of Medicine,* Jan. 1994; 96: 63–76.

Riis B, Thomsen K, Christinsen C. Does calcium supplementation prevent postmenopausal bone loss? *The New England Journal of Medicine,* 1987; 316: 173.

Seelig, MS. Interrelationship of magnesium and estrogen in cardiovascular and bone disorders, eclampsia, migraine and premenstrual syndrome. *Journal of the American College of Nutrition,* 1993; 12(4).

Seelig, MS. Adverse stress reactions and magnesium deficiency: preventive and therapeutic implications. *Journal of the American College of Nutrition* 1992; 11:609/Abstract 40.

Teo, K, et al. Effect of intravenous magnesium on mortality in myocardial infarction. *Circulation,* 1990; 82: 111–393.

Weaver, K. Magnesium and its role in vascular reactivity and coagulation. *Contemporary Nutrition,* 1987; 12(3).

CHROMIUM

Anderson, RA. Chromium, glucose intolerance and diabetes. *Journal of the American College of Nutrition,* 1998; 17:548–555.

Anderson, RA, Bryden, NA, Polansky, MM. Dietary chromium intake. Freely chosen diets, institutional diet, and individual foods. *Biological Trace Element Research,* 1992; 32:117–121.

Anderson, RA, Bryden, NA, Polansky, MM. Lack of toxicity of chromium chloride and chromium picolinate in rats. *Journal of the American College of Nutrition,* 1997; 16:273–279.

Anderson, RA, Chen, N, Bryden, NA, et al. Elevated intakes of supplemental chromium improve glucose and insulin variables in individuals with type II diabetes. *Diabetes,* 1997; 46:1786–1791.

Anderson, RA, Kozlovsky, AS. Chromium intake, absorption and excretion of subjects consuming self-selected diets. *American Journal of Clinical Nutrition,* 1985; 41:1177–1183.

Anderson, RA, Polasky, MM, Bryden, NA, et al. Effects of supplemental chromium on patients with symptoms of reactive hypoglycemia. *Metabolism,* 1987; 36:351–355.

Cefalu, WT, Bell-Farrow, AD, Stegner, J, et al. Effect of chromium picolinate on insulin sensitivity in vivo. *The Journal of Trace Elements in Experimental Medicine,* 1999; 12:71–83.

Cheng, N, Zhu, X, Shi, H, et al. Follow-up survey of people in China with type II diabetes mellitus consuming supplemental chromium. *The Journal of Trace Elements in Experimental Medicine,* 1999; 12:55–60.

Evans, GW, Meyer, LK. Life span is increased in rats supplemented with a chromium-pyridine 2 carboxylate complex. *Advances in Scientific Research,* 1994; 1:19–23.

Evans, GW, Swenson, G, Walters, K. Chromium picolinate decreases calcium excretion and increases dehydroepiandrosterone (DHEA) in post menopausal women. *FASEB Journal,* 1995; 9:525.

Jovanovic-Petersen, L, Gutierrez, M, Peterson, CM. Chromium supplementation for gestational diabetic women improves glucose tolerance and decreases hyperinsulinemia. *Journal of the American College of Nutrition,* 1995; 14:530.

Kaats, GR, Blum, K, Pullin, D, et al. A randomized, double-masked, placebo-controlled study of the effects of chromium picolinate supplementation of body composition: a replication and extension of a previous study. *Current Therapeutic Research,* 1998; 59:379–388.

Kaats, GR, Keith, SC, Wise, JA, et al. Effects of baseline total cholesterol levels on diet and exercise interventions. *Journal of the American Nutraceutical Association,* 1999; 2:42–49.

Khan, A, Bryden, NA, Polansky, MM, et al. Insulin potentiating factor and chromium content of selected foods and spices. *Biological Trace Element Research,* 1990; 24:183–188.

Komoroski, J, Greenberg, D, Maki, KC, et al. Chromium picolinate with biotin attenuates elevation in blood glucose levels in people with type II diabetes ingesting medium carbohydrate nutritional beverages. Presented at the 2001 American College of Nutrition Annual Meeting, October 6, 2001, Orlando, Florida.

Lane, BC. Myopia prevention and reversal: new data confirms the interaction of accommodative stress and deficit-inducing nutrition. *Journal of the International Academy of Preventive Medicine,* 1982; VII:17–30.

Lee, NA, and Reasner, CA. Beneficial effect of chromium supplementation on serum triglyceride levels in NIDDM. *Diabetes Care,* 1994; 17:1449–1452.

McCarthy, M. High-chromium yeast for acne? *Medical Hypothesis,* 1984; 14:307–310.

McLeod, MN, Gaynes, BN, Golden, RN. Chromium potentiation of antidepressant pharmacotherapy for dysthymic disorder in 5 patients. *Journal of Clinical Psychiatry,* 1999; 60:237–240.

McLeod, MN, Golden, RN. Chromium treatment of depression. *International Journal of Neuropsychopharmacology,* 2000; 3:311–314.

Preuss, HG, Jarrell, ST, Scheckenbach, R, et al. Comparative effects of chromium, vanadium and gymnema sylvestre on sugar-induced blood pressure elevations in SHR. *Journal of the American College of Nutrition,* 1998; 17:116–123.

Ravina, A, Slezak, L, Mirsky, N, et al. Reversal of corticosteroid-induced diabetes mellitus with supplemental chromium. *Diabetic Medicine,* 1999; 16: 164–167.

Ravina, A, Slezak, L, Rubal, A, et al. Clinical use of the trace element chromium (III) in the treatment of diabetes mellitus. *The Journal of Trace Elements in Experimental Medicine,* 1995; 8:183–190.

GLUCOSAMINE & CHONDROITIN

Bourgeois, P, Chales, G, Dehais, J, et al. Efficacy and tolerability of chondroitin sulfate 1200 mg/day vs chondroitin sulfate 3 x 400 mg/day vs placebo. *Osteoarthritis and Cartilage,* 1998; 6SupplA:25–30.

Conrozier, T. Anti-arthrosis treatments: efficacy and tolerance of chondroitin sulfates (CS 4&6). *Presse Medicale,* 1998; 27:1862–1865.

Das, A, Hammad, TA. Efficacy of a combination of FCHG49® glucosamine hydrochloride, TRH122® low molecular weight sodium chondroitin sulfate and manganese ascorbate in the management of knee osteoarthritis. *Osteoarthritis and Cartilage,* 2000; 8:343–350.

Deal, CL, Moskowitz, RW. Nutraceuticals as therapeutic agents in osteoarthritis. *Rheumatic Diseases Clinics of North America,* 1999; 25:379–395.

Ezzo, J, Hadhazy, V, Birch, S, et al. Acupuncture for osteoarthritis of the knee: a systematic review. *Arthritis and Rheumatism,* 2001; 44:819–825.

Flynn, MA. The effect of folate and cobalamin on osteoarthritic hands. *Journal of the American College of Nutrition,* August 1994; 13:351–356.

Gaby, AR. Natural treatments for osteoarthritis. *Alternative Medicine Review,* 1999; 4:330–341.

Hoffer, LJ, Kaplan, LN, Hamadeh, MJ, et al. Sulfate could mediate the therapeutic effect of glucosamine sulfate. *Metabolism,* 2001; 50:767–770.

Jonas, WB, Rapoza, CP, Blair, WF. The effect of niacinamide on osteoarthritis: a pilot study. *Inflammation Research,* 1996; 45:330–344.

Kaufman, W. The use of vitamin therapy to reverse certain concomitants of aging. *Journal of the American Geriatric Society,* 1955; 3:927–936.

Leffler, CT, Philippi, AF, Leffler, SG, et al. Glucosamine, chondroitin, and manganese ascorbate for degenerative joint disease of the knee or low back: a randomized, double-blind, placebo-controlled pilot study. *Military Medicine,* 1999; 164:85–91.

Lippiello, L, Woodward, J, Karpman, R, et al. In vivo chondroprotection and metabolic synergy of glucosamine and chondroitin sulfate. *Clinical Orthopaedics and Related Research,* 2000; 381:229–240.

McAlindon, TE, LaValley, MP, Gulin, JP, et al. Glucosamine and chondroitin for treatment of osteoarthritis. *Journal of the American Medical Association,* 2000; 283:1469–1475.

McAlindon, TE, Jacques, P, Zhang, Y, et al. Do antioxidant micronutrients protect against the development and progression of knee osteoarthritis? *Arthritis & Rheumatism,* 1996; 39:648–656.

Reginster, JY, Deroisy, R, Rovati, L, et al. Long-term effects of glucosamine sulphate on osteoarthritis progression: a randomized, placebo-controlled clinical trial. *Lancet,* 2001; 357:251–256.

Russell, AL. Glycoaminoglycan (GAG) deficiency in protective barrier as an underlying, primary cause of ulcerative colitis, Crohn's disease, interstitial cystitis, and possibly Reiter's syndrome. *Medical Hypotheses,* 1999; 52: 297–301.

Tapadinhas, MJ, Rivera, IC, Binamini, AA. Oral glucosamine sulfate in the management of arthrosis: report on a multi-centre open investigation in Portugal. *Pharmatherapeutica,* 1982; 3:157–168.

Thie, NM, Prasad, NG, Major, PW. Evaluation of glucosamine sulfate compared to ibuprofen for the treatment of temporomandibular joint osteoarthritis: a randomized double-blind, placebo-controlled 3 month clinical trial. *Journal of Rheumatology,* 2001; 28: 1347–1355.

Towheed, TE, Anastassiades, TP, Shea, B, et al. Glucosamine therapy for treating osteoarthritis (Cochrane Review). *Cochrane Database of Systematic Reviews,* 2001; 1:CD002946.

ST. JOHN'S WORT

American Herbal Pharmacopoeia and Therapeutic Compendium. "St. John's Wort (*Hypericum Performatum*) Monograph." *Herbalgram: The Journal of the American Botanical Council and the Herb Research Foundation,* 1997; 40:1–16.

Barnes J, Anderson LA, Phillipson JD. "St. John's wort (*Hypericum perforatum* L.): a review of its chemistry, pharmacology and clinical properties." *Journal Pharm Pharmacol,* 2001; 53:583–600.

Brenner R, Azbel V, Madhusoodanan S, Pawlowska M. "Comparison of an extract of hypericum (LI 160) and sertraline in the treatment of depression: a double-blind, randomized pilot study." *Clin Ther,* 2000; 22:411–418.

Grube B, Walper A, Wheatley D. "St. John's wort extract: efficacy for menopausal symptoms of psychological origin." *Adv Ther,* 1999; 16:177–186.

Huebner WD, Kirste T. "Experience with St. John's wort (*Hypericum performatum*) in children under 12 years with symptoms of depression and psychovegetative disturbances." *Phytotherapy Research* 2001; 15:367–370.

Kalb R, Troutman-Sponsel RD, Kieser M. "Efficacy and tolerability of Hypericum extract WS 5572 versus placebo in mildly to moderately depressed patients." *Pharmacopsychiatry*, 2001; 34: 96–103.

Linde K, Ramirez G, Mulrow CD, Weidenhammer W, and Melchart D. "St. John's wort for depression—an overview and metaanalysis of randomized clinical trials." *British Medical Journal*, 1996; 313:253–258.

Philipp M, Kohnen R, Hiller KO. "Hypericum extract versus imipramine or placebo in patients with moderate depression: randomised multicentre study of treatment for eight weeks." *British Medical Journal*, 1999; 319:1534–1538.

Schrader E. "Equivalence of St. John's wort extract (Ze 117) and fluoxetine: a randomized, controlled study in mild-moderate depression." *Int Clin Psychopharmacol*, 2000; 15:61–68.

Stevinson C, Ernst E. "A pilot study of Hypericum perforatum for the treatment of premenstrual syndrome." *BJOG*, 2000; 107:870–876.

Woelk H. "Comparison of St. John's wort and imipramine for treating depression: randomised controlled trial." *British Medical Journal*, 2000; 321:536–539.

GINKGO BILOBA

Bauer, U. 6-Month double-blind randomized clinical trial of Ginkgo biloba extract versus placebo in two parallel groups in patients suffering from peripheral arterial insufficiency. *Arzneimittelforsch*, 1984; 34:716–720.

Bruno, C, et al. Regeneration of motor nerves in bilobalide-treated rats. *Planta Medica*, 1993; 59:302–307.

Chatterjee, SS, et al. Studies on the mechanism of action of an extract of ginkgo biloba, a drug used for treatment of ischemic vascular diseases. *Archives of Pharmacology*, 1982; 320:R52.

Chung, KF, et al. Effect of a ginkgolide mixture (BN 52063) in antagonising skin and platelet responses to platelet activating factor in man. *Lancet*, 1987; 1:248–251.

Clostre, F. From the body to cell membranes: the different levels of action of Ginkgo biloba extract. *Presse-Medicale*, 1986; 15:1529–1538.

Coles, R. Trial of an extract of Ginkgo biloba (EGB) for tinnitus and hearing loss. *Clinical Otolaryngology and Allied Sciences*, 1988; 13:501–504.

De Long, Xie, Ning, et al. Ginkgo biloba composition, method to prepare the same and uses thereof, U.S. Patent, 6,030,621, Feb 29, 2000.

Doly, M, et al. Effect of Ginkgo biloba extract on the electrophysiology of the isolated diabetic rat retina. *Presse-Medicale*, 1986; 15:1480–1483.

Dubreuil, C. Comparative therapeutic trial of Ginkgo biloba extract and nicergoline in acute cochlear deafness. *Presse-Medicale*, 1986; 15:1559–1561.

Dumont, E, et al. Protection of polyunsaturated fatty acids against iron-dependent lipid peroxidation by a Ginkgo biloba extract (EGb 761). *Methods and Findings in Experimental and Clinical Pharmacology*, 1995; 17(2):83–88.

Emerit, I, et al. Radiation-induced clastogenic factors: anti-clastogenic effect of Ginkgo biloba extract. *Free Radical Biology and Medicine*, 1995; 18:985–991.

Gebner, B, et al. Study of the long-term action of a Ginkgo biloba extract on vigilance and mental performance as determined by means of quantitative pharmaco-EEG and psychometric measurements. *Arzneimittelforsch*, 1985; 35:1459–1465.

Guillon, JM, et al. Effects of Ginkgo biloba extract on various in vitro and in vivo models of experimental myocardial ischaemia. *Presse-Medicale*, 1986; 15:1516–1519.

Haguenauer, JP, et al. Treatment of disturbances of equilibrium with Ginkgo biloba extract. A multicentre, double-blind, drug versus placebo study. *Presse-Medicale*, 1986; 15: 1569–1572.

Huguet, F., and Tarrade, T. Alpha2-Adrenoceptor changes during cerebral ageing. The effect of ginkgo biloba extract. *Journal of Pharmacy and Pharmacology*, 1992; 44:24–27.

Haramaki, N, et al. Effects of natural antioxidant Ginkgo biloba extract (EGb 761) on myocardial ischemia-reperfusion injury. *Free Radical Biology and Medicine*, 1994; 16:789–794.

Hofferberth, B. Effect of ginkgo biloba extract on neurophysiological and psychometric measurement results in patients with cerebro-organic syndrome. A double-blind study versus placebo. *Arzneimittelforsch*, 1989; 39:918–922.

Hofferberth, B. The Efficacy of EGb 761 (Ginkgo biloba extract) in Patients with Senile Dementia of the Alzheimer Type, A Double-Blind, Placebo-Controlled Study on Different Levels of Investigation. *Human Psychopharmacology*, 1994; 9:215–222.

Holgers, K-M, et al. Ginkgo biloba extract for the treatment of tinnitus. *Audiology*, 1994; 33:85–92.

Jung, F, et al. Effect of Ginkgo biloba on fluidity of blood and peripheral microcirculation in volunteers. *Arzneimittelforsch*, 1990; 40:589–593.

Kanowski, S, et al. Proof of efficacy of the Ginkgo biloba special extract EGb 761 in outpatients suffering from mild to moderate primary degenerative dementia of the Alzheimer type or multi-infarct dementia. *Pharmacopsychiatry*, 1996; 29: 47–56.

Kleijnen, J, Knipschild, P. Ginkgo biloba for cerebral insufficiency. *British Journal of Clinical Pharmacology*, 1992; 34:352–358.

Kleijnen, J., and Knipschild, P. Ginkgo biloba, intermittent claudication and cerebral insufficiency. *Lancet*, 1992; 340:1136–1139.

Lagrue, G, et al. Idiopathic cyclic oedema. Role of capillary hyperpermeability and its correction by Ginkgo biloba extract. *Presse-Medicale*, 1986; 15: 1550–1553.

Le Bars, P., Katz, M., Berman, N., et al. A placebo-controlled, double-blind, randomized trial of an extract of ginkgo biloba for dementia. *JAMA*, 1997; 278(16):1327–1332.

Lebuisson, DA, Leroy, L, Rigal, G. Treatment of senile macular degeneration with Ginkgo biloba extract. A preliminary double-blind, drug versus placebo study. *Presse-Medicale*, 1986; 15: 1556–1558.

Meyer, B. A multicentre, randomized, double-blind drug versus placebo study of Ginkgo biloba extract in the treatment of tinnitus. *Presse-Medicale*, 1986; 15:1562–1564.

Mouren, X, et al. Study of the anti-ischemic action of EGB 761 in the treatment of peripheral arterial occlusive disease by TcPO2 determination. *Angiology*, 1994; 45:413–417.

Oberpichler, H, et al. Effects of Ginkgo biloba constituents related to protection against brain damage caused by hypoxia. *Pharmacological Research and Communications*, 1988; 20:349–368.

Otamiri, T, et al. Ginkgo biloba extract prevents mucosal damage associated with small-intestinal ischaemia. *Scandinavian Journal of Gastroenterology*, 1989; 24:666–670.

Pidoux, B. Effects of Ginkgo biloba extract on functional activity of the brain. Results of clinical and experimental studies. *Presse-Medicale*, 1986; 15: 1588–1591.

Pincemail, J, et al. Anti-radical properties of Ginkgo biloba extract. *Presse-Medicale*, 1986; 15:1475–1479.

Racagni, G, et al. Variations of neuromediators in cerebral ageing. Effects of Ginkgo biloba extract. *Presse-Medicale*, 1986; 15:1488–1490.

Rai, GS, et al. A double-blind, placebo-controlled study of Ginkgo biloba extract ("Tanakan") in elderly outpatients with mild to moderate memory impairment. *Current Medical Research and Opinion*, 1991; 12:350–355.

Rapin, JR, et al. Local cerebral glucose consumption. Effects of Ginkgo biloba extract. *Presse-Medicale*, 1986; 15:1494–1497.

Schaffler, K, et al. Double-blind study of the hypoxia-protec-

tive effect of a standardised Ginkgo bilobae preparation after repeated administration in healthy volunteers. *Arzneimittelforsch*, 1985; 35: 1283–1286.

Schubert, H, Halama, P. Depressive episode primarily unresponsive to therapy in elderly patients: efficacy of Ginkgo biloba extract (EGB 761) in combination with antidepressants. *Geriatr Forsch*, 1993; 3:45–53.

Shen, J-G, Zhou, D-Y. Efficiency of Ginkgo biloba extract (EGb 761) in antioxidant protection against myocardial ischemia and reperfusion injury. *Biochemical and Molecular Biology International*, 1995; 35:125–134.

Sikora, R, et al. Ginkgo biloba extract in the therapy of erectile dysfunction. *Journal of Urology*, 1989; 141:188A.

Spinnewyn, B, et al. Effects of Ginkgo biloba extract on a cerebral ischaemia model in gerbils. *Presse-Medicale*, 1986; 15:1511–1515.

Taillandier, J, et al. Ginkgo biloba extract in the treatment of cerebral disorders due to aging. *Presse-Medicale*, 1986; 15:1583–1587.

Tamborini, A, Taurelle, R. Value of standardized Ginkgo biloba extract (EGB 761) in the management of congestive symptoms of premenstrual syndrome. *International Journal of Gynecology and Obstetrics*, 1993; 88:447–457.

Taylor, JE. Binding of neuromediators to their receptors in rat brain. Effect of chronic administration of Ginkgo biloba extract. *Presse-Medicale*, 1986; 15:1491–1493.

Vesper, J, Hansgen, K-D. Efficacy of Ginkgo biloba in 90 outpatients with cerebral insufficiency caused by old age. Results of a placebo-controlled double-blind trial. *Phytomedicine*, 1994; 1:9–16.

Vorberg, G. Ginkgo biloba extract (GBE): a long-term study of chronic cerebral insufficiency in geriatric patients. *Clinical Trials Journal*, 1985; 22: 149–157.

Yan, L-J, et al. Ginkgo biloba extract (EGb 761) protects human low density lipoproteins against oxidative modification mediated by copper. *Biochemical and Biophysical Research Communications*, 1995; 212:360–366.

SAW PALMETTO & MEN'S HEALTH

Adriazola Semino, M, Lozano Ortega, JL, Garcia Cobo, E, et al. Symptomatic treatment of benign hypertrophy of the prostate. Comparative study of prazosin and serenoa repens. *Archivas Espanol Urologia*, 1992; 45(3):211–3.

Barlet, A, Albrecht, J, Aubert, A, et al. Efficacy of Pygeum africanum extract in the medical therapy of urination disorders due to benign prostatic hyperplasia: evaluation of objective and subjective parameters. A placebo-controlled double-blind multicenter study. *Wien Klinische Wochenschrift*, 1990; 102(22):667–73.

Bogden, JD, Oleske, JM, Lavenhar, MA, et al. Effects of one year of supplementation with zinc and other micronutrients on cellular immunity in the elderly. *Journal of the American College of Nutrition*, 1990; 9(3):214–25.

Braeckman, J. The extract of Serenoa repens in the treatment of benign prostatic hyperplasia: a multicenter open study. *Current Therapy Research,* 1994; 55:776–85.

Carani, C, Salvioli, V, Scuteri, A, et al. Urological and sexual evaluation of treatment of benign prostatic disease using Pygeum africanum at high doses. *Archivas Italiano Urologia Nefrologia e Andrologia*, 1991; 63(3):341–5.

Champault, G, Bonnard, AM, Cauquil, J, Patel, JC. Actualite Therapeutique: The medical treatment of prostatic adenoma. *Annals of Urology* (Paris), 1984; 18(6):407-10.

Champault, G, Patel, JC, Bonnard, AM. A double-blind trial of an extract of the plant Serenoa repens in benign prostatic hyperplasia. *British Journal of Clinical Pharmacology*, 1984; 18(3): 461–2.

Chatenoud, L, Tavani, A, La Vecchia, C, et al. Whole grain food intake and cancer risk. *International Journal of Cancer*, 1998; 77(1):24–8.

Dufour, B, Choquenet, C, Revol, M, Faure, G, Jorest, R. Controlled study of the effects of Pygeum africanum extract on the functional symptoms of prostatic adenoma. *Annals of Urology* (Paris), 1984; 18(3):193–5.

Flamm, J, Kiesswetter, H. A urodynamic study of patients with benign prostatic hypertrophy treated conservatively with phytotherapy or testosterone. *Wien Klinische Wochenschrift,* 1979; 91 (18):622–7.

Food Drug Cosmetic Law Reports, New Developments, 1990; 1427:42,434–41.

Gerber, GS, Zagaja, GP, Bales, GT, Chodak, GW, Contreras, BA. Saw palmetto (Serenoa repens) in men with lower urinary tract symptoms: effects on urodynamic parameters and voiding symptoms. *Urology*, 1998; 51(6):1003–7.

Grasso, M, Montesano, A, Buonaguidi, A, et al. Comparative effects of alfuzosin versus Serenoa repens in the treatment of symptomatic benign prostatic hyperplasia. *Archivas Espanol Urologia*, 1995; 48(1):97–103.

Habib, FK, Hammond, GL, Lee, IR, et al. Metal-androgen interrelationships in carcinoma and hyperplasia of the human prostate. *Journal of Endocrinology*, 1976; 71(1):133–41.

Hayes RB, Ziegler RG, Gridley G, et al. Dietary factors and risks for prostate cancer among blacks and whites in the United States. *Cancer Epidemiology Biomarkers and Prevention*, 1999; 8(1): 25–34.

Keen, CL, Gershwin, ME. Zinc deficiency and immune function. *Annual Review of Nutrition*, 1990; 10:415–31.

Kortt, MA, Bootman, JL. The economics of benign prostatic hyperplasia treatment: a literature review. *Clinical Therapeutics*, 1996; 18(6):1227–41.

Krzeski, T, Kazon, M, Borkowski, A, Witeska, A, Kuczera, J. Combined extracts of Urtica dioica and Pygeum africanum in the treatment of benign prostatic hyperplasia: double-blind comparison of two doses. *Clinical Therapeutics*, 1993; 15(6): 1011–20.

Mossad, SB, Macknin, ML, Medendorp, SV, Mason, P. Zinc gluconate lozenges for treating the common cold. A randomized, double-blind, placebo-controlled study. *Annals of Internal Medicine*, 1996; 125(2):81–8.

Pfeifer, BL, Pirani, JF, Hamann, SR, Klippel, KF. PC-SPES, a dietary supplement for the treatment of hormone-refractory prostate cancer. *British Journal of Urology International*, 2000; 85(4):481–5.

Platz, EA, Kawachi, I, Rimm, EB, et al. Physical activity and benign prostatic hyperplasia. *Archives of Internal Medicine*, 1998; 158(21):2349–56.

Platz, EA, Rimm, EB, Kawachi, I, et al. Alcohol consumption, cigarette smoking, and risk of benign prostatic hyperplasia. *American Journal of Epidemiology*, 1999; 149(2):106–15.

Plosker, GL, Brogden, RN. Serenoa repens (Permixon). A review of its pharmacology and therapeutic efficacy in benign prostatic hyperplasia. *Drugs & Aging*, 1996; (5):379–95.

Schneider, HJ, Honold, E, Masuhr, T. Treatment of benign prostatic hyperplasia. Results of a treatment study with the phytogenic combination of Sabal extract WS 1473 and Urtica extract WS 1031 in urologic specialty practices. *Fortschrift Medizinische*, 1995; 113(3):37–40.

Wynder, EL, Rose, DP, Cohen, LA. Nutrition and prostate cancer: a proposal for dietary intervention, *Nutrition and Cancer*, 1994; 22(1): 1–9.

NUTRITION FOR WOMEN'S HEALTH

Colston, KW, Hansen, CM. Mechanisms implicated in the growth regulatory effects of vitamin D in breast cancer. *Endocrine-Related Cancer*, 2002; (1):45–59.

Feskanich, D, Willett, WC, Stampfer, MJ, Colditz, GA. Milk, dietary calcium, and bone fractures in women: a 12-year prospective study. *American Journal of Public Health*, 1997; 87(6):992–997.

Fischer-Rasmussen, W, Kjaer, SK, Dahl, C, et al. Ginger treatment of hyperemesis gravidarum. *European Journal of Obstetrics & Gynecology, and Reproductive Biology*, 1990; 38:19–24.

Gallo, M, Sarkar, M, Au, W, Pietrzak, K, et al. Pregnancy outcome following gestational exposure to echinacea: a prospective controlled study. *Archives of Internal Medicine*, 2000; 160(20):3141–3143.

Jacobson, TA. Combination lipid-altering therapy: an emerging treatment paradigm for the 21st century. *Current Atherosclerosis Report*, 2001; 3(5):373–382.

Kwasniewska, A, Tukendorf, A, Semczuk, M. Folate deficiency and cervical intraepithelial neoplasia. *European Journal of Gynaecological Oncology*, 1997; 18(6):526–530.

Maillard, V, Bougnoux, P, Ferrari, P, et. al. N-3 and N-6 fatty acids in breast adipose tissue and relative risk of breast cancer in a case-control study in Tours, France. *International Journal of Cancer*, 2002; (1):78–83.

Palan, PR, Mikhail, MS, Romney, SL. Placental and serum levels of carotenoids in preeclampsia. *Obstetrics and Gynecology*, 2001; 98(3):459–462.

Peters-Welte, C, Diessen, M, Albrecht, K. Menstrual abnormalities and PMS: *Vitex agnus-castus* in a study of application. *Gynakologie*, 1994; 7:49–52.

Stevinson, C, Ernst, E. A pilot study of Hypericum perforatum for the treatment of premenstrual syndrome. *British Journal of Obstetrics & Gynaecology*, 2000; 107:870–876.

Stolze, H. An alternative to treat menopausal complaints. *Gynakologie*, 1982; 3(1):14–16.

Thys-Jacobs, S. Micronutrients and the premenstrual syndrome: the case for calcium. *Journal of the American College of Nutrition*, 2000; 19(2): 220–227.

Zhang, S, Hunter, DJ, Forman, MR, et.al. Dietary carotenoids and vitamins A, C, and E and risk of breast cancer. *Journal of the National Cancer Institute*, 1999; 91(6):547–556.

SPORTS NUTRITION SUPPLEMENTS

Astrup, A, Lundsgaard, C, Madsen, J, et al. Enhanced thermogenic responsiveness during chronic ephedrine treatment in man. *The American Journal of Clinical Nutrition*, 1985; 42:83–94.

Bucci, L. Selected herbals and human exercise performance. *American Journal of Clinical Nutrition*, 2000; 72(suppl): 624S–636S.

Burke, E. *Optimal Muscle Recovery*. Garden City Park, NY: Avery Publishing Group, 1999.

Clarkson, P and Haymes, E. Trace mineral requirements for athletes. *International Journal of Sport Nutrition*, 1994; 4:104–119.

Dinan, L. Phytoecdysteroids: Biological aspects. *Phytochemistry*, 2001; 57:325–339.

Fahey, T and Pearl M. The hormonal and perceptive effects of phosphatidylserine administration during two weeks of resistive exercise-induced overtraining. *Biology of Sport*, 1998; 15:135–143.

Graham, T. Caffeine and exercise: metabolism, endurance and performance. *Sports Medicine*, 2001; 31(11):785–807.

Jacob, S., Lawrence, R., and Zucker, M. *The Miracle of MSM: The Natural Solution for Pain*. New York: Penguin Putnam, 1999.

Lemon, P. Do athletes need more dietary protein and amino acids? *International Journal of Sport Nutrition*, 1995; 5:S39–S61.

Sahelian, R, and Tuttle, D. *Creatine: Nature's Muscle Builder*. Garden City Park, NY: Avery Publishing Group, 1999.

Van Der Beek, E. Vitamin supplementation and physical exercise performance. *Journal of Sports Sciences*, 1991; 9:77–89.

Welbourne, T. Increased plasma bicarbonate and growth hormone after an oral glutamine load. *American Journal of Clinical Nutrition*, 1995; 61: 1058–1061

Witter, J., Gallagher, P., Williamson, D., et al. Effects of ribose supplementation on performance during repeated high-intensity cycle sprints. Abstract presented at the Midwest Regional Chapter of the American College of Sports Medicine, October 2000.

Other Books and Resources

GreatLife Magazine
Consumer magazine with articles on vitamins, minerals, herbs, and foods.
Available for free at many health and natural food stores.

Let's Live Magazine
Consumer magazine with emphasis on the health benefits of vitamins, minerals, and herbs.
Customer service:
1-800-676-4333
P.O. Box 74908
Los Angeles, CA 90004
Subscriptions: 12 issues per year, $19.95 in the U.S.; $31.95 outside the U.S.

Physical Magazine
Magazine oriented to body builders and other serious athletes.
Customer service:
1-800-676-4333
P.O. Box 74908
Los Angeles, CA 90004
Subscriptions: 12 issues per year, $19.95 in the U.S.; $31.95 outside the U.S.

The Nutrition Reporter™ newsletter
Monthly newsletter that summarizes recent medical research on vitamins, minerals, and herbs.
Customer service:
P.O. Box 30246
Tucson, AZ 85751-0246
e-mail: jack@thenutritionreporter.com
www.nutritionreporter.com
Subscriptions: $26 per year (12 issues) in the U.S.; $32 U.S. or $48 CNC for Canada; $38 for other countries

Vitamins & Minerals

Balch, JF and Balch, P. *Prescription for Nutritional Healing,* third edition. New York, New York: Avery Penguin Putnam, 2000.

Griffith, H Winter. *Minerals, Supplements & Vitamins.* Tucson, Arizona: Fisher Books, 2000.

Hudson, Tori. *Women's Encyclopedia of Natural Medicine.* Los Angeles, California: Keats Publishing, 1999.

Murray, Michael, and Pizzorno, Joseph. *Encyclopedia of Natural Medicine,* revised second edition. Rocklin, California: Prima Publishing, 1998.

Redmon, George L. *Minerals: What Your Body Really Needs and Why.* Garden City Park, New York: Avery Publishing, 1999.

MEDLINE
www.ncbi.nlm.nih.gov/entrez/query
For specific medical journal abstracts.

National Center for Complementary and Alternative Medicine, National Institutes of Health (NIH)
http://nccam.nih.gov/nccam/
Search a database of 180,000 bibliographic citations regarding complementary and alternative therapies extracted from MEDLINE.

Office of Dietary Supplements, National Institutes of Health
http://dietary-supplements.info.nih.gov/
Scientific resources (including recent research findings regarding supplements), general information about supplements, and programs and activities of the Office of Dietary Supplements.

Vitamin E

Challem, J, Berkson, B, and Smith, MD. *Syndrome X: The Complete Nutritional Program to Prevent and Reverse Insulin Resistance.* New York, NY: John Wiley & Sons, 2000.

Challem, J, and Dolby, V. *Homocysteine: The Secret Killer.* New Canaan, CT: Keats Publishing, 1997.

Murray, Michael, and Pizzorno, Joseph. *Encyclopedia of Natural Medicine,* revised second edition. Prima Publishing: Rocklin, CA, 1998.

Smith, MD. *Going Against the Grain.* Chicago, IL: Contemporary Publishing, 2002.

Centers for Disease Control and Prevention (CDC)

www.cdc.gov/

Learn about a wide range of diseases at this government website.

MEDLINE

www.ncbi.nlm.nih.gov/entrez/query

For specific medical journal abstracts.

National Center for Complementary and Alternative Medicine, National Institutes of Health (NIH)

http://nccam.nih.gov/nccam/

Search a database of 180,000 bibliographic citations regarding complementary and alternative therapies extracted from MEDLINE.

Office of Dietary Supplements, National Institutes of Health

http://dietary-supplements.info.nih.gov/

Scientific resources (including recent research findings regarding supplements), general information about supplements, and programs and activities of the Office of Dietary Supplements.

Vitamin E Research and Information Service (VERIS)

www.veris-online.org
Read abstracts of antioxidant research.

VITAMIN C

Cameron, Ewan, Linus Pauling (Contributor). *Cancer and Vitamin C: A Discussion of the Nature, Causes, Prevention, and Treatment of Cancer.* Philadelphia, PA: Camino Books, 1993.

Cheraskin, E. *Vitamin C: Who Needs It?* Brooklyn, NY: Arlington Press, 1993.

Packer, Lester, and Jurgen Fuchs (eds.). *Vitamin C in Health and Disease.* New York, NY: Marcel Dekker, Inc., 1997.

Pauling, Dr. Linus. *How to Live Longer and Feel Better,* Reissue Edition. New York, NY: Avon, 1996.

Stone, Irwin. *The Healing Factor: "Vitamin C" Against Disease.* New York, NY: Putnam Publishing Group, 1974.

WEBSITES

C For Yourself • www.cforyourself.com

The Linus Pauling Institute • www.orst.edu/dept/lpi/

Orthomolecular Oncology • www.canceraction.org.gg/diff.htm

Vitamin C: Orthomolecular Medicine • www.orthomed.com

COENZYME Q$_{10}$

Bliznakov, Emile, and Hunt, Gerald. *The Coenzyme Q10 Phenomenon.* New York, NY: Bantam Books, 1987.

Littarru, Gian Paolo. *Energy and Defense: Facts and Perspectives on Coenzyme Q10 in Biology and Medicine.* Rome, Italy: Casa Editrice Scientifica Internazionale, 1995.

Sinatra, Stephen. *The Coenzyme Q10 Phenomenon.* Chicago, IL: Keats NTC/Contemporary Publishing Group, 1998.

Coenzyme Q$_{10}$ Association

www.coenzymeq10.org
A worldwide group of researchers and clinicians with a special interest in CoQ$_{10}$.

MEDLINE

www.ncbi.nlm.nih.gov/entrez/query
For specific medical journal abstracts.

CALCIUM & MAGNESIUM

Gaby, Alan R., M.D. *Preventing and Reversing Osteoporosis.* Rocklin, CA: Prima Publishing, 1994.

Solid information on bone health with information on calcium-to-magnesium ratio for women of all ages.

Gittelman, Ann Louise. *Super Nutrition for Menopause.* Garden City Park, NY: Avery Publishing Group, 1998.

A comprehensive program for menopausal and postmenopausal women with guidelines for calcium and magnesium intake.

Kirschmann, Gayla J., and Kirschmann, John D. *Nutrition Almanac,* Fourth Edition. New York: McGraw-Hill, 1996.

Contains charts with vitamin and mineral content of common foods.

Women's Health Letter

Monthly newsletter written by health writer and nutritionist Nan Kathryn Fuchs, Ph.D., with cutting-edge information for women over age fifty.

Soundview Publications

1-800-728-2288
P.O. Box 467939
Atlanta, Georgia 31146-7939
Subscription: 12 issues per year; $39 in the U.S.; $52 outside the U.S.

CHROMIUM

Broadhurst, C. Leigh. *Diabetes: Prevention and Cure*. New York, NY: Kensington Books, 1999.
An easy-to-read book that offers a wealth of information for those with type II or type I diabetes. It outlines a diet and supplement approach to their treatment, which includes chromium supplements.

Challem, Jack, Berkson, Burton, and Smith, Melissa Diane. *Syndrome X: The Complete Nutritional Program to Prevent and Reverse Insulin Resistance*. New York, NY: John Wiley & Sons, 2000.
The definitive consumer guide to Syndrome X—the combination of insulin resistance with abdominal obesity, high cholesterol, high triglycerides, and high blood pressure—which sets the stage for heart disease, type II diabetes, and other degenerative diseases. The book includes therapeutic diets, recipes, and supplement plans involving chromium for this common condition.

Smith, Melissa Diane. *Going Against the Grain: How Reducing and Avoiding Grains Can Revitalize Your Health*. Chicago, Illinois: Contemporary Books, 2002.
A book that covers all the health problems that can result from eating too many grains (and sugars), including conditions such as Syndrome X, overweight, and diabetes, as well as gluten sensitivity, grain allergies, and autoimmune disorders. Three therapeutic diets are outlined, along with information on supplements (including chromium) that are helpful for various conditions.

The Chromium Information Bureau Website
A not-for-profit educational organization that provides information to consumers, health care providers, nutrition researchers, and the media about the clinical functions, effects, and actions of dietary chromium.
P.O. Box 107
Inglefield, IN 47618
www.chromiuminfo.org

GLUCOSAMINE & CHONDROITIN

Lininger, SL. (Editor-in-chief). *The Natural Pharmacy*. Prima Health, Rocklin, CA, 1999.

Somer, E. *Age-Proof Your Body*. William Morrow and Company, New York, 1998.

Arthritis Foundation
P.O. Box 7669
Atlanta, Georgia 30357-0669
1-800-283-7800
www.arthritis.org

National Institute of Arthritis and Musculoskeletal and Skin Diseases
Information Clearinghouse
National Institutes of Health
1 AMS Circle
Bethesda, Maryland 20892-3675
1-877-22-NIAMS (toll-free)
e-mail: niamsinfo@mail.nih.gov
www.nih.gov/niams

ST. JOHN'S WORT

Burns, D. *Feeling Good: The New Mood Therapy*. New York, NY: Whole Care Publishing, 1999.

Cass, H. *St. John's Wort: Nature's Blues Buster*. Garden City Park, NY: Avery Publishing Group, 1998.

Glenmullen, J. *Prozac Backlash: Overcoming the Dangers of Prozac, Zoloft, Paxil, and Other Antidepressants with Safe, Effective Alternatives*. New York, NY: Simon and Schuster, 2000.

Murray, M. and Pizzorno, J. *Encyclopedia of Natural Medicine*. Rocklin, CA: Prima Publishing, 1998.

Vukovic, L. *Herbal Healing Secrets for Women*. Paramus, NJ: Prentice Hall, 2000.

Vukovic, L. *Journal of Desires: A Daily Diary with Readings and Reflections Guiding You to Fulfillment of Your Lifelong Wishes and Dreams*. Paramus, NJ: Prentice Hall, 2001.

National Institute of Mental Health
Information Resources and Inquiries Branch
6001 Executive Boulevard
Bethesda, MD 20892-9663
1-800-421-4211
www.nimh.nih.gov

National Depressive and Manic Depressive Association
730 N. Franklin Street, Suite 501
Chicago, IL 60610
1-800-82-NDMA
www.ndmda.org

GINKGO BILOBA

Cass, Hyla. *Kava: Nature's Answer to Stress, Anxiety, and Insomnia*. Rocklin, CA: Prima Publishing, 1998.

Cass, Hyla. *St. John's Wort: Nature's Blues Buster*. Garden City Park, NY: Avery Publishing Group, 1998.

Cass, Hyla, and Patrick Holford. *Natural Highs: Supplements, Nutrition, and Mind/Body Techniques to Help You Feel Good All the Time*. New York, NY: Avery Penguin Putnam, 2002.

Ginkgo Biloba Extract: A Review
Alan R. Gaby, M.D.
www.thorne.com/altmedrev/fulltext/ginkgo1-4.html

Ohio State University Extension Fact Sheet
Human Nutrition and Food Management
1787 Neil Avenue, Columbus, OH 43210-1295
Herbals In Your Life
Herb and Drug Interactions
http://ohioline.osu.edu/hyg-fact/5000/5406.html

PubMed, National Library of Medicine
www.ncbi.nlm.nih.gov/entrez/query.fcgi

USDA, ARS, Genetic Resources Web Server
www.ars-grin.gov/duke/

U.S. Pharmacist
A Review of Herb-Drug Interactions: Documented and Theoretical
www.uspharmacist.com/NewLook/DisplayArticle.cfm?item_num=566

SAW PALMETTO & MEN'S HEALTH

Janson, Michael. *Dr. Janson's New Vitamin Revolution*. New York, NY: Penguin-Putnam-Avery, 2000.

Murray, Michael, Pizzorno, Joseph. *Encyclopedia of Natural Medicine*. Rocklin, CA: Prima Publishing, 1991.

Schachter, Michael. *The Natural Way to a Healthy Prostate*. New Canaan, CT: Keats Publishing, 1995.

Werbach, Melvin, Murray, Michael. *Botanical Influences on Illness*. Tarzana, CA: Third Line Press, 1994.

Dr. Michael Janson's Website: www.drjanson.com
Updates of the medical literature; editorials; answers to commonly asked questions, or individual questions of general interest; free monthly newsletter available by e-mail.

American College for Advancement in Medicine
www.acam.org
Information about conferences in complementary and alternative medicine and a referral source if you are looking for doctors who practice this medicine.

NUTRITION FOR WOMEN'S HEALTH

Murray, M, and Pizzorno, J. *Encyclopedia of Natural Medicine, revised second edition*. Rocklin, CA: Prima Publishing, 1998.

Northrup, C. *Women's Bodies, Women's Wisdom*. New York, NY: Bantam Books, 1998.

Vukovic, L. *Herbal Healing Secrets for Women*. Paramus, NJ: Prentice Hall, 2000.

Vukovic, L. *14-Day Herbal Cleansing*. Paramus, NJ: Prentice Hall, 1998.

National Women's Health Information Center
1-800-994-WOMAN (1-800-994-9662)
Website: www.4woman.gov

The American College of Obstetricians and Gynecologists
1-202-863-2518
Website: www.acog.org

SPORTS NUTRITION SUPPLEMENTS

Burke, E. *Optimal Muscle Recovery*. Garden City Park, NY: Avery Publishing Group, 1999.

Challem, J., and Brown, L. *User's Guide to Vitamins and Minerals*, North Bergen, New Jersey: Basic Health Publications, 2002.

Di Pasquale, M. *Amino Acids and Proteins and the Athlete: An Anabolic Edge*. [CITY:] CRC Press, 1997.

Sahelian, R., and Tuttle, D. *Creatine: Nature's Muscle Builder*. Garden City Park, NY: Avery Publishing Group, 1997.

Tuttle, D. *50 Ways to Build Muscle Fast*. Garden City Park, NY: Avery Publishing Group, 1999.

Wilmore, J., and Costill, D. *Physiology of Sport and Exercise*. Champaign, Illinois: Human Kinetics, 1999.

INDEX